MEDICAL TERMINOLOGY
An Illustrated Guide

FIFTH EDITION

BARBARA JANSON COHEN, MEd

 Wolters Kluwer | Lippincott Williams & Wilkins
Health

Philadelphia • Baltimore • New York • London
Buenos Aires • Hong Kong • Sydney • Tokyo

Senior Publisher: Julie K. Stegman
Executive Editor: John Goucher
Marketing Manager: Hilary Henderson
Senior Product Manager: Eric Branger
Managing Editors: Rebecca Kerins and Cecilia González
Designer: Armen Kojoyian
Compositor: Techbooks
Printer: R. R. Donnelley

DISCLAIMER

Care has been taken to confirm the accuracy of the information present and to describe generally accepted practices. However, the authors, editors, and publisher are not responsible for errors or omissions or for any consequences from application of the information in this book and make no warranty, expressed or implied, with respect to the currency, completeness, or accuracy of the contents of the publication. Application of this information in a particular situation remains the professional responsibility of the practitioner; the clinical treatments described and recommended may not be considered absolute and universal recommendations.

The authors, editors, and publishers have exerted every effort to ensure that drug selection and dosage set forth in this text are in accordance with current recommendations and practice at the time of publication. However, in view of ongoing research, changes in government regulations, and the constant flow of information relating to drug therapy and drug reactions, the reader is urged to check the package insert for each drug for any change in indications and dosage and for added warnings and precautions. This is particularly important when the recommended agent is a new or infrequently employed drug.

Some drugs and medical devices presented in this publication have Food and Drug Administration (FDA) clearance for limited use in restricted research settings. It is the responsibility of the health care provider to ascertain the FDA status of each drug or device planned for use in their clinical practice.

Library of Congress Cataloging-in-Publication Data

Cohen, Barbara J.
   Medical terminology : an illustrated guide / Barbara Janson Cohen. – 5th ed.
     p. ; cm.
   Includes bibliographical references and index.
   ISBN-13: 978-0-7817-7667-7 (pbk.)
   ISBN-10: 0-7817-7667-8 (pbk.)
  1. Medicine–Terminology. I. Title.
   [DNLM: 1. Terminology. W 15 C678m 2007]
   R123.C56 2007
   610.1'4–dc22

                       2007001944

PREFACE

Every career in health care begins with learning the vast and challenging language of medical terminology. Without adequate learning and teaching resources, it can be an overwhelming challenge for students and faculty. This fifth edition of *Medical Terminology: An Illustrated Guide* meets that challenge with clear organization, full-color illustrations with a strong clinical focus, a wide array of effective pedagogical features, a variety of activities, and useful ancillaries to make teaching and learning more effective. Because the content is so accessible and logically organized, the text can be used as part of classroom instruction, for independent study, or for distance learning.

Organization and Approach

Medical Terminology: An Illustrated Guide, 5th Edition, takes a stepwise approach to learning the language of medical terminology. Part 1 describes how medical terms are built from separate word parts, and Part 2 introduces body structure, disease, and treatment. Students should study these chapters before proceeding to Part 3, which describes each of the body systems. Individual chapters also build on knowledge in stages, with Key Terms sections listing those terms most commonly used and more specialized terms included in a later section entitled Supplementary Terms. Students may study the latter terms according to time available and their needs.

Each chapter opens with a chapter outline and a list of student objectives—goals to be accomplished by the completion of the chapter. In Part 3, the chapters begin with an overview of the normal structure and function of the system under study, followed by a list of key terms with definitions and mention of some roots. Word parts related to each topic are then presented and illustrated, along with exercises on the new material. Next, there is an overview of clinical information pertaining to the system, also followed by a list of key terms with definitions. Most chapters contain reference boxes that unify and simplify material on specific topics.

This edition also has information on complementary and alternative medicine and special interest boxes on health care professions, clinical topics, and word derivations and usage.

Learning Resources

Features of *Medical Terminology: An Illustrated Guide,* 5th Edition, have been designed to bring the content alive and to aid in understanding and retention (also see the User's Guide).

➤ **Illustrations**—Detailed, full-color anatomical drawings and photographs illuminate the text. The art program has been updated and many figures have been added, especially clinical photographs and micrographs of tissues.
➤ **Pronunciations**—This text places great emphasis on pronunciation, and phonetic pronunciations are included with all new terms. It is important to practice saying these words and to be able to recognize them when they are heard.
➤ **Pretests**—Short quizzes to test previous knowledge begin each chapter and are new with this edition. Students should take each quiz before starting the chapter and again after completing the chapter in order to measure progress.

v

➤ **Exercises**—Exercises accompany the introduction of all material, and review exercises conclude each chapter. Many of the illustrations have corresponding labeling exercises that include helpful alphabetical word lists. All answers are included in the Answer Key at the end of the book. Students are actively involved in the learning process by answering questions on new material, checking answers with the answer keys, correcting mistakes, and keeping track of progress with review exercises.

➤ **Case Studies**—Case studies that present terminology in the context of a medical report are included in all chapters, followed by related questions. Professionals in a variety of health occupations figure in these scenarios to represent the diverse work settings students may encounter. Because they may include information learned in a previous chapter, the case studies also serve as an excellent mode of review. Understanding these cases, especially those in the early parts of the book, may seem challenging for students, but much of the information needed to answer the questions is given in the histories, and students should make their best efforts to figure out the answers. These can be verified with the Answer Key in the back of the book.

➤ **Glossaries of Word Parts**—In working through the exercises, students can refer to complementary lists at the end of the text. Appendix 3 lists word parts and their meanings, and Appendix 4 lists meanings with corresponding word parts. New with this edition are lists of roots, suffixes, and prefixes alone in Appendices 5 through 7. The remaining appendices include symbols, abbreviations, and units of the metric system.

➤ **Use of Dictionaries**—Some information on medical dictionaries is given in Chapter 1. Appendix 9 provides a sample page from a medical dictionary with information on how it is used.

➤ **Crosswords**—Each chapter on the body systems includes a crossword puzzle so that students can exercise their newfound knowledge. The Answer Key in the back of the book has the answers to these puzzles.

➤ **Flashcards**—Because flashcards offer an excellent way to learn this new vocabulary, a section with more than 100 flashcards is included at the back of the text. Flashcard content is presented in chapter order so that the cards can be removed in sequence as students progress through the book. Of course, these cards represent only a portion of the necessary vocabulary, and students should add to the collection with their own cards. Flash cards can be made to match the cards in the book by cutting a 3 × 5 card in half.

➤ **Interactive CD-ROM**—A CD-ROM is included with the text that contains:
  ➤ Various practice question sets per chapter, including multiple choice, true-false, fill-in-the-blank question types
  ➤ Matching exercises and word-building exercises
  ➤ Image labeling exercises
  ➤ Spelling bee exercises
  ➤ Additional case studies exercises
  ➤ In-context exercises of medical reports giving definitions and audio pronunciations of terms to show them in context
  ➤ Interactive flashcards
  ➤ Audio pronunciation glossary

Students are also encouraged to create their own learning aids, such as devising a practice test by covering lists of words and testing themselves on the definitions, or by covering definitions and testing themselves on the words. The same can be done with the charts on word parts and their definitions. It is also helpful for students to keep a personal list of words that they find difficult to spell or pronounce.

Teaching Resources

A strong package of ancillary materials is available to instructors with this edition. These resources include:

- **Instructor Resource Center**—This resource is also available via thePoint (http://thepoint.lww.com/cohen5e) and consists of:
  - PowerPoint slides for each chapter organized by learning objectives
  - Lesson plans for each chapter
  - Additional word search activities
  - Crossword puzzle answer keys
  - Additional fill-in-the-blank exercises
  - Image bank
- **Instructor's Test Generator**—This valuable teaching resource is available via thePoint (http://thepoint.lww.com/cohen5e) and contains a test generator with more than 500 questions in different formats (multiple choice, true-false, fill-in-the-blank, and matching).
- **thePoint Site (LWW's exclusive learning management system), WebCT, and Blackboard Online Course**—Customized course content has been developed for use with your learning management system. The Web site (http://thepoint.lww.com/cohen5e) also provides access to an image bank containing the text illustrations, Instructor's Resource content, and conversion guides from the text that you have used in your course.

An understanding of medical terminology provides an essential foundation for any career in health care. *Medical Terminology: An Illustrated Guide,* 5th Edition, both the textbook and its ancillaries, makes learning and teaching medical terminology a rewarding and exciting process.

ACKNOWLEDGMENTS

Once again, I wish to thank the many skilled and dedicated staff members at Lippincott Williams & Wilkins who worked with me to prepare this fifth edition of *Medical Terminology: An Illustrated Guide*. Rebecca Kerins, Senior Managing Editor, worked most closely with me in manuscript and art preparation, and I appreciate her efforts. Senior Publisher Julie Stegman, Eric Branger, Senior Project Manager, and Cecilia González, Associate Managing Editor, also guided this project with great skill.

Dragonfly Media Group again did an outstanding job of revising illustrations and designing additional figures for this edition of the book.

I appreciate the assistance of all the reviewers who gave of their time and expertise in evaluating this text and making suggestions for improvements.

Heartfelt thanks to my major contributor, Jason James Taylor, who wrote many of the special interest boxes that appear in the text and has also created all of the student and instructor resource materials. Jason and I have worked together successfully on other projects, and I look forward to continuing collaborations in the future.

And always, thanks to my husband Matthew, an anatomy and physiology instructor, who continues to listen and advise.

REVIEWERS

Zubin Austin, PhD
OCP Professor in Pharmacy
Leslie Dan Faculty of Pharmacy, University of Toronto
Toronto, Canada

Joseph A. Cipriani, EdD, OTR/L
Professor
Department of Occupational Therapy
Misericordia University
Dallas, Pennsylvania, USA

Susan S. Erue, RN, BSN, MS, PhD
Chair, Division of Nursing
Iowa Wesleyan College
Mount Pleasant, Iowa,US

Marie A. Fenske, EdD, RRT
Faculty/ Director of Clinical Education – Respiratory Care
Coordinator – Health Care Core classes
Gate Way Community College
Phoenix, Arizona, USA

Josh Hamilton
Department of Nursing
Casper College
Casper, Wyoming, USA

Steven P. Lewis, PhD
Instructor
Lamar University
Department of Biology
Beaumont, Texas, USA

Laura Logan
Program Coordinator
Angelina College @ Lufkin
Community Services Division
Lufkin, Texas, USA

Jo Ellen Sefton
Adjunct Faculty
Athletic Training Department
Indiana state University
Terre Haute, Indiana, USA

USER'S GUIDE

Medical Terminology: An Illustrated Guide, 5th Edition was created and developed to help you master the language of medicine. The tools and features in the text will help you work through the material presented. Please take a few moments to look through this User's Guide, which will introduce you to the features that will enhance your learning experience.

Chapter Contents, Objectives, and Pretests

Chapter Contents & Objectives help you identify learning goals and familiarize yourself with the material covered in the chapter. Chapter Pretests are a great way to identify your strengths and weaknesses, so you know what to focus on as you work through the chapter content

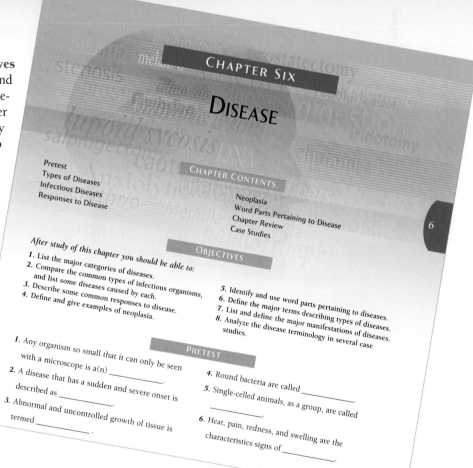

CHAPTER SIX

DISEASE

CHAPTER CONTENTS

Pretest
Types of Diseases
Infectious Diseases
Responses to Disease

Neoplasia
Word Parts Pertaining to Disease
Chapter Review
Case Studies

6

OBJECTIVES

After study of this chapter you should be able to:
1. List the major categories of diseases.
2. Compare the common types of infectious organisms, and list some diseases caused by each.
3. Describe some common responses to disease.
4. Define and give examples of neoplasia.
5. Identify and use word parts pertaining to diseases.
6. Define the major terms describing types of diseases.
7. List and define the major manifestations of diseases.
8. Analyze the disease terminology in several case studies.

PRETEST

1. Any organism so small that it can only be seen with a microscope is a(n) _____.
2. A disease that has a sudden and severe onset is described as _____.
3. Abnormal and uncontrolled growth of tissue is termed _____.
4. Round bacteria are called _____.
5. Single-celled animals, as a group, are called _____.
6. Heat, pain, redness, and swelling are the characteristics signs of _____.

Detailed Illustrations

Illustrations visually emphasize important terms and concepts

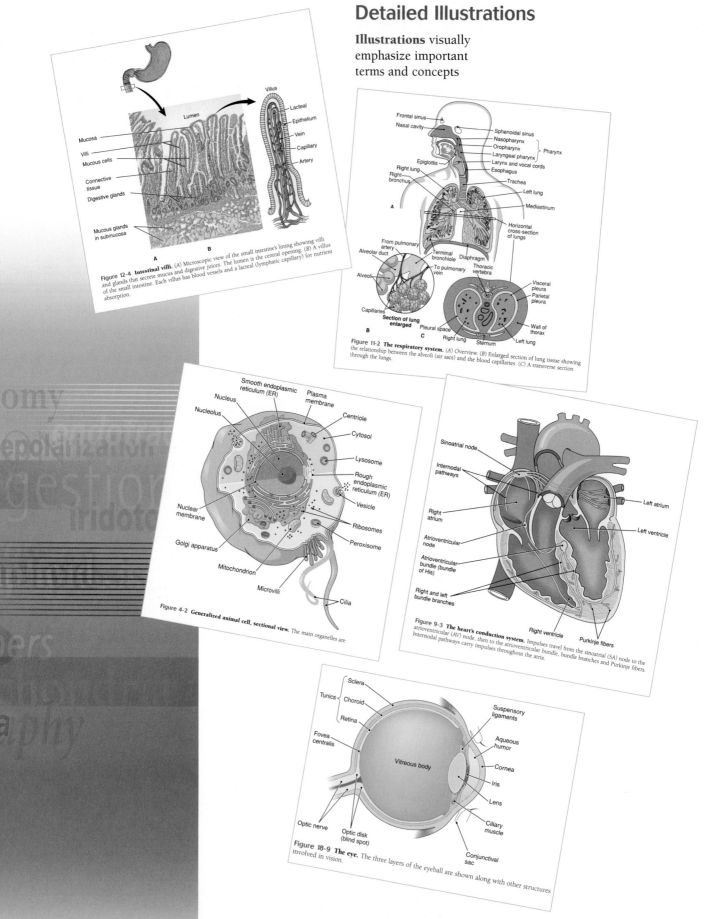

Figure 12-4 Intestinal villi. (A) Microscopic view of the small intestine's lining showing villi and glands that secrete mucus and digestive juices. The lumen is the central opening. (B) A villus of the small intestine. Each villus has blood vessels and a lacteal (lymphatic capillary) for nutrient absorption.

Figure 11-2 The respiratory system. (A) Overview. (B) Enlarged section of lung tissue showing the relationship between the alveoli (air sacs) and the blood capillaries. (C) A transverse section through the lungs.

Figure 4-2 Generalized animal cell, sectional view. The main organelles are

Figure 9-3 The heart's conduction system. Impulses travel from the sinoatrial (SA) node to the atrioventricular (AV) node, then to the atrioventricular bundle, bundle branches and Purkinje fibers. Internodal pathways carry impulses throughout the atria.

Figure 18-9 The eye. The three layers of the eyeball are shown along with other structures involved in vision.

Feature Boxes
Feature boxes call out important information:

Focus on Words provide historical or other interesting information on select terms within a chapter

Clinical Perspectives focus on body processes as well as techniques used in clinical settings

Health Professions focus on a variety of health careers, showing how the knowledge of medical terminology is applied in real-world jobs

For Your Reference provide supplemental information for terms within a chapter

---

Box 8·1 Focus on Words — *Where Do Drugs Get Their Names?*

Drug names are derived in a variety of ways. Some are named for their origin. Adrenaline, for example, is named for its source, the adrenal gland. Even its generic name, epinephrine, informs us that it comes from the gland that is above (epi-) the kidney (nephr/o). Pitocin, a drug used to induce labor, is named for its source, the pituitary gland, combined with the chemical name of the hormone, oxytocin. Botox, currently injected into the skin for cosmetic removal of wrinkles, is the toxin from the organism that causes botulism, a type of food poisoning. Aspirin (an anti-inflammatory agent), Taxol (an antitumor agent), digitalis (used to treat heart failure), and atropine (a smooth-muscle

relaxant) are all named for the plants they come from. For example, aspirin is named for the blossoms of Spiraea, from which it is derived. Taxol comes from a yew (evergreen) of the genus *Taxus*. Digitalis is from purple foxglove, genus *Digitalis*. Atropine comes from the plant *Atropa belladonna*.

Some names tell about the drug or its actions. The name for Humulin, a form of insulin made by genetic engineering, points out that this is human insulin and not a hormone from animal sources. Lomotil reduces intestin... and means...

Box 9·3 Clinical Perspectives — *Lymphedema: When Lymph Stops Flowing*

Fluid balance in the body requires appropriate distribution of fluid among the cardiovascular system, lymphatic system, and the tissues. **Edema** occurs when the balance is tipped toward excess fluid in the tissues. Often, edema is due to heart failure. However, blockage of lymphatic vessels (with resulting fluid accumulation in the tissues) can cause another form of edema, called **lymphedema**. The clinical hallmark of lymphedema is chronic swelling of an arm or leg, whereas heart failure usually causes swelling of both legs.

Lymphedema may be either primary or secondary. Primary lymphedema is a rare congenital condition caused by abnormal development of lymphatic vessels. Secondary lym... ...quired lymphedema, can develop as a res... ...ry radiation therapy, or inf... ...ngitis). One of th...

axillary lymph nodes during mastectomy, which disrupts lymph flow from the adjacent arm. Lymphedema may also occur following prostate surgery.

Therapies that encourage the flow of fluid through the lymphatic vessels are useful in treating lymphedema. These therapies may include elevation of the affected limb, manual lymphatic drainage through massage, light exercise, and firm wrapping of the limb to apply compression. In addition, changes in daily habits can lessen the effects of lymphedema. For example, further blockage of lymph drainage can be prevented by wearing loose clothing and jewelry, carrying a purse or handbag on the unaffected arm, and not crossing the legs when sitting. Lymphangitis requires the use of appropriate antibiotics. Prompt treatment is necessary because, in addition to swelling, other complications include poor wound healing, skin ulcers, and increased risk of infection.

Box 10·5 Health Professions — *Careers in Hematology*

Hematologists are physicians and other scientists who specialize in the study of blood and blood diseases. In medical practice, hematology is often combined with the study and treatment of blood cancers as the specialty hematology–oncology.

A hematology technician is usually a medical laboratory technician who specializes in blood studies. He or she may work in a clinical laboratory, blood banking, industry, or academic research. The job requires a BS or MS in biological science plus training in laboratory procedures, blood pathology, and testing methods. Hematology technicians perform a full range of blood studies for diagnosis of infections, allergies, anemia, leukemia, and other blood dis- eases. They als...

equipment used to analyze blood. In some cases, they may also draw blood or administer blood transfusions.

A phlebotomist draws blood for testing, transfusions, or research. The blood is often drawn from a vein (venipuncture), but may also be drawn from arteries and by skin puncture. Phlebotomists must be trained in sterile techniques and safety precautions to prevent the spread of infectious diseases. They must take specimens without harming the patient or interfering with medical care and must transport specimens to the proper laboratory. Educational requirements vary among states. Often, in... ...training with certi...

Box 11·2 For Your Reference — *Organisms That Infect the Respiratory System*

Organism	Disease
BACTERIA	
Streptococcus pneumoniae *strep-tō-KOK-us nū-MŌ-nē-ē*	Most common cause of pneumonia; streptococcal pneumonia
Haemophilus influenzae *hē-MOF-i-lus in-flū-EN-zē*	Pneumonia, especially in debilitated patients
Klebsiella pneumoniae *kleb-sē-EL-a nū-MŌ-nē-a*	Pneumonia in elderly and debilitated patients
Mycoplasma pneumoniae *mī-kō-PLAZ-ma nū-MŌ-nē-ē*	Mild pneumonia, usually in young adults and children; "walking pneumonia"
Legionella pneumophila *lē-ju-NEL-la nū-MO-fi-la*	Legionellosis (Legionnaire disease); respiratory disease spread through water sources, such as air conditioners, pools, humidifiers
Chlamydia psittaci *kla-MID-ē-a PSI-ta-sē*	Psittacosis (ornithosis); carried by birds
Streptococcus pyogenes *strep-tō-KOK-us pī-OJ-e-nēz*	"Strep throat," scarlet fever
Mycobacterium tuberculosis *mī-kō-bak-TĒR-ē-um tū-ber-kū-LŌ-sis*	Tuberculosis
Bordetella pertussis *bōr-de-TEL-a per-TUS-sis*	Pertussis (whooping cough)
Corynebacterium diphtheriae *kō-RĪ-nē-bak-tēr-ē-um dif-THĒ-rē-ē*	Diphtheria

Word Part Tables
Detailed Tables:

Present roots, prefixes, and suffixes covered in each chapter in an easy-to-reference format (with examples of their use in medical terminology).

Word Part Knowledge aids in the learning and understanding of common terminology

Roots Pertaining to Digestion

Table 12·1 Roots for the Mouth

ROOT	MEANING	EXAMPLE	DEFINITION OF EXAMPLE
bucc/o	cheek	buccoversion *buk-kō-VER-zhun*	turning toward the cheek
dent/o, dent/i	tooth, teeth	edentulous *ē-DEN-tū-lus*	without teeth
odont/o	tooth, teeth	periodontics *per-ē-ō-DON-tiks*	dental specialty that deals with the study and treatment of the tissues around the teeth
gingiv/o	gum (gingiva)	gingivectomy *jin-ji-VEK-tō-mē*	excision of gum tissue
gloss/o	tongue	glossoplegia *glos-ō-PLĒ-jē-a*	paralysis (-plegia) of the tongue
lingu/o	tongue	orolingual *or-ō-LING-gwal*	pertaining to the mouth and tongue
gnath/o	jaw	prognathous *PROG-na-thus*	having a projecting jaw
labi/o	lip	labium *LĀ-bē-um*	lip or liplike structure
or/o	mouth	circumoral *sir-kum-OR-al*	around the mouth
stoma, stomat/o	mouth	xerostomia *zē-rō-STŌ-mē-a*	dryness (xero-) of the mouth
palat/o		palatine *___-a-tin*	pertaining to the palate (also palatal)
sial/o			...diograph of the salivary glands and ducts
uvul/o			...vula

Exercise 10-2

Identify and define the root in the following words:

		Root	Meaning of Root
1.	panmyeloid (*pan-MĪ-e-loyd*)	myel/o	bone marrow
2.	prothrombin (*prō-THROM-bin*)	___	___
3.	preimmunization (*prē-im-ū-ni-ZĀ-shun*)	___	___
4.	ischemia (*is-KĒ-mē-a*)	___	___

Fill in the blanks:

5. Hemorrhage is a profuse flow (-rhage) of _____
6. Erythroclasis (*er-i-THROK-la-sis*) is the breaking (-clasis) of _____
7. The term *thrombocythemia* (*throm-bō-sī-THĒ-mē-a*) refers to an increase in the number of _____ in the blood.
8. Leukopoiesis (*lū-kō-poy-Ē-sis*) refers to the production of _____
9. An immunocyte (*im-ū-nō-SĪT*) is a cell active in _____
10. A hemocytometer (*hē-mō-sī-TOM-e-ter*) is a device for counting _____
11. Myelofibrosis (*mi-e-lō-fī-BRO-sis*) is formation of fibrous tissue in _____
12. Lymphokines (*LIM-fō-kīnz*) are chemicals active in immunity that are produced by _____.

Word building. Write a word for the following definitions:

13. Immature lymphocyte
14. Tumor of bone marrow _____
15. Decrease in red blood cells _____
16. Dissolving (-lysis) of a blood clot _____
17. Formation (-poiesis) of bone marrow _____

The suffix -osis added to a root for a type of cell means an increase in that type of cell in the blood. Use this suffix to write a word that means the same as the following:

18. Increase in granulocytes in the blood
19. Increase in lymphocytes in the blood _____ granulocytosis _____

Exercises

Exercises that are designed to test your knowledge before you move on to the next learning topic follow each table

Key Terms include the most commonly used words

TERMINOLOGY **Key Terms**

Normal Structure and Function

anus *Ā-nus*	The distal opening of the digestive tract (root: *an/o*)
appendix *a-PEN-diks*	An appendage; usually means the narrow tube of lymphatic tissue attached to the cecum, the vermiform (wormlike) appendix
bile *bīl*	The fluid secreted by the liver that emulsified fats and aids in their absorption (roots: *chol/e, bili*)
cecum *SĒ-kum*	A blind pouch at the beginning of the large intestine (root: *cec/o*)
colon *KŌ-lon*	The major portion of the large intestine: ⸺ rectum and is formed by ascen⸺ (root: *col/o, colon⸺*)
common bile duct	
duodenum	

Supplementary Terms list more specialized words

TERMINOLOGY **Supplementary Terms**

Continued

duodenal papilla	The raised area where the common bile duct and pancreatic duct enter the duodenum (see Fig. 12-14); papilla of Vater (FA-ter)
greater omentum *ō-MEN-tum*	A fold of the peritoneum that extends from the stomach over the abdominal organs
hepatic flexure	The right bend of the colon, forming the junction between the ascending colon and the transverse colon (see Fig. 12-1)
ileocecal valve *il-ē-ō-SĒ-kal*	A valvelike structure between the ileum of the small intestine and the cecum of the large intestine
mesentery *MES-en-ter-ē*	The portion of the peritoneum that folds over and supports the intestine
mesocolon *mes-ō-KŌ-lon*	The portion of the peritoneum that folds over and supports the colon
papilla of Vater	See duodenal papilla
⸺	The serous membrane that lines the abdominal cavity and supports the ⸺

Key Clinical Terms list medical terms pertinent to the body system under discussion

TERMINOLOGY **Key Clinical Terms**

Lymphatic Disorders

lymphadenitis *lim-fad-e-NĪ-tis*	Inflammation and enlargement of lymph nodes, usually as a result of infection
lymphangiitis *lim-fan-jē-Ī-tis*	Inflammation of lymphatic vessels as a result of bacterial infection. Appears as painful red streaks under the skin. (Also spelled *lymphangitis*.)
lymphedema *lim-fe-DĒ-ma*	Swelling of tissues with lymph caused by obstruction or excision of lymphatic vessels (see Box 9-3)
lymphoma *lim-FŌ-ma*	Any neoplastic disease of lymphoid tissue

Abbreviations for common terms

TERMINOLOGY **Abbreviations**

BE	Barium enema (for radiographic study of the colon)	HEV	Hepatitis E virus
		HCl	Hydrochloric acid
BM	Bowel movement	IBD	Inflammatory bowel disease
CBD	Common bile duct	IBS	Irritable bowel syndrome
ERCP	Endoscopic retrograde cholangiopancreatography	LES	Lower esophageal sphincter
		NG	Nasogastric (tube)
FAP	Familial adenomatous polyposis	N & V	Nausea and vomiting
GERD	Gastroesophageal reflux disease	N/V/D	Nausea, vomiting, and diarrhea
GI	Gastrointestinal	PONV	Postoperative nausea and vomiting
HAV	Hepatitis A virus	PPI	Proton-pump inhibitor
HBV	Hepatitis B virus	TPN	Total parenteral nutrition
HCV	Hepatitis C virus	UGI	Upper gastrointestinal (radiograph series)
HDV	Hepatitis D virus		

Chapter Review Exercises

Chapter Review Exercises are designed to test your knowledge of the chapter material and appear at the end of each chapter

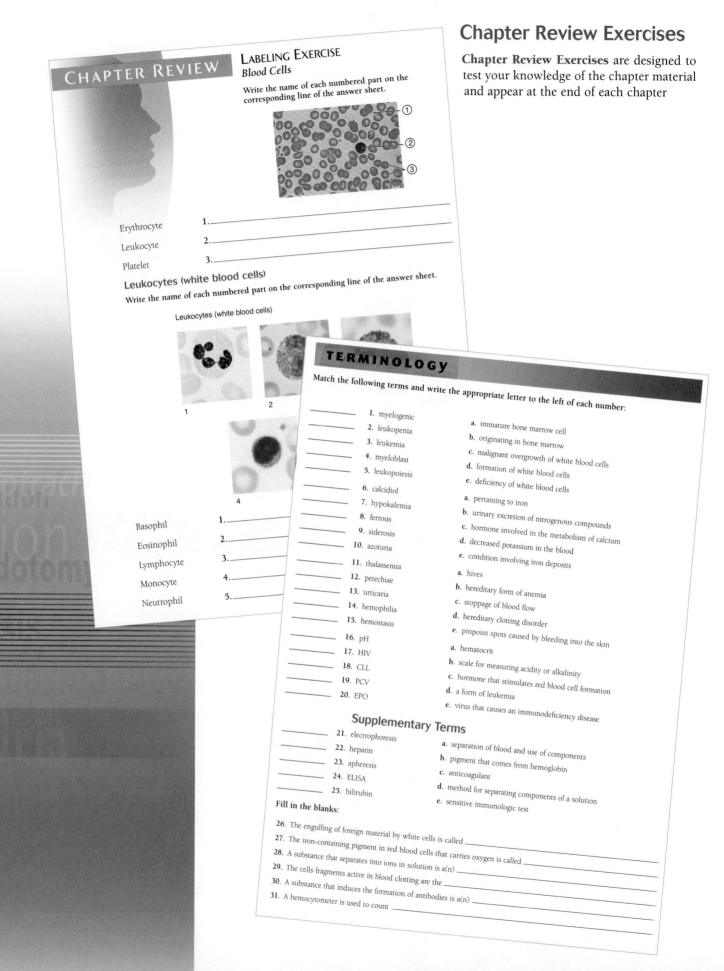

CHAPTER REVIEW

LABELING EXERCISE
Blood Cells

Write the name of each numbered part on the corresponding line of the answer sheet.

Erythrocyte 1._____

Leukocyte 2._____

Platelet 3._____

Leukocytes (white blood cells)

Write the name of each numbered part on the corresponding line of the answer sheet.

Leukocytes (white blood cells)

Basophil 1._____

Eosinophil 2._____

Lymphocyte 3._____

Monocyte 4._____

Neutrophil 5._____

TERMINOLOGY

Match the following terms and write the appropriate letter to the left of each number:

_____ 1. myelogenic
_____ 2. leukopenia
_____ 3. leukemia
_____ 4. myeloblast
_____ 5. leukopoiesis

  a. immature bone marrow cell
  b. originating in bone marrow
  c. malignant overgrowth of white blood cells
  d. formation of white blood cells
  e. deficiency of white blood cells

_____ 6. calcidiol
_____ 7. hypokalemia
_____ 8. ferrous
_____ 9. siderosis
_____ 10. azoturia

  a. pertaining to iron
  b. urinary excretion of nitrogenous compounds
  c. hormone involved in the metabolism of calcium
  d. decreased potassium in the blood
  e. condition involving iron deposits

_____ 11. thalassemia
_____ 12. petechiae
_____ 13. urticaria
_____ 14. hemophilia
_____ 15. hemostasis

  a. hives
  b. hereditary form of anemia
  c. stoppage of blood flow
  d. hereditary clotting disorder
  e. pinpoint spots caused by bleeding into the skin

_____ 16. pH
_____ 17. HIV
_____ 18. CLL
_____ 19. PCV
_____ 20. EPO

  a. hematocrit
  b. scale for measuring acidity or alkalinity
  c. hormone that stimulates red blood cell formation
  d. a form of leukemia
  e. virus that causes an immunodeficiency disease

Supplementary Terms

_____ 21. electrophoresis
_____ 22. heparin
_____ 23. apheresis
_____ 24. ELISA
_____ 25. bilirubin

  a. separation of blood and use of components
  b. pigment that comes from hemoglobin
  c. anticoagulant
  d. method for separating components of a solution
  e. sensitive immunologic test

Fill in the blanks:

26. The engulfing of foreign material by white cells is called _____

27. The iron-containing pigment in red blood cells that carries oxygen is called _____

28. A substance that separates into ions in solution is a(n) _____

29. The cells fragments active in blood clotting are the _____

30. A substance that induces the formation of antibodies is a(n) _____

31. A hemocytometer is used to count _____

Case Studies and Case Study Questions

Case Studies and Case Study Questions in every chapter present terminology in the context of a medical report. These are an excellent review tool as they test your cumulative knowledge of medical terminology, and put terminology into a real-world context

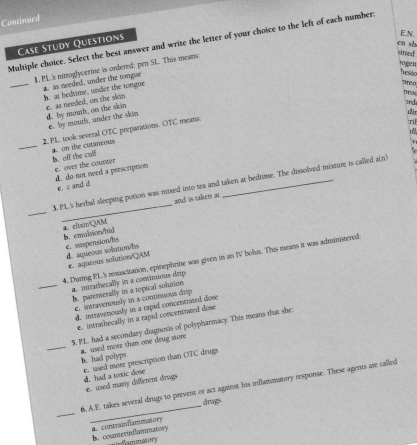

CASE STUDIES

CASE STUDY 8-1: Cardiac Disease and Crisis

P.L., who has a 4-year history of heart disease, was brought to the emergency room by ambulance with chest pain that radiated down her arm, dyspnea, and syncope. Her routine meds included Lanoxin to slow and strengthen her heart beat, Inderal to support her heart rhythm, Lipitor to decrease her cholesterol, Catapres to lower her hypertension, nitroglycerin prn for chest pain, Hydro DIURIL to eliminate fluid and decrease the workload of her heart, Diabinese for her diabetes, and Coumadin to prevent blood clots. She also took Tagamet for her stomach ulcer and several OTC preparations, including an herbal sleeping potion

that she mixed in tea, and Metamucil mixed in orange juice every morning for her bowels. Shortly after admission, P.L.'s heart rate deteriorated into full cardiac arrest. Immediate resuscitation was instituted with cardiopulmonary resuscitation (CPR), defibrillation, and a bolus of IV epinephrine. Between shocks she was given a bolus of lidocaine and a bolus of diltiazem plus repeated doses of epinephrine every 5 minutes. P.L. did not respond to resuscitation. On the death certificate, her primary cause of death was listed as cardiac arrest. Multiple secondary diagnoses were listed, including polypharmacy.

CASE STUDY 8-2: Inflammat... ...owel Disease

A.E., a 19-year-old college... ...age of 13 with C... ...ease th...

...dis-
...om
...el.
...-

suppressing the immune response. He takes Pentasa (mesalamine) 250 mg 4 caps po bid. Pentasa is of the 5-ASA (acetylsalicylic acid or aspirin) group of antiinflammatory agents, which work topically on the inner surface of the bowel. It has an enteric coating, which dissolves in the bowel environment. He also takes 6-mercaptopurine (Purinethol) 75 mg po qd and a therapeutic vitamin with breakfast. A.E. may take acetaminophen for pain but must avoid NSAIDs, which will irritate the intestinal mucosa (inner lining) and cause a flare-up of the disease.

E.N. stated that she has difficulty with her asthma ...en she is anxious and when she exercises. She also ...itted to occasional use of marijuana and ecstasy, a hal...ogen and mood-altering illegal recreational drug. The ...hesiologist wrote an order for lorazepam 4 mg IV 1 ...preop. The plastic surgeon recommended several ...products to complement her surgery and her recov... ...ordered a high-potency vitamin 3 tabs with break... ...dinner to support tissue health and healing. He ...ribed Bromelain, an enzyme from pineapple, to ...flammation, 1 po qid 3 days before surgery and ...ively for 2 weeks. Arnica Montana was pre... ...ecrease discomfort, swelling, and bruising; 3 ...al tid the evening after surgery and for the fol... ...rs.

CASE STUDIES

Continued

CASE STUDY QUESTIONS

Multiple choice. Select the best answer and write the letter of your choice to the left of each number:

_____ 1. P.L.'s nitroglycerine is ordered: prn SL. This means:
    a. as needed, under the tongue
    b. at bedtime, under the tongue
    c. as needed, on the skin
    d. by mouth, on the skin
    e. by mouth, under the skin

_____ 2. P.L. took several OTC preparations. OTC means:
    a. on the cutaneous
    b. off the cuff
    c. over the counter
    d. do not need a prescription
    e. c and d

_____ 3. P.L.'s herbal sleeping potion was mixed into tea and taken at bedtime. The dissolved mixture is called a(n) _____ and is taken at _____.
    a. elixir/QAM
    b. emulsion/bid
    c. suspension/hs
    d. aqueous solution/hs
    e. aqueous solution/QAM

_____ 4. During P.L.'s resuscitation, epinephrine was given in an IV bolus. This means it was administered:
    a. intrathecally in a continuous drip
    b. parenterally in a topical solution
    c. intravenously in a continuous drip
    d. intravenously in a rapid concentrated dose
    e. intrathecally in a rapid concentrated dose

_____ 5. P.L. had a secondary diagnosis of polypharmacy. This means that she:
    a. used more than one drug store
    b. had polyps
    c. used more prescription than OTC drugs
    d. had a toxic dose
    e. used many different drugs

_____ 6. A.E. takes several drugs to prevent or act against his inflammatory response. These agents are called _____ drugs.
    a. contrainflammatory
    b. counterinflammatory
    c. antiinflammatory
    d. proinflammatory
    e. hypoinflammatory

Flashcard Starter Set

More than 100 flashcards are included at the back of the text. Add to this collection with your own cards as you work through the text

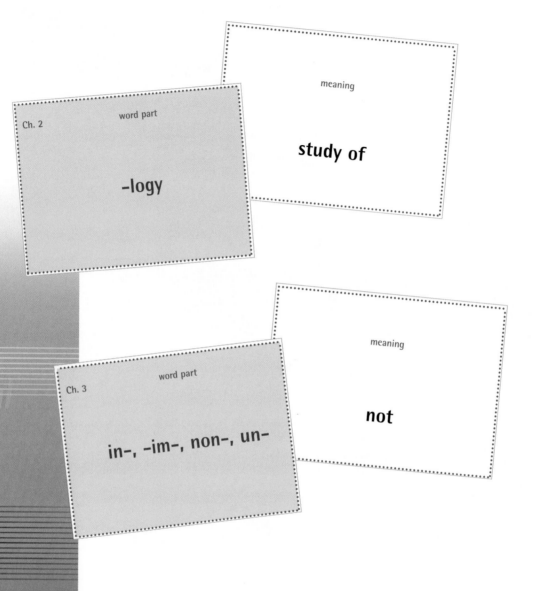

CD Icons

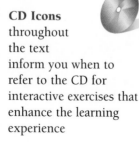

CD Icons throughout the text inform you when to refer to the CD for interactive exercises that enhance the learning experience

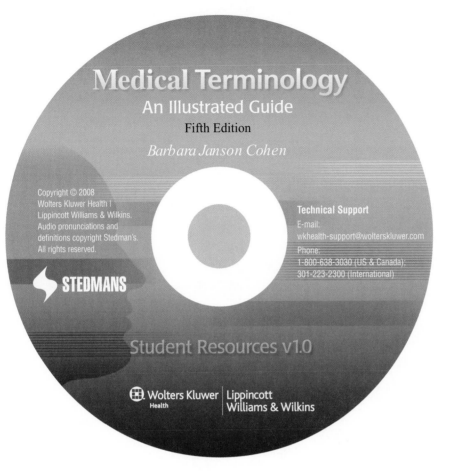

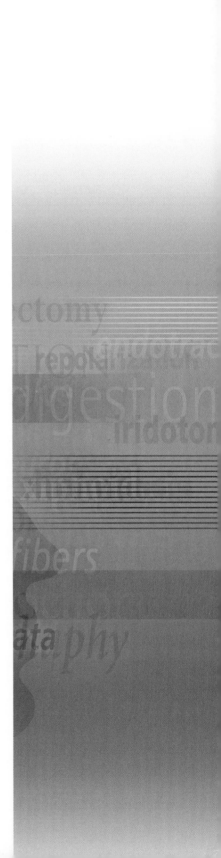

CD-ROM

Have FUN while you learn with the BONUS CD-ROM packaged with this text! This interactive learning resource includes exercises for every chapter (multiple choice, figure labeling, fill-in-the-blank, spelling bee, additional case studies, and more!), audio pronunciation glossary, electronic dictionary with STEDMAN'S audio pronunciations, and electronic flashcards. Use the CD in either Review or Test Taking mode to assess your knowledge!

CONTENTS

EXPANDED CONTENTS

PART ONE

INTRODUCTION TO MEDICAL TERMINOLOGY

Chapters 1 through 5, Part 1, present the basics of medical terminology and body structure. Chapters 6 through 8, Part 2, deal with disease and treatment. These beginning chapters form the basis for the chapters on the individual body systems in Part 3.

CONCEPTS OF MEDICAL TERMINOLOGY

1

OBJECTIVES

After study of this chapter you should be able to:

1. Explain the purpose of medical terminology.
2. Define the terms *root*, *suffix*, and *prefix*.
3. Explain what combining forms are and why they are used.
4. Name the languages from which most medical word parts are derived.

5. Pronounce words according to the pronunciation guide used in this text.
6. List some features of medical dictionaries.
7. Analyze some concepts of medical terminology in a case study.

PRETEST

1. The main part of a word is called the
   _____.

2. A word part at the beginning of a word is a(n)
   _____.

3. A word part at the end of a word is the
   _____.

4. Most medical words are derived from the
   languages _____ and _____.

5. The *ch* in the word *chemist* is pronounced like the
   letter _____.

6. The *ps* in the word *psychic* is pronounced like the
   letter _____.

Medical terminology is a special vocabulary used by health-care professionals for effective and accurate communication. Every health-related field requires an understanding of medical terminology, and this book will highlight selected health care occupations in special boxes (see Box 1-1). Because it is based mainly on Greek and Latin words, medical terminology is consistent and uniform throughout the world. It is also efficient; although some of the terms are long, they often reduce an entire phrase to a single word. The one word *gastroduodenostomy,* for example, stands for "a communication between the stomach and the first part of the small intestine" (Fig. 1-1). The part *gastr* means stomach; *duoden* stands for the duodenum, the first part of the small intestine; *ostomy* means a communication.

The medical vocabulary is vast, and learning it may seem like learning the entire vocabulary of a foreign language. Moreover, like the jargon that arises in all changing fields, it is always expanding. Think of the terms that have been added to our vocabulary with the development of computers, such as software, search engine, e-mail, chat room, and blog. The task may seem overwhelming, but there are methods to aid in learning and remembering words and even help to make informed guesses about unfamiliar words. Most medical terms can be divided into component parts—roots, prefixes, and suffixes—that maintain the same meaning whenever they appear. By learning these meanings, you can analyze and remember many words.

Word Parts

Word components fall into three categories:

1. The **root** is the fundamental unit of each medical word. It establishes the basic meaning of the word and is the part to which modifying prefixes and suffixes are added.
2. A **suffix** is a short word part or series of parts added at the end of a root to modify its meaning. This book indicates suffixes by a dash before the suffix, such as *-itis* (inflammation).
3. A **prefix** is a short word part added before a root to modify its meaning. This book indicates prefixes by a dash after the prefix, such as *pre-* (before).

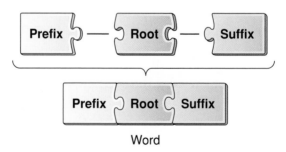

Words are formed from roots, suffixes, and prefixes.

The simple word *write* can be used as a root to illustrate. If we add the suffix *-er* to form *writer,* we have "one who writes." If we add the prefix *re-* to form *rewrite,* we have "to write again."

Not all roots are complete words. In fact, most medical roots are derived from other languages and are meant to be used in combinations. The Greek word *kardia,* for example, meaning "heart," gives us the root *cardi.* The Latin word *pulmo,* meaning "lung," gives us the root *pulm.* In a few instances, both the Greek and Latin roots are used. We find both the Greek root *nephr* and the Latin root *ren* used in words pertaining to the kidney (Fig. 1-2).

| Box 1·1 **Health Professions** | *Health Information Technicians* |

Every time a patient receives medical treatment, information is added to the patient's medical record, which includes data about symptoms, medical history, test results, diagnoses, and treatment. Health information technicians organize and manage these records, working closely with physicians, nurses, and other health professionals to ensure that they provide a complete and accurate basis for quality patient care.

Accurate medical records are essential for administrative purposes. Health information technicians assign a code to each diagnosis and procedure a patient receives, and this information is used for accurate patient billing. In addition, health information technicians analyze medical records to reveal trends in health and disease. This research can be used to improve patient care, manage costs, and help establish new medical treatments.

To read and interpret medical records, health information technicians need a thorough background in medical terminology. Most of these technicians work in hospitals and long-term–care facilities. Others may work in medical clinics, government agencies, insurance companies, and consulting firms. Because of the growing need for medical care, health information technology is projected to be one of the fastest-growing careers in the United States. For more information about this profession, contact the American Health Information Management Association.

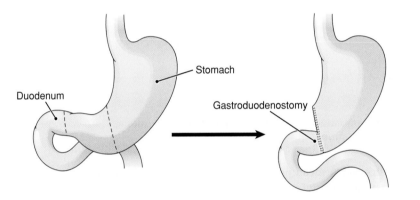

Figure 1-1 Gastroduodenostomy. A communication (-stomy) between the stomach (gastr) and the first part of the small intestine, or duodenum (duoden).

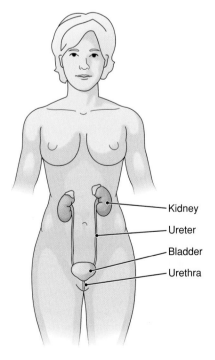

Figure 1-2 **Medical terminology uses both the Greek root *nephr* and the Latin root *ren* to refer to the kidney, an organ of the urinary system.**

Note that the same root may have different meanings in different fields of study, just as the words *spam, menu, browser, surfing,* and *cookie* have different meanings in common vocabulary than in "computerese." The root *myel* means "marrow" and may apply to either the bone marrow or the spinal cord. The root *scler* means "hard" but may also apply to the white of the eye. *Cyst* means "a filled sac or pouch" but also refers specifically to the urinary bladder. You will sometimes have to consider the context of a word before assigning its meaning.

Compound words contain more than one root. The words *eyeball, bedpan, frostbite,* and *wheelchair* are examples. Some compound medical words are *cardiovascular* (pertaining to the heart and blood vessels), *urogenital* (pertaining to the urinary and reproductive systems), and *lymphocyte* (a white blood cell found in the lymphatic system).

Combining Forms

When a suffix beginning with a consonant is added to a root, a vowel (usually an o) is inserted between the root and the suffix to aid in pronunciation, as seen in the previous example of gast**ro**duoden**o**stomy.

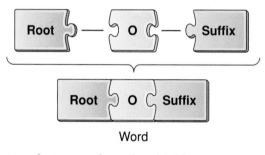

A combining vowel may be added between a root and a suffix.

Thus, when the suffix *-logy*, meaning "study of," is added to the root *neur,* meaning "nerve or nervous system," a combining vowel is added:

neur + o + logy = neurology (study of the nervous system)

Roots shown with a combining vowel are called **combining forms.**

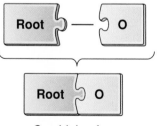

A root with a combining vowel is called a combining form.

This text gives roots with their most common combining vowels added after a slash and refers to them simply as roots, as in *neur/o.*

A combining vowel usually is not used if the ending begins with a vowel. For example, the root *neur* is combined with the suffix *-itis,* meaning "inflammation of," in this way:

neur + itis = neuritis (inflammation of a nerve)

This rule has some exceptions, particularly when they affect pronunciation or meaning, but you will observe these as you work.

Word Derivations

As mentioned, most medical word parts come from Greek (G) and Latin (L). The original words and their meanings are included in this text only occasionally. They are interesting, however, and may aid in learning. For example, *muscle* comes from a Latin word that means "mouse" because the movement of a muscle under the skin was thought to resemble the scampering of a mouse.

The coccyx, the tail end of the spine, is named for the cuckoo because it was thought to resemble the cuckoo's bill (Fig. 1-3). For those interested in the derivations of medical words, a good medical dictionary will provide this information.

Words Ending in *x*

When you add a suffix to a word ending in *x*, the *x* is changed to a *g* or a *c*. If there is a consonant before the *x*, such as *yx* or *nx*, the *x* is changed to a *g*. For example, *pharynx* (throat) becomes *pharyngeal* (*fa-RIN-jē-al*), to mean "pertaining to the throat"; *coccyx* (terminal portion of the spine) becomes *coccygeal* (*kok-SIJ-ē-al*), to mean "pertaining to the coccyx."

If a vowel comes before the *x*, such as *ax* or *ix*, you change the *x* to a *c*. Thus, *thorax* (chest) becomes *thoracotomy* (*thor-a-KOT-ō-mē*) to mean "incision into the chest" and *cervix* (neck) becomes *cervical* (*SER-vi-kal*) to mean "pertaining to a neck."

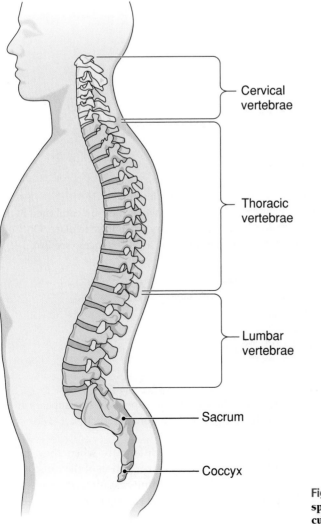

Cervical vertebrae

Thoracic vertebrae

Lumbar vertebrae

Sacrum

Coccyx

Figure 1-3 The coccyx of the spine looks like the bill of a cuckoo.

Suffixes Beginning with *rh*

When you add a suffix beginning with *rh* to a root, the *r* is doubled. For example:

hem/o (blood) + -**rh**age (bursting forth) = hemo**rr**hage (a bursting forth of blood)

men/o (menses) + -**rh**ea (flow, discharge) = meno**rr**hea (menstrual flow)

Pronunciation

This text provides phonetic pronunciations at every opportunity, even in the answer keys. The student CD that accompanies the text has a large auditory pronunciation dictionary. Take advantage of these aids. Repeat the word aloud as you learn to recognize it in print or hear it on the CD. The following pronunciation guidelines apply throughout the text.

A vowel (a, e, i, o, u) gets a short pronunciation if it has no pronunciation mark over it, such as:

a as in hat

e as in met

i as in bin

o as in some

u as in run

A short line over the vowel gives it a long pronunciation:

ā as in say

ē as in tea

ī as in lie

ō as in hose

ū as in sue

The accented syllable in each word is shown with capital letters.

Be aware that word parts may change in pronunciation when they are combined in different ways. Note also that accepted pronunciations may vary from place to place. Only one pronunciation for each word is given here, but be prepared for differences (see Box 1-2).

Soft and Hard *c* and *g*

➤ A soft *c*, as in *racer*, will be written as *s* (RĀ-ser).
➤ A hard *c*, as in *candy*, will be written as *k* (KAN-dē).
➤ A soft *g*, as in *page*, will be written as *j* (pāj).
➤ A hard *g*, as in *grow*, will be written as *g* (grō).

Silent Letters and Unusual Pronunciations

A silent letter or unusual pronunciation can be a problem, especially if it appears at the start of a word that you are trying to look up in the dictionary. See Box 1-3 for some examples.

The combinations in Box 1-3 may be pronounced differently when they appear within a word, as in dia**gn**osis (*dī-ag-NŌ-sis*), meaning determination of the cause of disease, in which the g is pronounced; **apn**ea (*AP-nē-a*), meaning cessation of breathing, in which the p is pronounced; nephro**pt**osis (*nef-rop-TŌ-sis*), meaning dropping of the kidney, in which the p is pronounced.

Box 1•2 Focus on Words   *Pronunciations*

When pronunciations are included in a text, it is sometimes difficult for authors to know which pronunciation of a term to use. Pronunciations may vary from country to country, and even in different regions of the same country. Think how easy it is to distinguish a southern accent and one from the Midwest or Northeast United States. The general rule is to use the most common pronunciation or to list that pronunciation first if more than one is given.

The word *gynecology* is usually pronounced with a hard g in the United States, but in many areas a soft g is used, as in jin-e-KOL-ō-jē. Words pertaining to the cerebrum (largest part of the brain) may have an accent on different syllables. The adjective is usually pronounced with the accent on the second syllable (se-RE-bral), but in cerebrum (SER-e-brum) and cerebrospinal (ser-e-brō-SPĪ-nal), the accented syllable differs.

The name for the first part of the small intestine (duodenum) is often pronounced dū-ō-DĒ-num, although the pronunciation dū-O-de-num is also acceptable. And the scientific term for the navel, umbilicus, is usually pronounced with the accent on the second syllable as um-BIL-i-kus, but um-bi-LĪ-kus is also used. When extreme, some alternative pronunciations can sound like a foreign language. The word we pronounce as SKEL-e-tal is pronounced in some other English-speaking countries as ske-LE-tal.

Box 1•3 For Your Reference   *Silent Letters and Unusual Pronunciations*

Letter(s)	Pronunciation	Example	Definition of Example
ch	k	chemistry *KEM-is-trē*	study of the elements and their interactions
dys	dis	dysfunction *dis-FUNK-shun*	difficult or abnormal function
eu	u	euphoria *ū-FOR-ē-a*	exaggerated feeling of well-being
gn	n	gnathic *NATH-ik*	pertaining to the jaw
ph	f	phantom *FAN-tom*	illusion or imaginary image
pn	n	pneumatic *nū-MAT-ik*	pertaining to air, lungs, or breathing
ps	s	pseudonym *SŪ-dō-nim*	false name
pt	t	ptosis *TŌ-sis*	dropping
rh	r	rhinitis *rī-NĪ-tis*	inflammation of the nasal (rhin/o) lining
x	z	xiphoid *ZIF-oyd*	pertaining to cartilage attached to the sternum

Learning Styles

The term "learning styles" describes how people differ in the senses they most depend on to learn. Visual learners want to see a word in print. They like diagrams, charts, and pictures. Auditory learners need to hear words pronounced. They like to talk over what they have learned and profit from listening again to recorded lessons. Tactile learners use touch, such as writing out answers or retyping notes. They like to follow demonstrations to learn a new skill. You can evaluate your own learning style with an inventory on the student CD or through the URL: http://thepoint.lww.com/cohen5e.

Of course, we use all of our senses to some degree in learning, and the more channels we use, the more likely it is that we will absorb and remember new information. This text, in combination with the student CD, calls on multiple senses to aid learning: seeing new words in print, writing out answers, using flashcards, listening to pronunciations, and completing exercises on the computer. Unlike the fashion magazines that use perfumed ads to sell products, the olfactory sense has not yet been incorporated into textbooks. Perhaps someday student CDs will have a smell feature!

Abbreviations

Symbols

Symbols are commonly used in case histories as a form of shorthand. Some examples are Ⓛ and Ⓡ for left and right; ↑ and ↓ for increase and decrease. A list of common symbols appears in Chapter 7 and in Appendix 1.

Word and Phrase Abbreviations

Like symbols, abbreviations can save time, but they can also cause confusion if they are not universally understood. Usage varies in different institutions, and the same abbreviation may have different meanings in different fields.

An **acronym** is an abbreviation formed from the first letter of each word in a phrase. Some everyday acronyms are ASAP (as soon as possible), ATM (automated teller machine), and a computer's RAM (random access memory). Acronyms have become popular for saving time and space in naming objects, organizations, and procedures.

Only the most commonly used acronyms and other abbreviations are given here. These are listed at the end of each chapter, but a more complete alphabetical list appears in Appendix 2. An abbreviation dictionary also is helpful.

Medical Dictionaries

With few exceptions, you can do all the exercises in this book without the aid of a dictionary, but medical dictionaries are valuable references for everyone in health-related fields. These include not only complete, unabridged versions, but also easy-to-carry short versions and dictionaries of medical acronyms and abbreviations. Many of these dictionaries are also available on CD. Dictionaries give information on meanings, pronunciation, synonyms, derivations, and related terms. Those intended for nursing and allied health professions include more complete clinical information, with notes on patient care.

Books vary in organization; in some, almost all terms are entered as nouns, such as disease, syndrome, procedure, or test. Those with a more clinical approach enter some terms according to their first word, which may be an adjective or proper name, for example biomedical engineering, Cushing disease, windchill factor. This format makes it easier to look up some terms. All dictionaries have directions on how to use the book and

TERMINOLOGY — Key Terms

acronym *AK-rō-nim*	An abbreviation formed from the first letter of each word in a phrase
combining form	A word root combined with a vowel to link the root with a suffix. Combining forms are shown with a slash between the root and the vowel, as in *neur/o*.
compound word	A word that contains more than one root
prefix *PRĒ-fix*	A word part added before a root to modify its meaning
root	The fundamental unit of a word
suffix *SU-fix*	A word part added to the end of a root to modify its meaning

Go to the pronunciation glossary in Chapter 1 on the CD-ROM to hear these words pronounced.

interpret the entries, as shown in Appendix 9, taken from *Stedman's Medical Dictionary*, 28th ed.

In addition to information on individual terms and phrases, medical dictionaries have useful appendices on measurements, clinical tests, drugs, diagnosis, body structure, information resources, and other topics.

CHAPTER REVIEW

Fill in the blanks:

1. A word part that comes after a root is a(n) _____.

2. A root with a vowel added to aid in pronunciation is called a(n) _____.

3. Combine the word parts *dia-*, meaning "through," and *-rhea*, meaning "flow," to form a word meaning "passage of fluid stool."_____.

4. Combine the root *cardi*, meaning "heart," with the suffix *-logy*, meaning "study of," to form a word meaning "study of the heart."_____.

Multiple choice. Select the best answer and write the letter of your choice to the left of each number:

_____ 5. Which of the following is a compound word?
    a. intestinal
    b. pharmacy
    c. urogenital
    d. muscular

_____ 6. The adjective for *pharynx* is
    a. pharynxic
    b. pharyngeal
    c. pharynal
    d. phargeal

_____ 7. The adjective for cervix is
    a. cervixal
    b. cervingeal
    c. cervical
    d. cervial

_____ 8. An acronym is formed from
    a. a proper name
    b. Latin or Greek
    c. two or more roots
    d. the first letter of each word in a phrase

Pronounce the following words:

9. dyslexia

10. rheumatism

11. pneumonia

12. chemotherapy

13. pharmacist

Pronounce the following phonetic forms, and write the words they represent:

14. *KAR-dē-ak* _____

15. *HĪ-drō-jen* _____

16. *OK-ū-lar* _____

17. *IN-ter-fās* _____

18. *rū-MAT-ik* _____

Go to the word exercises in Chapter 1 on the CD-ROM
for additional review exercises.

CASE STUDY 1-1: Multiple Health Problems Secondary to Injury

D.S., a 28-year-old woman, was treated for injuries sustained in a train-derailment accident. During the course of her treatment, she was seen by several specialists. For pain in her knee and hip joints, she was referred to an orthopedist. For migraine headaches and blurry vision, she consulted a neurologist. For pain on urination, occasional bloody urine, and possible nephritis, she saw a urologist. Later, for a persistent dry cough, pharyngitis, and problems resulting from a fractured nose, she was referred to an otorhinolaryngologist.

During D.S.'s initial course of treatment, she had a CT scan of her abdomen and brain and an MRI of her hip and knee. Her many visits also included respiratory endoscopic studies, pulmonary x-rays, and periodic blood tests in the hematology lab.

CASE STUDY QUESTIONS

Multiple choice. Select the best answer and write the letter of your choice to the left of each number:

_____ 1. The *de-* in the word *derailment* is a:
   a. suffix
   b. root
   c. prefix
   d. combining form

_____ 2. The *-ist* in the word *orthopedist* is a:
   a. root
   b. prefix
   c. derivation
   d. suffix

_____ 3. *MRI* stands for magnetic resonance imaging. This term represents a(n):
   a. combining form
   b. acronym
   c. prefix
   d. suffix

_____ 4. The root *nephr/o* in *nephritis* means:
   a. lung
   b. nerve
   c. joint
   d. kidney

_____ 5. The *rh* in the root *rhin/o* is pronounced as:
   a. r
   b. h
   c. er
   d. ro

Fill in the blanks:

6. Use Appendix 4 to find roots that mean *blood*. _____

7. Use the index to find the chapter that contains information on imaging techniques. _____

8. Use the flash cards at the back of this book to find the meaning of the prefix *endo-*. _____

9. Use Appendix 4 to find another word part with the same meaning as *endo-*. _____

10. Use Appendix 5 to look up the meaning of the roots in *otorhinolaryngology*.

ot/o _____

rhino _____

laryng/o _____

11. When the word *pharynx* has a suffix added, the *x* is changed to a _____

12. Appendix 2 tells you that the abbreviation *CT* in CT scan means _____

CHAPTER TWO

SUFFIXES

2

OBJECTIVES

After study of this chapter you should be able to:

1. Define a suffix.
2. Give examples of how suffixes are used.

3. Recognize and apply some general noun, adjective, and plural suffixes used in medical terminology.
4. Analyze the suffixes used in a case study.

PRETEST

1. The suffix in the word *studying* is _____.

2. Are the suffixes *-ism, -ia*, and *-ist* found in nouns, verbs, or adjectives? _____.

3. Are the suffixes *-ic, -ous*, and *-ile* found in nouns, verbs, or adjectives? _____.

4. The suffix *-oid* means _____.

5. The suffix *-logy* means _____.

6. The plural of *ovum* (egg) is _____.

7. The singular of *phenomena* is _____.

2

A suffix is a word ending that modifies a root. A suffix may indicate that the word is a noun or an adjective and often determines how the definition of the word will begin (Box 2-1). For example, using the root *myel/o,* meaning "bone marrow," the adjective ending *-oid* forms the word *myeloid,* which means "like or pertaining to bone marrow." The ending *-oma* produces *myeloma,* which is a tumor of the bone marrow. Adding another root, *gen,* which represents genesis or origin, and the adjective ending *-ous* forms the word *myelogenous,* meaning "originating in bone marrow."

The suffixes given in this chapter are general ones that are used throughout medical terminology. They include endings that form:

> ➤ Nouns: a person, place or thing
> ➤ Adjectives: words that modify nouns
> ➤ Plurals: endings that convert single nouns to multiples

Additional suffixes will be presented in later chapters, as they pertain to disease states, medical treatment, or specific body systems.

Noun Suffixes

The following general suffixes convert roots into nouns. Table 2-1 has suffixes that represent different conditions. Note that the ending *-sis,* may appear with different

Box 2•1	Focus on Words	*Meaningful Suffixes*

Suffixes sometimes take on a color of their own as they are added to different words. The suffix *-thon* is taken from the name of the Greek town Marathon, from which news of a battle victory was carried by a long-distance runner. It has been attached to various words to mean a contest of great endurance. We have bike-athons, dance-athons, telethons, and even major charity fund-raisers called thon-a-thons.

The adjective ending *-ish,* as in Scottish, can be added to imply that something is not right on target, as in largish, softish, oldish.

In science and medicine, the ending *-tech* is used to imply high technology, and *-pure* may be added to inspire confidence, as in the company name Genentech and the Multi-Pure water filter. The ending *-mate* suggests helping, as in *helpmate,* defined in the dictionary as a helpful companion, more specifically, a wife, or sometimes, a husband. The medical device HeartMate is a pump used to assist a damaged heart.

Table 2•1	Suffixes That Mean "Condition of"	
SUFFIX	**EXAMPLE**	**DEFINITION OF EXAMPLE**
-ia	dementia *dē-MEN-shē-a*	loss of (de-) intellectual function
-ism	egotism *Ē-gō-tizm*	exaggerated self-importance (from *ego*: self)
-sis	thrombosis *throm-BŌ-sis*	having a blood clot (thrombus) in a vessel (see Fig. 2-1)
-y	atony *AT-ō-nē*	lack of muscle tone

2

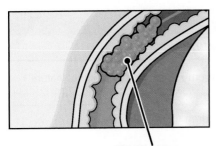

Blood clot
(thrombus)

Figure 2-1 Thrombosis (having a blood clot, or thrombus, in a vessel). The word *thrombosis* has the noun suffix *-sis*, meaning "condition of."

combining vowels as: *-osis*, *-iasis*, *-esis*, or *-asis*. The first two of these denote an abnormal condition.

Table 2-2 has endings that convert roots into medical specialties or specialists. The suffix *-logy* applies to many fields other than medicine. It contains the root *log/o* taken from the Greek word *logos*, which means "word," and generally means a field of study, as in *biology, archeology, terminology,* and *technology* (Box 2-2).

The two endings *-iatrics* and *-iatry* contain the root *-iatr/o*, based on a Greek word for healing and meaning "physician" or "medical treatment."

Exercise 2-1

Write the suffix that means "condition of" in the following words:

1. insomnia (inability to sleep; root somn/o)
   in-SOM-nē-a   _____ -ia _____

2. dysentery (intestinal disorder; root enter/o)
   DIS-en-ter-ē   _____

3. racism (discrimination based on race)
   RĀ-sizm   _____

4. psoriasis (skin disease)
   sō-RĪ-a-sis   _____

5. anesthesia (loss of sensation; root esthesi/o) (Fig. 2-2)
   an-es-THĒ-zē-a   _____

6. parasitism (infection with parasites or behaving as a parasite)
   PAR-a-sit-izm   _____

7. stenosis (narrowing of a canal)
   ste-NŌ-sis   _____

8. tetany (sustained muscle contraction)
   TET-a-nē   _____

9. diuresis (increased urination; root ur/o)
   dī-ū-rē-sis   _____

Table 2•2	Suffixes for Medical Specialties		
SUFFIX	**MEANING**	**EXAMPLE**	**DEFINITION OF EXAMPLE**
-ian	specialist in a field of study	physician *fi-ZISH-un*	practitioner of medicine (from root *physi/o,* meaning "nature")
-iatrics	medical specialty	pediatrics *pē-dē-AT-riks*	care and treatment of children (ped/o) (Fig. 2-3)
-iatry	medical specialty	psychiatry *sī-KĪ-a-trē*	study and treatment of mental (psych/o) disorders
-ics	medical specialty	orthopedics *or-thō-PĒ-diks*	study and treatment of the skeleton and joints (from root ped/o, meaning "child," and prefix ortho, meaning "straight")
-ist	specialist in a field of study	anesthetist *a-NES-the-tist*	one who administers anesthesia (see Fig. 2-2)
-logy	study of	dermatology *der-ma-TOL-ō-jē*	study and treatment of the skin (derma)

Box 2•2	Health Professions	*Medical Technology*

The field of medical technology includes a wide range of clinical laboratory sciences. Medical technologists test blood for abnormalities or infections and cross match it for transfusions. They analyze body fluids, looking for abnormal levels of various substances, such as cholesterol and glucose. They study the body's response to disease. They examine cells for signs of cancer and other diseases. A medical technologist working in a small lab may have to do tests in all these areas; those working in larger labs or hospitals usually specialize in one. Their work requires them to use microscopes, computers, and other complex instruments and equipment.

Most medical technologists have a bachelor's degree, which includes courses in mathematics and life sciences. Programs may also include on-the-job training. Advancement to supervisory positions requires advanced degrees. There are several accrediting agencies for medical technologists, and states vary in their licensing or registration policies. Medical technicians perform similar tasks in the laboratory, but generally are required to have a minimum of an associate (2-year) degree and to work under closer supervision.

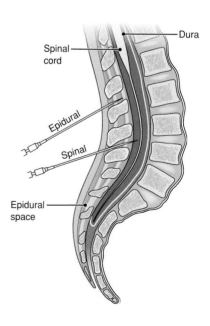

Figure 2-2 Injection sites for anesthesia. The word *anesthesia* uses the noun suffix *-ia,* meaning "condition of." The dura is a layer of the meninges, the membranes that cover the brain and spinal cord. One who administers anesthesia is an anesthetist or anesthesiologist.

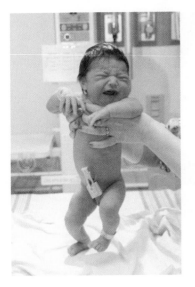

Figure 2-3 A practitioner of pediatrics, the care and treatment of children. The ending *-ics* indicates a medical specialty. This pediatrician, one who practices pediatrics, is testing an infant's reflexes.

Exercise 2-2

Write the suffix in the following words that means "study of," "medical specialty," or "specialist in a field of study":

1. cardiologist (specialist in the study and treatment of the heart; root cardi/o)   -ist
   kar-dē-OL-ō-jist

2. neurology (the study of the nervous system; root neur/o)
   nū-ROL-ō-jē

3. geriatrics (study and treatment of the aged; root ger/i) (Fig. 2-4)
   jer-ē-AT-riks

4. physiology (study of function in a living organism; root physi/o, meaning "nature")
   fiz-ē-OL-ō-jē

5. optician (one who makes and fits corrective lenses for the eyes; root opt/o)
   op-TISH-an

Write a word for a specialist in the following fields:

6. dermatology (study and treatment of the skin)
   der-ma-TOL-ō-je

7. pediatrics (care and treatment of children; root ped/o)
   pē-dē-AT-riks

8. radiology (use of radiation in diagnosis and treatment)
   rā-dē-OL-ō-jē

9. podiatry (study and treatment of the foot; root pod/o)
   pō-DĪ-a-trē

10. anatomy (study of body structure)
    a-NAT-ō-mē

11. technology (practical application of science)
    tek-NOL-ō-jē

2

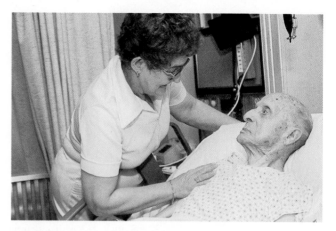

Figure 2-4 Geriatrics is the care and treatment of the aged. A specialist in this field, a geriatrician, is shown.

Adjective Suffixes

The suffixes below are all adjective endings that mean "pertaining to," "like," or "resembling" (Table 2-3). There are no rules for which ending to use for a given noun. Familiarity comes with practice. When necessary, tips on proper usage are given in the text.

Note that for words ending with the suffix *-sis*, the first *s* is changed to a *t* before adding *-ic* to form the adjective, as in genetic, pertaining to genesis (origin); psychotic, pertaining to psychosis (a mental disorder); or diuretic, pertaining to diuresis (increased urination).

Table 2·3	Suffixes That Mean "Pertaining to," "Like," or "Resembling"	
SUFFIX	**EXAMPLE**	**DEFINITION OF EXAMPLE**
-ac	cardiac *KAR-dē-ak*	pertaining to the heart
-al	vocal *VŌ-kal*	pertaining to the voice
-ar	nuclear *NŪ-klē-ar*	pertaining to a nucleus
-ary	salivary *SAL-i-var-ē*	pertaining to saliva
-form	epileptiform *ep-i-LEP-ti-form*	resembling epilepsy
-ic	neurotic *nū-ROT-ik*	pertaining to neurosis (a mental disorder)
-ical (ic + al)	anatomical *an-a-TOM-i-kl*	pertaining to anatomy (see Fig. 2-5)
-ile	virile *VIR-il*	pertaining to the male; masculine
-oid	lymphoid *LIM-foyd*	pertaining to the lymphatic system
-ory	respiratory *RES-pi-ra-tor-ē*	pertaining to respiration
-ous	venous *VĒ-nus*	pertaining to a vein (ven/o)

2

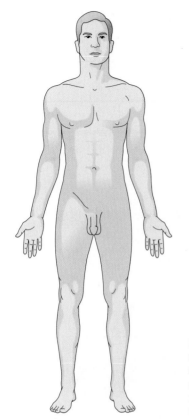

Figure 2-5 The anatomical position is standard in the study of anatomy. A person in this position is facing forward with arms at the side and palms forward (anterior). The adjective suffix *-ical* means "pertaining to."

Exercise 2-3

Identify the suffix meaning "pertaining to," "like," or "resembling" in the following words:

1. dietary (pertaining to the diet)
   DĪ-e-tar-ē   _____-ary_____

2. neuronal (pertaining to a nerve cell, or neuron) (Fig. 2-6)
   NŪR-ō-nal   _____

3. metric (pertaining to a meter or measurement)
   ME-trik   _____

4. cutaneous (pertaining to the skin; from L. *cutis*, skin)
   kū-TĀ-nē-us   _____

5. muciform (like or resembling mucus)
   MŪ-si-form   _____

6. toxoid (like or resembling a toxin, or poison)
   TOK-soyd   _____

7. topical (pertaining to a surface)
   TOP-i-kal   _____

8. febrile (pertaining to fever)
   FEB-rīl   _____

9. surgical (pertaining to surgery)
   SUR-ji-kal   _____

10. muscular (pertaining to a muscle)
    MUS-kū-lar   _____

11. urinary (pertaining to urine; root ur/o)
    Ū-ri-nar-ē   _____

12. circulatory (pertaining to circulation)
    SIR-kū-la-tor-ē   _____

13. pelvic (pertaining to the pelvis) (Fig. 2-7)
    PEL-vik   _____

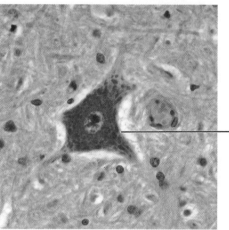

— Neuron

Figure 2-6 A neuron is a nerve cell. The adjective form of *neuron* is *neuronal.*

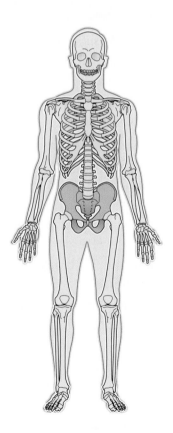

Figure 2-7 The pelvis is the bony hip girdle. The adjective form of *pelvis* is *pelvic.*

Forming Plurals

Many medical words have special plural forms based on the ending of the word. Table 2-4 gives some general rules for the formation of plurals along with examples. The plural endings listed in column 2 are substituted for the word endings in column 1. Note that both singular endings -*on* and -*um* change to -*a* for the plural. You have to learn which singular ending to use for specific words if you have to convert a plural ending in -*a* to the singular.

Some Exceptions to the Rules

There are exceptions to the rules given for forming plurals, some of which will appear in later chapters. For example, the plural of *virus* is *viruses*, and *serums* is sometimes used instead of *sera*. An -*es* ending may be added to words ending in -*ex* or -*ix* to form a plural, as in *appendixes*, *apexes*, and *indexes*.

Some incorrect plural forms are in common usage, for example *stigmas* instead of *stigmata*, *referendums* instead of *referenda*, *stadiums* instead of *stadia*. Often people use *phalange* instead of *phalanx* as the singular of *phalanges*. Words ending in -*oma*, meaning "tumor," should be changed to -*omata*, but most people just add an *s* to form the plural. For example, the plural of *carcinoma* (a type of cancer) should be *carcinomata*, but *carcinomas* is commonly used.

Table 2·4	Plural Endings		
WORD ENDING	**PLURAL ENDING**	**SINGULAR EXAMPLE**	**PLURAL EXAMPLE**
a	ae	vertebra (bone of the spine) *VER-te-bra*	vertebrae (Fig. 2-8) *VER-te-brē*
en	ina	lumen (central opening) *LŪ-men*	lumina (Fig. 2-9) *LŪ-min-a*
ex, ix, yx	ices	index (directory; list) *IN-deks*	indices *IN-di-sēz*
is	es	prognosis (prediction of disease outcome) *prog-NŌ-sis*	prognoses *prog-NŌ-sēz*
ma	mata	stigma (mark or scar) *STIG-ma*	stigmata *stig-MAT-a*
nx (anx, inx, ynx)	nges	phalanx (bone of finger or toe) *fa-LANKS*	phalanges (Fig. 2-10) *fa-LAN-jēz*
on	a	phenomenon (an occurrence or perception) *fe-NOM-e-non*	phenomena *fe-NOM-e-na*
um	a	serum (liquid) *SĒ-rum*	sera *SĒ-ra*
us	i	thrombus (see Fig. 2-1) *THROM-bus*	thrombi *THROM-bī*

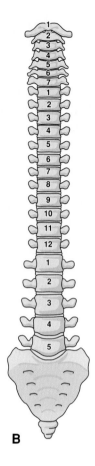

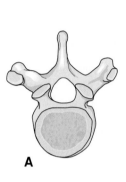

Figure 2-8 Each bone of the spine is a vertebra (*A*). The spinal column is made of 26 vertebrae (*B*).

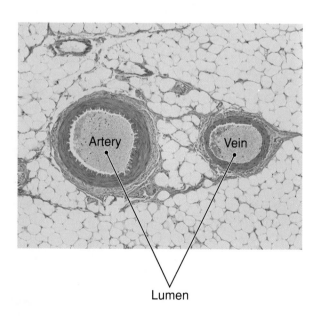

Figure 2-9 A lumen is the central opening of an organ or vessel. Two blood vessels are shown, an artery and a vein. The plural of *lumen* is *lumina*.

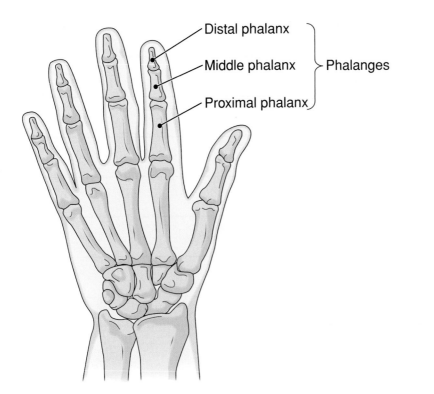

Figure 2-10 Bones of the right hand, anterior view. Each bone of a finger or toe is a phalanx. Each hand has 15 phalanges.

Exercise 2-4

Write the plural form of the following words. The word ending is underlined in each:

1. patell<u>a</u> (kneecap)
   pa-TEL-a

   _____ patellae _____

2. gangli<u>on</u> (mass of nervous tissue)
   GANG-lē-on

   _____

3. oment<u>um</u> (abdominal membrane)
   ō-MEN-tum

   _____

4. test<u>is</u> (male gonad)
   TES-tis

   _____

5. matr<u>ix</u> (background substance; mold)
   MĀ-triks

   _____

6. ov<u>um</u> (egg)
   Ō-vum

   _____

7. protozo<u>on</u> (single-celled animal)
   pro-tō-ZŌ-on

   _____

8. meni<u>nx</u> (membrane around the brain and spinal cord)
   ME-ninks

   _____

9. fung<u>us</u>
   fun-GUS

   _____

Write the singular form of the following words. The word ending is underlined in each:

10. spermatozo<u>a</u> (male reproductive cells)
    sper-ma-tō-ZŌ-a
    _____

11. append<u>ices</u> (things added)
    a-PEN-di-sēz
    _____

12. adeno<u>mata</u> (tumors of glands)
    ad-e-NŌ-ma-ta
    _____

13. embol<u>i</u> (circulating clots)
    EM-bō-lī
    _____

14. pelv<u>es</u>
    PEL-vēz
    _____

15. foram<u>ina</u> (openings, passageways)
    fō-RAM-i-na
    _____

16. curricul<u>a</u> (series of courses)
    kur-RIK-ū-la
    _____

CHAPTER REVIEW

Identify the suffix that means "condition of" in the following words:

1. alcoholism (*AL-kō-hol-izm*) _____

2. phobia (*FŌ-bē-a*) _____

3. acidosis (*as-i-DŌ-sis*) _____

4. dysentery (*DIS-en-ter-ē*) _____

5. paralysis (*pa-RAL-i-sis*) _____

6. insomnia (*in-SOM-nē-a*) _____

Give the suffix in the following words that means "specialty" or "specialist":

7. psychiatry (*sī-KĪ-a-trē*) _____

8. orthopedics (*or-thō-PĒ-diks*) _____

9. anesthesiologist (*an-es-thē-z ē-OL-ō-jist*) _____

10. technician (*tek-NISH-un*) _____

11. anatomist (*a-NAT-ō-mist*) _____

12. gynecology (*gī-ne-KOL- ō-jē*) _____

Give the name of a specialist in the following fields:

13. pediatrics (*pē-dē-A-triks*) _____

14. dermatology (*der-ma-TOL-ō-jē*) _____

15. cardiology (*kar-dē-OL- ō-jē*) _____

16. obstetrics (*ob-STET-riks*) _____

Identify the adjective suffix in the following words that means "pertaining to," "like," or "resembling":

17. physiologic (*fiz-ē-ō-LOJ-ik*) _____

18. skeletal (*SKEL-e-tal*) _____

19. fibrous (*FĪ-brus*) _____

20. ovoid (*OV-oyd*) _____

21. cellular (*SEL-ū-lar*) _____

22. basic (*BĀ-sik*) _____

23. binary (*BĪ-nar-ē*) _____

24. oral (*OR-al*) _____

25. rheumatoid (*RŪ-ma-toyd*) _____

26. febrile (*FEB-rīl*) _____

27. anatomical (*an-a-TOM-i-kal*) _____

28. circular (*SIR-ku-lar*) _____

29. exploratory (*ek-SPLOR-a-tor-ē*) _____

Write the plural for the following words. Each word ending is underlined:

30. gingiva (gums) _____
    JIN-ji-va

31. diagnosis (identification of disease) _____
    dī-ag-NŌ-sis

32. bacterium (type of microorganism) _____
    bak-TĒ-rē-um

33. foramen (opening) _____
    fō-RĀ-men

34. criterion (standard) _____
    kri-ter-ē-on

35. larynx (voicebox) _____
    LAR-inks

36. vertebra (bone of the spine) _____
    VER-te-bra

Write the singular form for the following words. Each word ending is underlined:

37. foci (centers) _____
    FŌ-sī

38. nuclei (centers; cores) _____
    NU-klē-ī

39. apices (high points, tips) _____
    Ā-pi-sēz

40. ganglia (small masses of nerve tissue) _____
    GANG-lē-a

41. lumina (central openings) _____
    LŪ-min-a

42. testes (male reproductive organs) _____
    TES-tēz

43. carcinomata (cancers) _____
    kar-si-NŌ-ma-ta

Go to the word exercises in Chapter 2 on the CD-ROM for additional exercises.

CASE STUDY

CASE STUDY 2-1: Health Problems on Return from the Rain Forest

E.G., a 39-year-old archaeologist returned from a 6-month expedition in the rain forest of South America suffering from a combination of physical symptoms and conditions that would not subside on their own. He was fatigued, yet unable to sleep through the night. He also had a mild fever, night sweats, occasional dizziness, double vision, and mild abdominal pain accompanied by intermittent diarrhea. In addition, he had a nonhealing wound on his ankle from an insect bite. He made an appointment with his family doctor, an internist.

On examination, E.G. was febrile (feverish) with a temperature of 101°F. His heart and lungs were normal, with a slightly elevated heart rate. His abdomen was tender, and his bowel sounds were active and gurgling. His skin was dry and warm. He had symmetrical areas of edema (swelling) around both knees and tenderness over both patellae (kneecaps). The ulceration on his left lateral ankle had a ring of necrosis (tissue death) surrounding an area of granulation tissue. There was a small amount of purulent (pus-containing) drainage.

E.G.'s doctor ordered a series of hematology lab studies and stool cultures for ova and parasites. The doctor suspected a viral disease, possibly carried by mosquitoes, native to tropical rain forests. He also suspected a form of dysentery typically caused by protozoa. E.G. was also possibly anemic, dehydrated, and septic (infected). The doctor was confident that after definitive diagnosis and treatment, E.G. would gain relief from his insomnia, diplopia (double vision), and dizziness.

CASE STUDY QUESTIONS

Multiple choice. Select the best answer and write the letter of your choice to the left of each number:

_____ 1. Diplopia, the condition of having double vision, has the suffix:
   a. lopia
   b. ia
   c. pia
   d. plopia

_____ 2. The adjective *septic* is formed from the noun:
   a. sepsis
   b. septosis
   c. septemia
   d. septery

_____ 3. E.G. was suspected to have anemia (diminished hemoglobin). The adjective form of the noun *anemia* is

   _____, and the field of health science devoted to the study of blood is called _____.
   a. anemic; hematology
   b. hematosis; hematism
   c. dehemia; hematomegaly
   d. anemic; parasitology

Write the suffix that means "condition of" in the following words:

4. necrosis _____

5. dysentery _____

6. insomnia _____

Write the adjective ending of the following words:

7. febrile _____

8. symmetrical _____

9. anemic _____

Write the singular form of the following words:

10. patellae _____

11. ova _____

12. protozoa _____

Write a word from the case study that means each of the following:

13. The word *virus* used as an adjective _____

14. The noun form of the adjective *necrotic* _____

15. Expert in the field of archeology _____

16. Expert in the field of internal medicine _____

17. The noun *abdomen* used as an adjective _____

PREFIXES

3

OBJECTIVES

After study of this chapter you should be able to:

1. Define a prefix and explain how prefixes are used.
2. Identify and define some of the prefixes used in medical terminology.
3. Use prefixes to form words used in medical terminology.

PRETEST

1. Where does a prefix appear in a word?

   _____

2. The prefix in the words prefix and *pretest* means _____.

3. The prefix in the word *microscopic* is _____.

4. The suffix in the word *microscopic* is _____.

5. The prefixes *mono-, tri,-* and *multi-* all refer to _____.

6. The prefixes *leuk/o-, melan/o-, and erythr/o-* all refer to _____.

7. The opposite of hyperglycemia (high blood sugar) is _____.

8. The opposite of postnatal (after birth) is _____.

A prefix is a short word part added before a word or word root to modify its meaning. For example, the word lateral means "side." Adding the prefix uni-, meaning "one," forms unilateral, which means "affecting or involving one side." Adding the prefix contra-, meaning "against or opposite," forms contralateral, which refers to an opposite side. The term equilateral means "having equal sides." Prefixes in this book will be followed by a hyphen to show that other parts will be added to the prefix to form a word.

This chapter introduces most of the prefixes used in medical terminology. Although the list is long, almost all of the prefixes you will need to work through this book are presented here. There is just one short additional table of prefixes related to position in Chapter 5 on body structure. The meanings of many of these prefixes will be familiar to you from words that are already in your vocabulary (see Box 3-1). You may not know all the words in the exercises, but make your best guess. The words in the tables are given as examples of usage. Almost all of them will reappear in later chapters. If you forget a prefix as you work, you may refer to this chapter or to the alphabetical lists of word parts and their meanings in Appendices 3 and 4. Appendix 7 lists prefixes only.

Box 3•1 Focus on Words   *Prefix Shorthand*

Many prefixes catch on rapidly as a form of shorthand. In everyday life, the prefix e- for electronic has spread to words such as e-mail, e-commerce, e-Bay, e-zine and others. X- for extreme appears in X-games and other X-sports.

The prefix endo- in the names of many surgical instruments signifies new endoscopic instruments that are longer and thinner and have smaller working tips to be used in areas where there is minimal access. Some examples are endoscissors, endosuture, endocautery, endograsper, and endosnare.

Health care products designed for specific age groups are also encoded by prefixes. Geri-, pertaining to old age, as in geriatrics, appears in geri-chair, geri-pads, geri-jacket, and the patent medicine Geritol, among others. Pedi- or pedia-, meaning "child," is found in the names pedi-cath, pedi-dose, pedi-set (instruments), and Pedialyte, a product used for children to replace fluid and electrolytes.

Common Prefixes

Table 3•1 Prefixes for Numbers*			
PREFIX	**MEANING**	**EXAMPLE**	**DEFINITION OF EXAMPLE**
prim/i-	first	primitive *PRIM-i-tiv*	occurring first in time
mon/o-	one	monoclonal *mon-ō-KLŌN-al*	describing a colony (clone) derived from one cell
uni-	one	unify *Ū-ni-fī*	make two or more parts into one
hemi-	half; one side	hemisphere *HEM-i-sfēr*	one half of a rounded structure (Fig. 3-1)

Table 3·1	Continued		
semi-	half; partial	semipermeable *sem-ē-PER-mē-a-bl*	partially permeable (capable of being penetrated)
bi-	two, twice	bisect *BĪ-sekt*	cut into two parts
di-	two, twice	diatomic *dī-a-TOM-ik*	having two atoms
dipl/o-	double	diplococci *dip-lō-KOK-sī*	round bacteria (cocci) that grow in groups of two
tri-	three	tricuspid *trī-KUS-pid*	having three points or cusps (Fig. 3-2)
quadr/i-	four	quadriplegia *kwa-dri-PLĒ-jē-a*	paralysis (-plegia) of all four limbs
tetra-	four	tetralogy *tet-RAL-ō-jē*	a group of four
multi-	many	multicellular *mul-tī-SEL-ū-lar*	consisting of many cells (Fig. 3-3)
poly-	many, much	polymorphous *pol-ē-MOR-fus*	having many forms (morph/o)

Prefixes pertaining to the metric system are in Appendix 1.

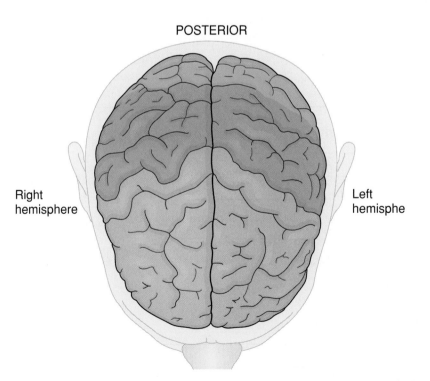

POSTERIOR

Right hemisphere

Left hemisphe

Figure 3-1 Brain hemispheres. Each half of the brain is a hemisphere. The prefix *hemi-* means half or one side.

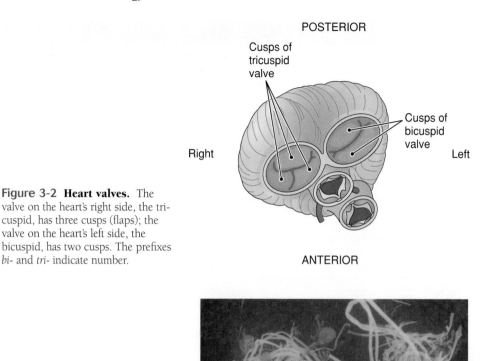

POSTERIOR

Cusps of tricuspid valve

Cusps of bicuspid valve

Right

Left

ANTERIOR

Figure 3-2 Heart valves. The valve on the heart's right side, the tricuspid, has three cusps (flaps); the valve on the heart's left side, the bicuspid, has two cusps. The prefixes *bi-* and *tri-* indicate number.

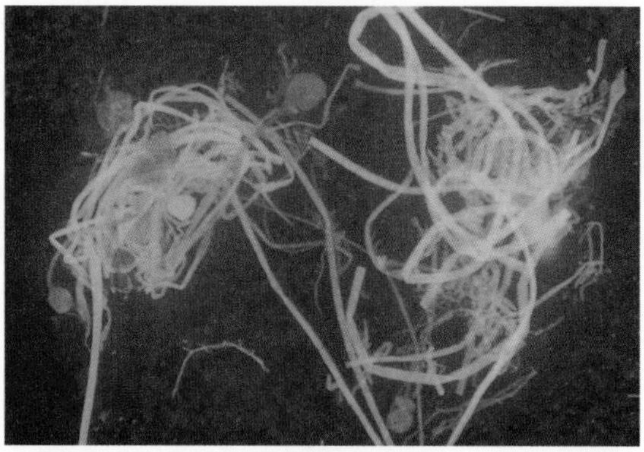

Figure 3-3 A multicellular organism has more than one cell. This fungus is a simple multicellular organism.

Exercise 3-1

Fill in the blanks:

1. Place the following prefixes in order according to increasing numbers:

   a. tri-   b. uni-   c. tetra-   d. bi- _____

2. A monocular (*mon-OK-ū-lar*) microscope has _____ lens(es).

3. A quadruped (*KWAD-rū-ped*) animal walks on _____ feet (ped/o).

4. The term unilateral (*ū-ni-LAT-e-ral*) refers to _____ side (later/o).

5. The term semilunar (*sem-ē-LŪ-nar*) means shaped like a _____ moon.

6. A diploid (*DIP-loyd*) organism has _____ sets of chromosomes (-ploid).

7. A tetrad (*TET-rad*) has _____ components.

8. A tripod (*TRĪ-pod*) has _____ legs (pod).

9. Bipolar means having _____ pole(s).

Give a prefix that is similar in meaning to each of the following:

10. di- _____

11. poly- _____

12. hemi- _____

13. mon/o- _____

Table 3·2	Prefixes for Colors		
PREFIX	**MEANING**	**EXAMPLE**	**DEFINITION OF EXAMPLE**
cyan/o-	blue	cyanosis *sī-a-NŌ-sis*	bluish discoloration of the skin due to lack of oxygen (Fig. 3-4)
erythr/o-	red	erythema *e-ri-THĒ-ma*	redness of the skin
leuk/o-	white, colorless	leukocyte *LŪ-kō-sīt*	white blood cell (-cyte)
melan/o-	black, dark	melanin *MEL-a-nin*	the dark pigment that colors the hair and skin
xanth/o-	yellow	xanthoma *zan-THŌ-ma*	yellow growth (-oma) on the skin

3

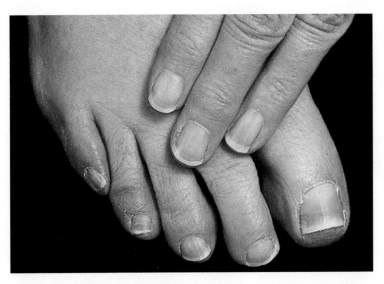

Figure 3-4 Cyanosis, a bluish discoloration. This abnormal coloration is seen in the toenails and toes, as compared to the normal coloration of the fingertips. The prefix *cyan/o-* means "blue."

Exercise 3-2

Match the following terms and write the appropriate letter to the left of each number:

_____ 1. melanocyte (*MEL-a-nō-sīt*)

_____ 2. xanthoderma (*zan-thō-DER-ma*)

_____ 3. cyanotic (*sī-a-NOT-ik*)

_____ 4. erythrocyte (*e-RITH-rō-sīt*)

_____ 5. leukoplakia (*lū-kō-PLĀ-kē-a*)

a. pertaining to bluish discoloration

b. red blood cell

c. yellow coloration of the skin

d. cell that produces dark pigment

e. white patches in the mouth

Table 3·3 Negative Prefixes

PREFIX	MEANING	EXAMPLE	DEFINITION OF EXAMPLE
a-, an-	not, without, lack of, absence	anhydrous *an-HĪ-drus*	lacking water (hydr/o)
anti-	against	antidote *AN-ti-dōt*	substance produced by the body that counteracts a foreign material
contra-	against, opposite	contraindicated *kon-tra-IN-di-kā-ted*	against recommendations; not advisable
de-	down, without, removal, loss	decalcify *dē-KAL-si-fī*	remove calcium (calc/i) from
dis-	absence, removal, separation	dissect *di-SEKT*	to separate tissues for anatomical study
in-*, im- (used before b, m, p)	not	incontinent *in-KON-ti-nent*	not able to contain or control discharge of excretions
non-	not	noncontributory *non-kon-TRIB-ū-tor-ē*	not significant; not adding information to a medical diagnosis
un-	not	uncoordinated *un-kō-OR-di-nā-ted*	not working together; not coordinated

May also mean "in" or "into" as in inject, inhale.

Exercise 3-3

Identify and define the prefix in the following words:

	Prefix	Meaning of Prefix
1. aseptic	a-	not, without, lack of, absence
2. antidote	_____	_____
3. amnesia	_____	_____
4. disintegrate	_____	_____
5. contraception	_____	_____
6. inadequate	_____	_____
7. depilatory	_____	_____
8. nonconductor	_____	_____

Add a prefix to form the negative of the following words:

9. conscious	unconscious
10. significant	_____
11. infect	_____
12. usual	_____
13. specific	_____
14. congestant	_____
15. compatible	_____

Table 3·4	Prefixes for Direction		
PREFIX	**MEANING**	**EXAMPLE**	**DEFINITION OF EXAMPLE**
ab-	away from	abduct *ab-DUKT*	to move away from the midline (Fig. 3-5)
ad-	toward; near	adduct *ad-DUKT*	to move toward the midline (see Fig. 3-5)
dia-	through	diarrhea *dī-a-RĒ-a*	frequent discharge of fluid fecal matter
per-	through	percutaneous *per-kū-TĀ-nē-us*	through the skin
trans-	through	transfusion *trans-FŪ-zhun*	introduction of blood or blood components into the bloodstream

3

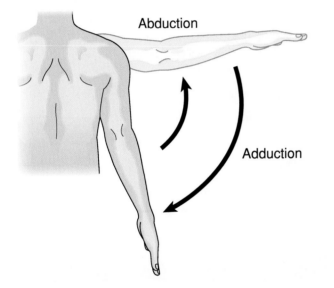

Figure 3-5 Abduction and adduction. The prefix *ab-* means "away from"; the arm is moved away from the body in abduction. The prefix *ad-* means "toward"; the arm is moved toward the body in adduction.

Exercise 3-4

Identify and define the prefix in the following words:

	Prefix	Meaning of Prefix
1. dialysis	dia-	through
2. percolate		
3. adjacent		
4. absent		
5. diameter		
6. transaction		

3

Table 3·5　Prefixes for Degree

PREFIX	MEANING	EXAMPLE	DEFINITION OF EXAMPLE
hyper-	over, excess, abnormally high, increased	hypertension *hī-per-TEN-shun*	high blood pressure
hypo-*	under, below, abnormally low, decreased	hypoglycemia *hī-pō-glī-SĒ-mē-a*	low blood sugar (glyc/o)
olig/o-	few, scanty	oligospermia *ol-i-gō-SPER-mē-a*	abnormally low number of sperm cells in semen
pan-	all	pandemic *pan-DEM-ik*	disease affecting an entire population
super-*	above, excess	supernumerary *su-per-NŪ-mer-ar-ē*	in excess number

*May also show position, as in hypodermic, superficial.

Exercise 3-5

Match the following terms and write the appropriate letter to the left of each number:

_____ 1. hyposecretion (*hi-pō-sē-KRĒ-shun*)

_____ 2. oligodontia (*ol-i-gō-DON-shē-a*)

_____ 3. panplegia (*pan-PLĒ-jē-a*)

_____ 4. superscript (*SŪ-per-skript*)

_____ 5. hyperventilation (*hī-per-ven-ti-LĀ-shun*)

a. excess breathing

b. something written above

c. underproduction of a substance

d. total paralysis

e. less than the normal number of teeth

Table 3·6　Prefixes for Size and Comparison

PREFIX	MEANING	EXAMPLE	DEFINITION OF EXAMPLE
equi-	equal, same	equilibrium *ē-kwi-LIB-rē-um*	a state of balance; state in which conditions remain the same
eu-	true, good, easy, normal	euthanasia *ū-tha-NĀ-zē-a*	easy or painless death (thanat/o)
hetero-	other, different, unequal	heterogeneous *het-er-ō-JĒ-nē-us*	composed of different materials; not uniform
homo, homeo-	same, unchanging	homograft *HŌ-mō-graft*	tissue transplanted to another of the same species
iso-	equal, same	isocellular *ī-sō-SEL-ū-lar*	composed of similar cells
macro-	large, abnormally large	macroscopic *mak-rō-SKOP-ik*	large enough to been seen without a microscope
mega-*, megalo-	large; abnormally large	megacolon *meg-a-KŌ-lon*	enlargement of the colon

Table 3·6	Continued			
micro-*	small	microcyte *MĪ-krō-sīt*	very small cell (-cyte)
neo-	new	neonate *NĒ-ō-nāt*	a newborn infant (Fig. 3-6)
normo-	normal	normovolemia *nor-mō-vol-Ē-mē-a*	normal blood volume
ortho-	straight, correct, upright	orthodontics *or-thō-DON-tiks*	branch of dentistry concerned with correction and straightening of the teeth (odont/o)
poikilo-	varied; irregular	poikilothermic *poy-ki-lō-THER-mik*	having variable body temperature (therm/o)
pseudo-	false	pseudoplegia *sū-dō-PLĒ-jē-a*	false paralysis (-plegia)
re-	again; back	reflux *RĒ-flux*	backward flow

*Mega- also means 1 million, as in megahertz. Micro- also means 1 millionth, as in microsecond.

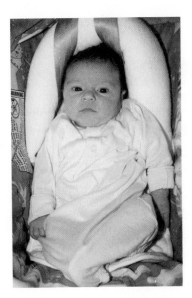

Figure 3-6 A neonate, or newborn. The prefix *neo-* means "new."

Exercise 3-6

Match the following terms and write the appropriate letter to the left of each number:

_____ 1. isograft (*Ī-sō-graft*)

_____ 2. orthotic (*or-THOT-ik*)

_____ 3. pseudoreaction (*sū-dō-rē-AK-shun*)

_____ 4. poikiloderma (*poy-kil-ō-DER-ma*)

_____ 5. homothermic (*hō-mō-THER-mik*)

a. having a constant body temperature

b. irregular, mottled condition of the skin

c. false response

d. tissue transplanted between identical individuals

e. straightening or correcting deformity

Identify and define the prefix in the following words:

	Prefix	Meaning of Prefix
6. homeostasis	homeo-	same, unchanging
7. equivalent		
8. orthopedics		
9. regurgitation		
10. euthyroidism		
11. neocortex		
12. megabladder		
13. isometric		
14. normothermic		

Write the opposite of the following words:

15. homogeneous (of uniform composition) _____
    hō-mō-JĒ-nē-us

16. microscopic (not visible with the naked eye) _____
    mī-krō-SKOP-ik

Table 3•7	Prefixes for Time and/or Position		
PREFIX	**MEANING**	**EXAMPLE**	**DEFINITION OF EXAMPLE**
ante-	before	antedate *AN-te-dāt*	to occur before the time of another event
pre-	before, in front of	prenatal *prē-NĀ-tal*	before birth (nat/i)
pro-	before, in front of	prodrome *PRŌ-drōm*	symptom that precedes a disease
post-	after, behind	postnasal *pōst-NĀ-sal*	behind the nose (nas/o)

Exercise 3-7

Match the following terms and write the appropriate letter to the left of each number:

_____ 1. postnatal (*pōst-NĀ-tal*)

_____ 2. antefebrile (*an-ti-FEB-ril*)

_____ 3. progenitor (*prō-JEN-i-tor*)

_____ 4. premature (*prē-ma-CHŪR*)

_____ 5. projectile (*prō-JEK-tīl*)

a. before a fever

b. occurring before the proper time

c. after birth

d. throwing or extending forward

e. ancestor; one who comes before

Identify and define the prefix in the following words:

	Prefix	Meaning of prefix
6. prediction (*prē-DIK-shun*)	pre-	before, in front of
7. postmenopausal (*pōst-men-ō-PAW-zal*)		
8. procedure (*prō-SĒD-ūr*)		
9. predisposing (*prē-dis-PŌ-zing*)		
10. antenatal (*an-ti-NĀ-tal*)		

3

Table 3•8	Prefixes for Position		
PREFIX	**MEANING**	**EXAMPLE**	**DEFINITION OF EXAMPLE**
dextr/o-	right	dextrogastria *deks-trō-GAS-trē-a*	displacement of the stomach (gastr/o) to the right
sinistr/o-	left	sinistromanual *sin-is-trō-MAN-ū-al*	left-handed
ec-, ecto-	out; outside	ectopic *ek-TOP-ik*	out of normal position
ex/o-	away from; outside	excise *ek-SĪZ*	to cut out
end/o-	in; within	endoderm *EN-dō-derm*	inner layer of a developing embryo
mes/o-	middle	mesencephalon *mes-en-SEF-a-lon*	middle portion of the brain (encephalon); midbrain
syn-, sym- (used before b, m, p,)	together	synapse *SIN-aps*	A junction between two nerve cells (Fig. 3-7)
tel/e-, tel/o-	end	telophase *TEL-ō-fāz*	the last stage of cell division (mitosis)

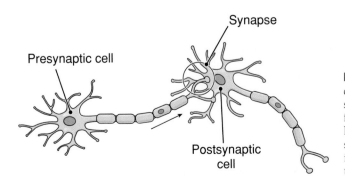

Figure 3-7 A synapse. Nerve cells come together at a synapse, as shown by the prefix *syn-*. The presynaptic cell is located before (prefix *pre-*) the synapse; the postsynaptic cell is located after (prefix *post-*) the synapse.

Exercise 3-8

Match the following terms and write the appropriate letter to the left of each number:

_____ 1. mesoderm (*MES-ō-derm*)

_____ 2. symbiosis (*sim-bī-ō-sis*)

_____ 3. dextrocardia (*deks-trō-KAR-dē-a*)

_____ 4. endoscope (*EN-dō-skōp*)

_____ 5. telencephalon (*tel-en-SEF-a-lon*)

a. displacement of the heart to the right

b. device for viewing the inside of a structure

c. two organisms living together

d. endbrain

e. middle layer of a developing embryo

Identify and define the prefix in the following words:

	Prefix	Meaning of Prefix
6. sympathetic *sim-pa-THET-ik*	sym-	together
7. extract *EKS-tract*		
8. ectocardia *ek-tō-KAR-dē-a*		
9. syndrome *SIN-drōm*		
10. endotoxin *en-dō-TOX-in*		

Write the opposite of the following words:

11. exogenous (outside the organism) _____
    eks-OJ-e-nus

12. dextromanual (right-handed) _____
    deks-trō-MAN-ū-al

13. ectoderm (outermost layer of the embryo) _____
    EK-tō-derm

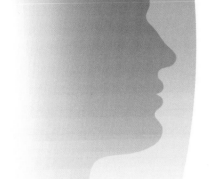

CHAPTER REVIEW

Match the following terms and write the appropriate letter to the left of each number:

_____	1. primary	**a.** one half or one side of the chest
_____	2. triceps	**b.** having two forms
_____	3. unite	**c.** a muscle with three parts
_____	4. dimorphous	**d.** form into one part
_____	5. hemithorax	**e.** first

_____	6. erythroderma	**a.** cell with yellow color
_____	7. melanoma	**b.** having a bluish discoloration
_____	8. xanthocyte	**c.** darkly pigmented tumor
_____	9. cyanotic	**d.** redness of the skin
_____	10. leukemia	**e.** overgrowth of white blood cells

_____	11. prophase	**a.** total paralysis
_____	12. mesoderm	**b.** final stage of cell division
_____	13. panplegia	**c.** double vision
_____	14. telophase	**d.** middle layer of tissue
_____	15. diplopia	**e.** first stage of cell division

Match each of the following prefixes with its meaning:

_____	16. poikilo-	**a.** good, true, easy
_____	17. eu-	**b.** straight, correct
_____	18. ortho-	**c.** false
_____	19. pseudo-	**d.** few, scanty
_____	20. oligo-	**e.** varied, irregular

Fill in the blanks:

21. A monocle has _____ lens(es).

22. A quadruplet is one of _____ babies born together.

(continued on next page)

23. Sinistrad means toward the _____ .

24. A disaccharide is a sugar composed of _____ subunits.

25. A contralateral structure is located on the side _____ to a given point.

26. A tetralogy is composed of _____ part(s).

Identify and define the prefix in the following words:

	Prefix	Meaning of Prefix
27. hyperactive	_____	_____
28. transfer	_____	_____
29. distant	_____	_____
30. regurgitate	_____	_____
31. exhale	_____	_____
32. adhere	_____	_____
33. unusual	_____	_____
34. detoxify	_____	_____
35. semisolid	_____	_____
36. premenstrual	_____	_____
37. perforate	_____	_____
38. dialysis (*dī-AL-i-sis*)	_____	_____
39. antibody	_____	_____
40. microsurgery	_____	_____
41. disease	_____	_____
42. ectoparasite	_____	_____
43. symbiotic (*sim-bī-OT-ik*)	_____	_____
44. prognosis (*prog-NŌ-sis*)	_____	_____
45. insignificant	_____	_____

True–False. Examine the following statements. If the statement is true, write T in the first blank. If the statement is false, write F in the first blank and correct the statement by replacing the underlined word in the second blank.

46. Immune cells are primed by their <u>first</u> exposure to a disease organism. __T__ _____

47. A unicellular organism is composed of <u>ten</u> cells. __F__ _____one_____

48. A binocular microscope has <u>two</u> lenses. _____ _____

49. In Latin, the oculus dexter (OD) is the <u>left</u> eye. _____ _____

50. The quadriceps muscle has <u>six</u> parts. _____ _____

51. A polygraph measures <u>many</u> physiologic responses. _____ _____

Opposites. Write a word that means the opposite of each of the following:

52. humidify _____

53. abduct _____

54. permeable _____

55. heterogeneous _____

56. exotoxin _____

57. macroscopic _____

58. hypoventilation _____

59. postsynaptic _____

Synonyms. Write a word that means the same as each of the following:

60. supersensitivity _____

61. megalocyte (extremely large red blood cell) _____

62. antenatal _____

63. isolateral (having equal sides) _____

Go to the word exercises in Chapter 3 on the CD-ROM
for additional review exercises.

CASE STUDY 3-1: Displaced Fracture of the Femoral Neck

While walking home from the train station, M.A., a 72-year-old woman with preexisting osteoporosis, tripped over a broken curb and fell. In the emergency department, she was assessed for severe pain in and swelling and bruising of her right thigh. A radiograph showed a fracture at the neck of the right femur (thigh bone) (Fig. 3-8). M.A. was prepared for surgery and given a preoperative injection of an analgesic to relieve her pain. During surgery, she was given spinal anesthesia and positioned on an operating room table, with her right hip elevated on a small pillow. Intravenous antibiotics were given before the incision was made. Her right hip was repaired with a bipolar hemi-arthroplasty (joint reconstruction). Postoperative care included maintaining the right hip in abduction, fluid replacement, physical therapy, and attention to signs of tissue degeneration and possible dislocation.

CASE STUDY 3-2: Sleep Study

The patient is a 58-year-old male 5'10", weighing 240 pounds, with a history of hypertension and previously treated for thymoma (thymus tumor) and melanoma. He reports excessive daytime sleepiness, snoring, and episodes of apnea (cessation of breathing). A full overnight polysomnography (sleep study) was arranged to evaluate for obstructive sleep apnea syndrome and upper airway resistance syndrome. The studies included electrical tracings of brain, heart, and muscle activity, along with measurement of eye movements and blood oxygen levels. Respiratory effort and airflow were also monitored.

Results showed multiple periods of wakefulness related to sleep-disordered breathing accompanied by recurrent and severe blood oxygen desaturation. Use of a mask to provide continuous positive airway pressure eliminated the respiratory distress, brought measurements to within normal limits, and eliminated snoring. Continued therapy was recommended, and the patient was also advised to lose weight. Assuming the patient complies with use of the mask, no further treatment or surgery should be necessary.

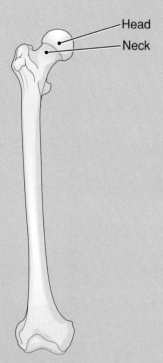

Head

Neck

Anterior view

Figure 3-8 The right femur (thigh bone). The femoral neck is the fracture site in Case Study 3-1.

CASE STUDIES

CASE STUDY QUESTIONS

Identify and define the prefixes in the following words:

	Prefix	Meaning of Prefix
1. preexisting	_____	_____
2. analgesic, anesthesia	_____	_____
3. dislocation, disordered	_____	_____
4. recurrent, replacement	_____	_____
5. bipolar	_____	_____
6. hemiarthroplasty	_____	_____
7. degeneration, desaturation	_____	_____
8. hypertension	_____	_____
9. apnea	_____	_____
10. polysomnography	_____	_____
11. syndrome	_____	_____

Fill in the blanks:

12. The suffixes in the words osteoporosis and anesthesia mean _____

13. The suffixes in the words intravenous, femoral, and analgesic mean _____

Find a word in the case histories that describes:

14. The time period before surgery _____

15. The time period after surgery _____

16. A position away from the midline of the body _____

17. A darkly pigmented tumor _____

CHAPTER FOUR

CELLS, TISSUES, AND ORGANS

4

OBJECTIVES

After study of this chapter you should be able to:

1. List the simplest to the most complex levels of a living organism.
2. Describe the main parts of a cell.
3. Label a diagram of a typical cell.
4. Name and give the functions of the four basic types of tissues in the body.

5. Define basic terms pertaining to the structure and function of body tissues.
6. Recognize and use roots and suffixes pertaining to cells, tissues, and organs.
7. Analyze case studies pertaining to cells and tissues.

PRETEST

1. The root that means "cell" is _____.

2. The root that means "tissue" is _____.

3. The control center of the cell is the _____.

4. The process of body cell division is called _____.

5. Compounds that speed up metabolism are the _____.

6. The substance that makes up the cell's genetic material is _____.

7. Chemicals—cells—tissues—_____—systems—organism. What belongs in the blank? _____

51

Body Organization

All organisms are built from simple to more complex levels (Fig. 4-1). Chemicals form the materials that make up cells, which are the body's structural and functional units. Groups of cells working together make up tissues, which in turn make up the organs with specialized functions. Organs become components of the various systems, which together comprise the whole organism. This chapter discusses the terminology related to cells, tissues, and organs, leading to the study of all the organ systems in Part 3.

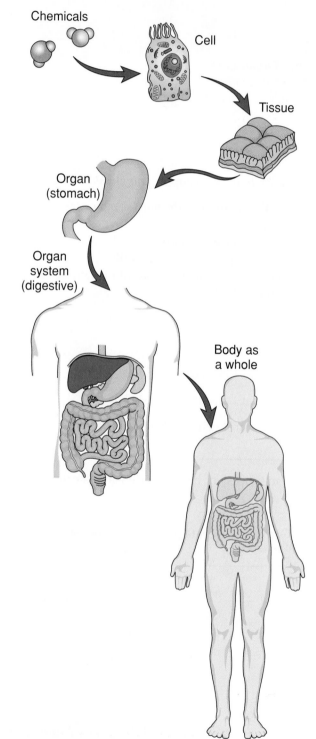

Figure 4-1 Levels of organization. The organ shown is the stomach, which is part of the digestive system

The Cell

The **cell** is the basic unit of living organisms (Fig. 4-2). Cells accomplish all the activities and produce all the components of the body. They carry out **metabolism**, the sum of all the body's physical and chemical activities. They provide the energy for metabolic reactions in the form of the chemical **ATP** (adenosine triphosphate), commonly described as the energy compound of the cell. The main categories of organic compounds contained in cells are:

➤ **Proteins**, which include the enzymes, some hormones, and structural materials.
➤ **Carbohydrates**, which include sugars and starches. The main carbohydrate is the sugar **glucose**, which circulates in the blood to provide energy for the cells.
➤ **Lipids**, which include fats. Some hormones are derived from lipids, and adipose (fat) tissue is designed to store lipids.

Within the **cytoplasm** that fills the cell are subunits called **organelles**, each with a specific function (see Fig. 4-2). The main cell structures are named and described in Box 4-1. Diseases may affect specific parts of cells. Cystic fibrosis and diabetes, for example, involve the plasma membrane. Other disorders center on mitochondria, ER, lysosomes, or peroxisomes (Box 4-2).

4

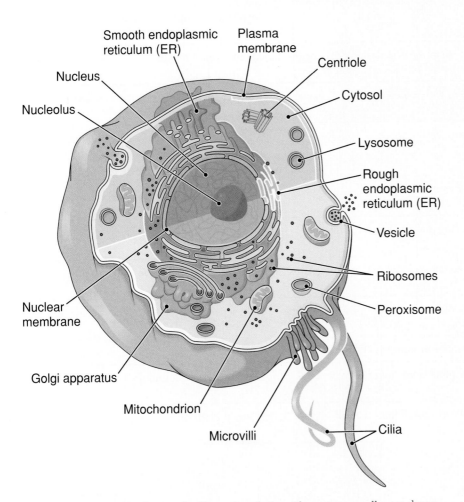

Figure 4-2 Generalized animal cell, sectional view. The main organelles are shown.

Box 4•1 **For Your Reference** *Cell Structures*

Name	Description	Function
Plasma membrane (PLAZ-ma)	Outer layer of the cell; composed mainly of lipids and proteins	Encloses the cell contents; regulates what enters and leaves the cell; participates in many activities, such as growth, reproduction, and interactions between cells.
Microvilli (mī-krō-VIL-ī)	Short extensions of the cell membrane	Absorb materials into the cell.
Nucleus (NŪ-klē-us)	Large, dark-staining organelle near the center of the cell, composed of DNA and proteins	Contains the chromosomes, the hereditary units that direct all cellular activities.
Nucleolus (nū-KLĒ-ō-lus)	Small body in the nucleus; composed of RNA, DNA, and protein	Makes ribosomes
Cytoplasm (SĪ-tō-plazm)	Colloidal suspension that fills the cell from the nuclear membrane to the plasma membrane	Site of many cellular activities. Consists of cytosol and organelles.
Cytosol (SĪ-tō-sol)	The fluid portion of the cytoplasm	Surrounds the organelles.
Endoplasmic reticulum (ER) (en-dō-PLAZ-mik re-TIK-ū-lum)	Network of membranes within the cytoplasm. Rough ER has ribosomes attached to it; smooth ER does not.	Rough ER sorts proteins and forms them into more complex compounds. Smooth ER is involved with lipid synthesis.
Ribosomes (RĪ-bō-sōmz)	Small bodies free in the cytoplasm or attached to the ER; composed of RNA and protein	Manufacture proteins
Mitochondria (mī-tō-KON-drē-a)	Large organelles with folded membranes inside	Convert energy from nutrients into ATP
Golgi apparatus (GŌL-jē)	Layers of membranes	Makes compounds containing proteins; sorts and prepares these compounds for transport to other parts of the cell or out of the cell.
Lysosomes (LĪ-sō-sōmz)	Small sacs of digestive enzymes	Digest substances within the cell
Peroxisomes (per-OKS-i-sōmz)	Membrane-enclosed organelles containing enzymes	Break down harmful substances
Vesicles (VES-i-klz)	Small membrane-bound sacs in the cytoplasm	Store materials and move materials into or out of the cell in bulk
Centrioles (SEN-trē-ōlz)	Rod-shaped bodies (usually two) near the nucleus	Help separate the chromosomes during cell division
Surface projections	Structures that extend from the cell	Move the cell or the fluids around the cell
Cilia (SIL-ē-a)	Short, hairlike projections from the cell	Move the fluids around the cell
Flagellum (fla-JEL-um)	Long, whip-like extension from the cell	Moves the cell

Box 4•2 Clinical Perspectives — *Cell Organelles and Disease*

Two organelles that play a vital role in cellular disposal and recycling may also be involved in disease. **Lysosomes** contain enzymes that break down carbohydrates, lipids, proteins, and nucleic acids. In a process called **autophagy** (aw-TOF-ah-je), lysosomes safely recycle cellular structures. They fuse with and digest worn out organelles then return the digested products to the cytoplasm for reuse. Lysosomes may also digest the cell itself in the process of **autolysis** (aw-TOL-ih-sis), a normal part of development. Cells that are no longer needed "self-destruct" by releasing lysosomal enzymes into their own cytoplasm.

Peroxisomes resemble lysosomes but contain different kinds of enzymes. They break down toxic substances that enter the cell, such as drugs and alcohol, as well as harmful by-products of normal metabolism.

In Tay–Sachs disease, the lysosomes in nerve cells lack an enzyme that breaks down certain kinds of lipids. These lipids build up inside the cells, causing malfunction that leads to brain injury, blindness, and death. Disease may also result if lysosomes or peroxisomes destroy cells when they should not. This may be true in the case of autoimmune diseases, in which the body develops an immune response to its own cells. The joint disease rheumatoid arthritis is one such example.

The **nucleus** is the control region of the cell. It contains the **chromosomes**, which carry genetic information (Fig. 4-3) . Each human cell, except for the sex cells, contains 46 chromosomes. These threadlike structures are composed of a complex organic substance, **DNA (deoxyribonucleic acid)**, which is organized into separate units called **genes**. Genes control the formation of proteins, most particularly **enzymes**, the catalysts needed for metabolic reactions. To help manufacture proteins, the cells use a compound called **RNA (ribonucleic acid)**, which is chemically related to DNA. Changes (mutations) in the genes or chromosomes are the source of hereditary diseases, as described in Chapter 15.

When a body cell divides, by the process of **mitosis**, the chromosomes are doubled and then equally distributed to the two daughter cells. The stages in mitosis are shown in Figure 4-4. When a cell is not dividing, it remains in a stage called *interphase*. In cancer, cells multiply without control causing cellular overgrowth and tumors. Sex cells (egg and sperm) divide by another process (meiosis) that halves the chromosomes in

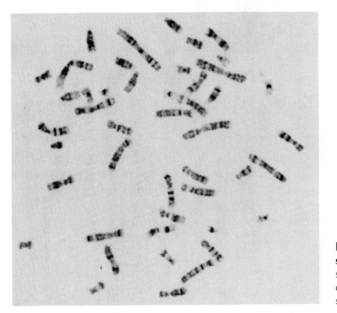

Figure 4-3 Human chromosomes. There are 46 chromosomes in each human cell, except the sex cells (egg and sperm).

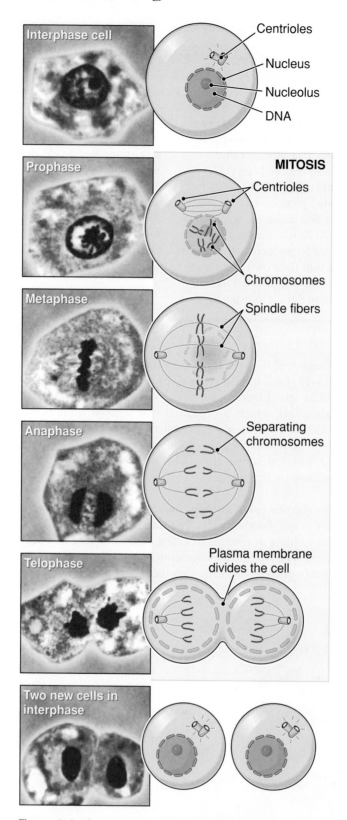

Figure 4-4 The stages in cell division (mitosis). When it is not undergoing mitosis, the cell is in interphase. The cell shown is for illustration only. It is not a human cell, which has 46 chromosomes.

preparation for fertilization. The role of meiosis in reproduction is further explained in Chapter 14.

The study of cells is **cytology** (*sī-TOL-ō-jē*), based on the root *cyt/o*, meaning "cell."

Tissues

Cells are organized into four basic types of **tissues** that perform specific functions:

> Epithelial (*ep-i-THĒ-lē-al*) tissue covers and protects body structures and lines organs, vessels, and cavities (Fig. 4-5). Simple epithelium, composed of cells in a single layer, functions to absorb substances from one system to another, as in the respiratory and digestive tracts. Stratified epithelium, with cells in multiple layers, protects deeper tissues, as in the mouth and vagina. Most of the active cells in glands are epithelial cells. Glands are described in more detail in Chapter 16.

> Connective tissue supports and binds body structures (Fig. 4-6). It contains fibers and other nonliving material between the cells. Included are adipose (fat) tissue, cartilage, bone (Chapter 19), and blood (Chapter 10).

> Muscle tissue (root: *my/o*) contracts to produce movement (Fig. 4-7). There are three types of muscle tissue:
>> Skeletal muscle moves the skeleton. It has visible cross-bands, or striations, that are involved in contraction. Because it is under conscious control, it is also called voluntary muscle. Skeletal muscle is discussed in greater detail in Chapter 20.
>> Cardiac muscle forms the heart. It functions without conscious control and is described as involuntary. Chapter 9 describes the heart and its actions.
>> Smooth, or visceral, muscle forms the walls of the abdominal organs; it is also involuntary. Many organs described in later chapters on the systems have walls made of smooth muscle. The walls of ducts and blood vessels also are composed mainly of smooth muscle.

> Nervous tissue (root *neur/o*) makes up the brain, spinal cord, and nerves (Fig. 4-8). It coordinates and controls body responses by the transmission of electrical impulses. The basic cell in nervous tissue is the neuron, or nerve cell. The nervous system and senses are discussed in Chapters 17 and 18.

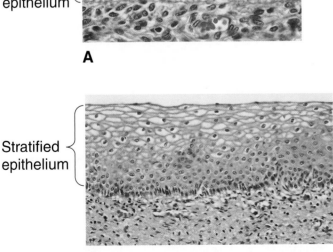

Simple epithelium

A

Stratified epithelium

B

Figure 4-5 Epithelial tissue. The cells in simple epithelium (*A*) are in a single layer and absorb materials from one system to another. The cells in stratified epithelium (*B*) are in multiple layers and protect deeper tissues.

4

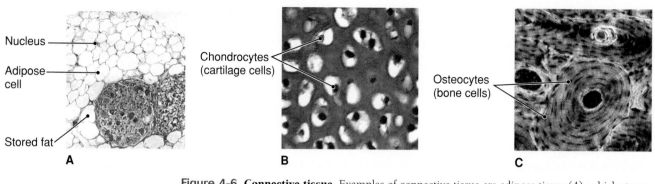

Figure 4-6 Connective tissue. Examples of connective tissue are adipose tissue (*A*), which stores fat; cartilage (*B*), which is used for protection and reinforcement; and bone (*C*), which makes up the skeleton.

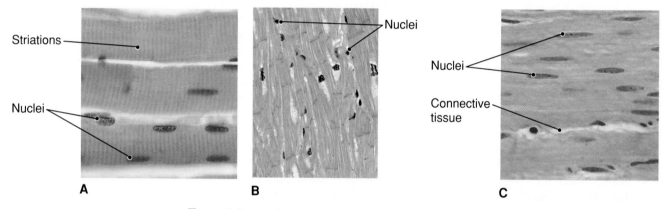

Figure 4-7 Muscle tissue. Skeletal muscle (*A*) moves the skeleton. It has visible bands (striations) that produce contraction. Cardiac muscle (*B*) makes up the wall of the heart. Smooth muscle (*C*) makes up the walls of hollow organs, ducts, and vessels.

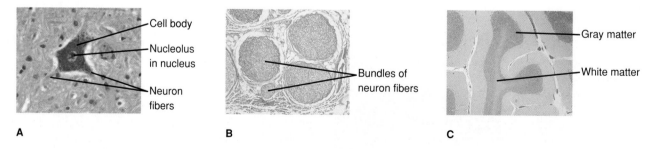

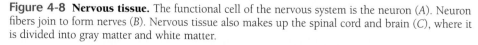

Figure 4-8 Nervous tissue. The functional cell of the nervous system is the neuron (*A*). Neuron fibers join to form nerves (*B*). Nervous tissue also makes up the spinal cord and brain (*C*), where it is divided into gray matter and white matter.

Box 4•3 Health Professions *Histotechnologist*

In the clinical laboratory, the histotechnologist is the health-care professional who prepares tissue samples for microscopic examination. When a tissue sample arrives at the laboratory, the histotechnologist cuts it into very thin slices, called sections, mounts the sections on glass slides, and treats them with various chemicals to preserve and prepare them for staining. The histotechnologist then stains the preserved sections with specific dyes to emphasize cellular details that a disease specialist (pathologist) might look for. To perform these tasks, histotechnologists require a strong clinical background and a thorough understanding of chemistry, anatomy, and physiology.

Most histotechnologists work in hospital and medical clinic laboratories, although some find employment in research laboratories, pharmaceutical companies, and government agencies. Job prospects are promising because of the growing need for health care and the development of new laboratory tests and technologies. For more information about careers in histotechnology, contact the American Society for Clinical Laboratory Science.

Membranes

The simplest tissues are membranes. Mucous membranes secrete **mucus**, a thick fluid that lubricates surfaces and protects underlying tissue, as in the lining of the digestive tract and respiratory passages. Serous membranes, which secrete a thin, watery fluid, line body cavities and cover organs. These include the membranes around the heart and lungs. Fibrous membranes cover and support organs, as found around the bones, the brain, and spinal cord.

The study of tissues is **histology** (*his-TOL-ō-jē*), based on the root *hist/o*, meaning "tissue." Focus Boxes 4-3 and 4-4 describe a profession involved in tissue study and some terms used in histology.

Box 4•4 Clinical Perspectives *Laboratory Study of Tissues*

Biopsy is the removal and examination of living tissue to determine a diagnosis. The term is also applied to the specimen itself. *Biopsy* comes from the Greek word *bios*, meaning "life," plus *opsis*, meaning "vision." Together they mean the visualization of living tissue.

Some other terms that apply to cells and tissues come from Latin. *In vivo* means "in the living body," as contrasted with *in vitro*, which literally means "in glass," and refers to procedures and experiments done in the labora- tory, as compared with studies done in living organisms. *In situ* means "in its original place," and is used to refer to tumors that have not spread.

In toto means "whole" or "completely," as in referring to a structure or organ removed totally from the body. *Postmortem* literally means "after death," as in referring to an autopsy performed to determine the cause of death.

Organs and Organ Systems

Tissues are arranged into **organs**, which serve specific functions, and organs, in turn, are grouped into systems. Figure 4-9 shows the organs of the digestive system as an example. Grouped according to functions, the body systems are:

- ➤ Circulation:
  - ➤ Cardiovascular system, consisting of the heart and blood vessels
  - ➤ Lymphatic system, organs and vessels that aid circulation and help protect the body from foreign materials
- ➤ Nutrition and fluid balance:
  - ➤ Respiratory system, which obtains the oxygen needed for metabolism and eliminates carbon dioxide, a by-product of metabolism
  - ➤ Digestive system, which takes in, breaks down, and absorbs nutrients and eliminates undigested waste
  - ➤ Urinary system, which eliminates soluble waste and balances the volume and composition of body fluids
- ➤ Production of offspring:
  - ➤ The male and female reproductive systems
- ➤ Coordination and control:
  - ➤ Nervous system, consisting of the brain, spinal cord, and nerves, and including the sensory system. This system receives and processes stimuli and directs responses.
  - ➤ Endocrine system, individual glands that produce hormones.

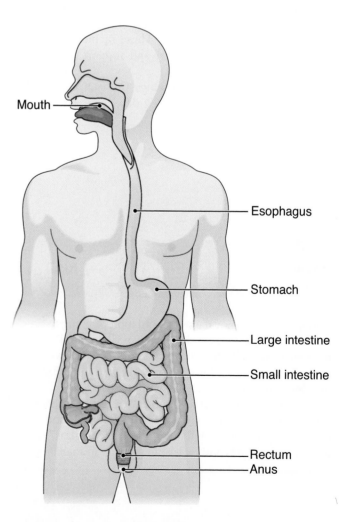

Figure 4-9 Organs of the digestive tract. Other organs and glands contribute to digestion, as described in Chapter 12.

Mouth

Esophagus

Stomach

Large intestine

Small intestine

Rectum

Anus

➤ Body structure and movement:
  ➤ Skeletal system, the bones and joints
  ➤ Muscular system, which moves the skeleton and makes up organs. The muscular system and skeleton protect vital organs.
➤ Body covering:
  ➤ The skin, or integumentary system, which functions in protection and also helps to regulate body temperature

Each of the body systems is discussed in Part 3. Bear in mind, however, that the body functions as a whole—no system is independent of the others. They work together to maintain the body's state of internal stability, termed **homeostasis**.

4

TERMINOLOGY — Key Terms

ATP	The energy compound of the cell; stores energy needed for cell activities. ATP stands for adenosine triphosphate (*a-DEN-ō-sēn trī-FOS-fāt*).
carbohydrate *kar-bō-HĪ-drāt*	The category of organic compounds that includes sugars and starches
cell *sel*	The basic structural and functional unit of the living organism; a microscopic unit that combines with other cells to form tissues (root *cyt/o*)
chromosome *KRŌ-mō-sōm*	A threadlike body in a cell's nucleus that contains genetic information
cytology *sī-TOL-ō-jē*	Study of cells
cytoplasm *SĪ-tō-plazm*	The fluid that fills a cell and holds the organelles
DNA	The genetic compound of the cell; makes up the genes. DNA stands for deoxyribonucleic (*dē-ok-sē-rī-bō-nū-KLĒ-ik*) acid.
enzyme *EN-zīm*	An organic substance that speeds the rate of metabolic reactions
gene *jēn*	A hereditary unit composed of DNA and combined with other genes to form the chromosomes
glucose *GLŪ-kōs*	A simple sugar that circulates in the blood; the main energy source for metabolism (roots: *gluc/o, glyc/o*)
histology *his-TOL-ō-jē*	Study of tissues
homeostasis *hō-mē-ō-STĀ-sis*	A steady state; a condition of internal stability and constancy
lipid *LIP-id*	A category of organic compounds that includes fats (root *lip/o*)
metabolism *me-TA-bō-lizm*	The sum of all the physical and chemical reactions that occur within an organism
mitosis *mī-TŌ-sis*	Cell division
mucus *MŪ-kus*	A thick fluid secreted by cells in membranes and glands that lubricates and protects tissues (roots: *muc/o, myx/o*); the adjective is *mucous*.

TERMINOLOGY Key Terms

Continued

nucleus *NŪ-klē-us*	The cell's control center; directs all cell activities based on the information contained in its chromosomes (roots *nucle/o, kary/o*)
organ *OR-gan*	A part of the body with a specific function. A component of a body system.
organelle *OR-ga-nel*	A specialized structure in the cytoplasm of a cell
protein *PRŌ-tēn*	A category of organic compounds that includes structural materials, enzymes, and some hormones
RNA	An organic compound involved in the manufacture of proteins within cells. RNA stands for ribonucleic (*rī-bō-nū-KLĒ-ik*) acid.
tissue *TISH-ū*	A group of cells that acts together for a specific purpose (root: *hist/o, histi/o*)

Go to the pronunciation glossary in Chapter 4 on the CD-ROM to hear these words pronounced.

Word Parts Pertaining to Cells, Tissues, and Organs

Table 4·1   Roots for Cells and Tissues

ROOT	MEANING	EXAMPLE	DEFINITION OF EXAMPLE
morph/o	form	amorphous *a-MOR-fus*	without form
cyt/o, -cyte	cell	cytogenesis *sī-tō-JEN-e-sis*	formation (-genesis) of cells
nucle/o	nucleus	nucleoplasm *NŪ-klē-ō-plazm*	substance that fills the nucleus
kary/o	nucleus	karyotype *KAR-ē-ō-tīp*	picture of a cell's chromosomes organized according to size (Fig. 4-10)
hist/o, histi/o	tissue	histologic *his-tō-LOJ-ik*	pertaining to tissues
fibr/o	fiber	fibrosis *fī-BRŌ-sis*	abnormal formation of fibrous tissue
reticul/o	network	reticulum *re-TIK-ū-lum*	a network

Table 4·1	Continued		
aden/o	gland	adenoma *ad-e-NO-ma*	tumor (-oma) of a gland
papill/o	nipple	papilla *pa-PIL-a*	projection that resembles a nipple
myx/o	mucus	myxadenitis *miks-ad-e-NĪ -tis*	inflammation (-itis) of a mucus-secreting gland
muc/o	mucus, mucous membrane	mucorrhea *mū-kō-RĒ-a*	increased flow (-rhea) of mucus
somat/o, -some	body, small body	chromosome *KRŌ-mō-sōm*	small body that takes up color (dye) (chrom/o)

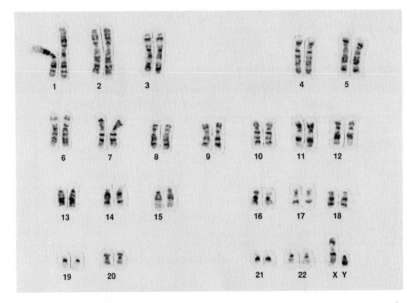

Figure 4-10 Human karyotype. The 46 chromosomes are in 23 pairs arranged according to size. The XY sex chromosomes, the 23rd pair at the lower right, indicate that the cell is from a male; a female cell has XX sex chromosomes.

Exercise 4-1

Fill in the blanks:

1. A fibril (*FĪ-bril*) is a small _____.

2. A histologist studies _____.

3. A polymorphic (*pol-ē-MOR-fik*) organism has many _____.

4. Karyomegaly (*kar-ē-ō-MEG-a-lē*) is enlargement (-megaly) of the _____.

5. The term *nuclear* means pertaining to a(n) _____.

6. Adenitis (*ad-e-NĪ-tis*) is inflammation (-itis) of a _____.

7. A papillary (*PAP-i-lar-ē*) structure resembles a(n) _____.

8. A myxoma (*mik-SŌ-ma*) is a tumor of tissue that secretes _____.

9. A reticulocyte (*re-TIK-ū-lō-sīt*) is a cell that contains a(n) _____.

10. The term *mucosa* (*mu-KŌ-sa*) is used to describe a membrane that secretes _____.

11. Somatotropin (*sō-ma-tō-TRŌ-pin*), also called growth hormone, has a general stimulating effect on the _____.

_____.

Use the suffix -logy to build a word with each of the following meanings:

12. The study of form _____

13. The study of cells _____

14. The study of tissues _____

The roots in Table 4-2 are often combined with a simple noun suffix (*-in*, *-y*, or *-ia*) or an adjective suffix (*-ic*) and used as word endings. Such combined forms that routinely appear as word endings will simply be described and used as suffixes in this book. Examples from the above list are *-trophy*, *-plasia*, *-tropin*, *-philic*, *-genic*.

Table 4·2 Roots for Cell Activity

ROOT	MEANING	EXAMPLE	DEFINITION OF EXAMPLE
blast/o, -blast	immature cell, productive cell, embryonic cell	blastocyte *BLAS-tō-sīt*	an early embryonic cell
gen	origin, formation	histogenesis *his-tō-JEN-e-sis*	origin or formation of tissues
phag/o	eat, ingest	autophagy *aw-TOF-a-jē*	self-destruction of a cell's organelles
phil	attract, absorb	basophilic *bā-sō-FIL-ik*	attracting basic stain
plas	formation, molding, development	hypoplasia *hī-pō-PLĀ-zē-a*	underdevelopment of an organ or tissue
trop	act on, affect	chronotropic *kron-o-TROP-ik*	affecting rate or timing (chron/o)
troph/o	feeding, growth, nourishment	hypertrophy *hī-PER-trō-fē*	overdevelopment of tissue

Exercise 4-2

Match the following terms and write the appropriate letter to the left of each number:

_____ 1. phagocyte (*FAG-ō-sīt*)

_____ 2. karyogenesis (*kar-ē-ō-JEN-e-sis*)

_____ 3. leukoblast (*LŪ-kō-blast*)

_____ 4. papilliform (*pa-PIL-i-form*)

_____ 5. atrophy (*A-trō-fē*)

a. wasting of tissue

b. resembling a nipple

c. formation of a nucleus

d. cell that ingests waste

e. immature white blood cell

_____ 6. neoplasia (nē-ō-PLĀ-jē-a)

_____ 7. gonadotropin (gon-a-dō-TRŌ-pin)

_____ 8. aplasia (a-PLĀ-jē-a)

_____ 9. somatic (sō-MAT-ik)

_____ 10. chromophilic (krō-mō-FIL-ik)

a. attracting color

b. pertaining to the body

c. substance that acts on the sex glands

d. new formation of tissue

e. lack of development

Identify and define the root in the following words:

	Root	Meaning of Root
11. genetics (je-NET-iks)	_____	_____
12. esophagus (e-SOF-a-gus)	_____	_____
13. normoblast (NOR-mō-blast)	_____	_____
14. aplastic (a-PLAS-tik)	_____	_____
15. dystrophy (DIS-trō-fē)	_____	_____

Table 4·3 Suffixes and Roots for Body Chemistry

WORD PART	MEANING	EXAMPLE	DEFINITION OF EXAMPLE
Suffixes			
-ase	enzyme	lipase *LĪ-pās*	enzyme that digests fat (lipid)
-ose	sugar	fructose *FRŪK-tōs*	fruit sugar
Roots			
hydr/o	water, fluid	hydrophilic *hī-drō-FIL-ik*	attracting water
gluc/o	glucose	glucogenesis *glū-kō-JEN-e-sis*	production of glucose
glyc/o	sugar, glucose	normoglycemia *nor-mō-glī-SĒ-mē-a*	normal blood sugar level
sacchar/o	sugar	polysaccharide *pol-ē-SAK-a-rīd*	compound containing many simple sugars
amyl/o	starch	amyloid *AM-i-loyd*	resembling starch
lip/o	lipid, fat	lipogenesis *lip-ō-JEN-e-sis*	formation of fat
adip/o	fat	adiposuria *ad-i-pō-SŪR-ē-a*	presence of fat in the urine (ur/o)
steat/o	fatty	steatorrhea *stē-a-tō-RĒ-a*	discharge (-rhea) of fatty stools
prote/o	protein	protease *PRŌ-tē-ās*	enzyme that digests protein

Exercise 4-3

Fill in the blanks:

1. A disaccharide (*dī-SAK-a-rīd*) is a compound that contains two _____.

2. The ending -*ose* indicates that sucrose is a(n) _____.

3. Hydrophobia (*hī-drō-FŌ-bē-a*) is an aversion (-phobia) to _____.

4. Amylase (*AM-i-lās*) is an enzyme that digests _____.

5. Liposuction (*LIP-ō-suk-shun*) is the surgical removal of _____.

6. A glucocorticoid (*glū-kō-KOR-ti-koyd*) is a hormone that controls the metabolism of
_____.

7. An adipocyte (*AD-i-pō-sīt*) is a cell that stores _____.

Identify and define the root in the following words:

	Root	Meaning of Root
8. asteatosis (*as-tē-a-TŌ-sis*)	_____	_____
9. lipoma (*lī-PŌ-ma*)	_____	_____
10. hyperglycemia (*hī-per-glī-SĒ-mē-a*)	_____	_____
11. glucolytic (*glū-kō-LIT-ik*)	_____	_____

TERMINOLOGY Supplementary Terms

amino acids *a-MĒ-nō*	The nitrogen-containing compounds that make up proteins
anabolism *a-NAB-ō-lizm*	The type of metabolism in which body substances are made; the building phase of metabolism
catabolism *ka-TAB-ō-lizm*	The type of metabolism in which substances are broken down for energy and simple compounds
collagen *KOL-a-jen*	A fibrous protein found in connective tissue
cortex *KOR-tex*	The outer region of an organ
glycogen *GLĪ-kō-jen*	A complex sugar compound stored in liver and muscles; broken down into glucose when needed for energy
interstitial *in-ter-STISH-al*	Between parts, such as the spaces between cells in a tissue
medulla *me-DUL-la*	The inner region of an organ; marrow (root: *medull/o*)

TERMINOLOGY
Continued

Supplementary Terms

parenchyma *par-EN-ki-ma*	The functional tissue of an organ
parietal *pa-RĪ-e-tal*	Pertaining to a wall; describes a membrane that lines a body cavity
soma *SŌ-ma*	The body
stem cell	An immature cell that has the capacity to develop into any of a variety of different cell types. A precursor cell.
visceral *VIS-er-al*	Pertaining to the internal organs; describes a membrane on the surface of an organ

4

 Go to the pronunciation glossary in Chapter 4 on the CD-ROM to hear these words pronounced.

CHAPTER REVIEW

LABELING EXERCISE
Diagram of a Typical Animal Cell

Write the name of each numbered part on the corresponding line of the answer sheet.

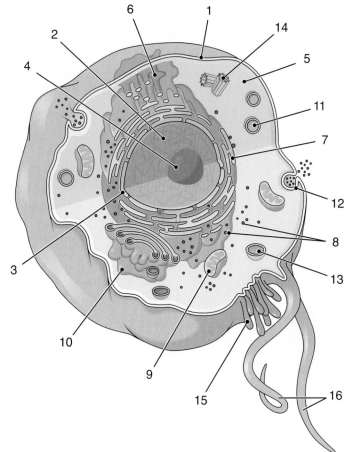

Centriole	1. _____
Cilia	2. _____
Cytosol	3. _____
Golgi apparatus	4. _____
Lysosome	5. _____
Microvilli	6. _____
Mitochondrion	7. _____
Nuclear membrane	8. _____
Nucleolus	9. _____
Nucleus	10. _____
Peroxisome	11. _____

Plasma membrane	12. _____
Ribosomes	13. _____
Rough ER	14. _____
Smooth ER	15. _____
Vesicle	16. _____

TERMINOLOGY

Match the following terms and write the appropriate letter to the left of each number:

_____	1. liposomes	**a.** state of internal stability
_____	2. DNA	**b.** small bodies that store fat
_____	3. ribosomes	**c.** energy compound of the cells
_____	4. homeostasis	**d.** genetic material
_____	5. ATP	**e.** organelles that contain RNA
_____	6. mitosis	**a.** immature cell
_____	7. nucleoplasm	**b.** organelles that produce ATP
_____	8. mitochondria	**c.** material that fills the nucleus
_____	9. blastocyte	**d.** material that holds the organelles
_____	10. cytoplasm	**e.** cell division
_____	11. reticulocyte	**a.** resembling a gland
_____	12. adenoid	**b.** fibrous tumor
_____	13. fibroma	**c.** cell with a very large nucleus
_____	14. megakaryocyte	**d.** cell that contains a network
_____	15. chromosome	**e.** structure that contains genes
_____	16. autotroph	**a.** like a nipple
_____	17. papillary	**b.** wasting of tissue
_____	18. amorphous	**c.** without form
_____	19. atrophy	**d.** acting on body cells
_____	20. somatotrophic	**e.** organism that can manufacture its own food
_____	21. amyloid	**a.** resembling mucus
_____	22. hyperplasia	**b.** enzyme that digests fat
_____	23. mucoid	**c.** overdevelopment of an organ or tissue
_____	24. protease	**d.** resembling starch
_____	25. lipase	**e.** enzyme that digests protein

_____	26. glucosuria	a.	formation of fibrous tissue
_____	27. proteolytic	b.	presence of glucose in the urine
_____	28. fibroplasia	c.	treatment using water
_____	29. polysaccharide	d.	compound composed of many simple sugars
_____	30. hydrotherapy	e.	destroying or dissolving protein

Supplementary Terms

_____	31. amino acid	a.	inner region of an organ
_____	32. collagen	b.	building block of protein
_____	33. glycogen	c.	fibrous protein in connective tissue
_____	34. medulla	d.	complex sugar stored in liver and muscles
_____	35. anabolism	e.	building phase of metabolism

Fill in the blanks:

36. All the activity of a cell make up its _____.

37. The four basic tissue types are _____.

38. The simple sugar that is the main energy source for metabolism is _____.

39. The control center of the cell is the _____.

40. An organic compound that speeds the rate of metabolic reactions is a(n) _____.

41. A cytotoxic substance is poisonous or damaging to _____.

42. The term *hydration* refers to the relative amount of _____.

43. Liposuria (lip-ō-SŪ-rē-a) is the presence in the urine of _____.

44. A myxocyte is found in tissue that secretes _____.

True–False. Examine the following statements. If the statement is true, write T in the first blank. If the statement is false, write F in the first blank, and correct the statement by replacing the <u>underlined</u> word in the second blank.

45. An adipocyte is a cell that stores <u>proteins</u>. _____ _____

46. Hydrophobia is an aversion to <u>fats</u>. _____ _____

47. A megakaryocyte is a cell with a large <u>nucleus</u>. _____ _____

48. There are <u>46</u> chromosomes in each human cell, aside from the sex cells. _____ _____

49. A whiplike extension of a cell is a <u>flagellum</u>. _____ _____

Word building. Write a word for each of the following definitions:

50. The study of form and structure _____

51. The study of tissues _____

52. The formation of cells (use *-genesis* as an ending) _____

53. An enzyme that digests starch _____

Go to the word exercises in Chapter 4 on the CD-ROM for additional review exercises.

CASE STUDY 4-1: Hematology Laboratory Studies

J.E. had a blood test as required for preoperative anesthesia assessment in preparation for scheduled plastic surgery on her breasts. The report read as follows:

Complete blood count (CBC) and differential
Red blood cell count (RBC)—4.5 million/μL
Hemoglobin (Hgb)—12.6 g/dL
Hematocrit (Hct)—38%
White blood cell count (WBC)—8500/μL
   Neutrophils—58%
   Lymphocytes—34%

   Monocytes—6%
   Eosinophils—1.5%
   Basophils—0.5%
Platelet count—200,000/μL
Prothrombin time (PT)—11.5 seconds
Partial thromboplastin time (PTT)—65 seconds
Blood glucose—84 mg/dL

The surgeon reviewed these results and concluded that they were within normal limits (WNL).

CASE STUDY 4-2: Pathology Laboratory Tests

R.C., the manager of the clinical and pathology laboratory, received several surgical specimens taken from a 26-year-old female patient with a 4-week history of nonspecific pelvic pain. The specimens included several small containers of pink-tinged cloudy fluid labeled *pelvic lavage* (washing) *for cytology,* which R.C. took to the cytology laboratory to be made into slides and checked microscopically for abnormal cells. R.C. also received a tissue specimen labeled *uterine myoma,* a wedge biopsy of right ovarian neoplasm, and four jars each labeled *pelvic lymph nodes.* She took all of the tissue specimens to the pathology laboratory for gross and microscopic evaluation. A test tube half-filled with a cloudy gel and a cotton-tipped applicator labeled *swab of pelvic fluid for culture and sensitivity and Gram stain* was taken to the microbiology laboratory to be streaked on a culture plate and incubated to look for growth. Any organisms that grew out would be Gram-stained and tested for sensitivity to antibiotics that might be used in treatment.

The laboratory form was accompanied by a surgeon's note stating that the patient's preoperative diagnosis was cervical dysplasia with atypical cells and a positive urine leukocyte esterase, indicating a urinary tract infection. R.C. placed a copy of the laboratory forms and surgeon's note on the desk of the pathologist who was involved in carcinogenesis (cancer) research.

CASE STUDY QUESTIONS

Multiple choice. Select the best answer and write the letter of your choice to the left of each number:

_____ 1. J.E.'s blood test results were within normal limits. She could be described as being in a state of:
   a. normosmosis
   b. dysplasia
   c. homeostasis
   d. hematophilia
   e. myogenesis

_____ 2. The suffix in *glucose* indicates that this compound is a:
   a. cervix
   b. enzyme
   c. protein
   d. sugar
   e. fat

4

_____ **3.** The suffix in *esterase* indicates that this compound is a:
   a. sugar
   b. carbohydrate
   c. cell
   d. enzyme
   e. lipid

_____ **4.** The root *gen* in carcinogenesis refers to a cancer's:
   a. origin
   b. treatment
   c. location
   d. laboratory results
   e. severity

Identify and give the meaning of the prefixes in the following words:

	Prefix	Meaning of Prefix
5. monocytes	_____	_____
6. prothrombin	_____	_____
7. neoplasm	_____	_____
8. atypical	_____	_____
9. leukocyte	_____	_____

Find words in the case studies for the following:

10. Three words that contain a root that means *attract, absorb*: _____
_____
_____

11. Three words with a root that means *formation, molding, development*: _____
_____
_____

12. Four words with a root that means *cell*: _____
_____
_____

BODY STRUCTURE

5

CHAPTER CONTENTS

OBJECTIVES

After study of this chapter you should be able to:

1. Define the main directional terms used in anatomy.
2. Describe division of the body along three different planes.
3. Locate the dorsal and ventral body cavities.
4. Locate the nine divisions of the abdomen.
5. Locate the four quadrants of the abdomen.
6. Describe the main body positions used in medical practice.
7. Define basic terms describing body structure.
8. Recognize and use roots pertaining to body regions.
9. Recognize and use prefixes pertaining to position and direction.
10. Analyze terms pertaining to body structure in a case study.

PRETEST

1. In humans, *ventral* is another term for _____.

2. A plane that divides the body into left and right parts is a(n) _____.

3. The scientific name for the chest cavity is _____.

4. The brain and spinal cord are in the _____ cavity.

5. The root *cephal/o* refers to the _____.

6. The root *brachi/o* refers to the _____.

7. The prefix *peri-* means _____.

8. The prefix *juxta-* means _____.

Directional Terms

All health-care fields require knowledge of body directions and orientations. Physicians, surgeons, nurses, occupational therapists, and physical therapists, for example, must be thoroughly familiar with the terms used to describe body locations and positions. Radiologic technologists, must be able to position a person and direct x-rays to obtain suitable images for diagnosis, as noted in Box 5-1.

In describing the location or direction of a given point in the body, it is always assumed that the subject is in the **anatomical position**, that is, upright, with face front, arms at the sides with palms forward, and feet parallel, as shown in Figure 5-1. In this

---

Box 5•1 **Health Professions** *Radiologic Technologist*

Radiologic technologists help in the diagnosis of medical disorders by taking x-ray images (radiographs) of the body. They must prepare patients for radiologic procedures, place patients in appropriate positions, and then adjust equipment to the correct angle, height, and settings for taking the x-ray image. They must position the x-ray film correctly and, after exposure, remove and develop the film. They are also required to keep patient records and maintain equipment. Radiologic technologists must minimize radiation hazards by using protective equipment for themselves and patients and by delivering the minimum possible amount of radiation. They wear badges to monitor radiation levels and keep records on their exposure.

Specialists in the field may be employed for more complex procedures, such as computerized tomography (CT) or magnetic resonance imaging (MRI), as described in later chapters. They may also administer materials, such as contrast media, to aid in imaging and diagnosis.

The majority of radiologic technologists work in hospitals, but they may also be employed in physicians' offices, diagnostic imaging centers (doing mammograms, for example), and outpatient care centers. Most have a 2-year associate degree, but a higher degree is needed for a supervisory or teaching position. The Joint Review Committee on Education in Radiologic Technology accredits most of the training programs, and the American Registry of Radiologic Technologists offers voluntary registration. Job opportunities in this field are currently good.

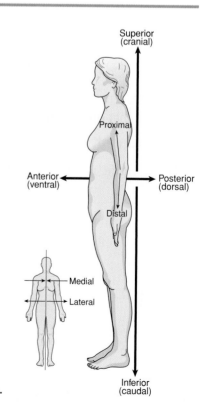

Figure 5-1 Directional terms.

Box 5•2 **For Your Reference**   *Anatomical Directions*

Term	Definition
anterior (ventral)	toward the front (belly) of the body
posterior (dorsal)	toward the back of the body
medial	toward the midline of the body
lateral	toward the side of the body
proximal	nearer to the point of attachment or to a given reference point
distal	farther from the point of attachment or from a given reference point
superior	above; in a higher position
inferior	below; in a lower position
cranial (cephalad)	toward the head
caudal	toward the lower end of the spine (Latin *cauda* means "tail"); in humans, in an inferior direction
superficial (external)	closer to the surface of the body
deep (internal)	closer to the center of the body

stance, the terms illustrated in Figure 5-1 and listed in Box 5-2 are used to designate relative position.

Figure 5-2 illustrates planes of section, that is, directions in which the body can be cut. A **frontal plane**, also called a coronal plane, is made at right angles to the midline and divides the body into anterior and posterior parts. A **sagittal** (*SAJ-i-tal*) **plane** passes

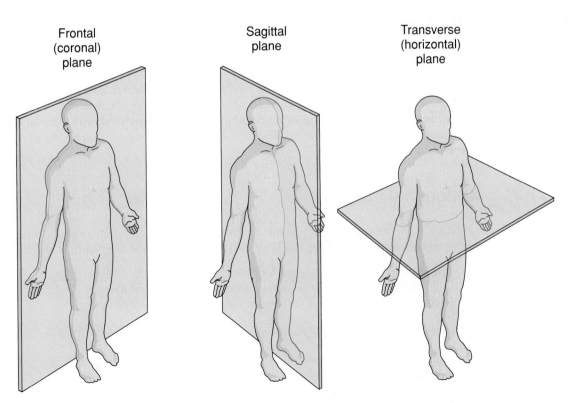

Frontal
(coronal)
plane

Sagittal
plane

Transverse
(horizontal)
plane

Figure 5-2 Planes of division.

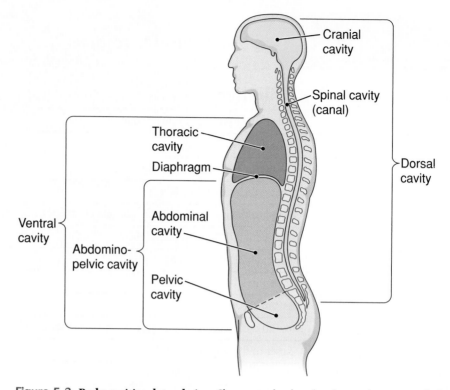

Figure 5-3 Body cavities, lateral view. Shown are the dorsal and ventral cavities with their subdivisions.

from front to back and divides the body into right and left portions. If the plane passes through the midline, it is a midsagittal or medial plane. A **transverse plane** passes horizontally, dividing the body into superior and inferior parts.

Body Cavities

Internal organs are located within dorsal and ventral cavities (Fig. 5-3). The dorsal cavity contains the brain in the **cranial cavity** and the spinal cord in the **spinal cavity (canal)**. The uppermost ventral space, the **thoracic cavity**, is separated from the **abdominal cavity** by the **diaphragm**. There is no anatomical separation between the abdominal cavity and the **pelvic cavity**, which together make up the **abdominopelvic cavity**. The large membrane that lines the abdominopelvic cavity and covers the organs within it is the **peritoneum** (*per-i-tō-NĒ-um*).

Abdominal Regions

For orientation, the abdomen can be divided by imaginary lines into nine regions, three medial regions and six lateral regions (Fig. 5-4). The sections down the midline are the:

> ➤ epigastric (*ep-i-GAS-trik*) region, located above the stomach
> ➤ umbilical (*um-BIL-i-kal*) region, named for the umbilicus, or navel
> ➤ hypogastric (*hī-pō-GAS-trik*) region, located below the stomach

The lateral regions have the same name on the left and right sides (Box 5-3). They are the:

> ➤ right and left hypochondriac (*hī-pō-KON-drē-ak*) regions, named for their position near the ribs, specifically near the cartilages (root *chondr/o*) of the ribs,
> ➤ right and left lumbar (*LUM-bar*) regions, which are located near the small of the back (lumbar region of the spine)

5

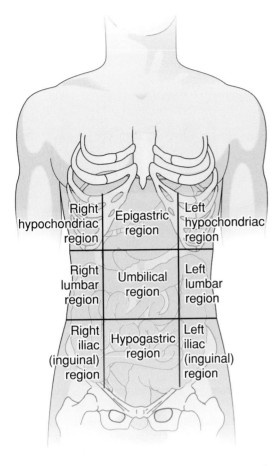

Figure 5-4 The nine regions of the abdomen.

> right and left iliac (*IL-ē-ak*) regions, named for the upper bone of the hip, the ilium. These regions are also called the inguinal (*ING-gwi-nal*) regions, with reference to the groin.

More simply, but less precisely, the abdomen can be divided into four sections by a single vertical line and a single horizontal line that intersect at the umbilicus (navel) (Fig. 5-5). The sections are the right upper quadrant (RUQ), left upper quadrant (LUQ), right lower quadrant (RLQ), and left lower quadrant (LLQ).

Additional terms for body regions are shown in Figures 5-6 and 5-7. You may need to refer to these illustrations as you work through the book.

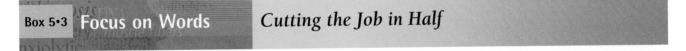

Box 5•3 Focus on Words   *Cutting the Job in Half*

A beginning student in medical science may be surprised by the vast number of names and terms that he or she is required to learn. This responsibility is lightened somewhat by the fact that we are bilaterally symmetrical; that is, aside from some internal organs such as the liver, spleen, stomach, pancreas, and intestine, nearly everything on the right side can be found on the left as well. The skeleton can be figuratively split down the center, giving equal structures on both sides of the midline. Many blood vessels and nerves are paired. This cuts the learning in half.

In addition, many of the blood vessels and nerves in a region have the same name. The radial artery, radial vein, and radial nerve are parallel, and all are located along the radius of the forearm. Vessels are commonly named for the organ they supply: the hepatic artery and vein of the liver, the pulmonary artery and vein of the lungs, the renal artery and vein of the kidney.

No one could say that the learning of medical terminology is a snap, but it could be harder!

5

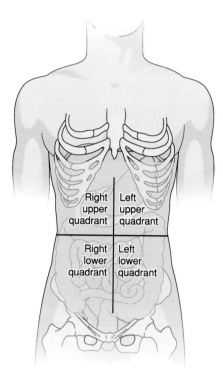

Figure 5-5 Quadrants of the abdomen. Some organs within the quadrants are indicated.

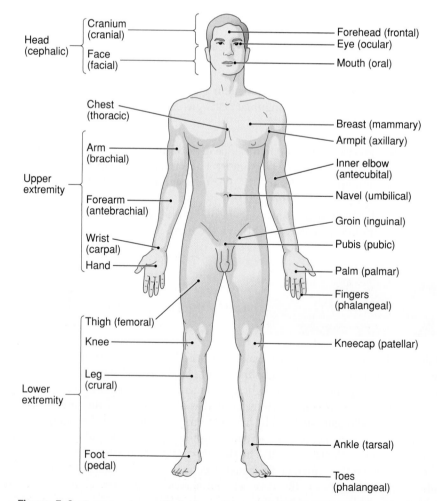

Figure 5-6 Common terms for body regions, anterior view. Anatomical terms for regions are in parentheses.

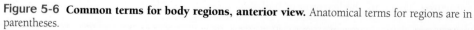

5

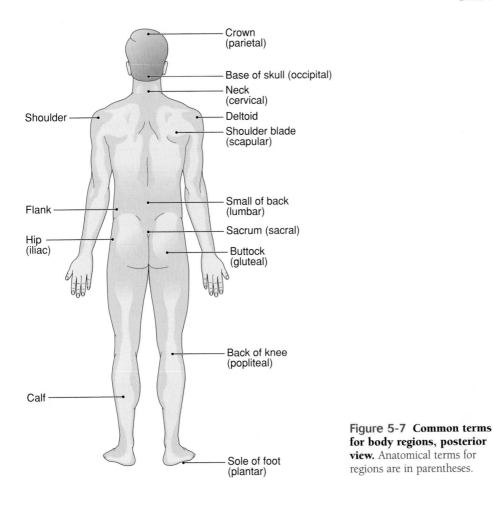

Figure 5-7 Common terms for body regions, posterior view. Anatomical terms for regions are in parentheses.

Positions

In addition to the anatomical position, there are other standard positions in which the body is placed for special purposes, such as examination, tests, surgery, or fluid drainage. The most common of these positions and some of their uses are described in Box 5-4.

Box 5•4 For Your Reference	*Body Positions*

Position	Description
anatomical position	standing erect, facing forward, arms at sides, palms forward, legs parallel, toes pointed forward. Used for descriptions and studies of the body.
decubitus position *dē-KŪ-bi-tus*	lying down, specifically according to the part of the body resting on a flat surface, as in left or right lateral decubitus, or dorsal or ventral decubitus
dorsal recumbent position	on back, with legs bent and separated, feet flat. Used for obstetrics and gynecology
Fowler position	on back, head of bed raised about 18 inches, knees elevated. Used to ease breathing and for drainage
jackknife position *JAK-nīf*	on back with shoulders elevated, legs flexed and thighs at right angles to the abdomen. Used to introduce a tube into the urethra.
knee–chest position	on knees, head and upper chest on table, arms crossed above head. Used in gynecology and obstetrics and for flushing the intestine

5

Box 5•4	For Your Reference	*Continued*

lateral recumbent position	on the side with one leg flexed; arm position may vary
lithotomy position *li-THOT-ō-mē*	on back, legs flexed on abdomen, thighs apart. Used for gynecologic and urologic surgery.
prone	lying face down
Sims position	on left side, right leg drawn up high and forward, left arm along back, chest forward resting on bed. Used for kidney and uterine surgery, colon examination, and enemas
supine* *SŪ-pīn*	lying face up
Trendelenburg position *tren-DEL-en-berg*	on back with head lowered by tilting bed back at 45° angle. Used for pelvic and abdominal surgery, treatment of shock

*To remember the difference between prone and supine, look for the word up in supine.

TERMINOLOGY Key Terms

abdominal cavity *ab-DOM-i-nal*	The large ventral cavity below the diaphragm and above the pelvic cavity
abdominopelvic cavity *ab-dom-i-nō-PEL-vik*	The large ventral cavity between the diaphragm and pelvis that includes the abdominal and pelvic cavities
anatomical position *an-a-TOM-ik-al*	Standard position for anatomical studies, in which the body is erect and facing forward, the arms are at the sides with palms forward, and the feet are parallel
cranial cavity *KRĀ-nē-al*	The dorsal cavity that contains the brain
diaphragm *DĪ-a-fram*	The muscle that separates the thoracic from the abdominal cavity
frontal (coronal) plane *ko-RŌN-al*	Plane of section that separates the body into anterior (front) and posterior (back) portions
pelvic cavity *PEL-vik*	The ventral cavity that is below the abdominal cavity
peritoneum *per-i-tō-NĒ-um*	The large serous membrane that lines the abdominopelvic cavity and covers the organs within it
sagittal plane *SAJ-i-tal*	Plane that divides the body into right and left portions
spinal cavity (canal) *SPĪ-nal*	Dorsal cavity that contains the spinal cord
thoracic cavity *thō-RAS-ik*	The ventral cavity above the diaphragm; the chest cavity
transverse (horizontal) plane *trans-VERS*	Plane that divides the body into superior (upper) and inferior (lower) portions

Go to the pronunciation glossary in Chapter 5 on the CD-ROM to hear these words pronounced.

Word Parts Pertaining to Body Structure

Table 5·1	Roots for Regions of the Head and Trunk		
ROOT	**MEANING**	**EXAMPLE**	**DEFINITION OF EXAMPLE**
cephal/o	head	microcephaly *mī-krō-SEF-a-lē*	abnormal smallness of the head
cervic/o	neck	cervicofacial *ser-vi-kō-FĀ-shal*	pertaining to the neck and face
thorac/o	chest, thorax	intrathoracic *in-tra-thō-RAS-ik*	within the thorax
abdomin/o	abdomen	intraabdominal *in-tra-ab-DOM-i-nal*	within the abdomen
celi/o	abdomen	celiac *SĒ-lē-ak*	pertaining to the abdomen
lapar/o	abdominal wall	laparoscope *LAP-a-rō-skōp*	instrument for viewing the peritoneal cavity through the abdominal wall
lumb/o	lumbar region, lower back	thoracolumbar *thō-rak-ō-LUM-bar*	pertaining to the chest and lumbar region
periton, peritone/o	peritoneum	peritoneal *per-i-tō-NĒ-al*	pertaining to the peritoneum

Exercise 5-1

Write the adjective for each of the following definitions. The correct suffix is given in parentheses:

1. Pertaining to (-al) the abdomen   _____abdominal_____

2. Pertaining to (-al) the neck   _____

3. Pertaining to (-ic) the chest   _____

4. Pertaining to (-ar) the lower back   _____

5. Pertaining to (-ic) the head   _____

Fill in the blanks:

6. Peritonitis (*per-i-tō-NĪ-tis*) is inflammation (-itis) of the _____.

7. Celiocentesis (*sē-lē-ō-sen-TĒ-sis*) is surgical puncture (centesis) of the _____.

8. Cephalad means toward the _____.

5

5

Table 5·2	Roots for the Extremities		
ROOT	**MEANING**	**EXAMPLE**	**DEFINITION OF EXAMPLE**
acro	extremity, end	acrocyanosis *ak-rō-sī-a-NŌ-sis*	bluish discoloration of the extremities
brachi/o	arm	antebrachium *an-tē-BRĀ-kē-um*	forearm
dactyl/o	finger, toe	dactylospasm *DAK-til-ō-spazm*	spasm (cramp) of a finger or toe
ped/o	foot	pedometer *pe-DOM-e-ter*	instrument that measures footsteps
pod/o	foot	podiatric *pō-dē-AT-rik*	pertaining to study and treatment of the foot

Exercise 5-2

Fill in the blanks:

1. Acrokinesia (*ak-rō-kī-NĒ-sē-a*) is excess motion (-kinesia) of the _____.

2. Animals that brachiate (*BRĀ-kē-āt*), such as monkeys, swing from place to place using their

   _____.

3. Polydactyly (*pol-ē-DAK-til-ē*) is having more than the normal number of _____.

4. The term brachiocephalic (*brā-kē-ō-se-FAL-ik*) refers to the _____.

5. Dextropedal (*desk-TROP-e-dal*) refers to the use of the right _____.

Table 5·3	Prefixes for Position and Direction		
PREFIX	**MEANING**	**EXAMPLE**	**DEFINITION OF EXAMPLE**
circum-	around	circumoral *ser-kum-OR-al*	around the mouth
peri-	around	periorbital *per-ē-OR-bit-al*	around the orbit (eye socket)
intra-	in, within	intravascular *in-tra-VAS-kū-lar*	within a vessel (vascul/o)
epi-	on, over	epithelium *ep-i-THĒ-lē-um*	tissue that covers surfaces
extra-	outside	extrathoracic *eks-tra-thō-RAS-ik*	outside the thorax

Table 5·3	Continued		
infra-*	below	infracostal *in-fra-KOS-tal*	below the ribs (cost/o)
sub-*	below, under	sublingual *sub-LING-gwal*	under the tongue (lingu/o)
inter-	between	interscapular *in-ter-SKAP-ū-lar*	between the scapulae (shoulder blades)
juxta-	near, beside	juxtaposition *juks-ta-pō-ZI-shun*	a location near or beside another structure
para-	near, beside	parasagittal *par-a-SAJ-i-tal*	near or beside a sagittal plane
retro-	behind, backward	retrouterine *re-trō-Ū-ter-in*	behind the uterus
supra-	above	suprapatellar *su-pra-pa-TEL-ar*	above the patella (kneecap)

*Also indicates degree.

Exercise 5-3

Synonyms. *Write a word that means the same as each of the following:*

1. perioral   <u>   circumoral   </u>

2. infrascapular   <u>   </u>

3. circumvascular   <u>   </u>

4. subcostal   <u>   </u>

5. periorbital   <u>   </u>

Opposites. *Write a word that means the opposite of each of the following:*

6. subpatellar   <u>   suprapatellar   </u>

7. extracellular   <u>   </u>

8. infrascapular   <u>   </u>

Define the following words:

9. paranasal (*par-a-NĀ-zal*) _____

10. retroperitoneal (*re-trō-per-i-tō-NĒ-al*) _____

11. supra-abdominal (*sū-pra-ab-DOM-i-nal*) _____

12. intrauterine (*in-tra-Ū-ter-in*) _____

Refer to Figures 5-6 and 5-7 to define the following terms:

13. epitarsal (*ep-i-TAR-sal*) _____

14. intergluteal (*in-ter-GLŪ-tē-al*) _____

15. periumbilical (*per-ē-um-BIL-i-kal*) _____

16. parasacral (*par-a-SĀ-kral*) _____

17. intrathoracic (*in-tra-thō-RAS-ik*) _____

5

TERMINOLOGY — Supplementary Terms

digit *DIJ-it*	A finger or toe (adjective, digital)
epigastrium *ep-i-GAS-trē-um*	The epigastric region
fundus *FUN-dus*	The base or body of a hollow organ; the area of an organ farthest from its opening
hypochondrium *hī-pō-KON-drē-um*	The hypochondriac region (left or right)
lumen *LŪ-men*	The central opening within a tube or hollow organ
meatus *mē-Ā-tus*	A passage or opening
orifice *OR-i-fis*	The opening of a cavity
os	Mouth; any body opening
septum *SEP-tum*	A wall dividing two cavities
sinus *SĪ-nus*	A cavity, as within a bone
sphincter *SFINK-ter*	A circular muscle that regulates an opening

Go to the pronunciation glossary in Chapter 5 on the CD-ROM to hear these words pronounced.

TERMINOLOGY — Abbreviations

LLQ	Left lower quadrant
LUQ	Left upper quadrant
RLQ	Right lower quadrant
RUQ	Right upper quadrant

CHAPTER REVIEW

LABELING EXERCISE
Directional Terms

Write the name of each numbered part on the corresponding line of the answer sheet.

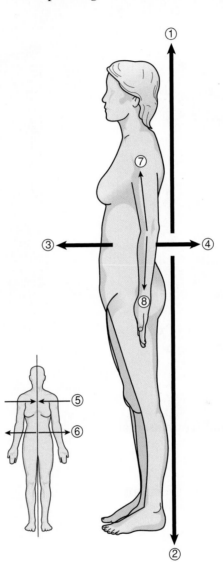

Anterior (ventral)	1. _____
Distal	2. _____
Inferior (caudal)	3. _____
Lateral	4. _____
Medial	5. _____
Posterior (dorsal)	6. _____
Proximal	7. _____
Superior (cranial)	8. _____

5

Planes of Division

Write the name of each numbered part on the corresponding line of the answer sheet.

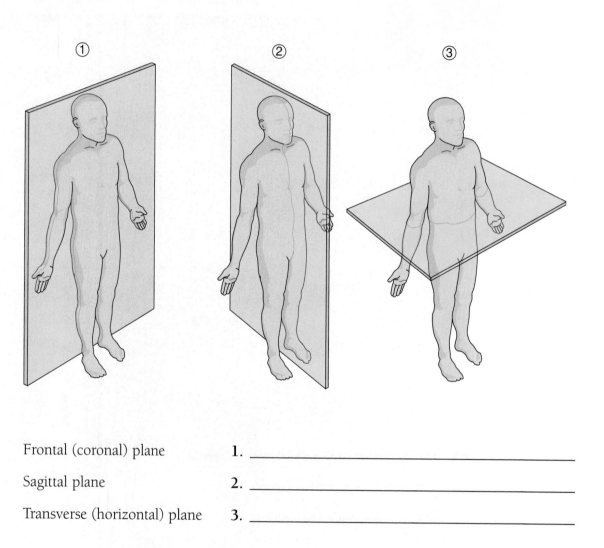

Frontal (coronal) plane   **1.** _____

Sagittal plane   **2.** _____

Transverse (horizontal) plane   **3.** _____

Body Cavities, Lateral View

Write the name of each numbered part on the corresponding line of the answer sheet.

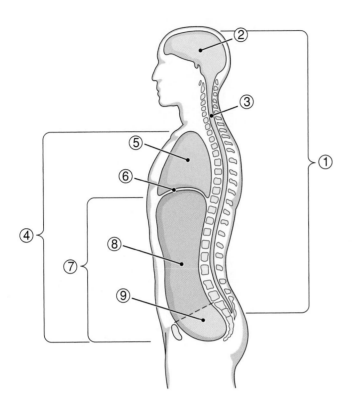

Abdominal cavity	1. _____
Abdominopelvic cavity	2. _____
Cranial cavity	3. _____
Dorsal cavity	4. _____
Diaphragm	5. _____
Pelvic cavity	6. _____
Spinal cavity (canal)	7. _____
Thoracic cavity	8. _____
Ventral cavity	9. _____

The Nine Regions of the Abdomen

Write the name of each numbered part on the corresponding line of the answer sheet.

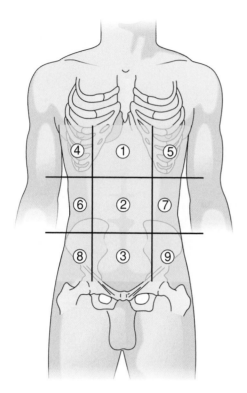

Epigastric region   1. _____

Hypogastric region   2. _____

Left hypochondriac region   3. _____

Left iliac (inguinal) region   4. _____

Left lumbar region   5. _____

Right hypochondriac region   6. _____

Right iliac (inguinal) region   7. _____

Right lumbar region   8. _____

Umbilical region   9. _____

TERMINOLOGY

Matching. Match the following terms and write the appropriate letter to the left of each number:

_____	1. syndactyly	a. incision into the chest
_____	2. acrodermatitis	b. skin inflammation of the extremities
_____	3. laparotomy	c. absence of a finger or toe
_____	4. adactyly	d. incision through the abdominal wall
_____	5. thoracotomy	e. fusion of fingers or toes
_____	6. macrocephaly	a. circular cut
_____	7. celiocentesis	b. excessive size of the feet
_____	8. macropodia	c. outer layer of the skin
_____	9. epidermis	d. abnormal largeness of the head
_____	10. circumcision	e. surgical puncture of the abdomen

Supplementary Terms

_____	11. sphincter	a. dividing wall
_____	12. lumen	b. circular muscle that regulates an opening
_____	13. sinus	c. central opening of a tube
_____	14. septum	d. cavity, as in a bone
_____	15. fundus	e. base of a hollow organ

True–False. Examine each of the following statements. If the statement is true, write T in the first blank. If the statement is false, write F in the first blank and correct the statement by replacing the <u>underlined</u> word in the second blank.

16. The cranial and spinal cavities are the <u>ventral</u> body cavities.   F   _____ dorsal _____

17. The wrist is <u>distal</u> to the elbow.   _____   _____

18. A <u>midsagittal</u> plane divides the body into equal right and left parts.   _____   _____

19. A <u>transverse</u> plane divides the body into anterior and posterior parts.   _____   _____

20. The thoracic cavity is <u>inferior</u> to the abdominal cavity.   _____   _____

21. The epigastric region is <u>superior</u> to the umbilical region.   _____   _____

22. In the <u>supine</u> position, a person is lying face-down.   _____   _____

23. The <u>left</u> hypochondriac region is in the LUQ.   _____   _____

Adjectives. Name the part of the body referred to in the following adjectives:

24. phalangeal _____

25. cervical _____

26. cephalic _____

27. popliteal _____

28. brachial _____

29. celiac _____

Define the following words:

30. infraumbilical _____

31. retroperitoneal _____

32. sublingual _____

33. intercostal _____

34. bipedal _____

Synonyms. Write a word that means the same as each of the following:

35. circumocular _____

36. submammary _____

37. dorsal _____

38. anterior _____

Opposites. Write a word that means the opposite of each of the following:

39. macrocephaly _____

40. intracellular _____

41. distal _____

42. inferior _____

43. infrapubic _____

44. superficial _____

Eliminations. In each of the sets below, underline the word that does not fit in with the rest and explain the reason for your choice:

45. thoracic cavity – abdominopelvic cavity – pelvic cavity – abdominal cavity – spinal cavity

_____

46. umbilical region – hypochondriac region – epigastric region – cephalic region – iliac region

_____

47. jackknife – sagittal – supine – decubitus – prone

_____

48. lumb/o – dactyl/o – brachi/o – acro – pod/o

_____

Go to the word exercises in Chapter 5 on the CD-ROM for additional practice exercises.

CASE STUDIES

CASE STUDY 5–1: Emergency Care

During a triathlon, paramedics responded to a scene with multiple patients involved in a serious bicycle accident. B.R., a 20-year-old woman, lost control of her bike while descending a hill at approximately 40 mph. As she fell, two other cyclists collided with her, sending all three crashing to the ground.

At the scene, B.R. reported pain in her head, back, chest, and leg. She also had numbness and tingling in her legs and feet. Other injuries included a cut on her face and on her right arm and an obvious deformity to both her shoulder and knee. She had slight difficulty breathing.

The paramedic did a rapid cephalocaudal assessment and immobilized B.R.'s neck in a cervical collar. She was secured on a backboard and given oxygen. After her bleeding was controlled and her injured extremities were immobilized, she was transported to the nearest emergency department.

During transport, the paramedic in charge radioed ahead to provide a prehospital report to the charge nurse. His report included the following information: occipital and frontal head pain; laceration to right temple, superior and anterior to right ear; lumbar pain; bilateral thoracic pain on inspiration at midclavicular line on the right and midaxillary line on the left; dull aching pain of the posterior proximal right thigh; bilateral paresthesia (numbness and tingling) of distal lower legs circumferentially; varus (knock-knee) adduction deformity of left knee; and posterior displacement deformity of left shoulder.

At the hospital, the emergency department physician ordered radiographs for B.R. Before the procedure, the radiology technologist positioned a lead gonadal shield centered on the midsagittal line above B.R.'s symphysis pubis to protect her ovaries from unnecessary irradiation by the primary beam. The technologist knew that gonadal shielding is important for female patients undergoing imaging of the lumbar spine, sacroiliac joints, acetabula, pelvis, and kidneys. Shields should not be used for any examination in which an acute abdominal condition is suspected.

CASE STUDY QUESTIONS

Multiple choice. Select the best answer and write the letter of your choice to the left of each number:

_____ 1. The term for the time span between injury and admission to the emergency department is:
   a. preoperative
   b. prehospital
   c. pre-emergency
   d. pretrauma
   e. intrainjury

_____ 2. A cephalocaudal assessment goes from _____.
   a. stem to stern
   b. front to back
   c. head to toe
   d. side to side
   e. skin to bone

_____ 3. The victim's injured extremities were immobilized before transport. Immobilized means:
   a. abducted as far as possible
   b. internally rotated and flexed
   c. adducted so that the limbs are crossed
   d. rotated externally
   e. held in place to prevent movement

_____ 4. A cervical collar was placed on the victim to stabilize and immobilize the _____.
  a. uterus
  b. shoulders
  c. chin
  d. neck
  e. pelvis

_____ 5. The singular form of acetabula is:
  a. acetyl
  b. acetabulum
  c. acetabia
  d. acetab
  e. acetabulae

Draw or shade the appropriate area(s) on one or both diagrams for each question:

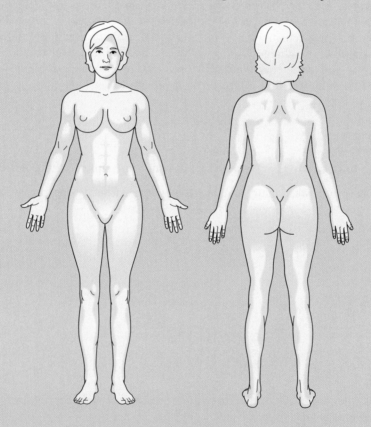

6. Draw dots over the areas of the victim's occipital and frontal head pain.

7. Draw a dash (—) over the area of the right temporal laceration—superior and anterior to the right ear.

8. Cross-hatch the area of lumbar pain.

9. Place an X over the area of thoracic pain at the anterior left midaxillary line.

10. Draw a star at the area of the pain on the right proximal posterior thigh.

11. Shade the area of the bilateral paresthesia of the distal lower legs, circumferentially.

12. Draw an arrow to show the direction of the varus adduction of the left knee.

13. Draw an arrow to show the direction of the posterior displacement of the left shoulder.

14. Draw a fig leaf to show the gonadal shield on the midsagittal line above the symphysis pubis.

15. Draw a circle around the area of the sacroiliac joints.

5

PART TWO

DISEASE AND TREATMENT

Chapters 6 through 8 in Part 2 cover general terminology related to diseases, diagnosis, and treatment, including information on drugs. More specific information about how diseases affect individual systems and how these diseases are treated will be presented in Part 3.

CHAPTER SIX

DISEASE

CHAPTER CONTENTS

Pretest
Types of Diseases
Infectious Diseases
Responses to Disease

Neoplasia
Word Parts Pertaining to Disease
Chapter Review
Case Studies

6

OBJECTIVES

After study of this chapter you should be able to:

1. List the major categories of diseases.
2. Compare the common types of infectious organisms, and list some diseases caused by each.
3. Describe some common responses to disease.
4. Define and give examples of neoplasia.
5. Identify and use word parts pertaining to diseases.
6. Define the major terms describing types of diseases.
7. List and define the major manifestations of diseases.
8. Analyze the disease terminology in several case studies.

PRETEST

1. Any organism so small that it can only be seen with a microscope is a(n) _____.

2. A disease that has a sudden and severe onset is described as _____.

3. Abnormal and uncontrolled growth of tissue is termed _____.

4. Round bacteria are called _____.

5. Single-celled animals, as a group, are called _____.

6. Heat, pain, redness, and swelling are the characteristics signs of _____.

Types of Diseases

A disease is any disorder of normal body function. Diseases can be grouped into a number of different but often overlapping categories. These include:

> Infectious diseases—caused by certain harmful microorganisms and other **parasites** that live at the expense of another organism. Any disease-causing organism is described as a **pathogen**.
> Degenerative diseases—resulting from wear and tear, aging, or **trauma** (injury) that can result in a **lesion** (wound) and perhaps **necrosis** (death of tissue). Common examples include arthritis, cardiovascular problems, and certain respiratory disorders such as emphysema. Structural malformations such as congenital malformations, **prolapse** (dropping), or **hernia** (rupture) may also result in degenerative changes.
> Neoplasia—abnormal and uncontrolled growth of tissue.
> Immune disorders—This category includes failures of the immune system, allergies, and autoimmune diseases, in which the body makes antibodies to its own tissues. (Immune disorders receive more detailed discussion in Chapter 10.)
> Metabolic disorders—resulting from lack of enzymes or other factors needed for cellular functions. Many hereditary disorders fall into this category. Malnutrition caused by inadequate intake of nutrients or inability of the body to absorb and use nutrients also upsets metabolism. (Metabolic disorders are discussed in more detail in Chapter 12, and hereditary disorders are discussed in Chapter 15.)
> Hormonal disorders—caused by underproduction or overproduction of hormones or by inability of the hormones to function properly. One example is diabetes mellitus. (Chapter 16 has more detail on hormonal disorders.)
> Mental and emotional disorders—disorders that affect the mind and adaptation of an individual to his or her environment. (Chapter 17 has further discussion on behavioral disorders.)

The cause of a disease is its **etiology** (ē-tē-OL-ō-jē), although many diseases have multiple interacting causes. *An* **acute** disease is sudden and severe and of short duration. A **chronic** disease is of long duration and progresses slowly. One health profession that deals with the immediate effects of acute disease is the Emergency Medical Technician (EMT) (Box 6-2).

Box 6•1 Focus on Words *Name That Disease*

Diseases get their names in a variety of ways. Some are named for the places where they were first found, such as Lyme disease for Lyme, Connecticut; West Nile disease and Rift Valley fever for places in Africa; and hantavirus fever for a river in Korea. Others are named for the people who first described them, such as Cooley anemia; Crohn disease, an inflammatory bowel disease; and Hodgkin disease of the lymphatic system.

Many diseases are named on the basis of the symptoms they cause. Tuberculosis causes small lesions known as tubercles in the lungs and other tissues. Skin anthrax produces lesions that turn black, and its name comes from the same root as anthracite coal. In sickle cell anemia, red blood cells become distorted into a crescent shape when they give up oxygen. Having lost their smooth, round form, the cells jumble together, blocking small blood vessels and depriving tissues of oxygen.

Bubonic plague causes painful and enlarged lymph nodes called buboes. Lupus erythematosus, a systemic autoimmune disorder, is named for the Latin term for wolf, because the red rash that may form on the face of people with this disease gives them a wolf-like appearance. Yellow fever, scarlet fever, and rubella (German measles) are named for colors associated with the pathology of these diseases.

| Box 6•2 | Health Professions | *Emergency Medical Technicians* |

Emergency medical technicians (EMTs) are the first health professionals to arrive at the scene of an automobile accident, heart attack, or other emergency situation. EMTs must assess and respond rapidly to a medical crisis, taking a medical history, performing a physical examination, stabilizing the patient, and, if necessary, transporting the patient to the nearest medical facility.

To perform their life-saving duties, EMTs need extensive training, including a thorough understanding of anatomy and physiology. EMTs must know how to use specialized equipment, such as backboards to immobilize injuries, electrocardiographs to monitor heart activity, and defibrillators to treat cardiac arrest, and they must also be proficient at giving intravenous fluids, oxygen, and certain life-saving medications. At medical facilities, EMTs work closely with physicians and nurses, reporting on histories, physical examinations, and measures taken to stabilize the patient. Most EMTs receive their training from a college or technical school and must be certified in the state where they are employed.

As the American population ages and becomes concentrated in urban centers, the rate of accidents and other emergencies is expected to rise. Thus, the need for EMTs remains high. For more information about this career, contact the National Association of Emergency Medical Technicians.

Infectious Diseases

Infectious diseases are caused by viruses, bacteria, fungi (yeasts and molds), protozoa (single-celled animals), and worms (Box 6-3). Infecting organisms can enter the body through several routes, or portals of entry, including damaged skin, the respiratory tract, digestive system, and the urinary and reproductive tracts. An infected person's bodily discharges may contain organisms that spread infection through the air, food, water, or direct contact. Microorganisms often produce disease by means of the **toxins** (poisons) they release. The presence of harmful microorganisms or their toxins in the body is termed **sepsis**.

| Box 6•3 | For Your Reference | *Common Infectious Organisms* |

Type of Organism	Description	Examples of Diseases Caused
bacteria *bak-TĒ-rē-a*	simple microscopic organisms that are widespread throughout the world, which can produce disease; singular, bacterium (*bak-TĒ-rē-um*)	
cocci *KOK-sī*	round bacteria; may be in clusters (staphylococci), chains (streptococci), and other formations; singular, coccus (*KOK-us*)	pneumonia, rheumatic fever, food poisoning, septicemia, urinary tract infections, gonorrhea
bacilli *ba-SIL-ī*	rod-shaped bacteria; singular, bacillus (*ba-SIL-us*)	typhoid, dysentery, salmonellosis, tuberculosis, botulism, tetanus
vibrios *VIB-rē-ōz*	short curved rods	cholera, gastroenteritis
spirochetes *SPĪ-rō-kētz*	corkscrew-shaped bacteria that move with a twisting motion	Lyme disease, syphilis, Vincent disease
chlamydia *kla-MID-ē-a*	extremely small bacteria that, like viruses, grow in living cells, but are susceptible to antibiotics	conjunctivitis, trachoma, pelvic inflammatory disease (PID), and other sexually transmitted infections (STIs)

Box 6•3 For Your Reference Continued

rickettsia *ri-KET-sē-a*	extremely small bacteria that grow in living cells but are susceptible to antibiotics	typhus, Rocky Mountain spotted fever
viruses *VĪ-rus-es*	submicroscopic infectious agents that can live and reproduce only within living cells	colds, herpes, hepatitis, measles, varicella (chickenpox), influenza, AIDS
fungi *FUN-jī*	simple, nongreen plants, some of which are parasitic; includes yeasts and molds; singular, fungus (*FUN-gus*)	candidiasis, skin infections (tinea, ringworm), valley fever
protozoa *prō-tō-ZŌ-a*	single-celled animals; singular, protozoon (*prō-tō-ZŌ-on*)	dysentery, *Trichomonas* infection, malaria
helminths *HEL-minths*	worms	trichinosis; infestations with roundworms, pinworms, hookworms

Bacteria

In shape, bacteria are:

> ➤ Round, or cocci, shown in Figure 6-1
> ➤ Rod-shaped, or bacilli, shown in Figure 6-2
> ➤ Curved, including vibrios and spirochetes, shown in Figure 6-3

Bacteria may be named according to their shape and also by the arrangements they form (see Fig. 6-1). They also are described according to the dyes they take up when stained in the laboratory. The most common laboratory bacterial stain is the **Gram stain**, with which gram-positive organisms stain purple and gram-negative organisms stain red (see Fig. 6-1).

Chlamydia and rickettsia are two bacterial groups that are smaller than typical bacteria and can grow only within living host cells (see Box 6-3).

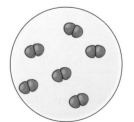

A Diplococci

B Streptococci

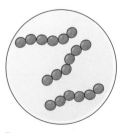

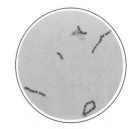

Figure 6-1 Cocci, round bacteria, Gram-stained. (*A*) Cells growing in pairs, diplococci. (*B*) Cells in chains, streptococci. (*C*) Cells in clusters, staphylococci. (*D*) Streptococci viewed under a microscope in a photomicrograph.

C Staphylococci

D Streptococci, photomicrograph

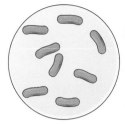

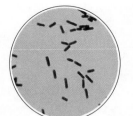

A Bacilli

B Bacilli, photomicrograph

Figure 6-2 Bacilli, rod-shaped bacteria. (*A*) Drawing of bacilli. (*B*) Photomicrograph of bacilli.

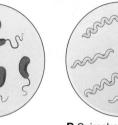

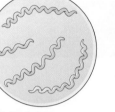

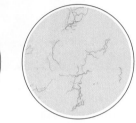

A Vibrios

B Spirochetes

C Spirochetes, photomicrograph

Figure 6-3 Curved bacteria. (*A*) Vibrios are short curved rods. (*B*) Spirochetes are spiral-shaped. (*C*) Spirochetes shown in a photomicrograph.

Responses to Disease

Inflammation

A common response to infection and to other forms of disease is **inflammation**. When cells are injured, they release chemicals that allow blood cells and fluids to move into the tissues. This inflow of blood results in the four signs of inflammation:

➤ heat
➤ pain
➤ redness
➤ swelling

The suffix *-itis* indicates inflammation, as in appendicitis (inflammation of the appendix) and tonsillitis (inflammation of the tonsils).

Inflammation is one possible cause of **edema**, a swelling or accumulation of fluid in the tissues (Fig 6-4). Other causes of edema include blockage of fluid, heart failure, and imbalance in body fluid composition, as described in later chapters.

Phagocytosis

The body uses **phagocytosis** to get rid of invading microorganisms, damaged cells, and other types of harmful debris. Certain white blood cells are capable of engulfing these materials and destroying them internally (Fig. 6-5). Phagocytic cells are found circulating in the blood, in the tissues, and in the lymphatic system (see Chapters 9 and 10). The remains of phagocytosis consist of fluid and white blood cells; this mixture is called **pus**.

Immunity

Immunity refers to all our defenses against infectious disease. Inflammation and phagocytosis are examples of inborn or innate protective mechanisms, which are based on a person's genetic makeup and do not require any previous exposure to a disease organism. Other defenses that fall into this category are mechanical barriers, such as intact skin and mucous membranes, as well as body secretions, such as stomach acid and enzymes in saliva and tears.

Immunity that we acquire during life from exposure to disease organisms is termed *adaptive immunity*. This type of immunity is specific for particular diseases encountered

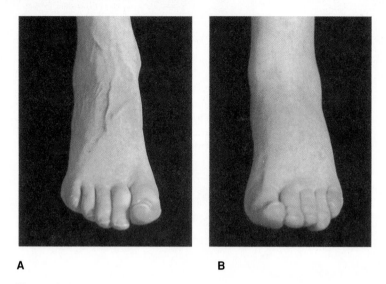

A **B**

Figure 6-4 Edema. (*A*) A normal foot showing veins, tendons, and bones. (*B*) Edema (swelling) obscures surface features.

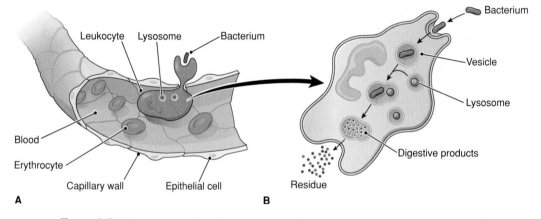

A **B**

Figure 6-5 Phagocytosis. (*A*) A phagocytic white blood cell squeezes through a capillary wall to engulf a bacterium. (*B*) Lysosomal enzymes destroy the bacterium, and the waste products are eliminated.

by natural exposure or by the administration of vaccines (see Chapter 10). The system responsible for adaptive immunity consists of cells in the blood, lymphatic system, and other tissues. These cells recognize different foreign invaders and get rid of them by direct attack and by production of circulating antibodies that immobilize and help to destroy them. The immune system also monitors the body continuously for abnormal and malfunctioning cells, such as cancer cells. The immune system may overreact to produce allergies, and may react to one's own tissues to cause autoimmune diseases.

Neoplasia

As noted earlier, a **neoplasm** is an abnormal and uncontrolled growth of tissue—a tumor or growth. A **benign** neoplasm does not spread, or **metastasize**, to other tissues, although it may cause damage at the site where it grows. A neoplasm that metastasizes to other tissues is termed **malignant**, and is commonly called *cancer*. A malignant tumor that involves epithelial tissue is a **carcinoma**. If the tumor arises in glandular epithelium, it is an adenocarcinoma (the root *aden/o* means "gland"); a cancer of pigmented epithelial cells (melanocytes) is a melanoma. A neoplasm that involves connective tissue or muscle is a **sarcoma**. Cancers of the blood, lymphatic system, and nervous system are classified according to the cell types involved and other clinical features. Further descriptions of these cancers appear in Chapters 10 and 17.

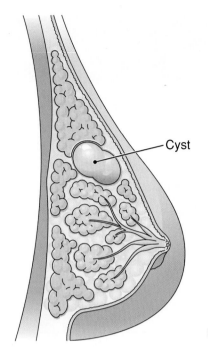

Figure 6-6 Cyst in the breast.

Often mistaken for a malignancy is a **cyst**, a sac or pouch filled with fluid or semi-solid material that is usually abnormal but not cancerous (Fig. 6-6). Common sites for cyst formation are the breasts, the sebaceous glands of the skin, and the ovaries. Causes of cyst formation include infection or blockage of a duct.

TERMINOLOGY	Key Terms
acute a-KŪT	Sudden, severe; having a short course
benign bē-NĪN	Not recurrent or malignant; favorable for recovery; describing tumors that do not spread
carcinoma kar-si-NŌ-ma	A malignant neoplasm composed of epithelial cells (from Greek root *carcino*, meaning "crab") (adjective: carcinomatous)
chronic KRON-ik	Of long duration; progressing slowly
cyst sist	A filled sac or pouch that is usually abnormal (see Fig. 6-6). Used as a root meaning a normal bladder or sac, such as the urinary bladder or gallbladder (root *cyst/o, cyst/i*).
edema e-DĒ-ma	Accumulation of fluid in the tissues; swelling. Adjective edematous (e-DĒ-ma-tus) (see Fig. 6-4)
etiology ē-tē-OL-ō-jē	The cause of a disease
Gram stain	A laboratory staining procedure that divides bacteria into two groups: gram-positive, which stain blue, and gram-negative, which stain red (see Fig. 6-1).
hernia HER-nē-a	Protrusion of an organ through an abnormal opening; a rupture (Fig. 6-7)

TERMINOLOGY **Key Terms**

Continued

inflammation *in-fla-MĀ-shun*	A localized response to tissue injury characterized by heat, pain, redness, and swelling
lesion *LĒ-zhun*	A distinct area of damaged tissue; an injury or wound
malignant *ma-LIG-nant*	Growing worse; harmful; tending to cause death; describing tumors that spread (metastasize)
metastasize *me-TAS-ta-sīz*	To spread from one part of the body to another; characteristic of cancer (noun: metastasis [*me-TAS-ta-sis*])
necrosis *ne-KRŌ-sis*	Death of tissue
neoplasm *NĒ-ō-plazm*	An abnormal and uncontrolled growth of tissue, namely, a tumor; may be benign or malignant. From prefix *neo-* meaning "new" and root *plasm* meaning "formation." The root *onc/o* and the suffix *-oma* refer to neoplasms.
parasite *PAR-a-sīt*	An organism that grows on or in another organism (the host), causing damage to it
pathogen *PATH-ō-jen*	An organism capable of causing disease (root *path/o* means "disease")
phagocytosis *fag-ō-sī-TŌ-sis*	The ingestion of organisms, such as invading bacteria or small particles of waste material by a cell; ingested material is then destroyed by the phagocytic cell, or phagocyte (root *phag/o* means "to eat") (see Fig. 6-5)
prolapse *PRŌ-laps*	A dropping or downward displacement of an organ or part; ptosis
pus	A product of inflammation consisting of fluid and white blood cells (root: *py/o*)
sarcoma *sar-KŌ-ma*	A malignant neoplasm arising from connective tissue (from Greek root *sarco*, meaning "flesh") (adjective: sarcomatous)
sepsis *SEP-sis*	The presence of harmful microorganisms or their toxins in the blood or other tissues (adjective: septic)
toxin *TOKS-in*	A poison (adjective, toxic) (roots: *tox/o, toxic/o*)
trauma *TRAW-ma*	A physical or psychological wound or injury

See also Box 6-3 on infectious diseases.

Go to the pronunciation glossary in Chapter 6 on the CD-ROM to hear these words pronounced.

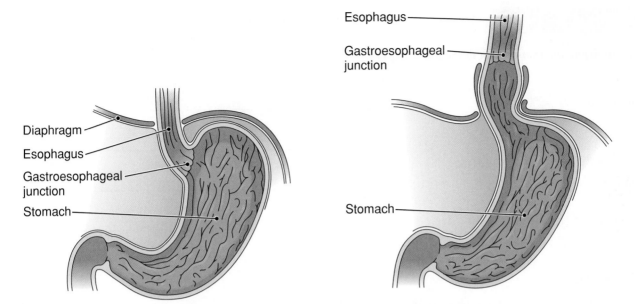

Figure 6-7 Hernia (A) A normal stomach (B) Hiatal hernia. The stomach protrudes through the diaphragm into the thoracic cavity, raising the level of the junction between the esophagus and the stomach.

Word Parts Pertaining to Disease

Table 6·1	Roots for Disease		
ROOT	**MEANING**	**EXAMPLE**	**DEFINITION OF EXAMPLE**
alg/o, algi/o, algesi/o	pain	algesia *al-JĒ-zē-a*	condition of having pain
carcin/o	cancer, carcinoma	carcinoid *KAR-si-noyd*	resembling a carcinoma
cyst/o, cyst/i	filled sac or pouch, cyst, bladder	cystic *SIS-tik*	pertaining to or having cysts
lith	calculus, stone	lithiasis *lith-Ī-a-sis*	stone formation
onc/o	tumor	oncogenic *on-kō-JEN-ik*	causing a tumor
path/o	disease	pathogen *PATH-ō-jen*	organism that produces disease
py/o	pus	pyoderma *pī-ō-DER-ma*	pus-containing skin disease
pyr/o, pyret/o	fever, fire	pyrexia *pī-REK-sē-a*	fever
scler/o	hard	sclerosis *skle-RŌ-sis*	hardening of tissue
tox/o, toxic/o	poison	endotoxin *en-dō-TOK-sin*	toxin within bacterial cells

Exercise 6-1

Identify and define the root in each of the following words:

	Root	Meaning of Root
1. antipyretic *an-tē-pī-RET-ik*	_____	_____
2. pathology *pa-THOL-ō-jē*	_____	_____
3. empyema *em-pī-Ē-ma*	_____	_____
4. intoxicate *in-TOK-si-kāt*	_____	_____

Fill in the blanks:

5. A carcinogen (*kar-SIN-ō-jen*) is a substance that causes _____.

6. A urolith (*Ū-rō-lith*) is a(n) _____ in the urinary tract (*ur/o*).

7. A pyocyst (*PĪ-ō-sist*) is a sac filled with _____.

8. A pyrogenic (*pī-rō-JEN-ik*) agent induces _____.

9. The term *pathogenic* (*path-ō-JEN-ik*) means producing _____.

10. Arteriosclerosis (*ar-tē-rē-ō-skle-RŌ-sis*) is a(n) _____ of the arteries.

11. An exotoxin (*ek-sō-TOK-sin*) is a(n) _____ secreted by bacterial cells.

12. An algesimeter (*al-je-SIM-e-ter*) is used to measure sensitivity to _____.

13. An oncogene (*ON-kō-jēn*) is a gene that causes a(n) _____.

Table 6·2	Prefixes for Disease		
PREFIX	**MEANING**	**EXAMPLE**	**DEFINITION OF EXAMPLE**
brady-	slow	bradycardia *brad-i-KAR-dē-a*	slow heart (cardi-) rate
dys-	abnormal, painful, difficult	dystrophy *DIS-trō-fē*	abnormal nourishment (troph/o) of tissue
mal-	bad, poor	malabsorption *mal-ab-SŌRP-shun*	poor absorption of nutrients
pachy-	thick	pachycephaly *pak-i-SEF-a-lē*	abnormal thickness of the skull
tachy-	rapid	tachypnea *tak-IP-nē-a*	rapid breathing (-pnea)
xero-	dry	xeroderma *zē-rō-DER-ma*	dryness of the skin

Exercise 6-2

Match the following terms and write the appropriate letter to the left of each number:

_____	1. dysplasia (*dis-PLĀ-jē-a*)	a. abnormal thickness of the fingers
_____	2. pachydactyly (*pak-ē-DAK-til-ē*)	b. abnormal development of tissue
_____	3. tachycardia (*tak-i-KAR-dē-a*)	c. difficulty in swallowing
_____	4. bradypnea (*brad-ip-NĒ-a*)	d. slow breathing
_____	5. dysphagia (*dis-FĀ-jē-a*)	e. rapid heart rate

Identify and define the prefix in each of the following words:

	Prefix	Meaning of Prefix
6. maladjustment (*ma-ad-JUST-ment*)	_____	_____
7. dysentery (*DIS-en-ter-ē*)	_____	_____
8. xerosis (*zē-RŌ-sis*)	_____	_____

Table 6·3 Suffixes for Disease

SUFFIX	MEANING	EXAMPLE	DEFINITION OF EXAMPLE
-algia, -algesia	pain	neuralgia *nū-RAL-jē-a*	pain in a nerve (neur/o)
-cele	hernia, localized dilation	gastrocele *GAS-trō-sēl*	hernia of the stomach (gastr/o)
-clasis, -clasia	breaking	karyoclasis *kar-ē-OK-la-sis*	breaking of a nucleus (kary/o)
-itis	inflammation	cystitis *sis-TĪ-tis*	inflammation of the urinary bladder (cyst/o)
-megaly	enlargement	hepatomegaly *hep-a-tō-MEG-a-lē*	enlargement of the liver (hepat/o)
-odynia	pain	urodynia *ū-rō-DIN-ē-a*	pain on urination (ur/o)
-oma*	tumor	lipoma *lī-PŌ-ma*	tumor of fat cells
-pathy	any disease of	nephropathy *nef-ROP-a-thē*	any disease of the kidney (nephr/o)
-rhage[†], -rhagia[†]	bursting forth, profuse flow, hemorrhage	hemorrhage *HEM-or-ij*	profuse flow of blood
-rhea[†]	flow, discharge	pyorrhea *pī-ō-RĒ-a*	discharge of pus

Table 6·3	Continued		
-rhexis†	rupture	amniorrhexis *am-nē-ō-REK-sis*	rupture of the amniotic sac (bag of waters)
-schisis	fissure, splitting	retinoschisis *ret-i-NOS-ki-sis*	splitting of the retina of the eye

*Plural: -omas, -omata.
†Remember to double the r when adding this suffix to a root.

Exercise 6-3

Match the following terms and write the appropriate letter to the left of each number:

_____ **1.** osteoclasis (*os-tē-OK-la-sis*)	**a.** tumor of immature cells
_____ **2.** blastoma (*blas-TŌ-ma*)	**b.** fissure of the chest
_____ **3.** melanoma (*mel-a-NŌ-ma*)	**c.** breaking of a bone
_____ **4.** thoracoschisis (*thō-ra-KOS-ki-sis*)	**d.** hernia containing fat
_____ **5.** adipocele (*AD-i-pō-sēl*)	**e.** tumor of pigmented cells
_____ **6.** menorrhagia (*men-ō-RĀ-jē-a*)	**a.** local dilation containing fluid
_____ **7.** hydrocele (*HĪ-drō-sēl*)	**b.** pain in a gland
_____ **8.** hepatorrhexis (*hep-a-tō-REK-sis*)	**c.** absence of pain
_____ **9.** adenodynia (*ad-e-nō-DIN-ē-a*)	**d.** profuse menstrual flow
_____ **10.** analgesia (*an-al-JĒ-zē-a*)	**e.** rupture of the liver

The root my/o means "muscle." Define the following terms:

11. myalgia (*mī-AL-jē-a*) _____ pain in a muscle _____

12. myorrhexis (*mī-ō-REK-sis*) _____

13. myopathy (*mī-OP-a-thē*) _____

14. myoma (*mī-ō-ma*) _____

15. myodynia (*mī-ō-DIN-ē-a*) _____

Some words pertaining to disease are used as suffixes in compound words. As previously noted, the term *suffix* is used in this book to mean any word part that consistently appears at the end of words. This may be a simple suffix (such as -y, -ia, -ic), a word, or a root–suffix combination, such as -megaly, -rhagia, -pathy (Table 6-4).

Table 6·4	Words for Disease Used as Suffixes		
WORD	**MEANING**	**EXAMPLE**	**DEFINITION OF EXAMPLE**
dilation*, dilatation*	expansion, widening	vasodilation *vas-ō-dī-LĀ-shun*	widening of blood vessels (vas/o)
ectasia, ectasis	dilation, dilatation, distension	gastrectasia *gas-trek-TĀ-sē-a*	dilatation of the stomach (gastr/o)
edema	accumulation of fluid, swelling	cephaledema *sef-al-e-DĒ-ma*	swelling of the head
lysis*	separation, loosening, dissolving, destruction	dialysis *dī-AL-i-sis*	separation of substances by passage through (dia-) a membrane
malacia	softening	osteomalacia *os-tē-ō-ma-LĀ-shē-a*	softening of a bone (oste/o)
necrosis	death of tissue	cardionecrosis *kar-dē-ō-ne-KRŌ-sis*	death of heart (cardi) tissue
ptosis	dropping, downward displacement, prolapse	blepharoptosis *blef-e-rop-TŌ-sis*	drooping of the eyelid (blephar/o; (Fig. 6-8)
sclerosis	hardening	phlebosclerosis *fleb-ō-skle-RŌ-sis*	hardening of veins (phleb/o)
spasm	sudden contraction, cramp	arteriospasm *ar-TĒR-ē-ō-spazm*	spasm of an artery
stasis*	suppression, stoppage	menostasis *men-OS-ta-sis*	suppression of menstrual (men/o) flow
stenosis	narrowing, constriction	bronchostenosis *brong-kō-ste-NŌ-sis*	narrowing of a bronchus (air passageway)
toxin	poison	nephrotoxin *nef-rō-TOK-sin*	substance poisonous or harmful for the kidneys

May also refer to treatment.

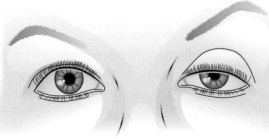

Normal lid   Drooping lid

Figure 6-8 Blepharoptosis (drooping of the eyelid). Ptosis means a downward displacement.

Exercise 6-4

Match the following terms and write the appropriate letter to the left of each number:

_____	**1.** myolysis (*mī-OL-i-sis*)	**a.**	destruction of blood cells
_____	**2.** craniomalacia (*kra-nē-ō-ma-LĀ-shē-a*)	**b.**	death of bone tissue
_____	**3.** osteonecrosis (*os-tē-ō-nē-KRŌ-sis*)	**c.**	stoppage of blood flow
_____	**4.** hemolysis (*hē-MOL-i-sis*)	**d.**	softening of the skull
_____	**5.** hemostasis (*hē-mō-STĀ-sis*)	**e.**	dissolving of muscle

The root splen/o means "spleen." Define the following words:

6. splenotoxin (*splē-nō-TOK-sin*) _____

7. splenoptosis (*splē-nop-TŌ-sis*) _____

8. splenomalacia (*splē-nō-ma-LĀ-shē-a*) _____

Table 6·5　Prefixes and Roots for Infectious Diseases

WORD PART	MEANING	EXAMPLE	DEFINITION OF EXAMPLE
Prefixes			
staphyl/o	grapelike cluster	staphylococcus *staf-i-lō-KOK-us*	a round bacterium that forms clusters
strept/o	twisted chain	streptobacillus *strep-tō-ba-SIL-us*	a rod-shaped bacterium that forms chains
Roots			
bacill/i, bacill/o	bacillus	bacilluria *bas-i-LŪ-rē-a*	bacilli in the urine (-uria)
bacteri/o	bacterium	bacteriostatic *bak-tēr-ē-ō-STAT-ik*	stopping (stasis) the growth of bacteria
myc/o	fungus, mold	mycotic *mī-KOT-ik*	pertaining to a fungus
vir/o	virus	viremia *vī-RĒ-mē-a*	presence of viruses in the blood (-emia)

Exercise 6-5

Fill in the blanks:

1. A bactericidal (*bak-tēr-i-SĪ-dal*) *agent kills* _____.

2. A mycosis (*mī-KŌ-sis*) is any disease caused by a(n) _____.

3. The term *bacillary* (*BAS-il-a-rē*) means pertaining to _____.

4. The prefix *staphyl/o*- means _____.

5. The prefix *strept/o*- means _____.

Use the suffix -logy to write a word that means the same as each of the following:

6. Study of bacteria _____

7. Study of viruses _____

8. Study of fungi _____

6

TERMINOLOGY Supplementary Terms

GENERAL TERMS PERTAINING TO DISEASE

acid-fast stain	A laboratory staining procedure used mainly to identify the tuberculosis organism
communicable *ko-MŪN-i-ka-bl*	Capable of passing from one person to another, such as an infectious disease
endemic *en-DEM-ik*	Occurring at a low level but continuously in a given region, such as the common cold
epidemic *ep-i-DEM-ik*	Affecting many people in a given region at the same time; a disease that breaks out in a large proportion of a population at a given time
exacerbation *eks-zas-er-BĀ-shun*	Worsening of disease; increase in severity of a disease or its symptoms
iatrogenic *ī-at-rō-JEN-ik*	Caused by the effects of treatment (from Greek root *iatro-*, meaning "physician")
idiopathic *id-ē-ō-PATH-ik*	Having no known cause (root *idio* means "self-originating")
in situ *in SĪ-tū*	Localized, noninvasive (literally "in position"); said of tumors that do not spread, such as carcinoma in situ (CIS)
normal flora *FLŌ-ra*	The microorganisms that normally live on or in the body. These organisms are generally harmless, and often are beneficial, but they can cause disease under special circumstances, such as injury or failure of the immune system.
nosocomial *nos-ō-KŌ-mē-al*	Describing an infection acquired in a hospital (root *nos/o* means "disease," and *comial* refers to a hospital). Such infections can be a serious problem, especially if they are resistant to antibiotics; for example, there are now strains of methicillin-resistant *Staphylococcus aureus* (MRSA) and vancomycin-resistant *S. aureus* (VRSA), which cause troublesome infections in hospital settings.
opportunistic *op-por-tū-NIS-tik*	Describing an infection that occurs because of a host's poor or altered condition
pandemic *pan-DEM-ik*	Describing a disease that is prevalent throughout an entire region or the world. AIDS is now pandemic in certain regions of the world.
remission *rē-MISH-un*	A lessening of disease symptoms; the period during which such lessening occurs

TERMINOLOGY   Supplementary Terms

Continued

septicemia *sep-ti-SĒ-mē-a*	Presence of pathogenic bacteria in the blood; blood poisoning
systemic *sis-TEM-ik*	Pertaining to the whole body

MANIFESTATIONS OF DISEASE

abscess *AB-ses*	A localized collection of pus
adhesion *ad-HĒ-zhun*	A uniting of two surfaces or parts that may normally be separated
anaplasia *a-na-PLĀ-jē-a*	Lack of normal differentiation, as shown by cancer cells
ascites *a-SĪ-tēz*	Accumulation of fluid in the peritoneal cavity
cellulitis *sel-ū-LĪ-tis*	A spreading inflammation of tissue
effusion *e-FŪ-zhun*	Escape of fluid into a cavity or other body part
exudate *EKS-ū-dāt*	Material that escapes from blood vessels as a result of tissue injury
fissure *FISH-ur*	A groove or split
fistula *FIS-tū-la*	An abnormal passage between two organs or from an organ to the surface of the body
gangrene *GANG-grēn*	Death of tissue, usually caused by lack of blood supply; may be associated with bacterial infection and decomposition
hyperplasia *hī-per-PLĀ-jē-a*	Excessive growth of normal cells in normal arrangement
hypertrophy *hī-PER-trō-fē*	An increase in size of an organ without increase in the number of cells; may result from an increase in activity, as in muscles
induration *in-dū-RĀ-shun*	Hardening; an abnormally hard spot or place
metaplasia *met-a-PLĀ-jē-a*	Conversion of cells to a form that is not normal for that tissue (prefix *meta-* means "change")

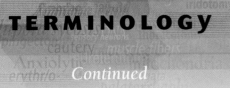

TERMINOLOGY — Supplementary Terms

Continued

polyp *POL-ip*	A tumor attached by a thin stalk
purulent *PUR-ū-lent*	Forming or containing pus
suppuration *sup-ū-RĀ-shun*	Pus formation

6

Go to the pronunciation glossary in Chapter 6 on the CD-ROM to hear these words pronounced.

TERMINOLOGY — Abbreviations

CA	Cancer	**staph**	Staphylococcus
CIS	Carcinoma in situ	**strep**	Streptococcus
FUO	Fever of unknown origin	**VRSA**	Vancomycin-resistant *Staphylococcus aureus*
MRSA	Methicillin-resistant *Staphylococcus aureus*		

CHAPTER REVIEW

TERMINOLOGY

Match the following terms and write the appropriate letter to the left of each number:

_____	1. hemorrhagic	a. pertaining to profuse flow of blood
_____	2. neuroma	b. cancer of glandular tissue
_____	3. encephalitis	c. tumor of a nerve
_____	4. adenocarcinoma	d. enlargement of the stomach
_____	5. gastromegaly	e. inflammation of the brain
_____	6. analgesia	a. stone formation
_____	7. oncolysis	b. dry
_____	8. sclerotic	c. destruction of a tumor
_____	9. lithiasis	d. absence of pain
_____	10. xerotic	e. hardened
_____	11. apyrexia	a. swelling of the fingers or toes
_____	12. dysphagia	b. thickness of the skin
_____	13. pachyderma	c. discharge of pus
_____	14. dactyledema	d. difficulty in swallowing
_____	15. pyorrhea	e. absence of fever
_____	16. carcinolysis	a. local wound or injury
_____	17. hemostasis	b. stoppage of blood flow
_____	18. ectasia	c. dilatation
_____	19. nephroptosis	d. destruction of cancer
_____	20. lesion	e. dropping of the kidney
_____	21. cardiorrhexis	a. any disease of a gland
_____	22. toxoid	b. hardening of a vessel
_____	23. venosclerosis	c. like a poison

_____	24. spasm	**d.**	sudden contraction or cramp
_____	25. adenopathy	**e.**	rupture of the heart

Supplementary Terms

_____	26. abscess	**a.**	a groove or split
_____	27. adhesion	**b.**	escape of fluid into a cavity
_____	28. fissure	**c.**	tumor attached by a thin stalk
_____	29. polyp	**d.**	localized collection of pus
_____	30. effusion	**e.**	union of two surfaces or parts

Fill in the blanks:

31. Heat, pain, redness, and swelling are the four major signs of _____.

32. Any abnormal and uncontrolled growth of tissue, whether benign or malignant, is called a(n) _____.

33. The spreading of cancer to other parts of the body is the process of _____.

34. Protrusion of an organ through an abnormal opening is a(n) _____.

35. Toxicology is the study of _____.

36. Death of tissue is called _____.

37. An oncoprotein is a protein associated with a(n) _____.

True–False. Examine the following statements. If the statement is true, write T in the first blank. If the statement is false, write F in the first blank and correct the statement by replacing the <u>underlined</u> word in the second blank.

38. A mycosis is an infection with a <u>fungus</u>.   _____ _____

39. Round bacteria in chains are <u>staphylococci</u>.   _____ _____

40. A sudden disease of short duration is <u>chronic</u>.   _____ _____

41. A tumor that does not metastasize is termed <u>benign</u>.   _____ _____

42. A slower than normal heart rate is <u>tachycardia</u>.   _____ _____

43. A tumor of connective tissue is classified as a <u>sarcoma</u>.   _____ _____

Eliminations. In each of the sets below, underline the word that does not fit in with the rest and explain the reason for your choice:

44. cocci – helminths – chlamydia – bacilli – vibrios

_____

45. neoplasm – tumor – carcinoma – pathogen – oncology

_____

46. septicemic – nosocomial – metastatic – opportunistic – epidemic

_____

Word building. Use the suffix -*genesis* to write words with the following meanings:

47. Formation of cancer   _____ carcinogenesis _____

48. Formation of pus   _____

49. Origin of any disease   _____

50. Formation of a tumor   _____

The root *bronch/o* pertains to a bronchus, an air passageway in the lungs. Add a suffix to this root to form words with the following meanings:

51. Sudden contraction of a bronchus   _____

52. Inflammation of a bronchus   _____

53. Narrowing of a bronchus   _____

54. Excessive flow or discharge from a bronchus   _____

Use the root *oste/o*, meaning "bone," to form words with the following meanings:

55. Death of bone tissue   _____

56. Softening of a bone   _____

57. Breaking of a bone   _____

58. Tumor of a bone   _____

59. Destruction of bone tissue   _____

Go to the word exercises in Chapter 6 on the CD-ROM for additional review exercises.

CASE STUDY 6–1: Esophageal Spasm

B.R., a 53-year-old woman, consulted with her primary physician because of occasional episodes of dysphagia with moderate to severe tight, gripping pain in her midthorax. She reported that the onset was sudden after ingestion of certain foods or beverages, beginning retrosternally and radiating to the cervical and dorsal regions. The pain was not relieved by assuming a supine position or holding her breath. B.R. also stated that she felt like her heart was racing and that she might be having a heart attack. She denied any dyspepsia, vomiting, or dyspnea. Her doctor suspected acute esophageal spasm or possibly a paraesophageal hiatal hernia and referred B.R. to a gastroenterologist for a gastroscopy and esophageal manometry study (pressure measurement). She also underwent a barium swallow study under fluoroscopic imaging.

CASE STUDY 6–2: HIV Infection and Tuberculosis

T.H., a 48-year-old man, was an admitted intravenous (IV) drug user and occasionally abused alcohol. Over 4 weeks, he had experienced fever, night sweats, malaise, a cough, and a 10-lb weight loss. He was also concerned about several discolored lesions that had erupted weeks before on his arms and legs.

T.H. made an appointment with a physician assistant (PA) at the neighborhood clinic. On examination, the PA noted bilateral anterior cervical and axillary lymphadenopathy and pyrexia. T.H.'s temperature was 39°C. The PA sent T.H. to the hospital for further studies.

T.H.'s chest radiograph (x-ray image) showed paratracheal adenopathy and bilateral interstitial infiltrates, suspicious of tuberculosis (TB). His blood study results were positive for human immunodeficiency virus (HIV) and showed a low lymphocyte count. Sputum and bronchoscopic lavage (washing) fluid were positive for an acid-fast bacillus (AFB); a PPD (purified protein derivative) skin test result was also positive. Based on these findings, T.H. was diagnosed with HIV, TB, and Kaposi sarcoma related to past IV drug abuse.

CASE STUDY 6–3: Endocarditis

D.A., a 37-year-old man, sought treatment after experiencing several days of high fever and generalized weakness on return from his vacation. D.A.'s family doctor suspected cardiac involvement because of D.A.'s history of rheumatic fever. The doctor was concerned because D.A.'s brother had died of acute malignant hyperpyrexia during surgery at the age of 12. D.A. was referred to a cardiologist, who scheduled an electrocardiogram (ECG) and a transesophageal echocardiogram (TEE).

D.A. was admitted to the hospital with subacute bacterial endocarditis (SBE) and placed on high-dose IV antibiotics and bed rest. He had also developed a heart murmur, which was diagnosed as idiopathic hypertrophic subaortic stenosis (IHSS).

CASE STUDY QUESTIONS

Multiple choice. Select the best answer and write the letter of your choice to the left of each number:

_____ 1. The cervical region is the region of the:
- a. heart
- b. uterus
- c. neck
- d. leg
- e. head

_____ 2. A word that has the same meaning as dorsal is:
- a. anterior
- b. posterior
- c. caudal
- d. inferior
- e. superior

6

_____ 3. In referring to tissues, the term *interstitial* means:
   a. around cells
   b. under cells
   c. between cells
   d. through cells
   e. within cells

_____ 4. The term *axillary* refers to the:
   a. bladder
   b. abdomen
   c. wrist
   d. armpit
   e. groin

_____ 5. The term *pyrexia* refers to a(n):
   a. fever
   b. stone
   c. tumor
   d. spasm
   e. poison

_____ 6. Dyspepsia refers to indigestion. Dysphagia and dyspnea refer to difficulty with:
   a. breathing and coughing
   b. swallowing and urinating
   c. walking and chewing gum
   d. swallowing and breathing
   e. sleeping and breathing

_____ 7. Paraesophageal and paratracheal refer to _____ the esophagus and trachea.
   a. under
   b. superior to
   c. near or beside
   d. in between
   e. within

_____ 8. The endocardium is the tissue lining the heart's chambers. Endocarditis refers to a(n) _____ of this lining.
   a. narrowing
   b. inflammation
   c. overgrowth of tissue
   d. cancerous growth
   e. thinning

_____ 9. D.A.'s heart murmur was caused by a stenosis, or _____ of the heart's aortic valve.
   a. narrowing
   b. inflammation
   c. overgrowth of tissue
   d. cancerous growth
   e. thinning

_____ 10. The term for a condition or disease of unknown etiology is:
    a. stenosis
    b. hypertrophic
    c. chronic
    d. acute
    e. idiopathic

Fill in the blanks:

11. The word in the case studies that means "protrusion of an organ through an abnormal body opening" is a(n)
    _____.

12. Adenopathy is any disease of a(n) _____.

13. Tuberculosis is caused by a rod-shaped bacterium described as a(n) _____.

14. A malignant neoplasm arising from muscle or connective tissue is a(n) _____.

15. A potentially fatal disease condition characterized by a very high fever is called
    _____.

Give the meaning of the following abbreviations:

16. HIV _____

17. PPD _____

18. ECG _____

19. AFB _____

DIAGNOSIS AND TREATMENT; SURGERY

CHAPTER CONTENTS

7

OBJECTIVES

After study of this chapter you should be able to:

1. List the main components of a patient history.
2. Describe the main methods used in patient examination.
3. Name and describe nine imaging techniques.
4. Name possible forms of treatment.
5. Describe theories of alternative and complementary medicine and some healing practices used in these fields.
6. Describe staging and grading as they apply to cancer.

7. Define basic terms pertaining to medical examination, diagnosis, and treatment.
8. Identify and use the roots and suffixes pertaining to diagnosis and surgery.
9. Interpret symbols and abbreviations used in diagnosis and treatment.
10. Interpret a case history containing terms related to diagnosis and treatment.

PRETEST

1. Determination of a disease's cause is called

   _____.

2. Measurements of the basic functions needed to maintain life, such as breathing and pulse, together are called _____.

3. The two phases recorded when measuring blood pressure are _____ and _____.

4. Prediction of a disease's outcome is a(n)

   _____.

5. Staging is a process used to evaluate the severity of _____.

6. An appendectomy is _____.

7. A tracheotomy is _____.

Diagnosis

Medical **diagnosis**, the determination of the nature and cause of an illness, begins with a patient history. This includes a history of the present illness with a description of **symptoms** (evidence of disease), a past medical history, and a family and a social history.

A physical examination, which includes a review of all systems and observation of any **signs** of illness, follows the history taking. Practitioners use the following techniques in performing physicals:

> ➤ **Inspection**: visual examination.
> ➤ **Palpation**: touching the surface of the body with the hands or fingers (Fig. 7-1).
> ➤ **Percussion**: tapping the body to evaluate tissue according to the sounds produced (Fig. 7-2).
> ➤ **Auscultation**: listening to body sounds with a **stethoscope** (Fig. 7-3).

Vital signs (VS) are also recorded for comparison with normal ranges. Vital signs are measurements that reflect basic functions necessary to maintain life and include:

> ➤ Temperature (T).
> ➤ Pulse rate, measured in beats per minute (bpm) (Fig. 7-4). Pulse rate normally corresponds to the heart rate (HR), the number of times the heart beats per minute.
> ➤ Respiration rate (R), measured in breaths per minute.
> ➤ Blood pressure (BP), measured in millimeters of mercury (mm Hg) and recorded when the heart is contracting (systolic pressure) and relaxing (diastolic pressure) (Fig. 7-5). An examiner typically uses a stethoscope and a blood pressure cuff, or **sphygmomanometer** (*sfig- mō-ma-NOM-e-ter*), to measure blood pressure. Newer devices that read blood pressure directly and give a digital reading are also in use. Chapter 9 has more information on blood pressure.

Additional tools used in physical examinations include the **ophthalmoscope** (Fig. 7-6A), for examination of the eyes; the **otoscope** (see Fig. 7-6B), for examination of the ears; and hammers, for testing reflexes.

The skin, hair, and nails provide easily observable indications of a person's state of health. Skin features such as color, texture, thickness, and presence of lesions (local injuries) are noted throughout the course of the physical examination. Chapter 21 contains a discussion of the skin and skin diseases.

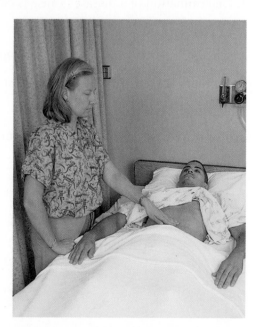

Figure 7-1 Palpation. The practitioner touches the body surface with the hands or fingers.

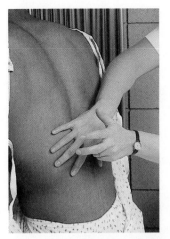

Figure 7-2 Percussion. The practitioner taps the body to evaluate tissues.

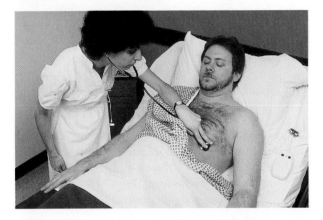

Figure 7-3 Auscultation. The practitioner uses a stethoscope to listen to body sounds.

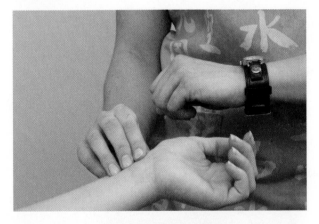

Figure 7-4 Pulse rate. The practitioner palpates an artery to measure pulse rate in beats per minute.

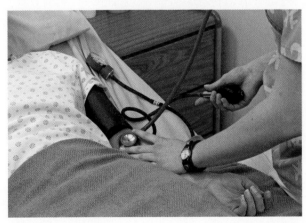

Figure 7-5 Blood pressure. The practitioner uses a blood pressure cuff (sphygmomanometer) and a stethoscope to measure systolic and diastolic pressures.

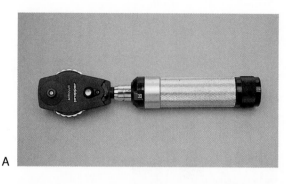

A

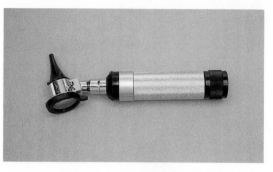

B

Figure 7-6 Examination tools.
(*A*) Ophthalmoscope for eye examination. (*B*) Otoscope for ear examination.

Diagnosis is further aided by laboratory test results. These may include tests on blood, urine, and other body fluids, and the identification of infectious organisms. Additional tests may include study of the electrical activity of tissues such as the brain and heart, examination of body cavities by means of an **endoscope** (Fig. 7-7), and imaging techniques. **Biopsy** is the removal of tissue for microscopic examination. Biopsy specimens can be obtained by:

➤ needle withdrawal (aspiration) of fluid, as from the chest or from a cyst
➤ a small punch, as of the skin
➤ endoscopy, as from the respiratory or digestive tract
➤ surgical removal, as of a tumor or node

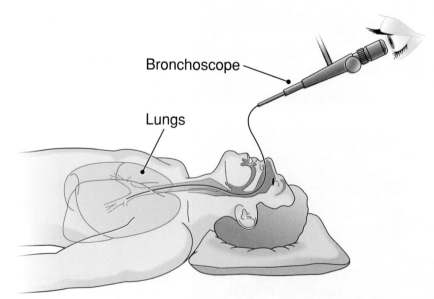

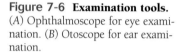

Figure 7-7 Endoscope. A bronchoscope is a type of endoscope used to examine the respiratory bronchi.

Box 7·1 Focus on Words   *Terminology Evolves with Medical Science*

The science of medicine never stands still, nor does its terminology. One can never say that his or her work in learning medical terminology is complete because vocabulary is constantly being added as new diagnoses, treatments, and technologies are discovered or developed.

A generation ago, gene therapy, genetic engineering, in vitro fertilization, cloning, and stem-cell research were unknown to the public. PET scans, MRI, DNA fingerprinting, radioimmunoassay, bone-density scans for identifying osteoporosis, and other diagnostic techniques were not in use. Some of the new categories of drugs, such as statins for reducing cholesterol, antiviral agents, histamine antagonists for treating ulcers, ACE inhibitors for treating hypertension, and breast cancer preventives were undiscovered. The genes associated with certain forms of cancer and with certain hereditary abnormalities had yet to be isolated.

Each of these advances brings new terminology into use. Anyone who wants to keep current with medical terminology has a lifetime of learning ahead.

When new tests appear, as in all other areas of health sciences, new terminology is added to the medical vocabulary (see Box 7-1).

Imaging Techniques

Imaging techniques employ various physical forces to produce visual images of the body. The most fundamental imaging method is **radiography** (Fig. 7-8), which uses x-rays to produce a picture (radiograph) on sensitized film. Radiography is best at showing dense tissues, such as bone, but views of soft tissue can be enhanced by using a contrast medium, such as a barium mixture, to outline the tissue. Other forms of energy used to produce diagnostic images include sound waves, radioactive isotopes, radio waves, and magnetic fields. See Box 7-2 for a description of the most commonly used imaging methods and Reference Box 7-3 for a summary of these and other imaging techniques in use.

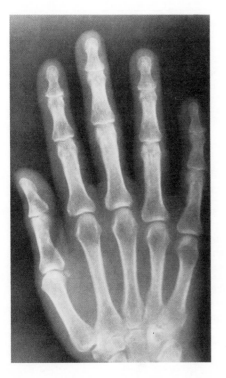

Figure 7-8 Radiography. The action of x-rays on sensitized film produced this image (radiograph) of a normal right hand.

Box 7•2 Clinical Perspectives *Medical Imaging*

Three imaging techniques that have revolutionized medicine are radiography, computed tomography, and magnetic resonance imaging. With them, physicians today can "see" inside the body without making a single cut.

The oldest technique is radiography (*rā-dē-OG-ra-fē*), in which a machine beams x-rays (a form of radiation) through the body onto a piece of film. The resulting picture is called a radiograph. Dark areas indicate where the beam passed through the body and exposed the film, whereas light areas show where the beam did not pass through. Dense tissues (bone, teeth) absorb most of the x-rays, preventing them from exposing the film. For this reason, radiography is commonly used to visualize bone fractures and tooth decay as well as abnormally dense tissues like tumors. Radiography does not provide clear pictures of soft tissues because most of the beam passes through and exposes the film, but contrast media can help make structures like blood vessels and hollow organs more visible. For example, barium sulfate (which absorbs x-rays) coats the digestive tract when ingested.

During a computed tomography (CT) scan, a machine revolves around the patient, beaming x-rays through the body onto a detector. The detector takes numerous pictures of the beam and a computer assembles them into transverse sections, or "slices." Unlike conventional radiography, CT produces clear images of soft structures such as the brain, liver, and lungs. It is commonly used to visualize brain injuries and tumors, and even blood vessels when used with contrast media.

Magnetic resonance imaging uses a strong magnetic field and radio waves. The patient undergoing MRI lies inside a chamber within a very powerful magnet. The molecules in the patient's soft tissues align with the magnetic field inside the chamber. When radio waves hit the soft tissue, the aligned molecules emit energy that the MRI machine detects, and a computer converts these signals into a picture. MRI produces even clearer images of soft tissue than does CT and can create detailed pictures of blood vessels without contrast media. MRI can visualize brain injuries and tumors that might be missed using CT.

Box 7•3 For Your Reference *Imaging Techniques*

Method	Description
cineradiography *sin-e-rā-dē-OG-ra-fē*	making of a motion picture of successive images appearing on a fluoroscopic screen
computed tomography (CT, CT scan) *tō-MOG-ra-fē*	use of a computer to generate an image from a large number of x-rays passed at different angles through the body; a three-dimensional picture of a cross-section of the body is obtained; reveals more about soft tissues than does simple radiography (Fig. 7-9A)
fluoroscopy *flū-ROS-kō-pē*	use of x-rays to examine deep structures; the shadows cast by x-rays passed through the body are observed on a fluorescent screen; the device used is called a fluoroscope
magnetic resonance imaging (MRI)	production of images through the use of a magnetic field and radio waves; the characteristics of soft tissue are revealed by differences in molecular properties; eliminates the need for x-rays and contrast media (see Fig. 7-9B)
positron emission tomography (PET)	production of sectional body images by administration of a natural substance, such as glucose, labeled with a positron-emitting isotope; the rays subsequently emitted are interpreted by computer to show the internal distribution of the substance administered; PET has been used to follow blood flow through an organ and to measure metabolic activity within an organ, such as the brain, under different conditions
radiography *rā-dē-OG-ra-fē*	use of x-rays passed through the body to make a visual record (radiograph) of internal structures on specially sensitized film. Also called roentgenography (*rent-ge-NOG-ra-fē*) after the developer of the technique.

Box 7•3 For Your Reference *Continued*

scintigraphy *sin-TIG-ra-fē*	production of an image of the radioactivity distribution in tissues after internal administration of a radioactive substance (radionuclide); the images are obtained with a scintillation camera; the record produced is a scintiscan (*SIN-ti-skan*) and usually specifies the part examined or the isotope used for the test, as in bone scan, gallium scan
single photon emission computed tomography (SPECT)	scintigraphic technique that permits visualization of a radioisotope's cross-sectional distribution
ultrasonography *ul-tra-son-OG-ra-fē*	generation of a visual image from the echoes of high-frequency sound waves traveling back from different tissues; also called sonography (*so-NOG-ra-fē*) and echography (*ek-OG-ra-fē*) (Fig. 7-10)

7

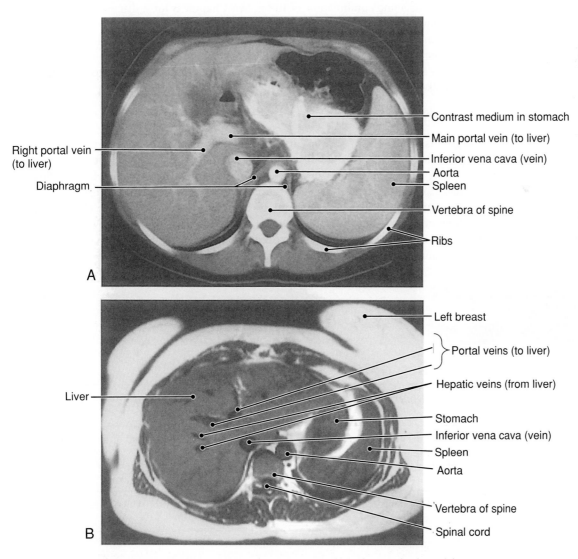

Right portal vein (to liver)

Diaphragm

Contrast medium in stomach

Main portal vein (to liver)

Inferior vena cava (vein)

Aorta

Spleen

Vertebra of spine

Ribs

A

Left breast

Portal veins (to liver)

Hepatic veins (from liver)

Liver

Stomach

Inferior vena cava (vein)

Spleen

Aorta

Vertebra of spine

Spinal cord

B

Figure 7-9 Imaging techniques. Shown are cross-sections through the liver and spleen. (*A*) Computed tomography (CT). (*B*) Magnetic resonance imaging (MRI).

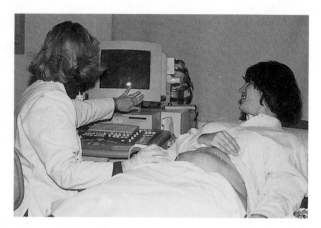

Figure 7-10 Ultrasonography.
The practitioner is using ultrasound to monitor pregnancy.

Treatment

If diagnosis so indicates, treatment, also termed **therapy**, is begun. This may consist of counseling, drugs, surgery, radiation, physical therapy, occupational therapy, psychiatric treatment, or some combination of these. See Chapter 8 for a discussion of drugs and their actions. **Palliative** therapy is treatment that provides relief but is not intended as a cure. Terminally ill patients, for example, may receive treatment that eases pain and pro-vides comfort but is not expected to change the outcome of their disease. During diagnosis and throughout the course of treatment, a patient is evaluated to establish a **prognosis**—that is, a prediction of the disease's outcome.

Surgery

Surgery is a method for treating disease or injury by manual operations. Surgery may be done through an existing body opening, but usually it involves cutting or punctur-ing tissue with a sharp instrument in the process of **incision**. See Reference Box 7-4 for descriptions of surgical instruments and Figure 7-11 for pictures of surgical instru-ments. Surgery usually requires some form of **anesthesia** to dull or eliminate pain. After surgery, incisions must be closed for proper healing. Traditionally, surgeons have used stitches or **sutures** to close wounds, but today they also use adhesive strips, staples, and skin glue.

Box 7•4 **For Your Reference** *Surgical Instruments*

Instrument	Description
bougie *BOO-zhē*	slender, flexible instrument for exploring and dilating tubes
cannula *KAN-ū-la*	tube enclosing a trocar (see below) that allows escape of fluid or air after removal of the trocar
clamp	instrument used to compress tissue
curet (curette) *KŪ-ret*	spoon-shaped instrument for removing material from the wall of a cavity or other surface (see Fig. 7-11)
elevator *EL-e-vā-tor*	instrument for lifting tissue or bone
forceps *FOR-seps*	instrument for holding or extracting (see Fig. 7-11)

Box 7•4 For Your Reference	*Continued*
Gigli saw *JĒL-yēz*	flexible wire saw
hemostat *HĒ-mō-stat*	small clamp for stopping blood flow from a vessel (see Fig. 7-11)
rasp	surgical file
retractor *rē-TRAK-tor*	instrument used to maintain exposure by separating a wound and holding back organs or tissues (see Fig. 7-11)
rongeur *ron-ZHUR*	gouge forceps
scalpel *SKAL-pel*	surgical knife with a sharp blade (see Fig. 7-11)
scissors *SIZ-ors*	a cutting instrument with two opposing blades
sound *sownd*	instrument for exploring a cavity or canal (see Fig. 7-11)
trocar *TRŌ-kar*	sharp pointed instrument contained in a cannula used to puncture a cavity

7

Many types of operations are now performed with a **laser**, an intense beam of light. Some procedures require destruction of tissue by a harmful agent, such as by heat or a chemical, in the process of **cautery** or cauterization.

Some of the purposes of surgery include:

➤ Treatment: For **excision** (cutting out) of diseased or abnormal tissue, such as a tumor or an inflamed appendix. Surgical methods are also used to repair wounds or injuries, as in skin grafting for burns or for realigning broken bones. Surgical methods are used to correct circulatory problems and to return structures to their normal position, as in raising a prolapsed organ, such as the bladder, in a surgical **fixation** procedure.

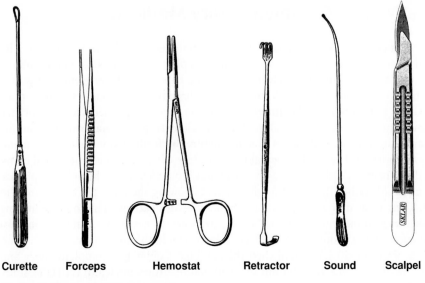

| Curette | Forceps | Hemostat | Retractor | Sound | Scalpel |

Figure 7-11 **Surgical instruments.**

Box 7•5 Health Professions *Surgical Technology*

Surgical technologists, also known as operating room technicians, prepare for and assist with surgical procedures under the supervision of surgeons and nurses. They prepare the operating room, surgical instruments, and equipment. They help the surgical team to scrub and put on gowns, gloves, and masks. They also prepare patients for surgery, helping to position them on the table and draping them with sterile linens. During an operation, surgical technologists hand instruments and other materials to the surgeon, maintain supplies, and operate special equipment. Finally, they help count materials to be sure that all have been removed from the patient at the conclusion of surgery, and they assist in suturing. They also take responsibility for specimens removed for laboratory testing.

A career in surgical technology requires training in a surgical technology program and certification. Preparation for this training should include courses in basic sciences, math, and computer applications. The job requires stamina, manual dexterity, and quick reaction time.

➤ Diagnosis: To remove tissue for laboratory study in a biopsy, as described above. Exploratory surgery to investigate the cause of symptoms is performed less frequently now because of advances in noninvasive diagnostic and imaging techniques.

➤ Restoration: Surgery may compensate for lost function, as when a section of the intestine is redirected in a colostomy; a tube is inserted to allow breathing in a tracheostomy; a feeding tube is inserted; or an organ is transplanted. Surgeons may perform plastic or reconstructive surgery to accommodate a prosthesis (substitute part), to restore proper appearance, or for cosmetic reasons.

➤ Relief: Palliative surgery relieves pain or discomfort, as by cutting the nerve supply to an organ or reducing the size of a tumor to relieve pressure.

Surgery may be done in an emergency or urgent situation under conditions of acute danger, as in traumatic injury or severe blockage. Other procedures, such as cataract removal from the eye, may be planned when convenient. Elective or optional surgery would not cause serious consequences if delayed or not done.

Over time, surgery has extended beyond the classic operating room of a hospital to other hospital areas and to private surgical facilities where people can be treated within 1 day as outpatients. Preoperative care is given before surgery and includes examination, obtaining the patient's informed consent for the procedure, and preadmission testing. Postoperative care includes recovery from anesthesia, follow-up evaluations, and instructions for home care.

Box 7-5 describes some aspects of careers in surgical technology.

Alternative and Complementary Medicine

During the past century, the leading causes of death in industrialized countries have gradually shifted from infectious diseases to chronic diseases of the cardiovascular and respiratory systems and cancer. In addition to advancing age, life habits and the environment greatly influence these conditions. As a result, many people have begun to consider healing practices from other philosophies and cultures as alternatives and complements to conventional Western medicine. Some of these philosophies include **osteopathy**, **naturopathy**, **homeopathy**, and **chiropractic**. Techniques of **acupuncture**, **biofeedback**, **massage**, and **meditation** may also be used, as well as herbal remedies (see Chapter 8) and nutritional counseling on diet, vitamins, and minerals. Complementary and alternative therapies emphasize maintaining health rather than treating disease and allowing the body the opportunity to heal itself. These ideas fit into the concept of **holistic health care**, which promotes treating an individual as a whole with emotional, social, and spiritual needs in addition to physical needs and encouraging people to be involved in their own health maintenance.

The U.S. government has established the National Center for Complementary and Alternative Medicine (NCCAM) within the National Institutes of Health (NIH) to study these therapies.

Cancer

Methods used in the diagnosis of cancer include physical examination, biopsy, imaging techniques, and laboratory tests for abnormalities, or "markers," associated with specific types of malignancies. Some cancer markers are by-products, such as enzymes, hormones, and cellular proteins, that are abnormal or are produced in abnormal amounts. Researchers are also linking specific genetic mutations to certain forms of cancer.

Oncologists (cancer specialists) use two methods, grading and staging, to classify cancers, to select and evaluate therapy, and to estimate disease outcome. **Grading** is based on histologic changes observed in tumor cells when they are examined microscopically. Grades increase from I to IV with increasing cellular abnormality.

Staging is a procedure for establishing the clinical extent of tumor spread, both at the original site and in other parts of the body (metastases). The TNM system is commonly used. These letters stand for primary tumor (T), regional lymph nodes (N), and distant metastases (M). Evaluation in these categories varies for each type of tumor. Based on TNM results, a stage ranging in severity from I to IV is assigned. Cancers of the blood, lymphatic system, and nervous system are evaluated by different standards.

The most widely used methods for treatment of cancer are surgery, radiation therapy, and **chemotherapy** (treatment with chemicals). Newer methods of **immunotherapy** use substances that stimulate the immune system as a whole or vaccines prepared specifically against a tumor. Hormone therapy may also be effective against certain types of tumors. When no active signs of the disease remain, the cancer is said to be in **remission**.

TERMINOLOGY — Key Terms

anesthesia *an-es-THĒ-zē-a*	Loss of the ability to feel pain, as by administration of a drug
auscultation *aws-kul-TĀ-shun*	Listening for sounds within the body, usually within the chest or abdomen (see Fig. 7-3)
biopsy *BĪ-op-sē*	Removal of a small amount of tissue for microscopic examination
cautery *KAW-ter-ē*	Destruction of tissue by a damaging agent, such as a harmful chemical, heat, or electric current (electrocautery); cauterization
chemotherapy *kē-mō-THER-a-pē*	The use of chemicals to treat disease. The term is often applied specifically to the treatment of cancer with chemicals.
diagnosis *dī-ag-NŌ-sis*	The process of determining the cause and nature of an illness
endoscope *EN-dō-skōp*	An instrument for examining the inside of an organ or cavity through a body opening or small incision; most endoscopes use fiberoptics for viewing (see Fig. 7-7)
excision *ek-SIZH-un*	Removal by cutting (suffix -*ectomy*)
fixation *fik-SĀ-shun*	Holding or fastening a structure in a fixed position (suffix: -*pexy*)
grading *GRĀ-ding*	A method for evaluating a tumor based on microscopic examination of the cells

TERMINOLOGY

Key Terms

Continued

immunotherapy *im-ū-nō-THER-a-pē*	Treatment that involves stimulation or suppression of the immune system, either specifically or nonspecifically
incision *in-SIZH-un*	A cut, as for surgery; also the act of cutting (suffix" -*tomy*)
inspection *in-SPEK-shun*	Visual examination of the body
laser *LĀ-zer*	A device that transforms light into a beam of intense heat and power; used for surgery and diagnosis
ophthalmoscope *of-THAL-mō-skōp*	An instrument for examining the interior of the eye (see Fig. 7-6A)
otoscope *Ō-tō-skōp*	Instrument used to examine the ears (see Fig. 7-6B)
palliative *PAL-ē-a-tiv*	Providing relief but not cure; a treatment that provides such relief
palpation *pal-PĀ-shun*	Examining by placing the hands or fingers on the surface of the body to determine characteristics such as texture, temperature, movement, and consistency (see Fig. 7-1)
percussion *per-KUSH-un*	Tapping the body lightly but sharply to assess the condition of the underlying tissue by the sounds obtained (see Fig. 7-2)
prognosis *prog-NŌ-sis*	Prediction of the course and outcome of a disease
radiography *rā-dē-OG-ra-fē*	Use of x-rays passed through the body to make a visual record (radiograph) of internal structures on specially sensitized film; roentgenography
remission *rē-MISH-un*	A lessening of disease symptoms; the period during which this decrease occurs or the period when no sign of a disease exists
sign *sīn*	An objective evidence of disease that can be observed or tested; examples are fever, rash, high blood pressure, and blood or urine abnormalities; an objective symptom.
sphygmomanometer *sfig-mō-ma-NOM-e-ter*	The blood pressure apparatus or blood pressure cuff; pressure is read in millimeters of mercury (mm Hg) when the heart is contracting (systolic pressure) and when the heart is relaxing (diastolic pressure) and is reported as systolic/diastolic (see Fig. 7-5)
staging *STĀ-jing*	The process of classifying malignant tumors for diagnosis, treatment, and prognosis
stethoscope *STETH-ō-skōp*	An instrument used for listening to sounds produced within the body (from the Greek root *steth/o*, meaning "chest") (see Fig. 7-3)
surgery *SUR-jer-ē*	A method for treating disease or injury by manual operations

TERMINOLOGY
Key Terms
Continued

suture *SŪ-chur*	To unite parts by stitching them together; also the thread or other material used in that process or the seam formed by surgical stitching (suffix -*rhaphy*)
symptom *SIM-tum*	Any evidence of disease; sometimes limited to subjective evidence of disease, as experienced by the individual, such as pain, dizziness, and weakness
therapy *THER-a-pē*	Treatment; intervention
vital signs	Measurements that reflect basic functions necessary to maintain life

ALTERNATIVE AND COMPLEMENTARY MEDICINE

acupuncture *AK-ū-punk-chur*	An ancient Chinese method of inserting thin needles into the body at specific points to relieve pain, induce anesthesia, or promote healing; similar effects can be obtained by using firm finger pressure at the surface of the body in the technique of *acupressure.*
biofeedback *bī-ō-FĒD-bak*	A method for learning control of involuntary physiologic responses by using electronic devices to monitor bodily changes and feeding this information back to a person
chiropractic *kī-rō-PRAK-tik*	A science that stresses the condition of the nervous system in diagnosis and treatment of disease; often, the spine is manipulated to correct misalignment. Most patients consult for musculoskeletal pain and headaches. (From Greek *cheir,* meaning "hand")
holistic health care *hō-LIS-tik*	Practice of treating a person as a whole entity with physical, emotional, social, and spiritual needs. It stresses comprehensive care, involvement in one's own care, and the maintenance of good health rather than the treatment of disease.
homeopathy *hō-mē-OP-a-thē*	A philosophy of treating disease by administering drugs in highly diluted form along with promoting healthy life habits and a healthy environment (from *home/o,* meaning "same," and *path,* meaning "disease")
massage *ma-SAHJ*	Manipulation of the body or portion of the body to calm, relieve tension, increase circulation, and stimulate muscles
meditation *med-i-TĀ-shun*	Process of clearing the mind by concentrating on the inner self while controlling breathing and perhaps repeating a word or phrase (mantra)
naturopathy *nā-chur-OP-a-thē*	A therapeutic philosophy of helping people to heal themselves by developing healthy lifestyles; naturopaths may use some of the methods of conventional medicine (from *nature* and *path/o,* meaning "disease").
osteopathy *os-tē-OP-a-thē*	A system of therapy based on the theory that the body can overcome disease when it has normal structure, a favorable environment, and proper nutrition. Osteopaths use standard medical practices for diagnosis and treatment but stress the identification and correction of faulty body structure (from *oste/o,* meaning "bone," and *path,* meaning "disease").

Go to the pronunciation glossary in Chapter 7 on the CD-ROM
to hear these words pronounced.

Word Parts Pertaining to Diagnosis and Treatment

Table 7·1 Roots for Physical Forces

ROOT	MEANING	EXAMPLE	DEFINITION OF EXAMPLE
aer/o	air, gas	aerobic *ār-Ō-bik*	pertaining to or requiring air (oxygen)
bar/o	pressure	barometer *ba-ROM-e-ter*	instrument used to measure pressure
chrom/o, chromat/o	color, stain	isochromatic *ī-sō-krō-MAT-ik*	having the same (iso-) color
chron/o	time	chronologic *kron-ō-LOJ-ik*	arranged according to the time of occurrence
cry/o	cold	cryoprobe *KRĪ-ō-prōb*	instrument used to apply extreme cold
electro/o	electricity	electrolyte *e-LEK-trō-līt*	substance that conducts an electrical current
erg/o	work	synergistic *sin-er-JIS-tik*	working together with increased effect, such as certain drugs in combination
phon/o	sound, voice	phonetics *fō-NET-iks*	study of sounds
phot/o	light	photography *fō-TOG-ră-fē*	using light to record an image on light-sensitive paper
radi/o	radiation, x-ray	radiology *rā-dē-OL-ō-jē*	study and use of radiation
son/o	sound	sonogram *SON-ō-gram*	record obtained by use of ultrasound
therm/o	heat, temperature	hyperthermia *hī-per-THER-mē-a*	abnormally high body temperature

Exercise 7-1

Match the following terms and write the appropriate letter to the left of each number:

_____ 1. radioactive (*rā-dē-ō-AK-tiv*)

_____ 2. hypothermia (*hī-pō-THER-mē-a*)

_____ 3. synchronous (*SIN-krō-nus*)

a. attracting color (stain)

b. abnormally low body temperature

c. pertaining to increased pressure

_____ 4. hyperbaric (hī-per-BAR-ik)　　　　　d. occurring at the same time

_____ 5. chromophilic (krō-mō-FIL-ik)　　　　e. giving off radiation

Identify and define the root in each of the following words:

	Root	Meaning of Root
6. ultrasonic (*ul-tra-SON-ik*)	son/o	sound
7. anaerobic (*an-er-Ō-bik*)	_____	_____
8. achromatous (*a-KRŌ-ma-tus*)	_____	_____
9. homeothermic (*hō-mē-ō-THER-mik*)	_____	_____
10. chronic (*KRON-ik*)	_____	_____
11. endergonic (*end-er-GON-ik*)	_____	_____

Fill in the blanks:

12. Barotrauma (*bar-ō-TRAW-ma*) is injury caused by _____.

13. Cryotherapy is treatment using _____.

14. A photoreaction (*fō-tō-rē-AK-shun*) is a response to _____.

15. The term electroconvulsive (*ē-lek-trō-con-VUL-siv*) means causing convulsions by means of
_____.

16. A phonograph (*FŌ-nō-graf*) is an instrument used to reproduce _____.

Table 7•2	**Suffixes for Diagnosis**		
SUFFIX	**MEANING**	**EXAMPLE**	**DEFINITION OF EXAMPLE**
-graph	instrument for recording data	polygraph POL-ē-graf	instrument used to record many physiologic responses simultaneously; lie detector
-graphy	act of recording data*	echography ek-OG-ra-fē	recording data obtained by ultrasound
-gram†	a record of data	electroencephalogram e-lek-trō -en-SEF-a-lō-gram	record of the brain's electrical activity
-meter	instrument for measuring	calorimeter kal-ō-RIM-e-ter	instrument for measuring the caloric energy of food
-metry	measurement of	audiometry aw-dē-OM-e-trē	measurement of hearing (*audi/o*)
-scope	instrument for viewing or examining	bronchoscope BRONG-kō-skōp	instrument for examining the bronchi (breathing passages) (see Fig. 7-7)
-scopy	examination of	celioscopy sē-lē-OS-kō-pē	examination of the abdominal cavity (*celi/o*)

*This ending is often used to mean not only the recording of data but also the evaluation and interpretation of the data.
†A picture taken simply using x-rays is called a radiograph. When special techniques are used to image an organ or region with x-rays, the ending -gram is used with the root for that area, as in urogram (urinary tract), angiogram (blood vessels), and mammogram (breast).

Exercise 7-2

Match the following terms and write the appropriate letter to the left of each number:

_____ 1. thermometer (*ther-MOM-e-ter*)

    a. instrument for examining very small objects

_____ 2. sonogram (*SON-ō-gram*)

    b. instrument for measuring temperature

_____ 3. laparoscopy (*lap-a-ROS-kō-pē*)

    c. measurement of work done

_____ 4. microscope (*MĪ-krō-skōp*)

    d. a record of sound

_____ 5. ergometry (*er-GOM-e-trē*)

    e. examination of the abdomen

_____ 6. chronometer (*kron-OM-e-ter*)

    a. a record of sound

_____ 7. phonogram (*FŌ-nō-gram*)

    b. instrument for measuring time

_____ 8. audiometer (*aw-dē-OM-e-ter*)

    c. instrument for viewing the inside of a cavity or organ

_____ 9. electrocardiograph (*e-lek-trō-KAR-dē-ō-graf*)

    d. instrument used to measure hearing

_____ 10. endoscope (*EN-dō-skōp*)

    e. instrument used to record the heart's electrical activity

Table 7·3 — Suffixes for Surgery

SUFFIX	MEANING	EXAMPLE	DEFINITION OF EXAMPLE
-centesis	puncture, tap	arthrocentesis *ar-thrō-sen-TĒ-sis*	puncture of a joint (*arthr/o*)
-desis	binding, fusion	pleurodesis *plū-ROD-e-sis*	binding of the pleura (membranes around the lungs)
-ectomy	excision, surgical removal	hepatectomy *hep-a-TEK-tō-mē*	excision of liver tissue (*hepat/o*)
-pexy	surgical fixation	hysteropexy *HIS-ter-ō-pek-sē*	surgical fixation of the uterus (*hyster/o*)
-plasty	plastic repair, plastic surgery, reconstruction	rhinoplasty *RĪ-nō-plas-tē*	plastic surgery of the nose (*rhin/o*)
-rhaphy	surgical repair, suture	herniorrhaphy *her-nē-OR-a-fē*	surgical repair of a hernia (*herni/o*)
-stomy	surgical creation of an opening	tracheostomy *trā-kē-OS-tō-mē*	creation of an opening into the trachea (*trache/o*)

Table 7·3	Continued			
-tome	instrument for incising (cutting)	microtome MĪ-krō-tōm	instrument for cutting thin sections of tissue for microscopic study
-tomy	incision, cutting	laparotomy lap-a-ROT-ō-mē	surgical incision of the abdomen (*lapar/o*)
-tripsy	crushing	neurotripsy nūr-ō-TRIP-sē	crushing of a nerve (*neur/o*)

Exercise 7-3

Match the following terms and write the appropriate letter to the left of each number:

_____	1. celiocentesis (*sē-lē-ō-sen-TĒ-sis*)	a.	puncture of the chest
_____	2. mammoplasty (*MAM-ō-plas-tē*)	b.	crushing of a stone
_____	3. lithotripsy (*LITH-ō-trip-sē*)	c.	puncture of the abdomen
_____	4. thoracentesis (*thor-a-sen-TĒ-sis*)	d.	excision of a gland
_____	5. adenectomy (*ad-e-NEK-tō-mē*)	e.	plastic surgery of the breast

The root cyst/o means "urinary bladder." Use this root to write a word that means each of the following:

6. Creation of an opening into the bladder _____ cystostomy _____

7. Surgical repair of the bladder _____

8. Plastic repair of the bladder _____

9. Incision into the bladder _____

10. Surgical fixation of the bladder _____

The root arthr/o means "joint." Use this root to write a word that means each of the following:

11. Puncture of a joint _____ arthrocentesis _____

12. Plastic repair of a joint _____

13. Fusion of a joint _____

14. Instrument for incising a joint _____

15. Incision of a joint _____

Build a word for each of the following definitions using the roots given:

16. Creation of an opening into the colon (*col/o*) _____

17. Incision into the trachea (*trache/o*) _____

18. Surgical fixation of the stomach (*gastr/o*) _____

TERMINOLOGY | Supplementary Terms

SYMPTOMS

clubbing *KLUB-ing*	Enlargement of the ends of the fingers and toes because of soft-tissue growth of the nails; seen in a variety of diseases, especially lung and heart diseases (Fig. 7-12)
colic *KOL-ik*	Acute abdominal pain associated with smooth-muscle spasms
cyanosis *sī-a-NŌ-sis*	Bluish discoloration of the skin due to lack of oxygen
diaphoresis *dī-a-fō-RĒ-sis*	Profuse sweating
malaise *ma-LĀZ*	A feeling of discomfort or uneasiness, often indicative of infection
nocturnal *nok-TUR-nal*	Pertaining to or occurring at night (roots *noct/i* and *nyct/o* mean "night")
pallor *PAL-or*	Paleness; lack of color
prodrome *PRŌ-drōm*	A symptom indicating an approaching disease
sequela *se-KWEL-a*	A lasting effect of a disease (plural, sequelae)
syncope *SIN-kō-pē*	A temporary loss of consciousness because of inadequate blood flow to the brain; fainting

DIAGNOSIS

alpha-fetoprotein (AFP) *AL-fa fē-to-PRŌ-tēn*	A fetal protein that appears in the blood of adults with certain types of cancer
bruit *brwē*	A sound, usually abnormal, heard in auscultation
facies *FĀ-shē-ēz*	The expression or appearance of the face
febrile *FEB-ril*	Pertaining to fever
nuclear medicine	The branch of medicine concerned with the use of radioactive substances (radionuclides) for diagnosis, therapy, and research
radiology *rā-dē-OL-ō-jē*	The branch of medicine that uses radiation, such as x-rays, in the diagnosis and treatment of disease; a specialist in this field is a radiologist.
radionuclide *rā-dē-ō-NŪ-klīd*	A substance that gives off radiation; used for diagnosis and treatment; also called radioisotope or radiopharmaceutical
speculum *SPEK-ō-lum*	An instrument for examining a canal (Fig. 7-13)

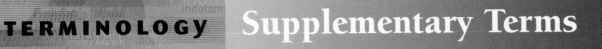

TERMINOLOGY Supplementary Terms
Continued

syndrome *SIN-drŏm*	A group of signs and symptoms that together characterize a disease condition

TREATMENT

catheter *KATH-e-ter*	A thin tube that can be passed into the body; used to remove fluids from or introduce fluids into a body cavity (Fig. 7-14).
clysis *KLĪ-sis*	The introduction of fluid into the body, other than orally, as into the rectum or abdominal cavity; also refers to the solution thus used
irrigation *ir-i-GĀ-shun*	Flushing of a tube, cavity, or area with a fluid (see Fig, 7-14)
lavage *la-VAJ*	The washing out of a cavity; irrigation
normal saline solution (NSS) *SĀ-lēn*	A salt (NaCl) solution compatible with living cells; also called physiologic saline solution (PSS)
paracentesis *par-a-sen-TĒ-sis*	Puncture of a cavity for removal of fluid
prophylaxis *prō-fi-LAK-sis*	Prevention of disease

SURGERY

drain	Device for allowing matter to escape from a wound or cavity; common types include Penrose (cigarette), T-tube, Jackson–Pratt (J-P), and Hemovac
ligature *LIG-a-chur*	A tie or bandage; the process of binding or tying (also called ligation)
resection *rē-SEK-shun*	Partial excision of a structure
stapling *STĀ-pling*	In surgery, the joining of tissue by using wire staples that are pushed through the tissue and then bent
surgeon *SUR-jun*	One who specializes in surgery

Go to the pronunciation glossary in Chapter 7 on the CD-ROM
to hear these words pronounced.

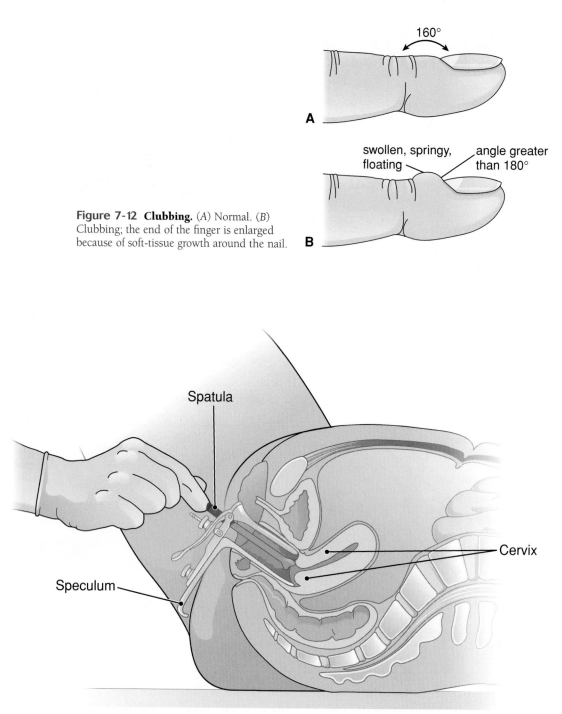

Figure 7-12 Clubbing. (*A*) Normal. (*B*) Clubbing; the end of the finger is enlarged because of soft-tissue growth around the nail.

Figure 7-13 A vaginal speculum. This instrument is used to examine the vagina and cervix and to obtain a cervical sample for testing

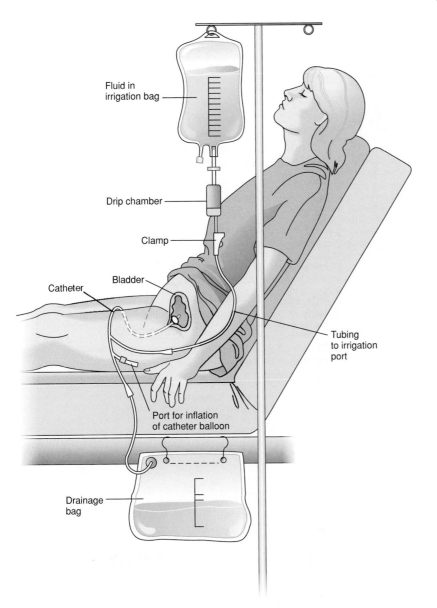

Figure 7-14 **Continuous bladder irrigation using a catheter.**

TERMINOLOGY   Symbols

1°	primary		>	greater than
2°	secondary (to)		<	less than
Δ	change		∧	above
Ⓛ	left		∨	below
Ⓡ	right		=	equal to
↑	increase(d)		≠	not equal to
↓	decrease(d)		±	doubtful, slight
♂	male		~	approximately
♀	female		×	times
°	degree		#	number, pound

TERMINOLOGY Abbreviations

HISTORY AND PHYSICAL EXAMINATION

ADL	Activities of daily living
BP	Blood pressure
bpm	Beats per minute
C	Celsius (centigrade)
CC	Chief complaint
c/o	Complains of
EOMI	Extraocular muscles intact
ETOH	Alcohol (ethyl alcohol)
F	Fahrenheit
HEENT	Head, eyes, ears, nose, and throat
h/o	History of
H & P	History and physical
HPI	History of present illness
HR	Heart rate
Hx	History
I & O	Intake and output
IPPA	Inspection, palpation, percussion, auscultation
IVDA	Intravenous drug abuse
NAD	No apparent distress
NKDA	No known drug allergies
P	Pulse
PE	Physical examination
PE(R)RLA	Pupils equal (regular) react to light and accommodation
PMH	Past medical history
pt	Patient
R	Respiration
R/O	Rule out
ROS	Review of systems
T	Temperature
TPR	Temperature, pulse, respiration
VS	Vital signs
WD	Well developed
WNL	Within normal limits
w/o	Without

DIAGNOSIS AND TREATMENT

ABC	Aspiration biopsy cytology
AFP	Alpha-fetoprotein
BS	Bowel sounds
bx	Biopsy
CAM	Complementary and alternative medicine
Ci	Curie (unit of radioactivity)
C & S	Culture and (drug) sensitivity (of bacteria)
CT	Computed tomography
D/C, dc	Discontinue, discharge
Dx	Diagnosis
EBL	Estimated blood loss
ICU	Intensive care unit
I & D	Incision and drainage
MET	Metastasis
MRI	Magnetic resonance imaging
NCCAM	National Center for Complementary and Alternative Medicine
NS, N/S	Normal saline
NSS	Normal saline solution
PCA	Patient-controlled analgesia
PET	Positron emission tomography
PICC	Peripherally inserted central catheter
postop	Postoperative
preop	Preoperative
PSS	Physiologic saline solution
RATx	Radiation therapy
Rx	Drug, prescription, therapy
SPECT	Single-photon emission-computed tomography
TNM	(Primary) tumor, (regional lymph) nodes, (distant) metastases
UV	Ultraviolet

VIEWS FOR RADIOGRAPHY

AP	Anteroposterior
LL	Left lateral
PA	Posteroanterior
RL	Right lateral

ORDERS

AMA	Against medical advice
AMB	Ambulatory
BRP	Bathroom privileges
CBR	Complete bed rest
DNR	Do not resuscitate
KVO	Keep vein open
NPO	Nothing by mouth (Latin, *non per os*)
OOB	Out of bed
QNS	Quantity not sufficient
QS	Quantity sufficient
STAT	Immediately
TKO	To keep open

Drug abbreviations are located in Chapter 8.

CHAPTER REVIEW

Match the following terms and write the appropriate letter to the left of each number:

_____ 1. electrolysis

_____ 2. symptom

_____ 3. staging

_____ 4. biopsy

_____ 5. suture

a. evidence of disease

b. classification of malignant tumors

c. destruction by means of electrical current

d. to unite parts by stitching them together

e. removal of tissue for microscopic examination

_____ 6. cautery

_____ 7. lithotripsy

_____ 8. cryalgesia

_____ 9. scintiscan

_____ 10. syndrome

a. a group of symptoms that characterizes a disease

b. pain caused by cold

c. destruction of tissue with a damaging agent

d. image obtained with a radionuclide

e. crushing of a stone

_____ 11. achromatous

_____ 12. osteotome

_____ 13. biofeedback

_____ 14. acupuncture

_____ 15. ergometer

a. instrument used to cut bone

b. colorless

c. instrument to measure work output

d. method for controlling involuntary responses

e. treatment by insertion of thin needles

Supplementary Terms

_____	16. nocturnal	a.	enlargement of the ends of the fingers and toes
_____	17. resection	b.	occurring at night
_____	18. clubbing	c.	prevention of disease
_____	19. bruit	d.	partial excision
_____	20. prophylaxis	e.	a sound heard on auscultation
_____	21. diaphoresis	a.	thin tube
_____	22. colic	b.	feeling of discomfort
_____	23. malaise	c.	acute abdominal pain
_____	24. catheter	d.	washing out of a cavity
_____	25. lavage	e.	profuse sweating

Identify and define the root in each of the following words:

	Root	Meaning of Root
26. chronology	_____	_____
27. thermal	_____	_____
28. ultrasonic	_____	_____
29. allergy	_____	_____
30. radiology	_____	_____
31. anaerobic	_____	_____

Word building. Use the root *-hepat/o*, meaning "liver," to write a word for each of the following:

32. Surgical repair of the liver _____

33. Incision of the liver _____

34. Surgical fixation of the liver _____

35. Excision of liver tissue _____

True–False. Examine the following statements. If the statement is true, write T in the first blank. If the statement is false, write F in the first blank and correct the statement by replacing the <u>underlined</u> word in the second blank.

36. Adenectomy is surgical removal of a <u>gland</u>. _____ _____

37. An image produced by x-rays is a <u>radiogram</u>. _____ _____

38. Prediction of the outcome of disease is a <u>diagnosis</u>. _____ _____

39. An echogram is produced by <u>ultrasound</u>. _____ _____

40. An arthroscope is used to examine a <u>joint</u>. _____ _____

41. A baroreceptor is sensitive to <u>temperature</u>. _____ _____

Eliminations. In each of the sets below, underline the word that does not fit in with the rest and explain the reason for your choice:

42. palpation – remission – auscultation – inspection – percussion

_____

43. ophthalmoscope – stethoscope – syncope – endoscope – otoscope

_____

44. curette – forceps – prodrome – scalpel – hemostat

_____

45. TNM – SPECT – PET – CT– MRI

_____

Word analysis. Define each of the following words, and give the meaning of the word parts in each. Use a dictionary if necessary.

46. synchrony (*SIN-kro-nē*) _____

    a. syn- _____

    b. chron/o _____

    c. -y _____

47. phonocardiography (*fō-nō-kar-dē-OG-ra-fē*) _____

    a. phon/o _____

    b. cardi/o _____

    c. -graphy _____

48. chromogenesis (*krō-mō-JEN-e-sis*) _____

    a. chrom/o _____

    b. gen/e _____

    c. –sis _____

Go to the word exercises in Chapter 7 on the CD-ROM
for additional review exercises.

CASE STUDY 7-1: Comprehensive History and Physical

C.F., a 46-year-old married Asian woman, works as an office manager for an insurance company. This morning, she had a follow-up visit with her oncologist and was sent to the hospital for immediate admission for possible recurrence or sequelae of her ovarian cancer. She is alert, articulate, and a reliable reporter.

CC: C.F. presents with mild, low, aching pelvic pain and low abdominal fullness. She states, "I feel like I have cramps and am bloated. Sometimes I'm so tired I cannot do my work without a short nap."

HPI: C.F. has been in remission for 14 months from aggressively treated ovarian carcinoma. She presents with mild abdominal distention and tenderness on deep palpation of the lower pelvis. C.F. claims a feeling of fullness in the lower abdomen, loss of appetite, and inability to sleep through the night. She is afraid that her cancer was not cured. Sometimes her heart races and she cannot catch her breath, but with two children in college, she cannot afford to miss work.

MEDS: Therapeutic vitamin × 1/day. Valium 5 mg every 6 hours (q6h) as needed (prn) for anxiety. Benadryl 25 mg at bedtime (hs) prn for insomnia. Echinacea tea 3 cups per day to prevent colds or flu. Ginkgo biloba 3 caps/day for energy.

ALLERGIES: NKDA; no food allergies

PMH: C.F. was diagnosed with ovarian CA 4 years ago and treated with surgery, radiation, and chemotherapy. A total abdominal hysterectomy (removal of the uterus) with bilateral removal of the oviducts and ovaries was performed. At the time of surgery, the pelvic lymph nodes tested negative for disease. Chemotherapy and radiation therapy occurred after surgical recovery. C.F. has been well and capable of full ADL until 4 weeks ago. Childhood history is unremarkable, with normal childhood diseases, including measles, mumps, and chicken pox. C.F. was born and raised in this country. She has no other adult diseases, surgery, or injuries.

CURRENT HEALTH Hx: Denies tobacco, ETOH, or recreational drugs or substances. She exercises 3 to 5 times per week with aerobic exercise class and treadmill. She is a vegetarian and drinks 1 to 5 cups of green tea per day. Immunizations are up to date; unsure of last tetanus booster. Recent negative mammogram and negative TB test (PPD).

FAMILY Hx: Both parents alive and well. Maternal aunt died of "stomach tumor" at age 37.

TPR & BP & PAIN: 37C-96-22 126/72 in no acute distress

HEENT: WNL. Normocephalic, fundi benign, PERRLA, uncorrected 20/20 vision, mouth clear, good dental health, neck supple w/o rigidity, thyromegaly, or cervical lymphadenopathy; trachea midline. No carotid bruits (sounds).

LUNGS: All lobes clear to auscultation and percussion

HEART: Rate 96 bpm, regular; no murmurs, gallops, or rubs

BREASTS: Symmetrical, w/o masses or discharge

ABDOMEN: Skin intact with healed suprapubic midline surgical incision and a symmetrical area of discoloration and dermal thickness from radiation therapy. Bowel sounds active and normal. Suprapubic tenderness on palpation. No hepatosplenomegaly. Absence of inguinal lymph nodes on palpation. Kidneys palpable. Rectal exam WNL. Hemoccult test (stool test for blood) result negative.

GU: Unremarkable. Surgical menopause.

MUSCULOSKELETAL: WNL. No weakness, limitation of mobility, joint pain, stiffness, or edema.

NEUROLOGIC: All reflexes intact. No syncope, paralysis, numbness.

DIAGNOSTIC IMPRESSION: Possible recurrence of ovarian CA, ascites

TREATMENT PLAN: Send blood for CA-125 [genetic marker for ovarian cancer]. Schedule abdominal paracentesis and second-look diagnostic laparoscopy with biopsy and tissue staging. D/C all herbal supplements.

CASE STUDY 7-2: Diagnostic Laparoscopy

For a laparoscopy, C.F. was given general anesthesia and her trachea was intubated. She was placed in lithotomy position with arms abducted. Her abdomen was insufflated with carbon dioxide (CO_2) through a thin needle placed below the umbilicus. Three trocar punctures were made to insert the telescope with camera and the cutting and grasping instruments. Biopsies were taken of several pelvic lymph nodes and sent to the pathology laboratory. There were many adhesions from prior surgery, which were lysed to mobilize her organs and enhance visualization. A loop of small bowel, which had adhered to the anterior abdominal wall, had been punctured when the trocar was introduced. The surgeon repaired the defect with an endoscopic stapler and irrigated the abdomen with 3 L of NSS mixed with antibiotic solution.

CASE STUDY 7–3: Postoperative Care

After surgery, C.F. reported numbness and tingling in her right arm and bilateral subscapular discomfort when she stood. The retained CO_2 was eventually absorbed. The subscapular discomfort decreased and was judged to have originated from hyperabduction of the arms during surgery.

Biopsy results were negative, there was no fluid found on paracentesis to explain the abdominal symptoms, and the CA-125 was below 35 U/mL, which is negative for recurrence. Psychological counseling was recommended to help C.F. verbalize her fears and gain a sense of control. She will call her oncologist to schedule a follow-up visit for reevaluation.

CASE STUDY QUESTIONS

Write the word from the case study that completes each of the following statements:

1. Secondary conditions, complications, or lasting effects of C.F.'s cancer would be called

   _____.

2. Examination by touching the surface of the body is _____.

3. The size and shape of C.F.'s head was described as _____.

4. A collection of abdominal fluid (ascites) would be drained by a cavity puncture and drainage procedure called a(n)

   _____.

5. Removal of tissue for microscopic examination is _____.

6. A surgical procedure in which an endoscope is inserted through the abdominal wall to visualize the abdominal cavity and determine the cause of a disorder is a(n) _____.

7. Extreme or overextension of an arm or leg away from the midline of the body is

   _____.

Multiple choice. Select the best answer and write the letter of your choice to the left of each number:

_____ 8. C.F.'s cancer was in a state of apparent cure with no active signs of disease. This state is called:
   a. exacerbation
   b. syndrome
   c. remission
   d. sequelae
   e. tumor staging

_____ 9. C.F. claimed that her heart races and she cannot catch her breath. The terms for these conditions are:
   a. tachypnea and dyspnea
   b. tachycardia and dyspnea
   c. dyspnea and tachycardia
   d. tachycardia and bradypnea
   e. bradycardia and tachypulmono

_____ 10. Hepatosplenomegaly means:
   a. removal of the liver and spleen
   b. prolapse of the heart and spleen
   c. hemorrhage of the liver and spleen
   d. enlargement of the liver and spleen
   e. surgical repair of the kidney and liver

_____ 11. C.F.'s abdominal cavity and organs were bound with fibrous tissue bands, which had to be lysed during surgery. These bands are called:
   a. prodromes
   b. sequelae
   c. adhesions
   d. ascites
   e. fibroids

_____ 12. The accidental puncture of the intestine was not an expected outcome of surgery. It was an incident that occurred despite attempts to protect her from harm. The term for this type of disorder is (see Chapter 6):
   a. iatrogenic
   b. nosocomial
   c. idiopathic
   d. etiologic
   e. surgical misadventure

Give the meaning of each of the following abbreviations:

13. HPI _____

14. CA _____

15. TPR _____

16. bpm _____

17. WNL _____

18. D/C _____

19. NSS _____

DRUGS

8

OBJECTIVES

After study of this chapter you should be able to:

1. Explain the difference between over-the-counter and prescription drugs.
2. List some potential adverse side effects of drugs.
3. Explain ways in which drugs can interact.
4. Explain the difference between the generic name and the trade name of a drug.
5. List several drug references.
6. Describe some of the issues involved in the use of herbal medicines.
7. Identify and use word parts pertaining to drugs.

8. Recognize the major categories of drugs and how they act.
9. List some common herbal medicines and how they act.
10. List common routes for drug administration.
11. List standard forms in which liquid and solid drugs are prepared.
12. Define abbreviations related to drugs and their use.
13. Analyze the terminology related to drugs in several case studies.

PRETEST

1. What federal agency approves drugs for sale?

_____

2. A reason for not using a specific drug is a(n)

_____

3. A manufacturer's registered name for a drug is its

_____

4. A written and signed order for a drug is a(n)

_____

5. The word root for drug or medicine is

_____

6. The abbreviation *IV* means _____

8

Drugs

A drug is a substance that alters body function. Traditionally, drugs have been derived from natural plant, animal, and mineral sources. Today, most are manufactured synthetically by pharmaceutical companies. A few, such as certain hormones and enzymes, have been produced by genetic engineering.

Many drugs, described as over-the-counter (OTC) drugs, are available without a signed order, or **prescription**. Others require a health-care provider's prescription for use. Responsibility for the safety and **efficacy** of all drugs sold in the United States lies with the Federal Food and Drug Administration (FDA), which must approve all drugs before they are sold.

Adverse Drug Effects

An unintended effect of a drug or other form of treatment is a **side effect**. Most drugs have potential adverse side effects that must be evaluated before they are prescribed. In addition, there may be **contraindications**, or reasons not to use a particular drug for a specific individual based on that person's medical conditions, current medications, sensitivity, or family history. While a patient is under treatment, it is important to be alert for signs of adverse effects such as digestive upset, changes in the blood, or signs of allergy, such as hives or skin rashes. **Anaphylaxis** is an immediate and severe allergic reaction that may be caused by a drug. It can lead to life-threatening respiratory distress and circulatory collapse.

Because drugs given in combination may interact, the prescriber must know of any drugs the patient is taking before prescribing another. In some cases, a combination may result in **synergy** or **potentiation**, meaning that the drugs together have a greater effect than either of the drugs acting alone. In other cases, one drug may act as an **antagonist** of another, interfering with its action. Drugs may also react adversely with certain foods or substances used socially, such as alcohol and tobacco.

Drugs that act on the central nervous system may lead to a psychological or physical **substance dependence**, in which a person has a chronic or compulsive need for a drug regardless of its bad effects. With repeated use, a drug **tolerance** may develop, whereby a constant dose has less effect and the dose must be increased to produce the original response. Cessation of the drug then leads to symptoms of substance **withdrawal**, a state that results from reduction of the dose or removal of a drug. Certain symptoms are associated with withdrawal from specific drugs.

Drug Names

Drugs may be cited by either their generic or their trade names. (Box 8-1 has information on drug naming.) The **generic name** is usually a simple version of the chemical

---

Box 8•1 Focus on Words   *Where Do Drugs Get Their Names?*

Drug names are derived in a variety of ways. Some are named for their origin. Adrenaline, for example, is named for its source, the adrenal gland. Even its generic name, epinephrine, informs us that it comes from the gland that is above (epi-) the kidney (nephr/o). Pitocin, a drug used to induce labor, is named for its source, the pituitary gland, combined with the chemical name of the hormone, oxytocin. Botox, currently injected into the skin for cosmetic removal of wrinkles, is the toxin from the organism that causes botulism, a type of food poisoning. Aspirin (an anti-inflammatory agent), Taxol (an antitumor agent), digitalis (used to treat heart failure), and atropine (a smooth-muscle

relaxant) are all named for the plants they come from. For example, aspirin is named for the blossoms of Spiraea, from which it is derived. Taxol comes from a yew (evergreen) of the genus *Taxus*. Digitalis is from purple foxglove, genus *Digitalis*. Atropine comes from the plant *Atropa belladonna*.

Some names tell about the drug or its actions. The name for Humulin, a form of insulin made by genetic engineering, points out that this is human insulin and not a hormone from animal sources. Lomotil reduces intestinal motility and is used to treat diarrhea. The name *belladonna* is from Italian and means "fair lady," because this drug dilates the pupils of the eyes, making women appear more beautiful.

| Box 8·2 | Health Professions | *Pharmacists and Pharmacy Technicians* |

Medications are chemicals designed to treat illness and improve quality of life. The role of pharmacists and pharmacy technicians is to ensure that patients receive the correct medication and the education they need to use it effectively and derive its intended health benefits.

As key members of the health-care team, pharmacists need a strong clinical background with a thorough understanding of chemistry, anatomy, and physiology. Pharmacists not only dispense prescription medications and monitor patients' responses to them, they also educate patients about appropriate use of medications and share their expertise with other health professionals. Pharmacists also participate in clinical research on drugs and their effects.

Pharmacy technicians assist pharmacists with their duties. State rules and regulations vary, but pharmacy technicians may perform many of the tasks related to dispensing medications, such as preparing drugs and packaging them with appropriate labels and instructions for use.

Most pharmacists and pharmacy technicians work in retail pharmacies; others work in hospitals and long-term–care facilities. Job prospects are promising because of the growing need for health care. In fact, pharmacy is projected to be one of the fastest-growing careers in the United States. For more information about careers in pharmacy, contact the American Association of Colleges of Pharmacy.

name for the drug and is not capitalized. The **trade name** (brand name, proprietary name) is a registered trademark of the manufacturer and is written with an initial capital letter. For example, Tylenol is the trade name for the analgesic compound acetaminophen; the antidepressant Prozac is fluoxetine. Reference Box 8-3, which appears later in this chapter, has many more examples of generic and trade names. Note that the same drug may be marketed by different companies under different trade names. Both Motrin and Advil, for example, are the generic antiinflammatory agent ibuprofen.

Drug Information

In the United States, the standard for drug information is the *United States Pharmacopeia* (USP). This reference is published by a national committee of pharmacologists and other scientists. It contains formulas for drugs sold in the United States; standards for testing the strength, quality, and purity of drugs; and standards for the preparation and dispensing of drugs. The American Society of Health System Pharmacists (ASHP) publishes extensive drug information; The *Physicians' Desk Reference*, published yearly by Thomson Healthcare, contains information supplied by drug manufacturers. An enormous amount of drug information is available online through the Web sites for these publications and others. Another excellent source of up-to-date information on drugs is a community or hospital pharmacist. See Box 8-2 for information on careers in pharmacy.

Herbal Medicines

For hundreds of years, people have used plants to treat diseases, a practice described as herbal medicine or **phytomedicine**. Many people in industrialized countries are now turning to herbal products as alternatives or complements to conventional medicines. Although plants are the source of many conventional drugs, pharmaceutical companies usually purify, measure, and often modify or synthesize the active ingredients in these plants rather than presenting them in their natural state.

Some issues have arisen with the increased use of herbal medicines, including questions about their purity, safety, concentration, and efficacy. Another issue is drug interactions. Health-care providers should ask about the use of herbal remedies when taking a patient's drug history, and patients should report any herbal medicines they take when under treatment. The FDA does not test or regulate herbal medicines, and there are no requirements to report adverse effects. There are, however, restrictions on the health claims that can be made by the manufacturers of herbal medicines. The U.S. government has established the Office of Dietary Supplements (ODS) to support and coordinate research in this field.

TERMINOLOGY — Key Terms

anaphylaxis *an-a fi-LAK-sis*	An extreme allergic reaction that can lead to respiratory distress, circulatory collapse, and death
antagonist *an-TAG-o-nist*	A substance that interferes with or opposes the action of a drug
contraindication *kon-tra-in-di-KĀ-shun*	A factor that makes the use of a drug undesirable or dangerous
drug	A substance that alters body function
efficacy *EF-i-ka-sē*	The power to produce a specific result; effectiveness
generic name *je-NER-ik*	The nonproprietary name of a drug; that is, a name that is not privately owned or trademarked; usually a simplified version of the chemical name; not capitalized
phytomedicine *fī-tō-MED-i-sin*	Another name for herbal medicine
potentiation *pō-ten-shē-Ā-shun*	Increased potency created by two drugs acting together
prescription (Rx) *prē-SKRIP-shun*	Written and signed order for a drug with directions for its administration
side effect	A result of drug therapy or other therapy that is unrelated to or an extension of its intended effect. The term usually applies to an undesirable effect of treatment.
substance dependence	A condition that may result from chronic use of a drug, in which a person has a chronic or compulsive need for a drug regardless of its adverse effects; dependence may be psychological or physical
synergy *SIN-er-jē*	Combined action of two or more drugs working together to produce an effect greater than any of the drugs could produce when acting alone; also called synergism (*SIN-er-jizm*); adj. synergistic (*sin-er-JIS-tik*)
tolerance	A condition in which chronic use of a drug results in loss of effectiveness and the dose must be increased to produce the original response
trade name	The brand name of a drug, a registered trademark of the manufacturer; written with a capital letter
withdrawal	A condition that results from cessation or reduction of a drug that has been used regularly

Go to the pronunciation glossary in Chapter 8 of the CD-ROM to hear these words pronounced.

Table 8·1	Word Parts Pertaining to Drugs		
	MEANING	**EXAMPLE**	**DEFINITION OF EXAMPLE**

SUFFIXES

	MEANING	EXAMPLE	DEFINITION OF EXAMPLE
-lytic	dissolving, reducing, loosening	thrombolytic *throm-bō-LIT-ik*	agent that dissolves a blood clot (thrombus)
-mimetic	mimicking, simulating	sympathomimetic *sim-pa-thō-mi-MET-ik*	mimicking the effects of the sympathetic nervous system
-tropic	acting on	psychotropic *sī-kō-TROP-ik*	acting on the mind (psych/o)

PREFIXES

	MEANING	EXAMPLE	DEFINITION OF EXAMPLE
anti-	against	antiemetic *an-tē-e-MET-ik*	drug that prevents vomiting (emesis)
contra-	against, oppose	contraceptive *kon-tra-SEP-tiv*	preventing conception
counter-	opposite, against	countertransport *kown-ter-TRANS-port*	movement in an opposite direction

ROOTS

	MEANING	EXAMPLE	DEFINITION OF EXAMPLE
alg/o, algi/o, algesi/o	pain	algesia *al-JĒ-zē-a*	sense of pain
chem/o	chemical	chemotherapy *kē-mō-THER-a-pē*	treatment with drugs
hypn/o	sleep	hypnotic *hip-NŌT-ik*	inducing sleep
narc/o	stupor	narcosis *nar-KŌ-sis*	state of stupor with decreased sensation
pharm, pharmac/o	drug, medicine	pharmacy *FAR-ma-sē*	the science of preparing and dispensing drugs, or the place where these activities occur
pyr/o, pyret/o	fever	antipyretic *an-ti-pī-RET-ik*	counteracting fever
tox/o, toxic/o	poison, toxin	toxicity *tok-SIS-i-tē*	state of being poisonous
vas/o	vessel	vasoconstriction *vas-ō-kon-STRIK-shun*	narrowing of a vessel

Exercise 8-1

Identify and define the suffix in each of the following words:

	Suffix	Meaning of Suffix
1. anxiolytic (*ang-zī-ō-LIT-ik*)	_____	_____
2. chronotropic (*kron-ō-TROP-ik*)	_____	_____
3. parasympathomimetic (*par-a-sim-pa-thō-mi-MET-ik*)	_____	_____

Using the prefixes listed in Table 8-1, write the opposite of each of the following words:

4. inflammatory _____ _____
5. indicated _____ _____
6. septic _____ _____
7. act _____ _____
8. toxin _____ _____
9. pyretic _____ _____

Identify and define the root in each of the following words:

	Root	Meaning of Root
10. hypnosis	_____	_____
11. toxic	_____	_____
12. analgesia	_____	_____
13. chemistry	_____	_____
14. narcotic	_____	_____

Define each of the following words:

15. vasodilation _____
16. pharmacology _____
17. mucolytic _____
18. gonadotropic _____

TERMINOLOGY Abbreviations

DRUGS AND DRUG FORMULATIONS

APAP	Acetaminophen	**ODS**	Office of Dietary Supplements
ASA	Acetylsalicylic acid (aspirin)	**OTC**	Over-the-counter
ASHP	American Society of Health System	**PDR**	*Physicians' Desk Reference*
	Pharmacists	**Rx**	Prescription
cap	Capsule	**supp**	Suppository
elix	Elixir	**susp**	Suspension
FDA	Food and Drug Administration	**tab**	Tablet
INH	Isoniazid (antituberculosis drug)	**tinct**	Tincture
MED(s)	Medicine(s), medication(s)	**ung**	Ointment
NSAID(s)	Nonsteroidal antiinflammatory drug(s)	**USP**	*United States Pharmacopeia*

DOSAGES AND DIRECTIONS

ā	Before (Latin, *ante*)	**po**	By mouth (Latin, *per os*)
āā	Of each (Greek, *ana*)	**pp**	Postprandial (after a meal)
ac	Before meals (Latin, *ante cibum*)	**prn**	As needed (Latin, *pro re nata*)
ad lib	As desired (Latin, *ad libitum*)	**qam**	Every morning (Latin, *quaque ante meridiem*)
aq	Water (Latin, *aqua*)		
bid	Twice a day (Latin, *bis in die*)	**qd**	Every day (Latin, *quaque die*)
c̄	With (Latin, *cum*)	**qh**	Every hour (Latin, *quaque hora*)
cc	Cubic centimeter	**q ___ h**	Every ____ hours
D/C, dc	Discontinue	**qid**	Four times a day (Latin, *quater in die*)
DS	Double strength	**qod**	Every other day (Latin, *quaque* [other] *die*)
gt(t)	Drop(s) (Latin, *gutta*)		
hs	At bedtime (Latin, *hora somni*)	**s̄**	Without (Latin, *sine*)
IM	Intramuscular(ly)	**SA**	Sustained action
IU	International unit	**SC, SQ, subcu**	Subcutaneous(ly)
IV	Intravenous(ly)	**SR**	Sustained release
LA	Long-acting	**s̄s̄**	Half (Latin, *semis*)
mcg	Microgram	**tid**	Three times per day (Latin, *ter in die*)
mg	Milligram	**U**	Unit(s)
p	After, post	**x**	Times
pc	After meals (Latin, *post cibum*)		

Reference Information on Drugs

So far, this chapter has been an overview of drugs and the terminology for drugs and drug usage. The next section of the chapter contains informational boxes that you can examine now and refer to again as you work through Part 3 of the text. Box 8-3 outlines the major categories of drugs and cites examples by both generic and trade names. Box 8-4 lists some common herbal medicines and their uses. Boxes 8-5 through 8-7 have information on routes of administration, drug preparations, and injectable drugs.

Box 8·3 For Your Reference *Common Drugs and Their Actions*

Category	Actions; Applications	Generic Name	Trade Name(s)
Adrenergics *ad-ren-ER-jiks* (sympathomimetics *[sim-pa-thō-mi-MET-iks]*)	Mimic the action of the sympathetic nervous system, which responds to stress; used to treat bronchospasms, allergic reactions, hypotension	epinephrine phenylephrine pseudoephedrine dopamine	Bronkaid Neo-Synephrine Sudafed Intropin
Analgesics *an-al-JĒ-siks*	Alleviate pain		
Narcotic *nar-KO-tik*	Decrease pain sensation in central nervous system; chronic use may lead to physical dependence	codeine morphine meperidine oxycodone	 Demerol Percodan, Percocet
Nonnarcotic *non-nar-KO-tik*	Act peripherally to inhibit prostaglandins (local hormones); they may also be antiinflammatory and antipyretic (reduce fever). Cox-2 inhibitors limit an enzyme that causes inflammation without affecting a related enzyme that protects the stomach lining.	aspirin (acetylsalicylic acid; ASA) acetaminophen (APAP) ibuprofen celecoxib (Cox-2 inhibitor)	 Tylenol Motrin, Advil Celebrex
Anesthetics *an-es-THET-iks*	Reduce or eliminate sensation (esthesi/o)	Local: lidocaine bupivacaine General: nitrous oxide midazolam thiopental	 Xylocaine Marcaine Versed Pentothal
Anticoagulants *an-ti-kō-AG-ū-lants*	Prevent coagulation and formation of blood clots	heparin warfarin	 Coumadin
Anticonvulsants *an-ti-kon-VUL-sants*	Suppress or reduce the number and/or intensity of seizures	phenobarbital phenytoin carbamazepine valproic acid	 Dilantin Tegretol Depakene
Antidiabetics *an-ti-dī-a-BET-iks*	Prevent or alleviate diabetes	insulin glyburide acarbose glipizide repaglinide glimepiride	Humulin (injected) Diabeta Precose Glucotrol Prandin Amaryl
Antiemetics *an-tē-e-MET-iks*	Relieve symptoms of nausea and prevent vomiting (emesis)	ondansetron dimenhydrinate prochlorperazine scopolamine promethazine	Zofran Dramamine Compazine TRANSDERM-SCŌP Phenergan
Antihistamines *an-ti-HIS-ta-mēnz*	Prevent responses mediated by histamine: allergic and inflammatory reactions	diphenhydramine fexofenadine loratadine cetirizine	Benadryl Allegra Claritin Zyrtec

Box 8•3 For Your Reference *Continued*

Antihypertensives *an-ti-hī-per-TEN-sivs*	Lower blood pressure by reducing cardiac output, dilating vessels, or promoting excretion of water by the kidneys; see also, calcium-channel blockers and beta-blockers under cardiac drugs and diuretics	amlodipine atenolol clonidine prazosin minoxidil (ACE inhibitors; see Chapter 9): captopril enalapril	Norvasc Tenormin Catapres Minipress Loniten Capoten Vasotec
Antiinflammatory drugs *an-tē-in-FLAM-a-tō-rē*	Counteract inflammation and swelling		
Corticosteroids *kor-ti-kō-STER-oyds*	Hormones from the cortex of the adrenal gland; used for allergy, respiratory, and blood diseases, injury, and malignancy; suppress the immune system	dexamethasone cortisone prednisone hydrocortisone fluticasone	Decadron Cortone Deltasone Hydrocortone, Cortef Flonase
Nonsteroidal antiinflammatory drugs (NSAIDs) *non-ster-OYD-al*	Reduce inflammation and pain by interfering with synthesis of prostaglandins; also antipyretic	aspirin ibuprofen indomethacin naproxen diclofenac celecoxib	Motrin, Advil Indocin Naprosyn, Aleve Voltaren Celebrex
Antiinfective agents	Kill or prevent the growth of infectious organisms		
Antibacterials; *an-ti-bak-TĒ-rē-als* antibiotics *an-ti-bī-OT-iks*	Effective against bacteria	amoxicillin penicillin V erythromycin vancomycin linezolid gentamicin clarithromycin cephalexin sulfisoxazole tetracycline ciprofloxacin (acts on ulcer-causing *Helicobacter pylori*) isoniazid (INH) (tuberculosis)	Polymox Pen-Vee K Erythrocin Vancocin Zyvox Garamycin Biaxin Keflex Gantrisin Achromycin Cipro Nydrazid
Antifungals *an-ti-FUNG-gals*	Effective against fungi	amphotericin B miconazole nystatin fluconazole itraconazole	Fungizone Monistat Nilstat Diflucan Sporanox
Antiparasitics *an-ti-par-a-SIT-iks*	Effective against parasites: protozoa, worms	iodoquinol (amebae) quinacrine	Yodoxin Atabrine
Antivirals *an-ti-VI-rals*	Effective against viruses	acyclovir amantadine zanamivir (influenza) zidovudine (HIV) indinavir (HIV protease inhibitor)	Zovirax Symmetrel Relenza Retrovir Crixivan

8

Box 8·3 For Your Reference *Continued*

Antineoplastics *an-ti-nē-ō-PLAS-tiks*	Destroy cancer cells; they are toxic for all cells but have greater effect on cells that are actively growing and dividing; hormones and hormone inhibitors also are used to slow tumor growth	cyclophosphamide doxorubicin methotrexate vincristine tamoxifen (estrogen inhibitor)	Cytoxan Adriamycin Folex Oncovin Nolvadex
Cardiac drugs *KAR-dē-ak*	Act on the heart		
Antiarrhythmics *an-tē-a-RITH-miks*	Correct or prevent abnormalities of heart rhythm	quinidine lidocaine digoxin	Quinidex Xylocaine Lanoxin
Beta-adrenergic blockers (beta-blockers) *bā-ta-ad-ren-ER-jik*	Inhibit sympathetic nervous system; reduce rate and force of heart contractions	propranolol metoprolol atenolol carvedilol	Inderal Toprol-XL Tenormin Coreg
Calcium-channel blockers *KAL-sē-um*	Dilate coronary arteries, slow heart rate, reduce contractions	diltiazem nifedipine verapamil nitroglycerin isosorbide	Cardizem Procardia Covera Nitrostat Isordil
Hypolipidemics *hī-pō-lip-i-DĒ-miks*	Lower cholesterol in patients with high serum levels that cannot be controlled with diet alone; hypocholesterolemics, statins	cholestyramine lovastatin pravastatin atorvastatin simvastatin	Questran Mevacor Pravachol Lipitor Zocor
Nitrates; *NĪ-trāts* **antianginal agents** *an-ti-AN-ji-nal*	Dilate coronary arteries and reduce workload of heart by lowering blood pressure and reducing venous return	nitroglycerin isosorbide	Nitrostat Isordil
CNS stimulants	Stimulate the central nervous system	methylphenidate amphetamine (chronic use may lead to drug dependence)	Ritalin Adderall, Dexedrine
Diuretics *dī-ū-RET-iks*	Promote excretion of water, sodium, and other electrolytes by the kidneys; used to reduce edema and blood pressure	bumetanide furosemide mannitol hydrochlorothiazide (HCTZ) triamterene + HCTZ	Bumex Lasix Osmitrol HydroDIURIL Dyazide
Gastrointestinal drugs *gas-trō-in-TES-tin-al*	Act on the digestive tract		
Antidiarrheals *an-ti-di-a-RĒ-als*	Treat or prevent diarrhea by reducing intestinal motility or absorbing irritants and soothing the intestinal lining	diphenoxylate loperamide attapulgite atropine	Lomotil Imodium Kaopectate
Histamine H₂ antagonists *HIS-ta-mēn*	Decrease secretion of stomach acid by interfering with the action of histamine at H₂ receptors; used to treat ulcers and other gastrointestinal problems	cimetidine ranitidine	Tagamet Zantac
Laxatives *LAK-sa-tivs*	Promote elimination from the large intestine; types include:		
stimulants		bisacodyl	Dulcolax
hyperosmotics (retain water)		lactulose	Constilac, Chronulac
stool softeners		docusate	Colace, Surfak
bulk-forming agents		psyllium	Metamucil

Box 8•3   For Your Reference   *Continued*

Hypnotics *hip-NOT-iks*	Induce sleep or dull the senses; see antianxiety agents (below, under psychotropics)		
Muscle relaxants *rē-LAK-sants*	Depress nervous system stimulation of skeletal muscles; used to control muscle spasms and pain	baclofen carisoprodol methocarbamol	Lioresal Soma Robaxin
Proton-pump inhibitors *PRŌ-ton*	Inhibit secretion of stomach acid by blocking the transport of hydrogen ions (protons) into the stomach	esomeprazole lansoprazole omeprazole	Nexium Prevacid Prilosec
Psychotropics *sī-kō-TROP-iks*	Affect the mind, altering mental activity, mental state, or behavior		
Antianxiety agents *an-tē-ang-ZĪ-e-tē*	Reduce or dispel anxiety; tranquilizers; anxiolytic agents	lorazepam chlordiazepoxide diazepam hydroxyzine alprazolam buspirone	Ativan Librium Valium Atarax Xanax BuSpar
Antidepressants *an-ti-dē-PRES-sants*	Relieve depression by raising brain levels of neurotransmitters (chemicals active in the nervous system)	amitriptyline imipramine fluoxetine paroxetine sertraline	Elavil Tofranil Prozac Paxil Zoloft
Antipsychotics *an-ti-sī-KOT-iks*	Act on nervous system to relieve symptoms of psychoses	chlorpromazine haloperidol clozapine risperidone olanzapine	Thorazine Haldol Clozaril Risperdal Zyprexa
Respiratory drugs	Act on the respiratory system		
Antitussives *an-ti-TUS-sivs*	Suppress coughing	dextromethorphan	Benylin DM
Asthma maintenance drugs	Used for prevention of asthma attacks and chronic treatment of asthma	fluticasone montelukast	Flovent Singulair
Bronchodilators *brong-kō-dī-LĀ-tors*	Prevent or eliminate spasm of the bronchi (breathing tubes) by relaxing bronchial smooth muscle; used to treat asthma attacks and bronchitis	albuterol epinephrine metaproterenol salmeterol theophylline	Proventil Sus-Phrine Alupent Serevent Theo-Dur
Expectorants *ek-SPEK-tō-rants*	Induce productive coughing to eliminate respiratory secretions	guaifenesin	Robitussin
Mucolytics *mū-kō-LIT-iks*	Loosen mucus to promote its elimination	acetylcysteine	Mucomyst
Sedatives/hypnotics *SED-a-tivs/hip-NOT-iks*	Induce relaxation and sleep; lower (sedative) doses promote relaxation leading to sleep; higher (hypnotic) doses induce sleep; antianxiety agents also used	phenobarbital zolpidem	 Ambien
Tranquilizers *tran-kwi-LĪZ-ers*	Reduce mental tension and anxiety; see Antianxiety agents (above, under Psychotropics)		

8

Box 8•4	For Your Reference	*Therapeutic Uses of Herbal Medicines*

Name	Part Used	Therapeutic Uses
Aloe	Leaf	Treatment of burns and minor skin irritations
Black cohosh	Root	Reduction of menopausal hot flashes
Chamomile	Flower	Antiinflammatory, gastrointestinal antispasmodic, sedative
Echinacea *e-ki-NĀ-shē-a*	All	May reduce severity and duration of colds; may stimulate the immune system; used topically for wound healing
Evening primrose oil	Seed	Source of essential fatty acids important for the health of the cardiovascular system; treatment of premenstrual syndrome (PMS), rheumatoid arthritis, skin disorders
Flax	Seed	Source of fatty acids important in maintaining proper lipids (e.g., cholesterol) in the blood
Ginkgo	Leaf	Improves blood circulation in and function of the brain; improves memory; used to treat dementia; antianxiety agent; protects the nervous system
Ginseng	Root	Stress reduction; lowers blood cholesterol and blood sugar
Green tea	Leaf	Antioxidant; acts against cancer of the gastrointestinal tract and skin; oral antimicrobial agent; reduces dental caries
Kava	Root	Antianxiety agent; sedative
Milk thistle	Seeds	Protects the liver against toxins; antioxidant
Saw palmetto	Berries	Used to treat benign prostatic hyperplasia (BPH)
Slippery elm	Bark	As lozenge for throat irritation; for gastrointestinal irritation and upset; protects irritated skin
Soy	Bean	Rich source of nutrients; protective estrogenic effects in menopausal symptoms, osteoporosis, cardiovascular disease, cancer prevention
St. John's wort	Flower	Treatment of anxiety and depression; antibacterial and antiviral properties (note: this product can interact with a variety of drugs)
Tea tree oil	Leaf	Antimicrobial; used to heal cuts, skin infections, burns
Valerian	Root	Sedative; sleep aid

Box 8•5	For Your Reference	*Routes of Drug Administration*

Route	Description
Absorption *ab-SORP-shun*	Drug taken into the circulation through the digestive tract or by transfer across another membrane
Inhalation *in-ha-LĀ-shun*	Administration though the respiratory system, as by breathing in an aerosol or nebulizer spray

Box 8•5 For Your Reference *Continued*

Instillation *in-stil-LĀ-shun*	Liquid is dropped or poured slowly into a body cavity or on the surface of the body, such as into the ear or onto the conjunctiva of the eye (Fig. 8-1)
Oral *OR-al*	Given by mouth; per os (po)
Rectal *REK-tal*	Administered by rectal suppository or enema
Sublingual (SL) *sub-LING-gwal*	Administered under the tongue
Topical *TOP-i-kal*	Applied to the surface of the skin
Transdermal *trans-DER-mal*	Absorbed through the skin, as from a patch placed on the surface of the skin
Injection (Fig. 8-2) *in-JEK-shun*	Administered by a needle and syringe (Fig. 8-3); described as parenteral (*pa-REN-ter-al*) routes of administration
Epidural *ep-i-DUR-al*	Injected into the space between the meninges (membranes around the spinal cord) and the spine
Intradermal (id) *in-tra-DER-mal*	Injected into the skin
Intramuscular (im) *in-tra-MUS-kū-lar*	Injected into a muscle
Intravenous *in-tra-VĒ-nus*	Injected into a vein
Spinal (intrathecal) *in-tra-THĒ-kal*	Injected through the meninges into the spinal fluid
Subcutaneous (sc) *sub-kū-TĀ-nē-us*	Injected beneath the skin; hypodermic

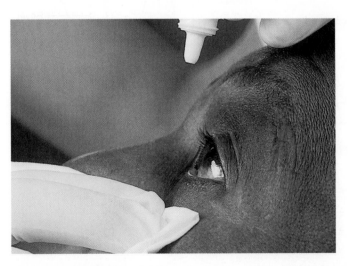

Figure 8-1 Instillation of a drug. A practitioner pulls down the lower lid to administer eye drops into the lower conjunctival sac.

8

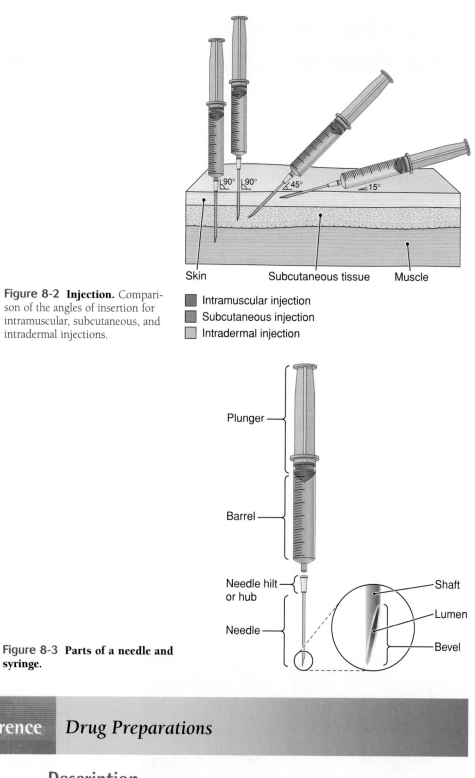

Figure 8-2 Injection. Comparison of the angles of insertion for intramuscular, subcutaneous, and intradermal injections.

Skin   Subcutaneous tissue   Muscle

■ Intramuscular injection
■ Subcutaneous injection
□ Intradermal injection

Plunger

Barrel

Needle hilt or hub

Needle

Shaft

Lumen

Bevel

Figure 8-3 Parts of a needle and syringe.

Box 8•6	For Your Reference	*Drug Preparations*

Form	Description
LIQUID	
Aerosol *AR-o-sol*	Solution dispersed as a mist to be inhaled
Aqueous solution *AK-wē-us*	Substance dissolved in water

Box 8•6 For Your Reference	*Continued*
Elixir (elix) *ē-LIK-sar*	A clear, pleasantly flavored and sweetened hydroalcoholic liquid intended for oral use
Emulsion *ē-MUL-shun*	A mixture in which one liquid is dispersed but not dissolved in another liquid
Lotion *LŌ-shun*	Solution prepared for topical use
Suspension (susp) *sus-PEN-shun*	Fine particles dispersed in a liquid; must be shaken before use
Tincture (tinct) *TINK-chur*	Substance dissolved in an alcoholic solution

SEMISOLID

Cream *krēm*	A semisolid emulsion used topically
Ointment (ung) *OYNT-ment*	Drug in a base that keeps it in contact with the skin

SOLID

Capsule (cap) *KAP-sūl*	Material in a gelatin container that dissolves easily in the stomach
Lozenge *LOZ-enj*	A pleasant-tasting medicated tablet or disk to be dissolved in the mouth, such as a cough drop
Suppository (supp) *su-POZ-i-tor-ē*	Substance mixed and molded with a base that melts easily when inserted into a body opening
Tablet (tab) *TAB-let*	A solid dosage form containing a drug in a pure state or mixed with a nonactive ingredient and prepared by compression or molding; also called a pill

Box 8•7 For Your Reference	*Terms Pertaining to Injectable Drugs*

Term	**Meaning**
Ampule *AM-pūl*	A small sealed glass or plastic container used for sterile intravenous solutions (Fig. 8-4)
Bolus *BŌ-lus*	A concentrated amount of a diagnostic or therapeutic substance given rapidly intravenously
Catheter *KATH-e-ter*	A thin tube that can be passed into a body cavity, organ, or vessel (Fig. 8-5)

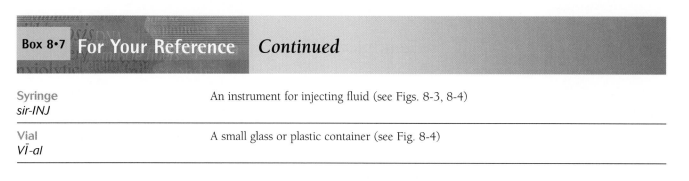

Box 8•7 For Your Reference *Continued*

Syringe *sir-INJ*	An instrument for injecting fluid (see Figs. 8-3, 8-4)
Vial *VĪ-al*	A small glass or plastic container (see Fig. 8-4)

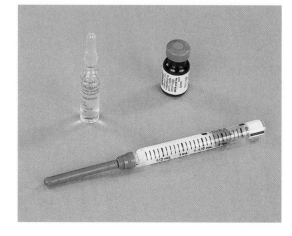

Figure 8-4 Injectable drug containers. An ampule (*top left*), a vial (*top right*), and a syringe (*bottom*) are shown.

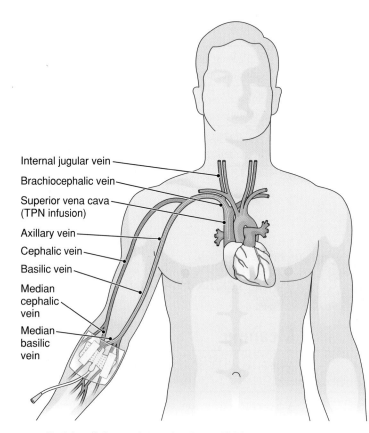

Internal jugular vein

Brachiocephalic vein

Superior vena cava
(TPN infusion)

Axillary vein

Cephalic vein

Basilic vein

Median
cephalic
vein

Median
basilic
vein

—— Peripherally inserted central catheter (PICC)

Figure 8-5 Catheter. Shown is placement of a peripherally inserted central catheter (PICC).

CHAPTER REVIEW

Match the following terms and write the appropriate letter to the left of each number:

_____ 1. diuretic

_____ 2. antiemetic

_____ 3. vasomotor

_____ 4. hyperpyrexia

_____ 5. potentiation

a. agent that prevents vomiting

b. pertaining to vessel movement

c. promoting excretion of water

d. combined drug action to greater effect

e. abnormally high body temperature

_____ 6. adrenergic

_____ 7. countercurrent

_____ 8. chronotropic

_____ 9. ampule

_____ 10. anaphylaxis

a. flowing in an opposite direction

b. affecting timing

c. extreme allergic reaction

d. small glass vial

e. sympathomimetic

_____ 11. po

_____ 12. prn

_____ 13. qam

_____ 14. s̄

_____ 15. qid

a. as needed

b. without

c. by mouth

d. four times a day

e. every morning

_____ 16. aloe

_____ 17. saw palmetto

_____ 18. tea tree oil

_____ 19. valerian

_____ 20. green tea

a. antimicrobial

b. antioxidant

c. treatment of burns, irritation

d. treatment of prostatic hyperplasia

e. sedative

Multiple choice. Select the best answer and write the letter of your choice to the left of each number:

_____ 21. Another term for trade name is:
  a. indicated name
  b. generic name
  c. prescription name
  d. chemical name
  e. brand name

8

_____ **22.** A drug that is administered topically is:
  a. swallowed
  b. injected
  c. applied to the skin
  d. placed under the tongue
  e. inserted with a catheter

_____ **23.** Drug administration by injection is described as:
  a. partial
  b. instilled
  c. encapsulated
  d. a bolus
  e. parenteral

_____ **24.** Another term for *hypodermic* is:
  a. intrathecal
  b. spinal
  c. epidural
  d. subcutaneous
  e. aqueous

_____ **25.** NSAIDs are used to treat:
  a. inflammation
  b. convulsions
  c. nausea
  d. hypertension
  e. diabetes

_____ **26.** Histamine H_2 antagonists are used to treat:
  a. cough
  b. ulcers
  c. muscle spasms
  d. anxiety
  e. depression

Fill in the blanks:

27. When a drug has lost its effect at a constant dose, the patient has developed _____.

28. An analgesic is used to treat _____.

29. An intravenous injection is given into a(n) _____.

30. Phytomedicine is the practice of treating with _____.

31. A transdermal route of administration is through the _____.

Eliminations. In each of the sets below, underline the word that does not fit in with the rest and explain the reason for your choice:

32. antineoplastics – nitrates – antiarrhythmics – calcium channel blockers – beta blockers

_____

33. anesthetic – analgesic – narcotic – adrenergic – sedative

_____

34. solution – elixir – tincture – emulsion – lozenge

_____

35. antitussive – hypolipidemic – expectorant – mucolytic – bronchodilator

_____

Define each of the following words:

36. anxiolytic _____

37. sublingual _____

38. psychotropic _____

39. bronchodilation _____

Opposites. Write a word that means the opposite of each of the following:

40. coagulant _____

41. vasodilation _____

42. convulsant _____

43. balance _____

44. indicated _____

45. toxin _____

Word building. Write a word for each of the following definitions:

46. One who studies poisons _____

47. Dissolving blood clots (root *thromb/o*) _____

48. Study of drugs _____

49. Counteracting fever _____

Define each of the following abbreviations:

50. IU _____

51. USP _____

52. ad lib _____

53. NSAIDs _____

54. Rx _____

55. mg _____

56. FDA _____

Word analysis. Define each of the following words, and give the meaning of the word parts in each. Use a dictionary if necessary.

57. adrenergic (*ad-ren-ER-jik*) _____

    a. adren/o _____

    b. erg/o _____

    c. -ic _____

58. pharmacokinetic (*far-ma-kō-ki-NET-ik*) _____

    a. pharmac/o _____

    b. kinet/o _____

    c. ic _____

Go to the word exercises in Chapter 8 of the CD-ROM for additional review exercises.

CASE STUDY 8-1: Cardiac Disease and Crisis

P.L., who has a 4-year history of heart disease, was brought to the emergency room by ambulance with chest pain that radiated down her arm, dyspnea, and syncope. Her routine meds included Lanoxin to slow and strengthen her heart beat, Inderal to support her heart rhythm, Lipitor to decrease her cholesterol, Catapres to lower her hypertension, nitroglycerin prn for chest pain, Hydro DIURIL to eliminate fluid and decrease the workload of her heart, Diabinese for her diabetes, and Coumadin to prevent blood clots. She also took Tagamet for her stomach ulcer and several OTC preparations, including an herbal sleeping potion that she mixed in tea, and Metamucil mixed in orange juice every morning for her bowels. Shortly after admission, P.L.'s heart rate deteriorated into full cardiac arrest. Immediate resuscitation was instituted with cardiopulmonary resuscitation (CPR), defibrillation, and a bolus of IV epinephrine. Between shocks she was given a bolus of lidocaine and a bolus of diltiazem plus repeated doses of epinephrine every 5 minutes. P.L. did not respond to resuscitation. On the death certificate, her primary cause of death was listed as cardiac arrest. Multiple secondary diagnoses were listed, including polypharmacy.

CASE STUDY 8-2: Inflammatory Bowel Disease

A.E., a 19-year-old college student, was diagnosed at the age of 13 with Crohn disease, a chronic inflammatory disease that can affect the entire gastrointestinal tract from mouth to anus. A.E.'s disease is limited to his large bowel. During a 9-month period of disease exacerbation, characterized by severe cramping and bloody stools, he took oral corticosteroids (prednisone) to reduce the inflammatory response. He experienced many of the drug's side effects, but has been in remission for 4 years. Currently, A.E.'s condition is managed on drugs that reduce inflammation by suppressing the immune response. He takes Pentasa (mesalamine) 250 mg 4 caps po bid. Pentasa is of the 5-ASA (acetylsalicylic acid or aspirin) group of antiinflammatory agents, which work topically on the inner surface of the bowel. It has an enteric coating, which dissolves in the bowel environment. He also takes 6-mercaptopurine (Purinethol) 75 mg po qd and a therapeutic vitamin with breakfast. A.E. may take acetaminophen for pain but must avoid NSAIDs, which will irritate the intestinal mucosa (inner lining) and cause a flare-up of the disease.

CASE STUDY 8-3: Asthma

E.N., a 20-year-old woman with asthma, visited the preadmission testing unit 1 week before her cosmetic surgery to meet with the nurse and anesthesiologist. Her current meds included several bronchodilators, which she takes by mouth and by inhalation, and a tranquilizer that she takes when needed for nervousness. She sometimes receives inhalation treatments with Mucomyst, a mucolytic agent. On E.N.'s preoperative note, the nurse wrote:

Theo-Dur 1 cap tid
Flovent inhaler 1 spray (50 mcg each nostril bid
Ativan (lorazepam) 1 mg po bid
Albuterol-metered dose inhaler 2 puffs (180 mcg) prn
   q4-6h for bronchospasm and before exercise

E.N. stated that she has difficulty with her asthma when she is anxious and when she exercises. She also admitted to occasional use of marijuana and ecstasy, a hallucinogen and mood-altering illegal recreational drug. The anesthesiologist wrote an order for lorazepam 4 mg IV 1 hour preop. The plastic surgeon recommended several herbal products to complement her surgery and her recovery. He ordered a high-potency vitamin 3 tabs with breakfast and dinner to support tissue health and healing. He also prescribed Bromelain, an enzyme from pineapple, to decrease inflammation, 1 po qid 3 days before surgery and postoperatively for 2 weeks. Arnica Montana was prescribed to decrease discomfort, swelling, and bruising; 3 tabs sublingual tid the evening after surgery and for the following 10 days.

CASE STUDY QUESTIONS

Multiple choice. Select the best answer and write the letter of your choice to the left of each number:

_____ 1. P.L.'s nitroglycerine is ordered: prn SL. This means:
   a. as needed, under the tongue
   b. at bedtime, under the tongue
   c. as needed, on the skin
   d. by mouth, on the skin
   e. by mouth, under the skin

_____ 2. P.L. took several OTC preparations. OTC means:
   a. on the cutaneous
   b. off the cuff
   c. over the counter
   d. do not need a prescription
   e. c and d

_____ 3. P.L.'s herbal sleeping potion was mixed into tea and taken at bedtime. The dissolved mixture is called a(n)
   _____ and is taken at _____.
   a. elixir/QAM
   b. emulsion/bid
   c. suspension/hs
   d. aqueous solution/hs
   e. aqueous solution/QAM

_____ 4. During P.L.'s resuscitation, epinephrine was given in an IV bolus. This means it was administered:
   a. intrathecally in a continuous drip
   b. parenterally in a topical solution
   c. intravenously in a continuous drip
   d. intravenously in a rapid concentrated dose
   e. intrathecally in a rapid concentrated dose

_____ 5. P.L. had a secondary diagnosis of polypharmacy. This means that she:
   a. used more than one drug store
   b. had polyps
   c. used more prescription than OTC drugs
   d. had a toxic dose
   e. used many different drugs

_____ 6. A.E. takes several drugs to prevent or act against his inflammatory response. These agents are called
   _____ drugs.
   a. contrainflammatory
   b. counterinflammatory
   c. antiinflammatory
   d. proinflammatory
   e. hypoinflammatory

8

_____ 7. A.E. presented with several untoward results or risks from the corticosteroid therapy. These sequelae are called:
  a. contraindications
  b. side effects
  c. antagonistic effects
  d. exacerbations
  e. synergy states

_____ 8. A.E. takes four 250-mg capsules of Pentasa po bid. How many capsules does he take in 1 day?
  a. 2000
  b. 1000
  c. 4
  d. 8
  e. 12

_____ 9. A.E. must avoid NSAIDs; therefore, these drugs are _____ in inflammatory bowel disease.
  a. contraindicated
  b. indicated
  c. complementary
  d. synergistic
  e. prescriptive

_____ 10. E.N. used a mucolytic drug when needed. This drug's action is to:
  a. increase secretions
  b. decrease spasm
  c. calm anxiety
  d. decrease mucus secretions
  e. simulate mucus

_____ 11. E.N.'s Flovent inhaler is indicated as 1 spray of 50 mcg in each nostril bid. How many micrograms (mcg) does she get in 1 day?
  a. 100 mcg
  b. 200 mcg
  c. 250 mcg
  d. 500 mcg
  e. 5000 mcg

_____ 12. The Ativan that E.N. takes for nervousness is a(n) _____ drug.
  a. anxiolytic
  b. potentiating
  c. antiemetic
  d. analgesic
  e. bronchodilator

_____ 13. The anesthesiologist ordered lorazepam (Ativan) to be given IV preop to decrease anxiety and to smooth E.N.'s anesthesia induction. The complementary way that lorazepam and anesthesia work together is called:
  a. antagonistic
  b. complementary medicine
  c. parasympathomimetic
  d. tolerance
  e. synergy

_____ 14. Bromelain and Arnica Montana are herbal products that can be described as all of the following except:
  a. phytopharmaceutical
  b. alternative
  c. herbal
  d. complementary
  e. chronotropic

_____ 15. Arnica Montana was prescribed 3 tabs SL tid. How many tabs would E.N. take in 1 day?
  a. 6
  b. 9
  c. 12
  d. 21
  e. 33

_____ 16. Flovent is administered as an inhalant. The form in which the drug is prepared is called a(n):
  a. emulsion
  b. elixir
  c. aerosol
  d. suspension
  e. unguent

PART THREE

BODY SYSTEMS

In this section, the basics of medical terminology are applied
to the body systems. Each chapter begins with a description of
normal structure and function because these form the basis
for all health-care studies.

CHAPTER NINE

CIRCULATION: THE CARDIOVASCULAR AND LYMPHATIC SYSTEMS

9

CHAPTER CONTENTS

OBJECTIVES

After study of this chapter you should be able to:

1. Label a diagram of the heart.
2. Trace the path of blood flow through the heart.
3. Trace the path of electrical conduction through the heart.
4. Identify the components of an electrocardiogram.
5. Differentiate among arteries, arterioles, capillaries, veins, and venules.
6. Explain blood pressure and describe how blood pressure is measured.
7. Identify and use the roots pertaining to the cardiovascular and lymphatic systems.

8. Describe the main disorders that affect the cardiovascular and lymphatic systems.
9. Define medical terms pertaining to the cardiovascular and lymphatic systems.
10. List the functions and components of the lymphatic system.
11. Interpret medical abbreviations referring to circulation.
12. Analyze case studies involving circulation.

PRETEST

1. The system that includes the heart and blood vessels is the _____.

2. The thick, muscular layer of the heart wall is the _____.

3. The lower chambers of the heart are the _____.

4. A vessel that carries blood away from the heart is a(n) _____.

5. The tonsils, spleen, thymus and nodes are part of the _____.

6. The medical term for a "heart attack" is _____.

7. The accumulation of fatty deposits in the lining of a vessel is called _____.

9

*B*lood circulates throughout the body in the **cardiovascular system**, which consists of the heart and the blood vessels (Fig. 9-1). This system forms a continuous circuit that delivers oxygen and nutrients to all cells and carries away waste products. The **lymphatic system** also functions in circulation. Its vessels drain fluid and proteins left in the tissues and return them to the bloodstream. The lymphatic system plays a part in immunity and in the digestive process as well, as explained in Chapters 10 and 12. This chapter discusses the circulatory system in detail, in both its normal and clinical aspects, and then proceeds to study of the lymphatic system.

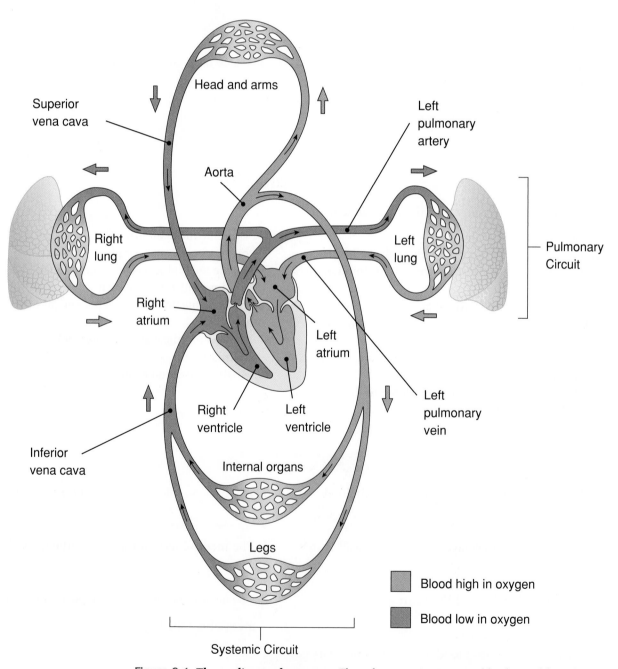

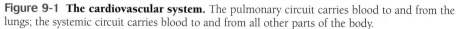

Figure 9-1 The cardiovascular system. The pulmonary circuit carries blood to and from the lungs; the systemic circuit carries blood to and from all other parts of the body.

The Heart

The **heart** is located between the lungs, with its point or **apex** directed toward the inferior and left (Fig. 9-2). The wall of the heart consists of three layers, all named with the root *cardi*, meaning "heart." Moving from the innermost to the outermost layer, these are the:

1. **Endocardium**—a thin membrane that lines the chambers and valves (the prefix *endo-* means "within")
2. **Myocardium**—the thick muscle layer that makes up most of the heart wall (the root *my/o* means "muscle")
3. **Epicardium**—a thin membrane that covers the heart (the prefix *epi-* means "on")

A fibrous sac, the **pericardium**, contains the heart and anchors it to surrounding structures, such as the sternum (breastbone) and diaphragm (the prefix *peri-* means "around")

Each of the upper receiving chambers of the heart is an **atrium** (plural: atria). Each of the lower pumping chambers is a **ventricle** (plural, ventricles). The chambers of the heart are divided by walls, each of which is called a **septum**. The interventricular septum separates the two ventricles; the interatrial septum divides the two atria. There is also a septum between the atrium and ventricle on each side.

The heart pumps blood through two circuits. The right side pumps blood to the lungs to be oxygenated through the **pulmonary circuit**. The left side pumps to the remainder of the body through the **systemic circuit** (see Fig. 9-1).

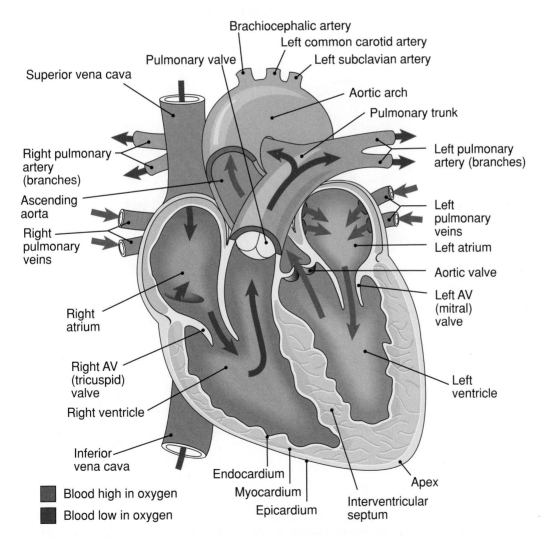

Figure 9-2 The heart and great vessels. AV = atrioventricular.

Blood Flow through the Heart

The pathway of blood through the heart is shown by the arrows in Figure 9-2. The sequence is as follows:

1. The right atrium receives blood low in oxygen, or deoxygenated, from all body tissues through the **superior vena cava** and the **inferior vena cava**.
2. The blood then enters the right ventricle and is pumped to the lungs through the **pulmonary artery**.
3. Blood returns from the lungs high in oxygen, or oxygenated, and enters the left atrium through the **pulmonary veins**.
4. Blood enters the left ventricle and is forcefully pumped into the **aorta** to be distributed to all tissues.

One-way **valves** in the heart keep blood moving in a forward direction. The valves between the atrium and ventricle on each side are the **atrioventricular (AV) valves** (see Fig. 9-2). The valve between the right atrium and ventricle is the **right AV valve**, also known as the tricuspid valve because it has three cusps (flaps). The valve between the left atrium and ventricle is the **left AV valve**, which is a bicuspid valve with two cusps; it is often called the **mitral valve** (so named because it resembles a bishop's miter).

The valves leading into the pulmonary artery and the aorta have three cusps. Each cusp is shaped like a half-moon, so these valves are described as *semilunar valves*. The valve at the entrance to the pulmonary artery is specifically named the **pulmonary valve**; the valve at the entrance to the aorta is the **aortic valve**.

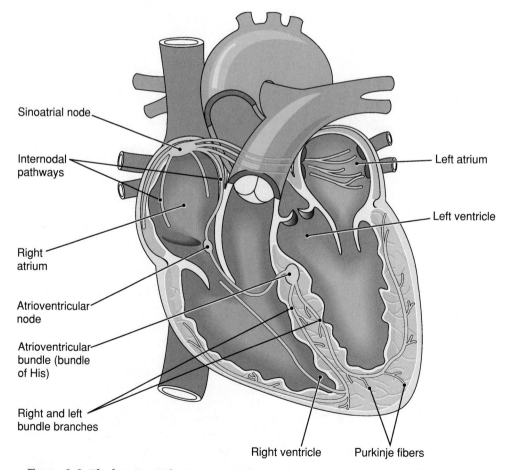

Figure 9-3 The heart's conduction system. Impulses travel from the sinoatrial (SA) node to the atrioventricular (AV) node, then to the atrioventricular bundle, bundle branches and Purkinje fibers. Internodal pathways carry impulses throughout the atria.

Heart sounds are produced as the heart functions. The loudest of these, the familiar lubb and dupp that can be heard through the chest wall, are produced by alternate closing of the valves. The first heart sound (S_1) is heard when the valves between the chambers close. The second heart sound (S_2) is produced when the valves leading into the aorta and pulmonary artery close. Any sound made as the heart functions normally is termed a **functional murmur**. (The word *murmur* used alone with regard to the heart describes an abnormal sound.)

The Heartbeat

Each contraction of the heart, termed **systole** (*SIS-tō-lē*), is followed by a relaxation phase, **diastole** (*dī-AS-tō-lē*), during which the chambers fill. Each time the heart beats, both atria contract and immediately thereafter both ventricles contract. The number of times the heart contracts per minute is the **heart rate**. The wave of increased pressure produced in the **vessels** each time the ventricles contract is the **pulse**. Pulse rate is usually counted by palpating a peripheral artery, such as the radial artery at the wrist or the carotid artery in the neck (see Fig. 7-4).

Heart contractions are stimulated by a built-in system that regularly transmits electrical impulses through the heart. The components of this conduction system are shown in Figure 9-3. In the sequence of action they include the:

1. **Sinoatrial (SA) node**, located in the upper right atrium and called the pacemaker because it sets the rate of the heartbeat
2. **Atrioventricular (AV) node**, located at the bottom of the right atrium near the ventricle. Internodal fibers between the SA and AV node carry stimulation throughout both atria.
3. **AV bundle** (bundle of His) at the top of the interventricular septum
4. Left and right **bundle branches**, which travel along the left and right sides of the septum
5. **Purkinje** (*pur-KIN-jē*) **fibers**, which carry stimulation throughout the walls of the ventricles. (See information on naming in Box 9-1.)

Box 9•1 | Focus on Words | *Name That Structure*

An eponym (*EP-o-nim*) is a name that is based on the name of a person, usually the one who discovered a particular structure, disease, principle, or procedure. Everyday examples are graham cracker, Ferris wheel, and boycott. In the heart, the bundle of His and Purkinje fibers are part of that organ's conduction system. Korotkoff sounds are heard in the vessels when taking blood pressure. Cardiovascular disorders named for people include the tetralogy of Fallot, a combination of four congenital heart defects; Raynaud disease of small vessels; and the cardiac arrhythmia known as Wolff–Parkinson–White syndrome. In treatment, Doppler echocardiography is named for a physicist of the 19th century. The Holter monitor and the Swan–Ganz catheter give honor to their developers.

In other systems, the islets of Langerhans are clusters of cells in the pancreas that secrete insulin. The graafian follicle in the ovary surrounds the developing egg cell. The eustachian tube connects the middle ear to the throat.

Many diseases names are eponymic: Parkinson and Alzheimer, which affect the brain; Graves, a disorder of the thyroid; Addison and Cushing, involving the adrenal cortex; and Down syndrome, a hereditary disorder. The genus and species names of microorganisms often are based on the names of their discoverers, *Escherichia, Salmonella, Pasteurella,* and *Rickettsia* to name a few.

Many reagents, instruments, and procedures are named for their developers. The original name for a radiograph was roentgenograph (*RENT-jen-ō-graf*), named for Wilhelm Roentgen, discoverer of x-rays. A curie is a measure of radiation, derived from the name of Marie Curie, a co-discoverer of radioactivity.

Although eponyms give honor to physicians and scientists of the past, they do not convey any information and may be more difficult to learn. There is a trend to replace these names with more descriptive ones; for example, auditory tube instead of eustachian tube, ovarian follicle for graafian follicle, pancreatic islets for islets of Langerhans, and trisomy 21 for Down syndrome.

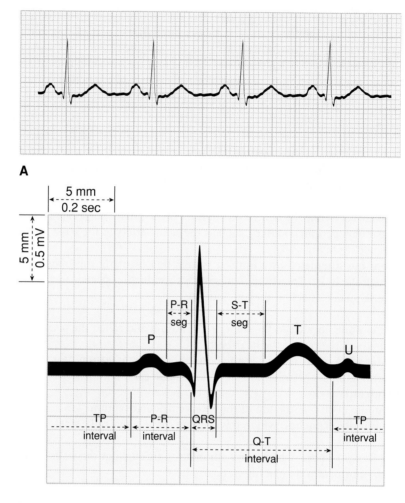

A

B

Figure 9-4 Electrocardiography (ECG). (*A*) ECG tracing showing a normal sinus rhythm. (*B*) Components of a normal ECG tracing. Shown are the P, QRS, T, and U waves, which represent electrical activity in different parts of the heart. Intervals measure from one wave to the next; segments are smaller components of the tracing.

Although the heart itself generates the heartbeat, factors such as nervous system stimulation, hormones, and drugs can influence the rate and the force of heart contractions.

Electrocardiography

Electrocardiography (ECG) measures the heart's electrical activity as it functions (Fig. 9-4). Electrodes (leads) placed on the body's surface detect the electrical signals, which are then amplified and recorded as a tracing. A normal, or **sinus rhythm**, which originates at the SA node, is shown in Figure 9-4A. Figure 9-4B shows the letters assigned to individual components of one complete cycle:

1. The P wave represents electrical change, or **depolarization**, of the atrial muscles
2. The QRS component shows depolarization of the ventricles
3. The T wave shows return, or **repolarization**, of the ventricles to their resting state. Repolarization of the atria is hidden by the QRS wave.
4. The small U wave, if present, follows the T wave. It is of uncertain origin.

An *interval* measures the distance from one wave to the next; a *segment* is a smaller component of the tracing. Many heart disorders, some of which are described later in the chapter, appear as abnormalities in the components of the ECG.

The Vascular System

The vascular system consists of:

1. **Arteries** that carry blood away from the heart (Fig. 9-5).
2. **Arterioles**, vessels smaller than arteries that lead into the capillaries.
3. **Capillaries**, the smallest vessels, through which exchanges take place between the blood and the tissues.
4. **Venules**, small vessels that receive blood from the capillaries and drain into the veins
5. **Veins** that carry blood back to the heart (Fig. 9-6)

9

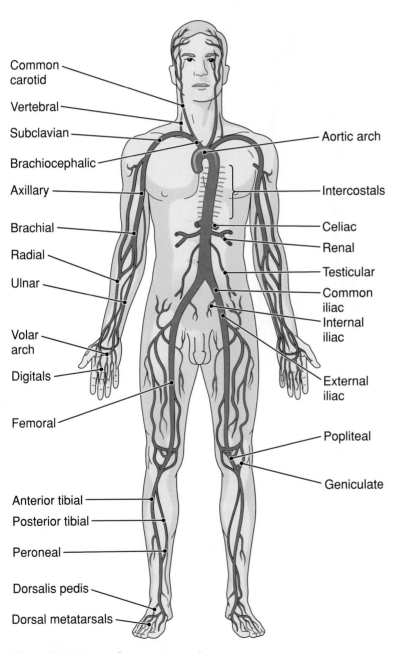

Common carotid
Vertebral
Subclavian
Brachiocephalic
Axillary
Brachial
Radial
Ulnar
Volar arch
Digitals
Femoral
Anterior tibial
Posterior tibial
Peroneal
Dorsalis pedis
Dorsal metatarsals

Aortic arch
Intercostals
Celiac
Renal
Testicular
Common iliac
Internal iliac
External iliac
Popliteal
Geniculate

Figure 9-5 Principal systemic arteries.

9

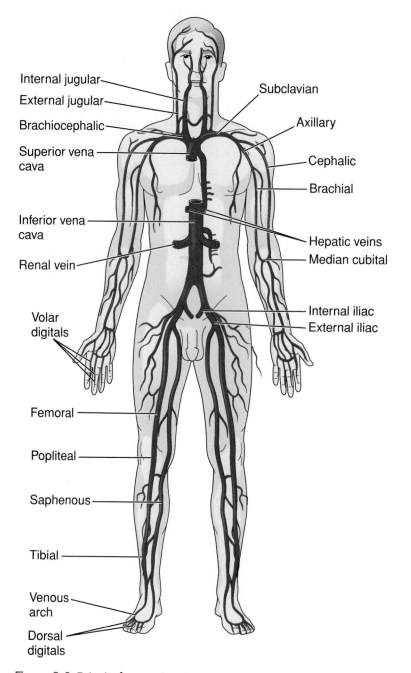

Figure 9-6 Principal systemic veins.

All arteries, except the pulmonary artery (and the umbilical artery in the fetus), carry oxygenated blood. They are thick-walled, elastic vessels that carry blood under high pressure. All veins, except the pulmonary vein (and the umbilical vein in the fetus), carry deoxygenated blood. Veins have thinner, less elastic walls and tend to give way under pressure. Like the heart, veins have one-way valves that keep blood flowing forward.

Nervous system stimulation can cause the diameter of a vessel to increase (vasodilation) or decrease (vasoconstriction). These changes alter blood flow to the tissues and affect blood pressure.

Blood Pressure

Blood pressure (BP) is the force exerted by blood against the wall of a blood vessel. It falls as the blood travels away from the heart, and is influenced by a variety of factors,

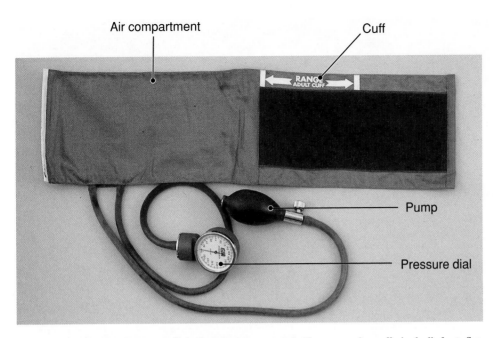

Air compartment

Cuff

Pump

Pressure dial

Figure 9-7 Blood pressure cuff (sphygmomanometer). Shown are the cuff, the bulb for inflating the cuff, and the manometer for measuring pressure.

including cardiac output, vessel diameters, and total blood volume. Vasoconstriction increases blood pressure in a vessel; vasodilation decreases pressure.

Blood pressure is commonly measured in a large artery with an inflatable cuff (Fig. 9-7) known as a blood pressure cuff or blood pressure apparatus, but technically called a **sphygmomanometer**. The cuff is inflated to stop blood flow in a vessel. Then a stethoscope is used to listen for blood flow in the vessel as the pressure is slowly released (see Fig. 7-5). The blood pressure reading includes both systolic pressure, measured while the heart is contracting, and diastolic pressure, measured when the heart relaxes. These are reported as systolic then diastolic separated by a slash, such as 120/80. Pressure is expressed as millimeters of mercury (mm Hg)—that is, the height to which the pressure can push a column of mercury in a tube. Blood pressure is a valuable diagnostic measurement that is easily obtained. (See Box 9-2 for more information on blood pressure measurement.)

Box 9•2 Clinical Perspectives *Cardiac Catheterization: Measuring Blood Pressure from Within*

Because arterial blood pressure decreases as blood flows further away from the heart, measurement of blood pressure with a simple inflatable cuff around the arm is only a reflection of the pressure in the heart and pulmonary arteries. Precise measurement of pressure in these parts of the cardiovascular system is useful in diagnosing certain cardiac and pulmonary disorders.

More accurate readings can be obtained using a catheter (thin tube) inserted directly into the heart and large vessels. One type commonly used is the pulmonary artery catheter (also known as the Swan–Ganz catheter), which has an inflatable balloon at the tip. This device is threaded into the right side of the heart through a large vein. Typically, the right internal jugular vein is used because it is the shortest

and most direct route to the heart, but the subclavian and femoral veins may also be used. The catheter's position in the heart is confirmed by a chest x-ray and, when appropriately positioned, the atrial and ventricular blood pressures are recorded. As the catheter continues into the pulmonary artery, pressure in this vessel can be read. When the balloon is inflated, the catheter becomes wedged in a branch of the pulmonary artery, blocking blood flow. The reading obtained is called the **pulmonary capillary wedge (PCW) pressure**. It gives information on pressure in the heart's left side and on resistance in the lungs. Combined with other tests, cardiac catheterization can be used to diagnose cardiac and pulmonary disorders such as shock, pericarditis, congenital heart disease, and heart failure.

TERMINOLOGY Key Terms

Cardiovascular System

NORMAL STRUCTURE AND FUNCTION

aorta *ā-OR-ta*	The largest artery. It receives blood from the left ventricle and branches to all parts of the body (root: *aort/o*).
aortic valve *ā-OR-tik*	The valve at the entrance to the aorta
apex *Ā-peks*	The point of a cone-shaped structure (adjective, apical). The apex of the heart is formed by the left ventricle and is pointed toward the inferior and left.
artery	A vessel that carries blood away from the heart. All except the pulmonary and umbilical arteries carry oxygenated blood (root: *arter, arteri/o*).
arteriole *ar-TĒ-rē-ōl*	A small vessel that carries blood from the arteries into the capillaries (root: *arteriol/o*)
atrioventricular (AV) node *ā-trē-ō-ven-TRIK-ū-lar*	A small mass in the lower septum of the right atrium that passes impulses from the sinoatrial (SA) node toward the ventricles
AV bundle	A band of fibers that transmits impulses from the atrioventricular (AV) node to the top of the interventricular septum. It divides into the right and left bundle branches, which descend along the two sides of the septum; the bundle of His.
atrioventricular (AV) valve	A valve between the atrium and ventricle on the right and left sides of the heart. The right AV valve is the tricuspid valve; the left is the mitral valve.
atrium *Ā-trē-um*	An entrance chamber, one of the two upper receiving chambers of the heart (root *atri/o*)
blood pressure	The force exerted by blood against the wall of a vessel
bundle branches	Branches of the AV bundle that divide to the right and left sides of the interventricular septum
capillary *KAP-i-lar-ē*	A microscopic blood vessel through which materials are exchanged between the blood and the tissues
cardiovascular system *kar-dē-ō-VAS-kū-lar*	The part of the circulatory system that consists of the heart and the blood vessels
depolarization *dē-pō-lar-i-ZĀ-shun*	A change in electrical charge from the resting state in nerves or muscles
diastole *dī-AS-tō-lē*	The relaxation phase of the heartbeat cycle; adjective, diastolic
electrocardiography (ECG) *ē-lek-trō-kar-dē-OG-ra-fē*	Study of the electrical activity of the heart as detected by electrodes (leads) placed on the surface of the body. Also abbreviated EKG from the German *electrokardiography*.
endocardium *en-dō-KAR-dē-um*	The thin membrane that lines the chambers of the heart and covers the valves

TERMINOLOGY   Key Terms
Continued

epicardium *ep-i-KAR-dē-um*	The thin outermost layer of the heart wall
functional murmur	Any sound produced as the heart functions normally
heart *hart*	The muscular organ with four chambers that contracts rhythmically to propel blood through vessels to all parts of the body (root: *cardi/o*)
heart rate	The number of times the heart contracts per minute; recorded as beats per minute (BPM)
heart sounds	Sounds produced as the heart functions. The two loudest sounds are produced by alternate closing of the valves and are designated S_1 and S_2.
inferior vena cava *VĒ-na KĀ-va*	The large inferior vein that brings blood back to the right atrium of the heart from the lower part of the body
left AV valve	The valve between the left atrium and the left ventricle; the mitral valve or bicuspid valve
mitral valve *MĪ-tral*	The valve between the left atrium and the left ventricle; the left AV valve or bicuspid valve
myocardium *mī-ō-KAR-dē-um*	The thick middle layer of the heart wall composed of cardiac muscle
pericardium *per-i-KAR-dē-um*	The fibrous sac that surrounds the heart
pulmonary artery *PUL-mō-nār-ē*	The vessel that carries blood from the right side of the heart to the lungs
pulmonary circuit	The system of vessels that carries blood from the right side of the heart to the lungs to be oxygenated and then back to the left side of the heart
pulmonary veins	The vessels that carry blood from the lungs to the left side of the heart
pulmonary valve *PUL-mō-nār-ē*	The valve at the entrance to the pulmonary artery
pulse *puls*	The wave of increased pressure produced in the vessels each time the ventricles contract
Purkinje fibers *pur-KIN-jē*	The terminal fibers of the conducting system of the heart. They carry impulses through the walls of the ventricles.
repolarization *rē-pō-lar-i-ZĀ-shun*	A return of electrical charge to the resting state in nerves or muscles
right AV valve	The valve between the right atrium and right ventricle; the tricuspid valve
septum *SEP-tum*	A wall dividing two cavities, such as the chambers of the heart

9

TERMINOLOGY   Key Terms

Continued

sinus rhythm *SĪ-nus*	Normal rhythm of the heart
sinoatrial (SA) node *sī-nō-Ā-trē-al*	A small mass in the upper part of the right atrium that initiates the impulse for each heartbeat; the pacemaker
sphygmomanometer *sfig-mō-man-OM-e-ter*	An instrument for determining arterial blood pressure (root *sphygm/o* means "pulse"); blood pressure apparatus or cuff
superior vena cava *VĒ-na KĀ-va*	The large superior vein that brings deoxygenated blood back to the right atrium from the upper part of the body
systemic circuit *sis-TEM-ik*	The system of vessels that carries oxygenated blood from the left side of the heart to all tissues except the lungs and returns deoxygenated blood to the right side of the heart
systole *SIS-tō-lē*	The contraction phase of the heartbeat cycle; adjective, systolic
valve *valv*	A structure that keeps fluid flowing in a forward direction (root *valv/o*, *valvul/o*)
vein *vān*	A vessel that carries blood back to the heart. All except the pulmonary and umbilical veins carry blood low in oxygen (root: *ven/o*, *phleb/o*).
ventricle *VEN-trik-l*	A small cavity. One of the two lower pumping chambers of the heart (root: *ventricul/o*).
venule *VEN-ūl*	A small vessel that carries blood from the capillaries to the veins
vessel *VES-el*	A tube or duct to transport fluid (root: *angi/o*, *vas/o*, *vascul/o*)

Go to the pronunciation glossary in Chapter 9 on the CD-ROM to hear these words pronounced.

Roots Pertaining to the Cardiovascular System

Table 9·1	Roots for the Heart		
ROOT	**MEANING**	**EXAMPLE**	**DEFINITION OF EXAMPLE**
cardi/o	heart	cardiomyopathy* *kar-dē-ō-mī-OP-a-thē*	any disease of the heart muscle
atri/o	atrium	interatrial *in-ter-Ā-trē-al*	between the atria
ventricul/o	cavity, ventricle	ventriculotomy *ven-trik-ū-LOT-ō-mē*	surgical incision of a ventricle
valv/o, valvul/o	valve	valvuloplasty *val-vū-lō-PLAS-tē*	plastic repair of a valve

Preferred over myocardiopathy.

Exercise 9-1

Fill in the blanks:

1. The word *cardiogenic* (*kar-dē-ō-GEN-ik*) means originating in the _____.

2. An atriotomy (*ā-trē-OT-ō-mē*) is surgical incision of a(n) _____.

3. Supraventricular (*sū-pra-ven-TRIK-ū-lar*) means above a(n) _____.

4. A valvulotome (*VAL-vū-lō-tōm*) is an instrument for incising a(n) _____.

Write the adjective for the following definitions. The proper suffix is given for each.

5. Pertaining to the heart (-ac) _____

6. Pertaining to the myocardium (-al; ending differs from adjective ending for the heart) _____

7. Pertaining to an atrium (-al) _____

8. Pertaining to a valve (-ar) _____

9. Pertaining to a ventricle (-ar) _____

10. Pertaining to the pericardium (-al) _____

Following the example, write a word for the following definitions pertaining to the tissues of the heart:

11. Inflammation of the lining of the heart (usually at a valve)   endocarditis

12. Inflammation of the heart muscle _____

13. Inflammation of the fibrous sac around the heart _____

Write a word for the following definitions:

14. Study (-logy) of the heart _____

15. Between (inter-) the ventricles _____

16. Pertaining to an atrium and a ventricle _____

17. Enlargement (-megaly) of the heart _____

18. Surgical incision of a valve _____

Table 9·2 Roots for the Blood Vessels

ROOT	MEANING	EXAMPLE	DEFINITION OF EXAMPLE
angi/o*	vessel	angiogram *AN-jē-ō-gram*	x-ray image (radiograph) of a vessel
vas/o, vascul/o	vessel, duct	vasoconstriction *vas-ō-kon-STRIK-shun*	narrowing of a blood vessel
arter/o, arteri/o	artery	endarterial *end-ar-TĒ-rē-al*	within an artery
arteriol/o	arteriole	arteriolar *ar-tē-rē-Ō-lar*	pertaining to an arteriole
aort/o	aorta	aortostenosis *ā-or-tō-ste-NŌ-sis*	narrowing of the aorta
ven/o, ven/i	vein	venous *VĒ-nus*	pertaining to a vein
phleb/o	vein	phlebotomy *fle-BOT-ō-mē*	incision of a vein to withdraw blood

*The root *angi/o* usually refers to a blood vessel but is used for other types of vessels as well. Hemangi/o refers specifically to a blood vessel.

Exercise 9-2

Fill in the blanks:

1. Vasospasm (*vas-ō-spazm*) means sudden contraction of a(n) _____.

2. Endarterectomy (*end-ar-ter-EK-tō-mē*) is removal of the inner lining of a(n)

   _____.

3. Arteriolitis (*ar-tē-rē-Ō-LĪ-tis*)is inflammation of a(n) _____

4. Angioedema (*an-jē-ō-e-DĒ-ma*) is localized swelling caused by changes in

   _____

5. Aortoptosis (*ā-or-tōp-TŌ-sis*) is downward displacement of the _____

6. Phlebectasia (*fleb-ek-TĀ-zē-a*) is dilatation of a(n) _____

7. The term *microvascular* (*mī-krō-VAS-kū-lar*) means pertaining to small

   _____

Define the following words:

8. angiitis (*an-jē-Ī-tis*) (note spelling); also angitis or vasculitis _____

9. cardiovascular (*kar-dē-ō-VAS-kū-lar*) _____

10. arteriorrhexis (*ar-tē-rē-ō-REK-sis*) _____

11. intraaortic (*in-tra-ā-OR-tik*) _____

12. phlebitis (*fleb-Ī-tis*) _____

Use the ending -gram to form a word for a radiograph of the following:

13. vessels (use angi/o) _____

14. aorta _____

15. veins _____

Use the root angi/o to write words with the following meanings:

16. Any disease (-pathy) of a vessel _____

17. Dilatation (-ectasis) of a vessel _____

18. Plastic repair (-plasty) of a vessel _____

19. Formation (-genesis) of a vessel _____

Use the appropriate root to write words with the following meanings:

20. Hardening (-sclerosis) of the aorta _____

21. Excision of a vein _____

22. Incision of an artery _____

23. Within (intra-) a vein _____

Clinical Aspects of the Cardiovascular System

Atherosclerosis

The accumulation of fatty deposits within the lining of an artery is termed **atherosclerosis** (Fig. 9-8). This type of deposit, called a **plaque** (*plak*), begins to form when a vessel receives tiny injuries, usually at a point of branching. Plaques gradually thicken and harden with fibrous material, cells, and other deposits, restricting the vessel's lumen (opening) and reducing blood flow to the tissues, a condition known as **ischemia**. A major risk factor for the development of atherosclerosis is **dyslipidemia**, abnormally high levels or imbalance in **lipoproteins** that are carried in the blood, especially high levels of cholesterol-containing, low-density lipoproteins (LDL). Other risk factors for atherosclerosis include smoking, high blood pressure, poor diet, inactivity, stress, and a family history of the disorder. Atherosclerosis may involve any arteries, but most of its effects are seen in the coronary vessels of the heart, the aorta, the carotid arteries in the neck, and vessels in the brain. The techniques described later for treating coronary artery disease are used for these other vessels as well.

Atherosclerosis is the most common form of a more general condition known as **arteriosclerosis**, in which vessel walls harden from any cause. In addition to plaque, calcium salts and scar tissue may contribute to a thickening of the arterial wall, with a narrowing of the lumen and loss of elasticity.

9

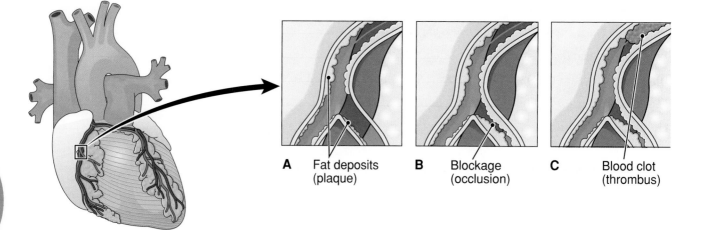

Figure 9-8 Coronary atherosclerosis. (*A*) Fat deposits (plaque) narrow an artery, leading to ischemia (lack of blood supply). (*B*) Plaque causes blockage (occlusion) of a vessel. (*C*) Formation of a blood clot (thrombus) in a vessel leads to myocardial infarction (MI).

Thrombosis and Embolism

Atherosclerosis predisposes a person to **thrombosis**, the formation of a blood clot within a vessel, (see Fig. 9-8). The clot, called a **thrombus**, interrupts blood flow to the tissues supplied by that vessel, resulting in necrosis (tissue death). Blockage of a vessel by a thrombus or other mass carried in the bloodstream is an **embolism**, and the mass itself is called an **embolus**. Usually the mass is a blood clot that breaks loose from the wall of a vessel, but it may also be air (as from injection or trauma), fat (as from marrow released after a bone break), bacteria, or other solid materials. Often a venous thrombus will travel through the heart and then lodge in an artery of the lungs, resulting in a life-threatening pulmonary embolism. An embolus from a carotid artery often blocks a cerebral vessel, causing a **cerebrovascular accident** (**CVA**), commonly called **stroke** (see Chapter 17).

Aneurysm

An arterial wall weakened by atherosclerosis, malformation, injury, or other changes may balloon out, forming an **aneurysm**. If an aneurysm ruptures, hemorrhage results. Rupture of a cerebral artery is another cause of stroke. The abdominal aorta and carotid arteries are also common sites of aneurysm. In a **dissecting aneurysm** (Fig. 9-9), blood hemorrhages into the thick middle layer of the arterial wall, separating the muscle as it spreads and sometimes rupturing the vessel. The aorta is most commonly involved. It may be possible to repair a dissecting aneurysm surgically with a graft.

Hypertension

High blood pressure, or **hypertension** (HTN), is a contributing factor in all of the conditions described above. In simple terms, hypertension is defined as a systolic pressure greater than 140 mm Hg or a diastolic pressure greater than 90 mm Hg. Hypertension causes the left ventricle to enlarge (hypertrophy) as a result of increased work. Some cases of HTN are secondary to other disorders, such as kidney malfunction or endocrine disturbance, but most of the time the causes are unknown, a condition described as primary, or essential, hypertension.

Changes in diet and life habits are the first line of defense in controlling HTN. Drugs that are used include diuretics to eliminate fluids, vasodilators to relax the blood vessels, and drugs that prevent the formation or action of angiotensin, a substance in the blood that normally acts to increase blood pressure.

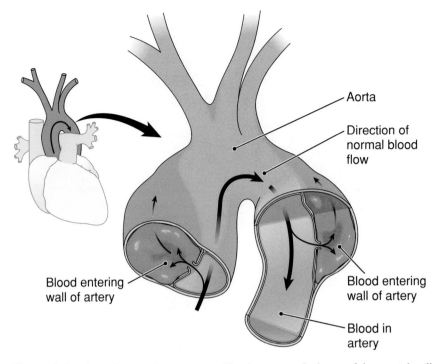

Aorta

Direction of normal blood flow

Blood entering wall of artery

Blood entering wall of artery

Blood in artery

Figure 9-9 Dissecting aortic aneurysm. Blood separates the layers of the arterial wall.

Heart Disease

Coronary Artery Disease

Coronary artery disease (CAD), which results from atherosclerosis in the vessels that supply blood to the heart muscle, is a leading cause of death in industrialized countries (see Fig. 9-8). An early sign of CAD is the type of chest pain known as **angina pectoris**. This is a feeling of constriction around the heart or pain that may radiate to the left arm or shoulder, usually brought on by exertion. Often there is anxiety, **diaphoresis** (profuse sweating), and **dyspnea** (difficulty in breathing). CAD is diagnosed by electrocardiography (ECG), **stress tests**, **coronary angiography** (imaging), **echocardiography**, and other tests.

CAD is treated by control of exercise and administration of nitroglycerin to dilate coronary vessels. Other drugs may be used to regulate the heartbeat, strengthen the force of heart contraction, or prevent formation of blood clots.

Patients with severe cases of CAD may be candidates for **angioplasty**, surgical dilatation of the blocked vessel by means of a balloon catheter, a procedure technically called percutaneous transluminal coronary angioplasty (PTCA) (Fig. 9-10). Angioplasty may include placement of a **stent**, a small mesh tube, to keep the vessel open (Fig. 9-11). Stents prevent recoil of the vessel, and newer versions release drugs to prevent vascular restenosis.

If further intervention is required, surgeons can bypass the blocked vessel or vessels with a vascular graft (Fig. 9-12). In this procedure, known as a **coronary artery bypass graft (CABG)**, another vessel or a piece of another vessel, usually the left internal mammary artery or part of the leg's saphenous vein, is grafted and used to carry blood from the aorta to a point past the obstruction in a coronary vessel.

Myocardial Infarction (MI)

Degenerative changes in the arteries predispose a person to thrombosis and sudden **occlusion** (obstruction) of a coronary artery. The resultant area of myocardial necrosis is termed an **infarct** (Fig. 9-13), and the process is known as **myocardial infarction** (MI), the "heart attack" that may cause sudden death. Symptoms of MI include pain over the heart (precordial pain) or upper part of the abdomen (epigastric pain) that may extend

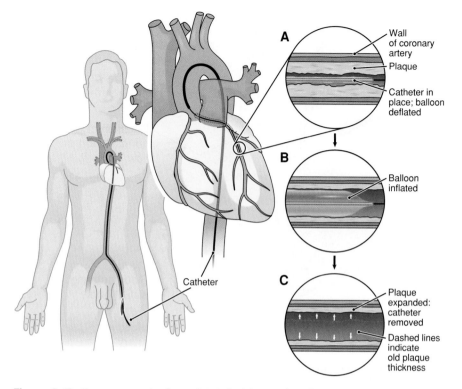

Figure 9-10 Coronary angioplasty (PTCA). (*A*) A guide catheter is threaded into the coronary artery. (*B*) A balloon catheter is inserted through the occlusion. (*C*) The balloon is inflated and deflated until plaque is flattened and the vessel is opened.

to the jaw or arms, pallor (paleness), diaphoresis, nausea, and dyspnea. There may be a burning sensation similar to indigestion or heartburn.

MI is diagnosed by electrocardiography and assays for specific substances in the blood. **Creatine kinase** (CK) is an enzyme normal to muscle cells. It is released in increased amounts when muscle tissue is injured. The form of CK specific to cardiac muscle cells is creatine kinase MB (CK-MB). **Troponin** (Tn) is a protein that regulates contraction in muscle cells. Increased serum levels, particularly the forms TnT and TnI, indicate MI.

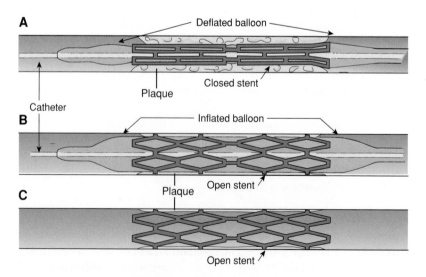

Figure 9-11 Arterial stent. (*A*) Stent closed, before balloon inflation (*B*) Stent open, balloon inflated; stent will remain expanded after balloon is deflated and removed. (*C*) Stent open, balloon removed.

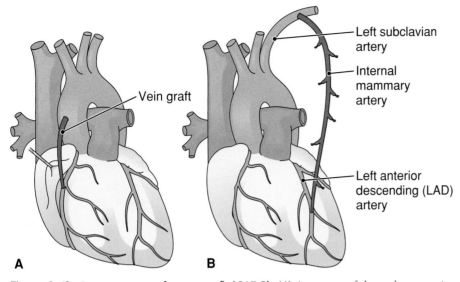

Figure 9-12 Coronary artery bypass graft (CABG). (*A*) A segment of the saphenous vein carries blood from the aorta to a part of the right coronary artery that is distal to an occlusion. (*B*) The mammary artery is used to bypass an obstruction in the left anterior descending (LAD) coronary artery.

Patient outcome is based on the degree of damage and the speed of treatment to dissolve the clot and to reestablish normal blood flow and heart rhythm.

Arrhythmia

Arrhythmia is any irregularity of heart rhythm, such as a higher- or lower-than-average heart rate, extra beats, or an alteration in the pattern of the beat. **Bradycardia** is a slower-than-average rate, and **tachycardia** is a higher-than-average rate.

Damage to cardiac tissue, as by myocardial infarction, may result in **heart block**, an interruption in the heart's electrical conduction system resulting in arrhythmia (Fig. 9-14). Heart block is classified in order of increasing severity as first-, second-, or third-degree heart block. Block in a bundle branch is designated as a left or right bundle branch block (BBB).

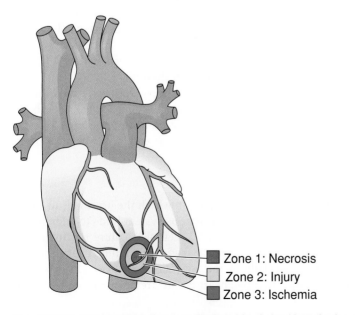

Zone 1: Necrosis
Zone 2: Injury
Zone 3: Ischemia

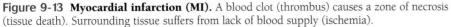

Figure 9-13 Myocardial infarction (MI). A blood clot (thrombus) causes a zone of necrosis (tissue death). Surrounding tissue suffers from lack of blood supply (ischemia).

9

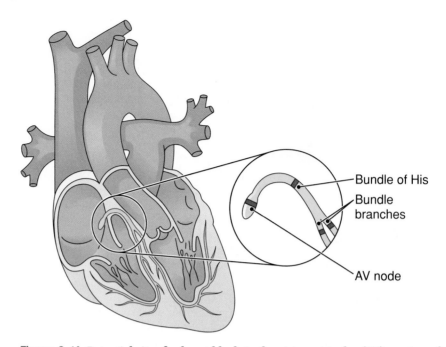

Figure 9-14 Potential sites for heart block in the atrioventricular (AV) portion of the heart's conduction system.

Bundle of His
Bundle branches
AV node

If, for any reason, the SA node is not generating a normal heartbeat or there is heart block, an **artificial pacemaker** may be implanted to regulate the beat (Fig. 9-15). Usually the pacemaker is inserted under the skin below the clavicle, and leads are threaded through veins into one or both of the right chambers. Some pacemakers act only when the heart is not functioning on its own, and some adjust to the need for a change in heart rate based on activity.

MI is also a common cause of **fibrillation**, an extremely rapid, ineffective beating of the heart, especially dangerous when it affects the ventricles. **Cardioversion** is the general term for restoration of a normal heart rhythm, either by drugs or application of electric current. Hospital personnel use external chest "paddles" for emergency electrical **defibrillation**. In addition to **cardiopulmonary resuscitation** (CPR), automated external defibrillators (AED) can help save lives when available for high-risk patients or in public places, such as malls, aircraft, and sports venues. The AED detects fatal arrhythmia and automatically delivers a correct preprogrammed shock. An implantable cardioverter–defibrillator (ICD), applied much like a pacemaker, detects potential fibrillation and automatically shocks the heart to restore normal rhythm.

A newer approach to the treatment of heart rhythm irregularities is **ablation**, or destruction, of the portion of the conduction pathway that is involved in the arrhythmia. Electrode catheter ablation (ECA) uses high-frequency sound waves, freezing (cryoablation), or electrical energy delivered through an intravascular catheter to ablate a defect in the conduction pathway.

Heart Failure

The general term **heart failure** refers to any condition in which the heart fails to empty effectively. The resulting increased pressure in the venous system leads to **edema**, justifying the description *congestive heart failure* (CHF). Left-side failure results in pulmonary edema with breathing difficulties (dyspnea); right-side failure causes peripheral edema with tissue swelling, especially in the legs, along with weight gain from fluid retention. Other symptoms of congestive heart failure are **cyanosis**, and **syncope** (fainting).

Heart failure is treated with rest, drugs to strengthen heart contractions, diuretics to eliminate fluid, and restriction of salt in the diet.

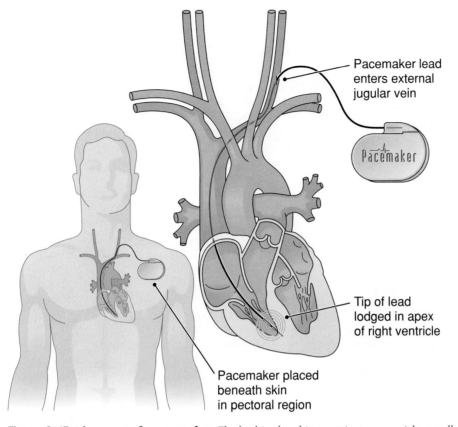

Pacemaker lead
enters external
jugular vein

Pacemaker

Tip of lead
lodged in apex
of right ventricle

Pacemaker placed
beneath skin
in pectoral region

Figure 9-15 Placement of a pacemaker. The lead is placed in an atrium or ventricle, usually on the right side. A dual-chamber pacemaker has leads in both chambers.

Heart failure is one cause of **shock**, a severe disturbance in the circulatory system resulting in inadequate blood delivery to the tissues. Shock is classified according to cause as:

➤ Cardiogenic shock, caused by heart failure
➤ Hypovolemic shock, caused by loss of blood volume
➤ Septic shock, caused by bacterial infection
➤ Anaphylactic shock, caused by severe allergic reaction

Congenital Heart Disease

A congenital defect is any defect that is present at birth. The most common type of congenital heart defect is a **septal defect**, a hole in the septum (wall) that separates the atria or the one that separates the ventricles (Fig. 9-16). An atrial septal defect often results from persistence of an opening, the foramen ovale, that allows blood to bypass the lungs in fetal circulation. A septal defect permits blood to shunt from the left to the right side of the heart and return to the lungs instead of flowing out to the body. The heart has to work harder to meet the tissues' needs for oxygen. Symptoms of septal defect include cyanosis (leading to the description "blue baby"), syncope, and **clubbing** of the fingers.

Another congenital defect that results from persistence of a fetal modification is **patent ductus arteriosus** (see Fig. 9-16D). In this case, a small bypass between the pulmonary artery and the aorta fails to close at birth. Blood then can flow from the aorta to the pulmonary artery and return to the lungs.

Malformation of a heart valve is another type of congenital heart defect. Failure of a valve to open or close properly is evidenced by a **murmur**, an abnormal sound heard as the heart cycles. A localized narrowing, or **coarctation of the aorta**, is a congenital

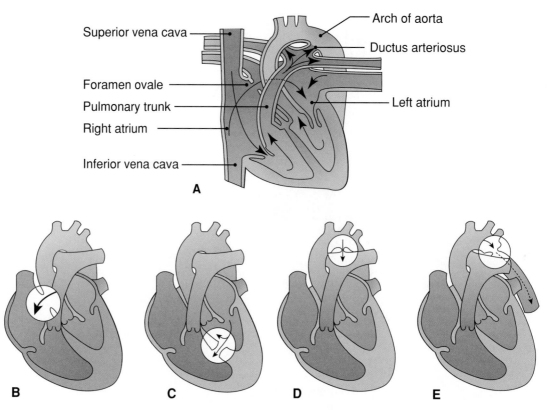

Figure 9-16 Congenital heart defects. (*A*) Normal fetal heart showing the foramen ovale and ductus arteriosus. (*B*) Persistence of the foramen ovale results in an atrial septal defect. (*C*) A ventricular septal defect. (*D*) Persistence of the ductus arteriosus (patent ductus arteriosus) forces blood back into the pulmonary artery. (*E*) Coarctation of the aorta restricts outward blood flow in the aorta.

defect that restricts blood flow through that vessel (see Fig. 9-16E). Most of the congenital defects described can be corrected surgically.

Rheumatic Heart Disease

In **rheumatic heart disease**, infection with a specific type of streptococcus sets up an immune reaction that ultimately damages the heart valves. The infection usually begins as a "strep throat," and most often it is the mitral valve that is involved. Scar tissue fuses the leaflets of the valve, causing a narrowing or **stenosis** that interferes with proper function. People with rheumatic heart disease are subject to repeated infections of the valves and must take antibiotics prophylactically (preventively) before any type of surgery and before even minor invasive procedures such as dental cleaning. Severe cases of rheumatic heart disease may require surgical correction or even valve replacement. The incidence of rheumatic heart disease has declined with the use of antibiotics.

Disorders of the Veins

A breakdown in the valves of the veins in combination with a chronic dilatation of these vessels results in **varicose veins** (Fig. 9-17). These appear twisted and swollen under the skin, most commonly in the legs. Contributing factors include heredity, obesity, prolonged standing, and pregnancy, which increases pressure in the pelvic veins. Varicosities can impede blood flow and lead to edema, thrombosis, hemorrhage, or ulceration. Treatment includes the wearing of elastic stockings and, in some cases, surgical removal of the varicose veins, after which collateral circulation is naturally established. A varicose vein in the rectum or anal canal is referred to as a **hemorrhoid**.

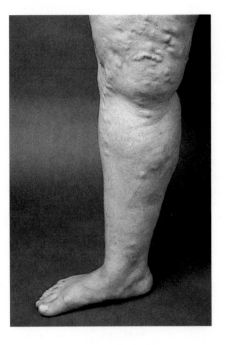

Figure 9-17 Varicose veins.

Phlebitis is any inflammation of the veins and may be caused by infection, injury, poor circulation, or damage to valves in the veins. Such inflammation typically initiates formation of a blood clot, resulting in **thrombophlebitis**. Any veins are subject to thrombophlebitis, but the more serious condition involves the deep veins as opposed to the superficial veins, in the condition termed **deep vein thrombosis** (DVT). The most common sites for DVT are the deep veins of the legs, causing serious reduction in venous drainage from these areas.

TERMINOLOGY Key Terms

CARDIOVASCULAR DISORDERS

aneurysm *AN-ū-rizm*	A localized abnormal dilation of a blood vessel, usually an artery, caused by weakness of the vessel wall; may eventually burst
angina pectoris *an-JĪ-na PEK-tō-ris*	A feeling of constriction around the heart or pain that may radiate to the left arm or shoulder, usually brought on by exertion; caused by insufficient blood supply to the heart
arrhythmia *a-RITH-mē-a*	Any abnormality in the rate or rhythm of the heartbeat (literally "without rhythm"; note doubled r). Also called *dysrhythmia*.
arteriosclerosis *ar-tēr-ē-ō-skler-Ō-sis*	Hardening (sclerosis) of the arteries, with loss of capacity and loss of elasticity, as from fatty deposits (plaque), deposit of calcium salts, or formation of scar tissue
atherosclerosis *ath-er-ō-skler-Ō-sis*	The development of fatty, fibrous patches (plaques) in the lining of arteries, causing narrowing of the lumen and hardening of the vessel wall. The most common form of arteriosclerosis (hardening of the arteries). The root *ather/o* means "porridge" or "gruel."
bradycardia *brad-ē-KAR-dē-a*	A slow heart rate, of less than 60 beats per minute

TERMINOLOGY   Key Terms
Continued

cerebrovascular accident (CVA) *ser-e-brō-VAS-kū-lar*	Sudden damage to the brain resulting from reduction of blood flow. Causes include atherosclerosis, embolism, thrombosis, or hemorrhage from a ruptured aneurysm; commonly called stroke.
clubbing *KLUB-ing*	Enlargement of the ends of the fingers and toes caused by growth of the soft tissue around the nails (see Fig. 7-12). Seen in a variety of diseases in which there is poor peripheral circulation.
coarctation of the aorta *kō-ark-TĀ-shun*	Localized narrowing on the aorta with restriction of blood flow (see Fig. 9-16E)
cyanosis *sī-a-NŌ-sis*	Bluish discoloration of the skin caused by lack of oxygen (see Fig. 3-4)
deep vein thrombosis (DVT)	Thrombophlebitis involving the deep veins
diaphoresis *dī-a-fō-RĒ-sis*	Profuse sweating
dissecting aneurysm	An aneurysm in which blood enters the arterial wall and separates the layers. Usually involves the aorta (see Fig. 9-9).
dyslipidemia *dis-lip-i-DĒ-mē-a*	Disorder in serum lipid levels, which is an important factor in development of atherosclerosis. Includes hyperlipidemia (high lipids), hypercholesterolemia (high cholesterol), and hypertriglyceridemia (high triglycerides).
dyspnea *DYSP-nē-a*	Difficult or labored breathing (*-pnea*)
edema *e-DĒ-ma*	Swelling of body tissues caused by the presence of excess fluid (see Fig. 6-4). Causes include cardiovascular disturbances, kidney failure, inflammation, and malnutrition.
embolism *EM-bō-lizm*	Obstruction of a blood vessel by a blood clot or other matter carried in the circulation
embolus *EM-bō-lus*	A mass carried in the circulation. Usually a blood clot, but also may be air, fat, bacteria, or other solid matter from within or from outside the body.
fibrillation *fi-bri-LĀ-shun*	Spontaneous, quivering, and ineffectual contraction of muscle fibers, as in the atria or the ventricles
heart block	An interference in the conduction system of the heart resulting in arrhythmia (see Fig. 9-14).
heart failure	A condition caused by the inability of the heart to maintain adequate circulation of blood
hemorrhoid *HEM-ō-royd*	A varicose vein in the rectum
hypertension *hī-per-TEN-shun*	A condition of higher-than-normal blood pressure. Essential (primary, idiopathic) hypertension has no known cause.

TERMINOLOGY *Continued*

Key Terms

9

infarct *in-FARKT*	An area of localized necrosis (death) of tissue resulting from a blockage or a narrowing of the artery that supplies the area
ischemia *is-KĒ-mē-a*	Local deficiency of blood supply caused by obstruction of the circulation (root: *hem/o*)
murmur	An abnormal heart sound
myocardial infarction (MI) *mī-ō-KAR-dē-al in-FARK-shun*	Localized necrosis (death) of cardiac muscle tissue resulting from blockage or narrowing of the coronary artery that supplies that area. Myocardial infarction is usually caused by formation of a thrombus (clot) in a vessel (see Fig. 9-13).
occlusion *ō-KLŪ-zhun*	A closing off or obstruction, as of a vessel
patent ductus arteriosus *PĀ-tent DUK-tus ar-tēr-ē-Ō-sus*	Persistence of the ductus arteriosus after birth. The ductus arteriosus is a vessel that connects the pulmonary artery to the descending aorta in the fetus to bypass the lungs (see Fig 9-16D)
phlebitis *fle-BĪ-tis*	Inflammation of a vein
plaque *plak*	A patch. With regard to the cardiovascular system, a deposit of fatty material and other substances on a vessel wall that impedes blood flow and may block the vessel. Atheromatous plaque.
rheumatic heart disease *rū-MAT-ik*	Damage to heart valves after infection with a type of streptococcus (group A hemolytic streptococcus). The antibodies produced in response to the infection produce scarring of the valves, usually the mitral valve.
septal defect *SEP-tal*	An opening in the septum between the atria or ventricles; a common cause is persistence of the foramen ovale (*for-Ā-men ō-VAL-ē*), an opening between the atria that bypasses the lungs in fetal circulation (see Figs. 9-16B and C)
shock	Circulatory failure resulting in an inadequate supply of blood to the tissues. Cardiogenic shock is caused by heart failure; hypovolemic shock is caused by a loss of blood volume; septic shock is caused by bacterial infection.
sinus rhythm *SĪ-nus*	A normal heart rhythm originating from the sinoatrial (SA) node
stenosis *ste-NŌ-sis*	Constriction or narrowing of an opening
stroke	See *cerebrovascular accident*
syncope *SIN-kō-pē*	A temporary loss of consciousness caused by inadequate blood flow to the brain; fainting
tachycardia *tak-i-KAR-dē-a*	An abnormally rapid heart rate, usually over 100 beats per minute

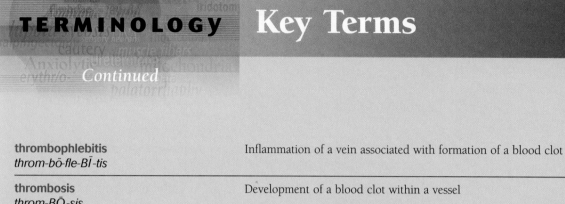

TERMINOLOGY Key Terms
Continued

thrombophlebitis *throm-bō-fle-BĪ-tis*	Inflammation of a vein associated with formation of a blood clot
thrombosis *throm-BŌ-sis*	Development of a blood clot within a vessel
thrombus *THROM-bus*	A blood clot that forms within a blood vessel (root: *thromb/o*)
varicose vein *VAR-i-kōs*	A twisted and swollen vein resulting from breakdown of the valves, pooling of blood, and chronic dilatation of the vessel (root: *varic/o*); also called varix (*VAR-iks*) or varicosity (*var-i-KOS-i-tē*) (see Fig. 9-17)

DIAGNOSIS AND TREATMENT

angioplasty *AN-jē-ō-plas-tē*	A procedure that reopens a narrowed vessel and restores blood flow. Commonly accomplished by surgically removing plaque, inflating a balloon within the vessel, or installing a device (stent) to keep the vessel open. (see Figs. 9-10 and 9-11)
artificial pacemaker	A battery-operated device that generates electrical impulses to regulate the beating of the heart. It may be external or implanted, may be designed to respond to need, and may have the capacity to prevent tachycardia (see Fig. 9-15).
cardiopulmonary resuscitation (CPR) *rē-sus-i-TĀ-shun*	Restoration of cardiac output and pulmonary ventilation after cardiac arrest using artificial respiration and chest compression or cardiac massage
cardioversion *KAR-dē-ō-ver-zhun*	Correction of an abnormal cardiac rhythm. May be accomplished pharmacologically, with antiarrhythmic drugs, or by application of electric current (see defibrillation).
coronary angiography *an-jē-OG-ra-fē*	Radiographic study of the coronary arteries after introduction of an opaque dye by means of a catheter
coronary artery bypass graft (CABG)	Surgical creation of a shunt to bypass a blocked coronary artery. The aorta is connected to a point past the obstruction with another vessel or a piece of another vessel, usually the left internal mammary artery or part of the leg's saphenous vein (see Fig. 9-12).
creatine kinase MB (CK-MB) *krē-a-tin KĪ-nāz*	Enzyme released in increased amounts from cardiac muscle cells following myocardial infarction (MI). Serum assays help diagnose MI and determine the extent of muscle damage.
defibrillation *dē-fib-ri-LĀ-shun*	Use of an electronic device (defibrillator) to stop fibrillation by delivering a brief electric shock to the heart. The shock may be delivered to the surface of the chest, as by an automated external defibrillator (AED), or directly into the heart through wire leads, using an implantable cardioverter defibrillator (ICD).
echocardiography (ECG) *ek-ō-kar-dē-OG-ra-fē*	A noninvasive method that uses ultrasound to visualize internal cardiac structures

TERMINOLOGY Key Terms

Continued

lipoprotein *lip-ō-PRŌ-tēn*	A compound of protein with lipid. Lipoproteins are classified according to density as very-low-density (VLDL), low-density (LDL), and high-density (HDL). Relatively higher levels of HDLs have been correlated with health of the cardiovascular system.
percutaneous transluminal coronary angioplasty (PTCA)	Dilatation of a sclerotic blood vessel by means of a balloon catheter inserted into the vessel and then inflated to flatten plaque against the artery wall (see Fig. 9-10)
stent	A small metal device in the shape of a coil or slotted tube that is placed inside an artery to keep the vessel open after balloon angioplasty (see Fig. 9-11).
stress test	Evaluation of physical fitness by continuous ECG monitoring during exercise. In a thallium stress test, a radioactive isotope of thallium is administered to trace blood flow through the heart during exercise.
troponin (Tn) *trō-PŌ-nin*	A protein in muscle cells that regulates contraction. Increased serum levels, primarily in the forms TnT and TnI, indicate recent myocardial infarction (MI).

Go to the pronunciation glossary in Chapter 9 on the CD-ROM
to hear these words pronounced.

The Lymphatic System

The **lymphatic system** is a widely distributed system with multiple functions (Fig. 9-18). Its role in circulation is to return excess fluid and proteins from the tissues to the bloodstream. Blind-ended lymphatic capillaries pick up these materials in the tissues and carry them into larger vessels (Fig. 9-19). The fluid carried in the lymphatic system is called **lymph**. Lymph drains from the lower part of the body and the upper left side into the **thoracic duct**, which travels upward through the chest and empties into the left subclavian vein near the heart (see Fig. 9-18). The **right lymphatic duct** drains the upper right side of the body and empties into the right subclavian vein.

Another major function of the lymphatic system is to protect the body from impurities and invading microorganisms (see discussion of immunity in Chapter 10). Along the path of the lymphatic vessels are small masses of lymphoid tissue, the **lymph nodes** (Fig. 9-20). Their function is to filter the lymph as it passes through. They are concentrated in the cervical (neck), axillary (armpit), mediastinal (chest), and inguinal (groin) regions. Other protective organs and tissues of the lymphatic system include the:

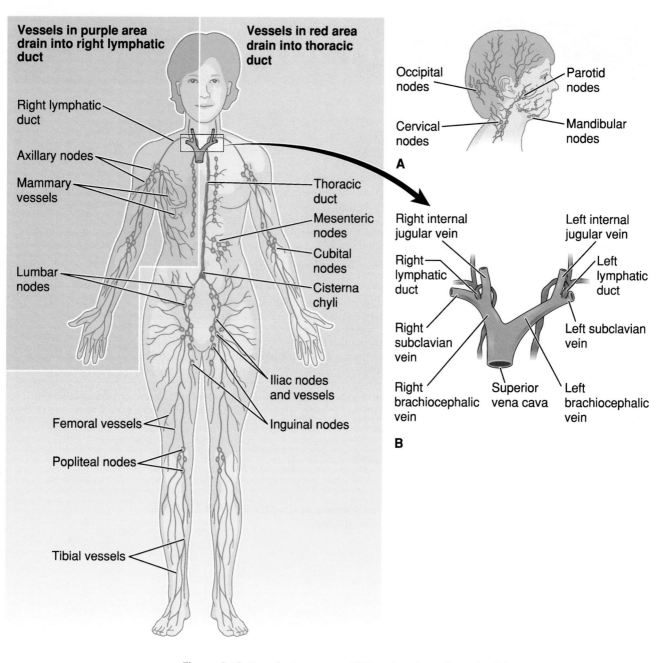

Figure 9-18 Lymphatic system. (*A*) Lymph nodes and vessels of the head. (*B*) Drainage of the right lymphatic duct and the thoracic duct into the subclavian veins.

> ➤ **Tonsils**, located in the throat (pharynx). They filter inhaled or swallowed materials and aid in immunity early in life. The tonsils are further discussed in Chapter 11.
> ➤ **Thymus gland** in the chest, above the heart. It processes and stimulates lymphocytes active in immunity.
> ➤ **Spleen** in the upper left region of the abdomen. It filters blood and destroys old red blood cells.
> ➤ **Appendix**, attached to the large intestine. It may aid in the development of immunity.

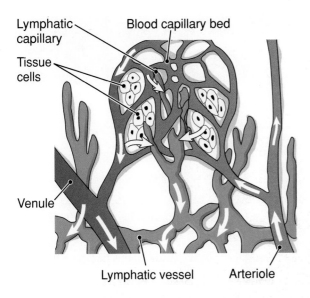

Figure 9-19 Lymphatic drainage in the tissues. Lymphatic capillaries pick up fluid and proteins left in the tissues and carry them back to the bloodstream.

➤ **Peyer patches**, in the lining of the intestine. They help protect against invading microorganisms.

A final function of the lymphatic system is to absorb digested fats from the small intestine (see Chapter 12). These fats are then added to the blood with the lymph that drains from the thoracic duct.

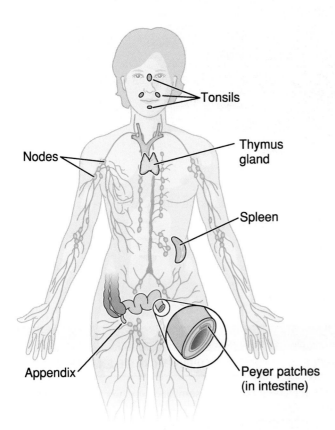

Figure 9-20 Location of lymphoid tissue.

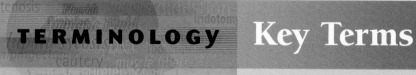

TERMINOLOGY Key Terms

Lymphatic System

NORMAL STRUCTURE AND FUNCTION

appendix *a-PEN-diks*	A small, fingerlike mass of lymphoid tissue attached to the first part of the large intestine
lymph *limf*	The thin plasmalike fluid that drains from the tissues and is transported in lymphatic vessels (root: *lymph/o*)
lymph node	A small mass of lymphoid tissue along the path of a lymphatic vessel that filters lymph (root: *lymphaden/o*)
lymphatic system *lim-FAT-ik*	The system that drains fluid and proteins from the tissues and returns them to the bloodstream. This system also participates in immunity and aids in absorption of fats from the digestive tract.
Peyer patches *PĪ-er*	Aggregates of lymphoid tissue in the lining of the intestine
right lymphatic duct	The lymphatic duct that drains fluid from the upper right side of the body
spleen	A large reddish-brown organ in the upper left region of the abdomen. It filters blood and destroys old red blood cells (root: *splen/o*).
thoracic duct	The lymphatic duct that drains fluid from the upper left side of the body and all of the lower portion of the body
thymus gland *THĪ-mus*	A gland in the upper part of the chest beneath the sternum. It functions in immunity (root: *thym/o*).
tonsils *TON-silz*	Small masses of lymphoid tissue located in regions of the throat (pharynx)

Go to the pronunciation glossary in Chapter 9 on the CD-ROM to hear these words pronounced.

Table 9·3 Roots for the Lymphatic System

ROOT	MEANING	EXAMPLE	DEFINITION OF EXAMPLE
lymph/o	lymph, lymphatic system	lymphoid *LIM-foyd*	resembling lymph or lymphatic tissue
lymphaden/o	lymph node	lymphadenectomy *lim-fad-e-NEK-tō-mē*	surgical removal of a lymph node

Table 9·3	Continued		
lymphangi/o	lymphatic vessel	lymphangiography *lim-fan-jē-OG-ra-fē*	x-ray study of lymphatic vessels
splen/o	spleen	splenalgia *splē-NAL-jē-a*	pain in the spleen
thym/o	thymus gland	athymia *a-THĪ-mē-a*	absence of the thymus gland
tonsill/o	tonsil	tonsillar *TON-sil-ar*	pertaining to a tonsil

9

Exercise 9-3

Fill in the blanks:

1. Lymphedema (*limf-e-DĒ-ma*) means swelling caused by obstruction of the flow of

   _____.

2. Lymphadenitis (*lim-fad-e-NĪ-tis*) is inflammation of a(n) _____.

3. A lymphangioma (*lim-fan-jē-Ō-ma*) is a tumor of _____.

4. The adjective *splenic* (*SPLEN-ik*) means pertaining to the _____.

5. Thymectomy (*thī-MEK-tō-mē*) is surgical removal of the _____.

6. Tonsillopathy (*ton-sil-OP-a-thē*) is any disease of the _____.

Identify and define the root in the following words:

		Root	**Meaning of Root**
7.	lymphangial (*lim-FAN-jē-al*)	lymphangi/o	lymphatic vessel
8.	lymphadenography (*lim-fad-e-NOG-ra-fē*)	_____	_____
9.	perisplenitis (*per-i-splē-NĪ-tis*)	_____	_____
10.	hypothymism (*hī-pō-THĪ-mizm*)	_____	_____
11.	tonsillectomy (*ton-sil-EK-tō-mē*)	_____	_____

Use the appropriate root to write words with the following meanings:

12. Inflammation of lymphatic vessels _____

13. A tumor (-oma) of lymphatic tissue _____

14. Any disease (-pathy) of the lymph nodes _____

15. Enlargement (-megaly) of the spleen _____

16. Pertaining to (-ic) the thymus gland _____

17. Inflammation of a tonsil _____

Clinical Aspects of the Lymphatic System

Changes in the lymphatic system often are related to infection and may consist of inflammation and enlargement of the nodes, called **lymphadenitis**, or inflammation of the vessels, called **lymphangiitis**. Obstruction of lymphatic vessels because of surgical excision or infection results in tissue swelling, or **lymphedema** (see Box 9-3). Any neoplastic disease involving lymph nodes is termed **lymphoma**. These neoplastic disorders affect the white cells found in the lymphatic system, and they are discussed more fully in Chapter 10.

Box 9•3 **Clinical Perspectives** *Lymphedema: When Lymph Stops Flowing*

Fluid balance in the body requires appropriate distribution of fluid among the cardiovascular system, lymphatic system, and the tissues. **Edema** occurs when the balance is tipped toward excess fluid in the tissues. Often, edema is due to heart failure. However, blockage of lymphatic vessels (with resulting fluid accumulation in the tissues) can cause another form of edema, called **lymphedema**. The clinical hallmark of lymphedema is chronic swelling of an arm or leg, whereas heart failure usually causes swelling of both legs.

Lymphedema may be either primary or secondary. Primary lymphedema is a rare congenital condition caused by abnormal development of lymphatic vessels. Secondary lymphedema, or acquired lymphedema, can develop as a result of trauma to a limb, surgery, radiation therapy, or infection of the lymphatic vessels (lymphangitis). One of the most common causes of lymphedema is the removal of axillary lymph nodes during mastectomy, which disrupts lymph flow from the adjacent arm. Lymphedema may also occur following prostate surgery.

Therapies that encourage the flow of fluid through the lymphatic vessels are useful in treating lymphedema. These therapies may include elevation of the affected limb, manual lymphatic drainage through massage, light exercise, and firm wrapping of the limb to apply compression. In addition, changes in daily habits can lessen the effects of lymphedema. For example, further blockage of lymph drainage can be prevented by wearing loose clothing and jewelry, carrying a purse or handbag on the unaffected arm, and not crossing the legs when sitting. Lymphangitis requires the use of appropriate antibiotics. Prompt treatment is necessary because, in addition to swelling, other complications include poor wound healing, skin ulcers, and increased risk of infection.

TERMINOLOGY Key Clinical Terms

LYMPHATIC DISORDERS

lymphadenitis *lim-fad-e-NĪ-tis*	Inflammation and enlargement of lymph nodes, usually as a result of infection
lymphangiitis *lim-fan-jē-Ī-tis*	Inflammation of lymphatic vessels as a result of bacterial infection. Appears as painful red streaks under the skin. (Also spelled *lymphangitis*.)
lymphedema *lim-fe-DĒ-ma*	Swelling of tissues with lymph caused by obstruction or excision of lymphatic vessels (see Box 9-3)
lymphoma *lim-FŌ-ma*	Any neoplastic disease of lymphoid tissue

Go to the pronunciation glossary in Chapter 9 on the CD-ROM to hear these words pronounced.

TERMINOLOGY   Supplementary Terms

NORMAL STRUCTURE AND FUNCTION

apical pulse	Pulse felt or heard over the apex of the heart. It is measured in the fifth left intercostal space (between the ribs) about 8 to 9 cm from the midline.
cardiac output	The amount of blood pumped from the right or left ventricle per minute
Korotkoff sounds *ko-rot-KOF*	Arterial sounds heard with a stethoscope during determination of blood pressure with a cuff
perfusion *per-FŪ-zhun*	The passage of fluid, such as blood, through an organ or tissue
precordium *prē-KOR-dē-um*	The anterior region over the heart and the lower part of the thorax; adjective, precordial
pulse pressure	The difference between systolic and diastolic pressure
stroke volume	The amount of blood ejected by the left ventricle with each beat
Valsalva maneuver *val-SAL-va*	Bearing down, as in childbirth or defecation, by attempting to exhale forcefully with the nose and throat closed. This action has an effect on the cardiovascular system.

SYMPTOMS AND CONDITIONS

bruit *brwē*	An abnormal sound heard in auscultation
cardiac tamponade *tam-pon-ĀD*	Pathologic accumulation of fluid in the pericardial sac. May result from pericarditis or injury to the heart or great vessels.
ectopic beat *ek-TOP-ik*	A heartbeat that originates from some part of the heart other than the SA node
extrasystole *eks-tra-SIS-tō-lē*	Premature contraction of the heart that occurs separately from the normal beat and originates from a part of the heart other than the SA node
flutter	Very rapid (200 to 300 beats per minute) but regular contractions, as in the atria or the ventricles
hypotension *hī-po-TEN-shun*	A condition of lower-than-normal blood pressure
intermittent claudication *claw-di-KĀ-shun*	Pain in a muscle during exercise caused by inadequate blood supply. The pain disappears with rest.
mitral valve prolapse	Movement of the cusps of the mitral valve into the left atrium when the ventricles contract
occlusive vascular disease	Arteriosclerotic disease of the vessels, usually peripheral vessels
palpitation *pal-pi-TĀ-shun*	A sensation of abnormally rapid or irregular heartbeat (Fig. 9-21)
pitting edema	Edema that retains the impression of a finger pressed firmly into the skin

Supplementary Terms

polyarteritis nodosa *nō-DŌ-sa*	Potentially fatal collagen disease causing inflammation of small visceral arteries. Symptoms depend on the organ affected.
Raynaud disease *rā-NŌ*	A disorder characterized by abnormal constriction of peripheral vessels in the arms and legs on exposure to cold
regurgitation *rē-gur-ji-TĀ-shun*	A backward flow, such as the backflow of blood through a defective valve
stasis *STĀ-sis*	Stoppage of normal flow, as of blood or urine. Blood stasis may lead to dermatitis and ulcer formation.
subacute bacterial endocarditis (SBE)	Growth of bacteria in a heart or valves previously damaged by rheumatic fever
tetralogy of Fallot *fal-Ō*	A combination of four congenital heart abnormalities: pulmonary artery stenosis, interventricular septal defect, displacement of the aorta to the right, and right ventricular hypertrophy
thromboangiitis obliterans	Inflammation and thrombus formation resulting in occlusion of small vessels, especially in the legs. Most common in young men and correlated with heavy smoking. Thrombotic occlusion of leg vessels may lead to gangrene of the feet. Patients show a hypersensitivity to tobacco. Also called *Buerger disease*.
vegetation	Irregular outgrowths of bacteria on the heart valves; associated with rheumatic fever
Wolff–Parkinson–White syndrome (WPW)	A cardiac arrhythmia consisting of tachycardia and a premature ventricular beat caused by an alternative conduction pathway

DIAGNOSIS

cardiac catheterization	Passage of a catheter into the heart through a vessel to inject a contrast medium for imaging, diagnosing abnormalities, obtaining samples, or measuring pressure
central venous pressure (CVP)	Pressure in the superior vena cava
cineangiocardiography *sin-e-an-jē-ō-kar-dē-OG-ra-fē*	The photographic recording of fluoroscopic images of the heart and large vessels using motion-picture techniques
Doppler echocardiography	An imaging method used to study the rate and pattern of blood flow
heart scan	Imaging of the heart after injection of a radioactive isotope. The PYP (pyrophosphate) scan using technetium-99m (^{99m}Tc) is used to test for myocardial infarction because the isotope is taken up by damaged tissue. The MUGA (multigated acquisition) scan gives information on heart function.
Holter monitor	A portable device that can record up to 24 hours of an individual's ECG readings during normal activity

TERMINOLOGY
Continued

Supplementary Terms

homocysteine *hō-mō-SIS-tēn*	An amino acid in the blood that at higher-than-normal levels is associated with increased risk of cardiovascular disease
phlebotomist *fle-BOT-ō-mist*	Technician who specializes in drawing blood
phonocardiography *fō-nō-kar-dē-OG-ra-fē*	Electronic recording of heart sounds
plethysmography *ple-thiz-MOG-ra-fē*	Measurement of changes in the size of a part based on the amount of blood contained in or passing through it. Impedance plethysmography measures changes in electrical resistance and is used in the diagnosis of deep vein thrombosis.
pulmonary capillary wedge pressure (PCWP)	Pressure measured by a catheter in a branch of the pulmonary artery. It is an indirect measure of pressure in the left atrium. (see Box 9-2)
Swan–Ganz catheter	A cardiac catheter with a balloon at the tip that is used to measure pulmonary arterial pressure. It is flow-guided through a vein into the right side of the heart and then into the pulmonary artery.
transesophageal echocardiography (TEE)	Use of an ultrasound transducer placed endoscopically into the esophagus to obtain images of the heart
triglycerides *trī-GLIS-er-īdz*	Simple fats that circulate in the bloodstream
ventriculography *ven-trik-ū-LOG-ra-fē*	X-ray study of the ventricles of the heart after introduction of an opaque dye by means of a catheter

TREATMENT AND SURGICAL PROCEDURES

atherectomy *ath-er-EK-tō-mē*	Removal of atheromatous plaque from the lining of a vessel. May be done by open surgery or through the lumen of the vessel.
commissurotomy *kom-i-shur-OT-ō-mē*	Surgical incision of a scarred mitral valve to increase the size of the valve opening
embolectomy *em-bō-LEK-tō-mē*	Surgical removal of an embolus
intraaortic balloon pump (IABP)	A mechanical-assist device that consists of an inflatable balloon pump inserted through the femoral artery into the thoracic aorta. It inflates during diastole to improve coronary circulation and deflates before systole to allow blood ejection from the heart.
left ventricular assist device (LVAD)	A pump that takes over the function of the left ventricle in delivering blood into the systemic circuit. These devices are used to assist patients awaiting heart transplantation or those who are recovering from heart failure.

9

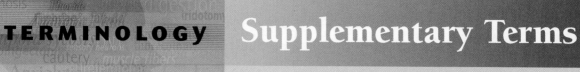

TERMINOLOGY

Supplementary Terms

Continued

MEDICATIONS

angiotensin-converting–enzyme (ACE) inhibitor	A drug that lowers blood pressure by blocking the formation in the blood of angiotensin II, a substance that normally acts to increase blood pressure
angiotensin II receptor antagonist	A drug that blocks tissue receptors for angiotensin II
antiarrhythmic agent	A drug that regulates the rate and rhythm of the heartbeat
beta-adrenergic blocking agent	Drug that decreases the rate and strength of heart contractions
calcium-channel blocker	Drug that controls the rate and force of heart contraction by regulating calcium entrance into the cells
digitalis *dij-i-TAL-is*	A drug that slows and strengthens heart muscle contractions
diuretic *dī-ū-RET-ik*	Drug that eliminates fluid by increasing the output of urine by the kidneys. Lowered blood volume decreases the workload of the heart.
hypolipidemic agent *hī-pō-lip-i-DĒ-mik*	Drug that lowers serum cholesterol
lidocaine *LĪ-dō-kān*	A local anesthetic that is used intravenously to treat cardiac arrhythmias
nitroglycerin *nī-trō-GLIS-er-in*	A drug used in the treatment of angina pectoris to dilate coronary vessels
statins	Drugs that act to lower lipids in the blood. The drug names end with -*statin*, such as lovastatin, pravastatin, atorvastatin.
streptokinase (SK) *strep-tō-KĪ-nās*	An enzyme used to dissolve blood clots
tissue plasminogen activator (tPA)	A drug used to dissolve blood clots. It activates production of a substance (plasmin) in the blood that normally dissolves clots.
vasodilator *vas-ō-dī-LĀ-tor*	A drug that widens blood vessels and improves blood flow

Go to the pronunciation glossary in Chapter 9 on the CD-ROM to hear these words pronounced.

A   **B**

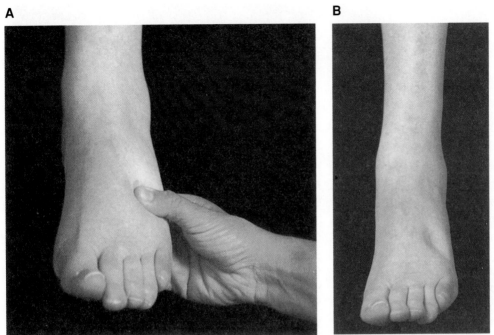

Figure 9-21 Pitting edema. When the skin is pressed firmly with the finger (*A*), a pit remains after the finger is removed (*B*).

TERMINOLOGY Abbreviations

ACE	Angiotensin-converting enzyme		**CK-MB**	Creatine kinase MB
AED	Automated external defibrillator		**CPR**	Cardiopulmonary resuscitation
AF	Atrial fibrillation		**CVA**	Cerebrovascular accident
AMI	Acute myocardial infarction		**CVD**	Cardiovascular disease
APC	Atrial premature complex		**CVI**	Chronic venous insufficiency
AR	Aortic regurgitation		**CVP**	Central venous pressure
AS	Aortic stenosis; arteriosclerosis		**DOE**	Dyspnea on exertion
ASCVD	Arteriosclerotic cardiovascular disease		**DVT**	Deep vein thrombosis
ASD	Atrial septal defect		**ECG (EKG)**	Electrocardiogram
ASHD	Arteriosclerotic heart disease		**HDL**	High-density lipoprotein
AT	Atrial tachycardia		**HTN**	Hypertension
AV	Atrioventricular		**IABP**	Intraaortic balloon pump
BBB	Bundle branch block (left or right)		**ICD**	Implantable cardioverter–defibrillator
BP	Blood pressure		**IVCD**	Intraventricular conduction delay
bpm	Beats per minute		**JVP**	Jugular venous pulse
CABG	Coronary artery bypass graft		**LAD**	Left anterior descending (coronary artery)
CAD	Coronary artery disease		**LAHB**	Left anterior hemiblock
CCU	Coronary/cardiac care unit		**LDL**	Low-density lipoprotein
CHD	Coronary heart disease		**LV**	Left ventricle
CHF	Congestive heart failure		**LVAD**	Left ventricular assist device

TERMINOLOGY Abbreviations

Continued

LVEDP	Left ventricular end-diastolic pressure	**PVD**	Peripheral vascular disease
LVH	Left ventricular hypertrophy	**PYP**	Pyrophosphate (scan)
MI	Myocardial infarction	**S$_1$**	First heart sound
mm Hg	Millimeters of mercury	**S$_2$**	Second heart sound
MR	Mitral regurgitation, reflux	**SA**	Sinoatrial
MS	Mitral stenosis	**SBE**	Subacute bacterial endocarditis
MUGA	Multigated acquisition (scan)	**SK**	Streptokinase
MVP	Mitral valve prolapse	**SVT**	Supraventricular tachycardia
MVR	Mitral valve replacement	**^{99m}Tc**	Technetium-99m
NSR	Normal sinus rhythm	**TEE**	Transesophageal echocardiography
P	Pulse	**Tn**	Troponin
PAC	Premature atrial contraction	**tPA**	Tissue plasminogen activator
PAP	Pulmonary arterial pressure	**VAD**	Ventricular assist device
PCI	Percutaneous coronary intervention	**VF, v fib**	Ventricular fibrillation
PCWP	Pulmonary capillary wedge pressure	**VLDL**	Very–low-density lipoprotein
PMI	Point of maximal impulse	**VPC**	Ventricular premature complex
PSVT	Paroxysmal supraventricular tachycardia	**VSD**	Ventricular septal defect
PTCA	Percutaneous transluminal coronary angioplasty	**VT**	Ventricular tachycardia
		VTE	Venous thromboembolism
PVC	Premature ventricular contraction	**WPW**	Wolff–Parkinson–White syndrome

Chapter Review

Labeling Exercise
The Cardiovascular System

Write the name of each numbered part on the corresponding line of the answer sheet:

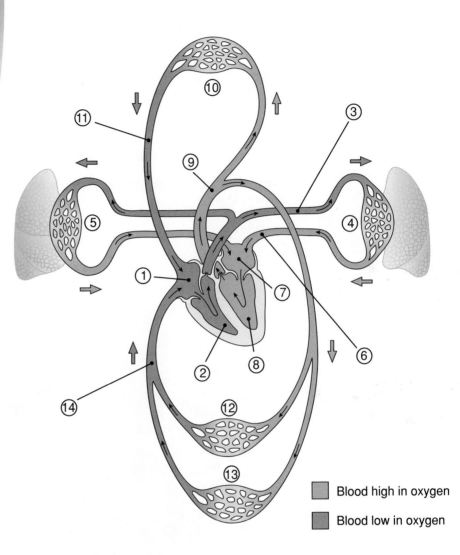

Blood high in oxygen

Blood low in oxygen

Aorta	1. _____
Head and arms	2. _____
Inferior vena cava	3. _____
Internal organs	4. _____
Left atrium	5. _____
Left lung	6. _____
Left pulmonary artery	7. _____
Left pulmonary vein	8. _____

(continued on next page)

Left ventricle   9. _____

Legs   10. _____

Right atrium   11. _____

Right lung   12. _____

Right ventricle   13. _____

Superior vena cava   14. _____

9

The Heart and Great Vessels

Write the name of each numbered part on the corresponding line of the answer sheet.

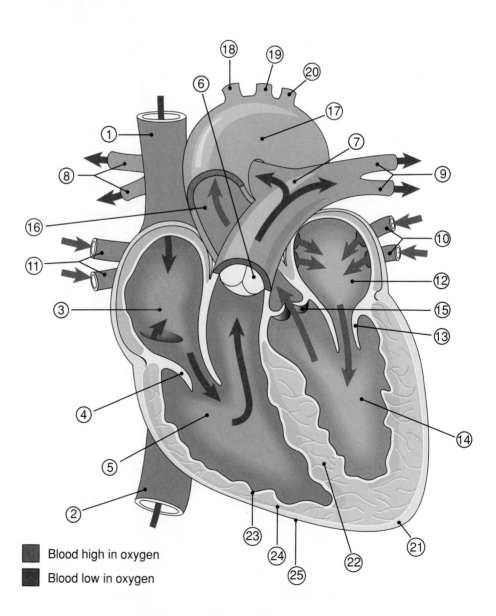

Blood high in oxygen

Blood low in oxygen

Aortic arch

Aortic valve

Apex

Ascending aorta

Brachiocephalic artery

Endocardium

Epicardium

Inferior vena cava

Interventricular septum

Left atrium

Left AV (mitral) valve

Left common carotid
artery

Left pulmonary artery
(branches)

Left pulmonary veins

Left subclavian artery

Left ventricle

Myocardium

Pulmonary artery

Pulmonary valve

Right atrium

Right AV (tricuspid) valve

Right pulmonary artery
(branches)

Right pulmonary veins

Right ventricle

Superior vena cava

1. _____

2. _____

3. _____

4. _____

5. _____

6. _____

7. _____

8. _____

9. _____

10. _____

11. _____

12. _____

13. _____

14. _____

15. _____

16. _____

17. _____

18. _____

19. _____

20. _____

21. _____

22. _____

23. _____

24. _____

25. _____

9

Location of Lymphoid Tissue

Write the name of each numbered part on the corresponding line of the answer sheet:

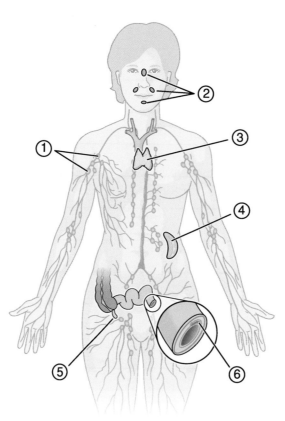

appendix	1. _____
nodes	2. _____
Peyer patches (in intestine)	3. _____
spleen	4. _____
thymus gland	5. _____
tonsils	6. _____

TERMINOLOGY

Match the following terms and write the appropriate letter to the left of each number:

_____	1. lumen	a.	vessel that empties into the right atrium
_____	2. vena cava	b.	fibrous sac around the heart
_____	3. pericardium	c.	fainting
_____	4. apex	d.	central opening of a vessel
_____	5. syncope	e.	lower pointed region of the heart

	6. ischemia	a. ineffective quivering of muscle
_____	7. occlusion	b. blockage
_____	8. fibrillation	c. accumulation of fatty deposits
_____	9. infarction	d. local deficiency of blood
_____	10. atherosclerosis	e. local death of tissue

	11. aneurysm	a. twisted and swollen vessel
_____	12. asystole	b. inflammation of the heart muscle
_____	13. thrombosis	c. absence of a heartbeat
_____	14. varix	d. localized dilatation of a vessel
_____	15. myocarditis	e. formation of a blood clot in a vessel

	16. CPR	a. surgery to bypass a blocked vessel
_____	17. CVA	b. study of the heart's electrical activity
_____	18. HTN	c. emergency cardiac care
_____	19. ECG	d. high blood pressure
_____	20. CABG	e. stroke

Supplementary Terms

	21. bruit	a. simple fat
_____	22. regurgitation	b. abnormal sound
_____	23. streptokinase	c. fluid in the pericardial sac
_____	24. triglyceride	d. drug used to dissolve blood clots
_____	25. cardiac tamponade	e. backward flow

Fill in the blanks:

26. A sinus rhythm originates in the _____.

27. Each lower pumping chamber of the heart is a(n) _____.

28. The heart muscle is the _____.

29. The microscopic vessels through which materials are exchanged between the blood and the tissues are the _____.

30. The largest artery is the _____.

31. Blood returning to the heart from the lungs enters the chamber called the _____.

32. The lymphoid organ in the chest is the _____.

33. At its termination in the abdomen, the aorta divides into the right and left (see Fig. 9-5) _____.

34. The large vein that drains the head is the (see Fig. 9-6) _____.

35. The term *varicoid* pertains to a(n) _____.

36. A phlebotomist (*fle-BOT-ō-mist*) is one who drains blood from a(n) _____.

37. The right lymphatic duct and the thoracic duct drain into vessels called the _____.

True–False. Examine the following statements. If the statement is true, write T in the first blank. If the statement is false, write F in the first blank and correct the statement by replacing the underlined word in the second blank.

38. The right AV valve is the bicuspid   _____   _____

39. The systemic circuit pumps blood to the lungs.   _____   _____

40. A vein is a vessel that carries blood away from the heart.   _____   _____

41. Diastole is the relaxation phase of the heart cycle.   _____   _____

42. The right ventricle pumps blood into the aorta.   _____   _____

43. The brachial artery supplies blood to the arm.   _____   _____

44. Peyer patches are in the intestine   _____   _____

45. Bradycardia is a lower-than-average heart rate.   _____   _____

Eliminations. In each of the sets below, underline the word that does not fit in with the rest and explain the reason for your choice:

46. AV bundle – Purkinje fibers – apex – AV node – SA node

_____

47. mm Hg – diastolic – sphygmomanometer – murmur – systolic

_____

48. U – S_1 – QRS – T – P

_____

49. thymus – cusp – tonsil – spleen – Peyer patches

_____

Define the following terms:

50. Atriotomy (*ā-trē-OT-ō-mē*) _____

51. Avascular (*ā-VAS-kū-lar*) _____

52. Lymphadenitis (*lim-fad-e-NĪ-tis*) _____

53. Splenectomy (*splē-NEK-tō-mē*) _____

54. Supraventricular (*sū-pra-ven-TRIK-ū-lar*) _____

55. Phlebectasis (*fleb-EK-ta-sis*) _____

56. Angioplasty (*an-jē-ō-PLAS-tē*) _____

Word building. Write words for the following definitions:

57. Physician who specializes in study and treatment of the heart _____

58. Suture (-rhaphy) of an artery _____

59. Surgical fixation (-pexy) of the spleen _____

60. An instrument (-tome) for incising a valve _____

61. Stoppage (-stasis) of lymph flow _____

62. Excision of a lymph node _____

Word building. Use the root *aort/o* to write words with the following meanings:

63. Downward displacement (-ptosis) of the aorta _____

64. Narrowing (-stenosis) of the aorta _____

65. Radiograph (-gram) of the aorta _____

66. Before or in front of (pre-) the aorta _____

Adjectives. Write the adjective form of the following words:

67. atrium _____

68. thymus _____

69. vein _____

70. septum _____

71. sclerosis _____

72. spleen _____

Plurals. Write the plural form of the following words:

73. thrombus _____

74. varix _____

75. stenosis _____

76. septum _____

Write the meaning of the following abbreviations as they apply to the cardiovascular system:

77. AED _____

78. LVAD _____

79. DVT _____

80. VF _____

81. BBB _____

82. PCTA _____

Word analysis. Define the following words, and give the meaning of the word parts in each. Use a dictionary if necessary.

83. Endarterectomy (*end-ar-ter-EK-tō-mē*) _____

   a. end/o- _____

   b. arteri/o _____

   c. ecto- _____

   d. -tomy _____

84. Telangiectasia (*tel-an-jē-ek-TĀ-zē-a*) _____

   a. tel- _____

   b. angi/o _____

   c. -ectasia _____

85. Lymphangiophlebitis (*lim-fan-jē-ō-fle-BĪ-tis*) _____

   a. lymph/o _____

   b. angi/o _____

   c. phleb/o _____

   d. -itis _____

Go to the word exercises in Chapter 9 on the CD-ROM for additional review exercises.

CASE STUDIES

CASE STUDY 9–1: PTCA and Echocardiogram

A.L., a 68-year-old woman, was admitted to the CCU with chest pain, dyspnea, diaphoresis, syncope, and nausea. She had taken three sublingual doses of nitroglycerin tablets within a 10-minute time span without relief before dialing 911. A previous stress test and thallium uptake scan suggested cardiac disease.

Her family history was significant for cardiovascular disease. Her father died at the age of 62 of an acute myocardial infarction. Her mother had bilateral carotid endarterectomies and a femoral–popliteal bypass procedure and died at the age of 72 of congestive heart failure. A.L.'s older sister died from a ruptured aortic aneurysm at the age of 65. A.L.'s ECG on admission showed tachycardia with a rate of 126 bpm with inverted T waves. A murmur was heard at S_1. Her skin color was dusky to cyanotic on her lips and fingertips. Her admitting diagnosis was possible coronary artery disease, acute myocardial infarction, and valvular disease.

Cardiac catheterization with balloon angioplasty (PTCA) was performed the next day. Significant stenosis of the left anterior descending coronary artery was shown and was treated with angioplasty and stent placement. Left ventricular function was normal.

Echocardiography, 2 days later, showed normal-sized left and enlarged right ventricular cavities. The mitral valve had normal amplitude of motion. The anterior and posterior leaflets moved in opposite directions during diastole. There was a late systolic prolapse of the mitral leaflet at rest. The left atrium was enlarged. The impression of the study was mitral prolapse with regurgitation. Surgery was recommended.

CASE STUDY 9–2: Mitral Valve Replacement Operative Report

A.L. was transferred to the operating room, placed in a supine position, and given general endotracheal anesthesia. Her pericardium was entered longitudinally through a median sternotomy. The surgeon found that her heart was enlarged, with a dilated right ventricle. The left atrium was dilated. Preoperative transesophageal echocardiography revealed severe mitral regurgitation with severe posterior and anterior prolapse. Extracorporeal circulation was established. The aorta was cross-clamped, and cardioplegic solution (to stop the heartbeat) was given into the aortic root intermittently for myocardial protection.

The left atrium was entered via the interatrial groove on the right, exposing the mitral valve. The middle scallop of the posterior leaflet was resected. The remaining leaflets were removed to the areas of the commissures and preserved for the sliding plasty. The elongated chordae were shortened to better anchor the valve cusps. The surgeon slid the posterior leaflet across the midline and sutured it in place. A no. 30 annuloplasty ring was sutured in place with interrupted no. 2-0 Dacron suture. The valve was tested by inflating the ventricle with NSS and proved to be competent. The left atrium was closed with continuous no. 4-0 Prolene suture. Air was removed from the heart. The cross-clamp was removed. Cardiac action resumed with normal sinus rhythm. After a period of cardiac recovery and attainment of normothermia, cardiopulmonary bypass was discontinued.

Protamine was given to counteract the heparin. Pacer wires were placed in the right atrium and ventricle. Silicone catheters were placed in the pleural and substernal spaces. The sternum and soft tissue wound was closed. A.L. recovered from her surgery and was discharged 6 days later.

CASE STUDY QUESTIONS

Write the word or phrase from the case study that means each of the following:

1. The state of profuse perspiration _____

2. Under the tongue _____

3. Test of cardiac function during physical exertion _____

4. Disease that includes both heart and blood vessel pathology _____

5. Excision of the inner lining along with atherosclerotic plaque from an artery (plural) _____

6. An abnormal heart sound _____

7. Bluish discoloration of the skin; sign of anoxia _____

8. The noun form of stenotic _____

9. Between the atria _____

10. Below the sternum _____

Multiple choice. Select the best answer and write the letter of your choice to the left of each number:

_____11. The word transluminal means:
    a. across a wall
    b. between branches
    c. through an outer layer
    d. through a central opening
    e. across a valve

_____12. The term that means backflow, as of blood, is:
    a. infarction
    b. regurgitation
    c. amplitude
    d. prolapse
    e. tourniquet

_____13. The term for a narrowing of the bicuspid valve is:
    a. atrial prolapse
    b. pulmonic stenosis
    c. mitral stenosis
    d. mitral prolapse
    e. atrial stenosis

_____14. Blowout of a dilated segment of the main artery is:
    a. left anterior diastole
    b. peritoneal infarction
    c. coarctation of the aorta
    d. cardiac tamponade
    e. ruptured aortic aneurysm

_____15. Sternotomy is:
    a. incision into the sternum
    b. removal of the sternum
    c. narrowing of the sternum
    d. plastic repair of the sternum
    e. surgical fixation of the sternum

_____16. Extracorporeal circulation occurs:
    a. within the brain
    b. within the pericardium
    c. within the body
    d. in the legs
    e. outside the body

9

_____17. Protamine was given to counteract the action of the heparin. This drug action is described as:
   a. antagonistic
   b. synergy
   c. potentiating
   d. similation
   e. addiction

Abbreviations. Define the following abbreviations:

18. CCU _____

19. AMI _____

20. CAD _____

21. LAD _____

22. CHF _____

23. TEE _____

24. MVR _____

Circulation

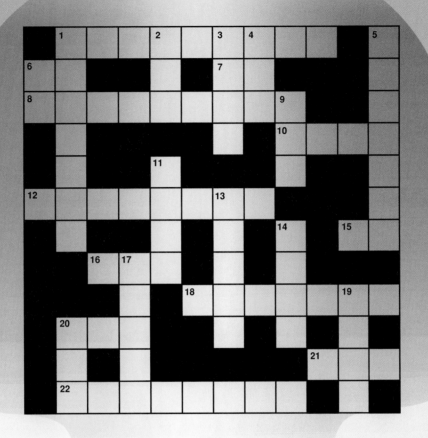

ACROSS

1. A microscopic vessel
6. Pacemaker of the heart: ____ ____ node
7. A route for injection (abbreviation)
8. The right AV valve
10. Vein: combining form
12. Relaxation phase of the heart cycle
15. Hardening of the arteries (abbreviation)
16. Substance used to dissolve blood clots (abbreviation)
18. Pulse: combining form, as in the name of blood pressure apparatus
20. Form of lipoprotein (abbreviation)
21. Heart disease associated with edema (abbreviation)
22. Part of the heart's conduction system; it receives impulses from the AV node

DOWN

1. Main artery in the neck
2. Hospital unit that cares for the critically ill (abbreviation)
3. Category of compounds that includes fats: combining form
4. Heart attack (abbreviation)
5. Obstruction circulating in the bloodstream
6. Segment of the ECG tracing
9. Thrombotic condition of the veins (abbreviation)
11. Procedure for dilating an obstructed vessel (abbreviation)
13. Fluid that circulates in the lymphatic system
14. Lymphoid organ in the chest: root
17. Vein: root
19. Units in which blood pressure is measured (abbreviation)
20. Mechanical device to assist the heart, ____ ____ ____ D (abbreviation)

CHAPTER TEN

BLOOD AND IMMUNITY

CHAPTER CONTENTS

OBJECTIVES

After study of this chapter you should be able to:

1. Describe the composition of the blood plasma.
2. Describe and give the functions of the three types of blood cells.
3. Label pictures of the blood cells.
4. Explain the basis of blood types.
5. Define immunity and list the possible sources of immunity.
6. Identify and use roots and suffixes pertaining to the blood and immunity.
7. Identify and use roots pertaining to blood chemistry.
8. List and describe the major disorders of the blood.
9. List and describe the major disorders of the immune system.
10. Describe the major tests used to study blood.
11. Interpret abbreviations used in blood studies.
12. Analyze several case studies involving the blood.

PRETEST

1. The scientific name for red blood cells is _____.

2. The scientific name for white blood cells is _____.

3. Platelets, or thrombocytes, are involved in _____.

4. The white blood cells active in adaptive immunity are the _____.

5. Substances produced by immune cells that counteract microorganisms and other foreign materials are called _____.

6. A deficiency of hemoglobin results in the disorder called _____.

7. A neoplasm involving overgrowth of white blood cells is called _____.

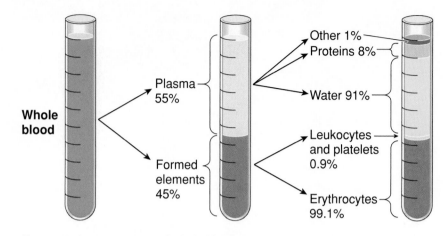

Figure 10-1 Composition of whole blood. Percentages show the relative proportions of the different components of plasma and formed elements.

Blood

Blood circulates through the vessels, bringing oxygen and nourishment to all cells and carrying away carbon dioxide and other waste products. The blood also distributes body heat and carries special substances, such as antibodies and hormones. The total adult blood volume is about 5 liters (5.2 quarts). Whole blood can be divided into two main components: the liquid portion, or **plasma** (55%), and **formed elements,** or blood cells (45%) (Fig. 10-1).

Blood Plasma

Plasma is about 90% water. The remaining 10% contains nutrients, **electrolytes** (dissolved salts), gases, **albumin** (a protein), clotting factors, antibodies, wastes, enzymes, and hormones. A multitude of these substances are tested for in blood chemistry tests. The pH (relative acidity) of the plasma remains steady at about 7.4.

Blood Cells

The blood cells (Fig. 10-2) are **erythrocytes,** or red blood cells (RBCs); **leukocytes,** or white blood cells (WBCs); and **platelets,** also called **thrombocytes.** All blood cells are produced in red bone marrow. Some white blood cells multiply in lymphoid tissue as well. Reference Box 10-1 summarizes the different types of blood cells; Box 10-2 discusses time-saving acronyms, such as RBC and WBC.

Erythrocytes

The major function of erythrocytes is to carry oxygen to cells. This oxygen is bound to an iron-containing pigment in the cells called **hemoglobin.** Erythrocytes are small, disk-shaped cells with no nucleus (Fig 10-3). Their concentration of about 5 million per µL (microliter; mcL) of blood makes them by far the most numerous of the blood cells. The

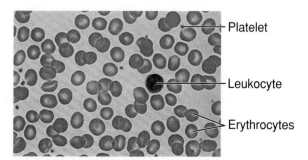

Figure 10-2 Blood cells. When viewed under a microscope, all three types of formed elements are visible.

Box 10·1 For Your Reference *Blood Cells*

Cells	Number per μL of Blood	Description	Function
Erythrocyte (red blood cell)	5 million	Tiny (7 μm diameter), biconcave disk without nucleus (anuclear)	Carries oxygen bound to hemoglobin; also carries some carbon dioxide and buffers blood
Leukocyte (white blood cell)	5,000 to 10,000	Larger than red cell with prominent nucleus that may be segmented (granulocyte) or unsegmented (agranulocyte); varies in staining properties	Protects against pathogens. Destroys foreign matter and debris. Some are active in the immune system. Located in blood, tissues, and lymphatic system.
Platelet	150,000 to 450,000	Fragment of large cell (megakaryocyte)	Hemostasis. Forms a platelet plug and starts blood clotting (coagulation).

hemoglobin that they carry averages 15 g per dL (100 mL) of blood. A red blood cell gradually wears out and dies in about 120 days, so these cells must be constantly replaced. Production of red cells in the bone marrow is regulated by the hormone **erythropoietin** (EPO), which is made in the kidneys.

Leukocytes

White blood cells all show prominent nuclei when stained (Fig. 10-4). They total about 5000 to 10,000 per μL, but their number may increase during infection. There are five types of leukocytes, which are identified by the size and appearance of the nucleus and by their staining properties:

➤ **Granulocytes,** or granular leukocytes, have visible granules in the cytoplasm when stained. The nucleus of a granulocyte is segmented. There are three types of granulocytes, named for the kind of stain (dye) they take up:

Box 10·2 Focus on Words *Acronyms*

Acronyms are abbreviations that use the first letters of the words in a name or phrase. They have become very popular because they save time and space in writing as the number and complexity of technical terms increases. Some examples that apply to studies of the blood are CBC (complete blood count) and RBC and WBC for red and white blood cells. Some other common acronyms are CNS (central nervous system), ECG (electrocardiograph), NIH (National Institutes of Health), and STI (sexually transmitted infection).

If the acronym has vowels and lends itself to pronunciation, it may be used as a word in itself, such as AIDS (acquired immunodeficiency syndrome); ELISA (enzyme-linked immunosorbent assay); JAMA (*Journal of the American Medical Association*); NSAID (nonsteroidal antiinflammatory agent), pronounced "en-sayd"; and CABG (coronary artery bypass graft), which inevitably becomes "cabbage." Few people even know that LASER is an acronym that means "light amplification by stimulated emission of radiation."

An acronym usually is introduced the first time a phrase appears in an article and is then used without explanation. If you have spent time searching back through an article in frustration for the meaning of an acronym, you probably wish, as does this author, that all the acronyms used and their meanings would be listed at the beginning of each article.

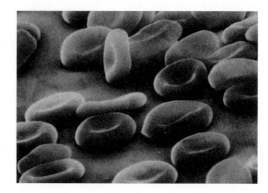

Figure 10-3 Erythrocytes (red blood cells). The cells are seen under a scanning electron microscope, which gives a three-dimensional view.

> **Neutrophils** stain with either acidic or basic dyes.
> **Eosinophils** stain with acidic dyes.
> **Basophils** stain with basic dyes.

> **Agranulocytes** do not show visible granules when stained. The nucleus of an agranulocyte is large and either round or curved. There are two types of agranulocytes:
>> **Lymphocytes,** which are the smaller agranulocytes.
>> **Monocytes,** which are the largest of all the white blood cells.

White blood cells protect against foreign substances. Some engulf foreign material by the process of **phagocytosis**; others function as part of the immune system. In diagnosis it is important to know not only the total number of leukocytes but also the relative number of each type because these numbers can change in different disease conditions. Reference Box 10-3 gives the relative percentage and functions of the different types of white cells.

The most numerous white blood cells, neutrophils, are called *polymorphs* because of their various-shaped nuclei. They are also referred to as *segs, polys,* or *PMNs* (polymorphonuclear leukocytes). A **band cell,** also called a *stab cell*, is an immature neutrophil with a solid curved nucleus (Fig. 10-5). Large numbers of band cells in the blood indicate an active infection.

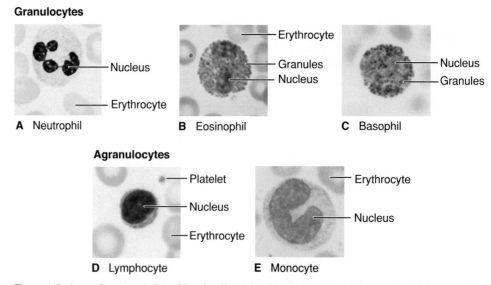

Granulocytes

A Neutrophil — Nucleus, Erythrocyte

B Eosinophil — Erythrocyte, Granules, Nucleus

C Basophil — Nucleus, Granules

Agranulocytes

D Lymphocyte — Platelet, Nucleus, Erythrocyte

E Monocyte — Erythrocyte, Nucleus

Figure 10-4 Leukocytes (white blood cells). The three types of granulocytes (*A–C*) have visible granules in the cytoplasm when stained. The two types of agranulocytes (*D, E*) do not show granules when stained.

Box 10•3 For Your Reference *White Blood Cells (Leukocytes)*

Type of Cell	Relative Percentage (Adult)	Function
GRANULOCYTES		
neutrophils *NŪ-trō-fils*	54%–62%	phagocytosis
eosinophils *ē-ō-SIN-ō-fils*	1%–3%	allergic reactions; defense against parasites
basophils *BĀ-sō-fils*	less than 1%	allergic reactions
AGRANULOCYTES		
lymphocytes *LIM-fō-sītz*	25%–38%	immunity (T cells and B cells)
monocytes *MON-ō-sītz*	3%–7%	phagocytosis

10

Platelets

The blood platelets (thrombocytes) are not complete cells, but fragments of large cells named **megakaryocytes,** which form in bone marrow (Fig. 10-6). They number from 200,000 to 400,000 per µL of blood. Platelets are important in **hemostasis,** the prevention of blood loss, one part of which is the process of blood clotting, or **coagulation.**

When a vessel is injured, platelets stick together to form a plug at the site. Substances released from the platelets and from damaged tissue then interact with clotting factors in the plasma to produce a wound-sealing clot. Clotting factors are inactive in the blood until an injury occurs. To protect against unwanted clot formation, 12 factors must interact before blood coagulates. The final reaction is the conversion of **fibrinogen** to threads of **fibrin** that trap blood cells and plasma to produce the clot (Fig. 10-7). What remains of the plasma after blood coagulates is **serum.**

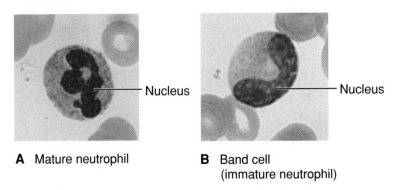

A Mature neutrophil

B Band cell (immature neutrophil)

Figure 10-5 Band cell. (*A*) A mature neutrophil. (*B*) A band cell, or stab cell, is an immature neutrophil with a thick curved nucleus.

10

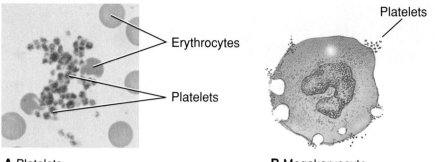

A Platelets   **B** Megakaryocyte

Figure 10-6 Platelets (thrombocytes). (A) Platelets seen in a blood smear under the microscope. (B) A megakaryocyte releases platelets.

Blood Types

Genetically inherited proteins on the surface of red blood cells determine blood type. More than 20 groups of these proteins have now been identified, but the most familiar are the ABO and Rh blood groups. The ABO system includes types A, B, AB, and O. The Rh types are Rh-positive (Rh^+) and Rh-negative (Rh^-).

In giving blood transfusions, it is important to use blood that is the same type as the recipient's blood or a type to which the recipient will not have an immune reaction, as described below. Compatible blood types are determined by **cross-matching** (Fig. 10-8). When a blood sample is mixed separately with different antisera, its red cells will agglutinate (clump) with the antiserum that corresponds to its blood type.

Whole blood may be used to replace a large volume of blood lost, but in most cases requiring blood transfusion, a blood fraction such as packed red cells, platelets, plasma, or specific clotting factors is administered.

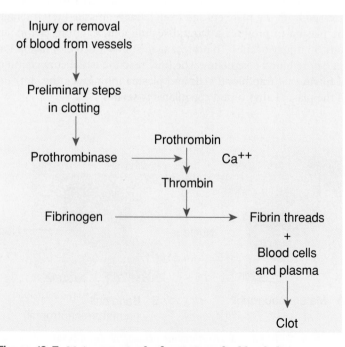

Figure 10-7 Main steps in the formation of a blood clot.

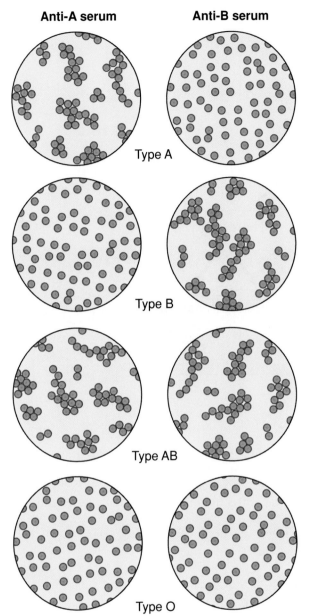

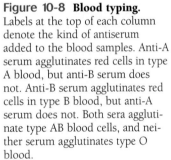

Figure 10-8 Blood typing. Labels at the top of each column denote the kind of antiserum added to the blood samples. Anti-A serum agglutinates red cells in type A blood, but anti-B serum does not. Anti-B serum agglutinates red cells in type B blood, but anti-A serum does not. Both sera agglutinate type AB blood cells, and neither serum agglutinates type O blood.

Immunity

Immunity is protection against disease. It includes defenses against harmful microorganisms, their products, or any other foreign substance. These defenses may be inborn or acquired during life (Fig. 10-9).

Innate Immunity

Innate defense mechanisms are inborn; they are based on the genetic makeup of the individual. Most of these defenses are physical mechanisms and are nonspecific (i.e., they protect against any intruder), and include:

➤ Unbroken skin, which acts as a barrier.
➤ Cilia, tiny cell projections that sweep impurities out of the body, as in the respiratory tract.
➤ Mucus that traps foreign material.

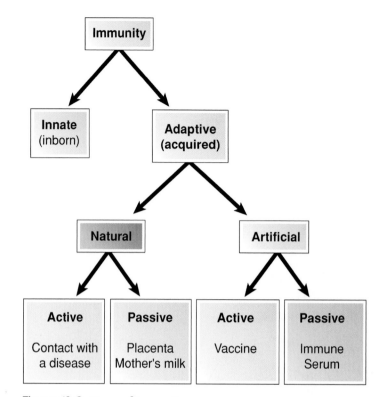

Figure 10-9 **Types of immunity.**

> Bactericidal body secretions, as found in tears, the skin, the digestive tract, and the reproductive tract.
> Reflexes, such as coughing and sneezing, which expel impurities.
> Lymphoid tissue, which filters impurities from blood and lymph, as described in Chapter 9.
> Phagocytes—cells that attack, ingest, and destroy foreign organisms.

Adaptive Immunity

Adaptive immunity is acquired during life and is specific, which means that it is directed toward a particular disease organism or other foreign substance. Thus, protection against measles, for example, will not protect against chickenpox or any other disease.

The specific immune response involves complex interactions between components of the lymphatic system and the blood. Any foreign particle, but mainly proteins, may act as an **antigen,** a substance that provokes an immune response. This response comes from two types of lymphocytes that circulate in the blood and lymphatic system:

> **T cells** (T lymphocytes), mature in the thymus gland. They are capable of attacking a foreign cell directly, producing *cell-mediated immunity.* **Macrophages,** descendants of monocytes, are important in the function of T cells. Macrophages take in and process foreign antigens. A T cell is activated when it contacts an antigen on the surface of a macrophage in combination with some of the body's own proteins.
> **B cells** (B lymphocytes) mature in bone marrow. When they meet a foreign antigen, they multiply rapidly and mature into **plasma cells.** These cells produce **antibodies,** also called **immunoglobulins** (Ig), that inactivate antigens (Fig. 10-10). Antibodies remain in the blood, often providing long-term immunity to the specific organism against which they were formed. Antibody-based immunity is referred to as *humoral immunity.*

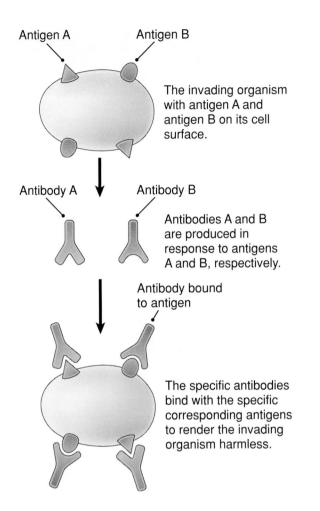

Figure 10-10 **The antigen-antibody reaction.** Antibodies produced by immune cells bind with specific antigens to aid in their inactivation and elimination.

Types of Adaptive Immunity

Adaptive immunity may be acquired either naturally or artificially (see Fig. 10-9). In addition, each avenue for acquiring immunity may be either active or passive. In active immunity, a person makes his or her own antibodies in response to contact with an antigen. In passive immunity, an antibody, known as an immune serum, is transferred from an outside source. Immune sera may come from other people or from immunized animals. The portion of the blood plasma that contains antibodies is the **gamma globulin** fraction. The types of adaptive immunity are:

➤ Natural adaptive immunity
  ➤ Active—from contact with a disease organism or other foreign antigen
  ➤ Passive—by transfer of antibodies from a mother to her fetus through the placenta or through the mother's milk

➤ Artificial adaptive immunity
  ➤ Active—by administration of a vaccine, which may be a killed or weakened organism, part of an organism, or an altered toxin (toxoid)
  ➤ Passive—by administration of an immune serum obtained from other people or animals

Immunology has long been a very active area of research. The above description is only the barest outline of the events that are known to occur in the immune response, and there is much still to be discovered. Some of the areas of research include autoimmune diseases, in which an individual produces antibodies to his or her own body tissues; hereditary and acquired immunodeficiency diseases; the relationship between cancer and immunity; and the development of techniques for avoiding rejection of transplanted tissue.

TERMINOLOGY Key Terms

NORMAL STRUCTURE AND FUNCTION

agranulocytes Ā-gran-ū-lō-sītz	White blood cells that do not have visible granules in their cytoplasm. Agranulocytes include lymphocytes and monocytes (see Fig. 10-4).
albumin al-BŪ-min	A simple protein found in blood plasma
antibody AN-ti-bod-ē	A protein produced in response to, and interacting specifically with, an antigen
antigen AN-ti-jen	A substance that induces the formation of an antibody
B cell	A lymphocyte that matures in lymphoid tissue and is active in producing antibodies; B lymphocyte (LIM-fō-sīt)
band cell	An immature neutrophil with a nucleus in the shape of a band; also called a stab cell. Band-cell counts are used to trace infections and other diseases (see Fig. 10-5).
basophil BĀ-sō-fil	A granular leukocyte that stains with basic dyes; active in allergic reactions
blood	The fluid that circulates in the cardiovascular system (root: *hem/o, hemat/o*)
coagulation kō-ag-ū-LĀ-shun	Blood clotting
cross-matching	Testing the compatibility of donor and recipient blood in preparation for a transfusion. Donor red cells are mixed with recipient serum, and red cells of the recipient are mixed with donor serum to look for an immunologic reaction. Similar tests are done on tissues before transplantation.
electrolyte ē-LEK-trō-līt	A substance that separates into charged particles (ions) in solution; a salt. Term also applied to ions in body fluids.
eosinophil ē-ō-SIN-ō-fil	A granular leukocyte that stains with acidic dyes; active in allergic reactions and defense against parasites
erythrocyte e-RITH-rō-sīt	A red blood cell (root: *erythr/o, erythrocyt/o*) (see Figs. 10-2 and 10-3)
erythropoietin (EPO) e-rith-rō-POY-e-tin	A hormone produced in the kidneys that stimulates red-blood-cell production in the bone marrow. This hormone is now made by genetic engineering for clinical use.
fibrin FĪ-brin	The protein that forms a clot in the process of blood coagulation
fibrinogen fi-BRIN-ō-jen	The inactive precursor of fibrin
formed elements	The cellular components of blood
gamma globulin GLOB-ū-lin	The fraction of the blood plasma that contains antibodies; given for passive transfer of immunity
granulocytes GRAN-ū-lō-sītz	White blood cells that have visible granules in their cytoplasm. Granulocytes include neutrophils, basophils, and eosinophils (see Fig 10-4).

TERMINOLOGY   Key Terms
Continued

10

hemoglobin (Hb, Hgb) *HĒ-mō-glō-bin*	The iron-containing pigment in red blood cells that transports oxygen
hemostasis *hē-mō-STĀ-sis*	The stoppage of bleeding
immunity	The state of being protected against a specific disease (root: *immun/o*)
immunoglobulin (Ig) *im-ū-nō-GLOB-ū-lin*	An antibody. Immunoglobulins fall into five classes, each abbreviated with a capital letter: IgG, IgM, IgA, IgD, IgE.
leukocyte *LŪ-kō-sīt*	A white blood cell (root: *leuk/o, leukocyt/o*)
lymphocyte *LIM-fō-sīt*	An agranular leukocyte active in immunity (T cells and B cells); found in both the blood and in lymphoid tissue (root: *lymph/o, lymphocyt/o*)
megakaryocyte *meg-a-KAR-ē-ō-sīt*	A large bone marrow cell that fragments to release platelets
macrophage *MAK-rō-faj*	A phagocytic cell derived from a monocyte; usually located within the tissues. Macrophages process antigens for T cells.
monocyte *MON-ō-sīt*	An agranular phagocytic leukocyte
neutrophil *NŪ-trō-fil*	A granular leukocyte that stains with acidic or basic dyes. The most numerous of the white blood cells. A type of phagocyte.
phagocytosis *fag-ō-sī-TŌ-sis*	The engulfing of foreign material by white blood cells
plasma *PLAZ-ma*	The liquid portion of the blood
plasma cell	A mature form of a B cell that produces antibodies
platelet *PLĀT-let*	A formed element of the blood that is active in hemostasis; a thrombocyte (root: *thrombocyt/o*)
serum *SĒR-um*	The fraction of the plasma that remains after blood coagulation; it is the equivalent of plasma without its clotting factors (plural: sera, serums).
T cell	A lymphocyte that matures in the thymus gland and attacks foreign cells directly; T lymphocyte
thrombocyte *THROM-bo-sit*	A blood platelet (root: *thrombocyt/o*)

Go to the pronunciation glossary in Chapter 10 on the CD-ROM to hear these words pronounced.

Word Parts Pertaining to Blood and Immunity

Table 10·1 Suffixes for Blood

SUFFIX	MEANING	EXAMPLE	DEFINITION OF EXAMPLE
-emia,* -hemia	condition of blood	erythremia *er-i-THRĒ-mē-a*	increase in red cells in the blood
-penia	decrease in, deficiency of	cytopenia *sī-tō-PĒ-nē-a*	deficiency of cells in the blood
-poiesis	formation, production	hemopoiesis *hē-mō-poy-Ē-sis*	production of blood cells

A shortened form of the root hem plus the suffix -ia.

Exercise 10-1

Define the following terms:

1. hypoproteinemia (*hī-pō-prō-tēn-Ē-mē-a*) _____ decreased protein in the blood

2. hyperalbuminemia (*hī-per-al-bū-mi-NĒ-mē-a*) _____

3. erythrocytopenia (*e-rith-rō-sī-tō-PĒ-nē-a*) _____

4. toxemia (*tok-SĒ-mē-a*) _____

5. bacteremia (*bak-ter-Ē-mē-a*) _____

6. erythropoiesis (*e-rith-rō-poy-Ē-sis*) _____

Word building. Use the suffix -emia to write words for the following definitions:

7. Presence of pus in the blood _____

8. Presence of viruses in the blood _____

9. Presence of excess white cells (*leuk/o-*) in the blood _____

Many of the words relating to blood cells can be formed either with or without including the root *cyt/o*, as in erythropenia or erythrocytopenia, leukopoiesis or leukocytopoiesis. The remaining types of blood cells are designated by easily recognized roots such as *agranulocyt/o, monocyt/o, granul/o,* and so on.

Table 10·2 Roots for Blood and Immunity

ROOT	MEANING	EXAMPLE	DEFINITION OF EXAMPLE
myel/o	bone marrow	myelogenous *mī-e-LOJ-e-nus*	originating in bone marrow
hem/o, hemat/o	blood	hematology *hē-ma-TOL-ō-jē*	study of blood
erythr/o, erythrocyt/o	red blood cell	erythropoiesis *e-rith-rō-poy-Ē-sis*	formation of blood cells
leuk/o, leukocyt/o	white blood cell	leukoblast *LŪ-kō-blast*	immature white blood cell

Table 10·2	Continued			
lymph/o, lymphocyt/o	lymphocyte	lymphocytic *lim-fō-SĪT-ik*		pertaining to lymphocytes
thromb/o	blood clot	thrombosis *throm-BŌ-sis*		formation of a blood clot
thrombocyt/o	platelet, thrombocyte	thrombocytopenia *throm-bō-sī-tō-PĒ-nē-a*		deficiency of platelets in the blood
immun/o	immunity, immune system	immunization *im-ū-ni-ZĀ-shun*		production of immunity

10

Exercise 10-2

Identify and define the root in the following words:

		Root	Meaning of Root
1.	panmyeloid (*pan-MĪ-e-loyd*)	myel/o	bone marrow
2.	prothrombin (*prō-THROM-bin*)	_____	_____
3.	preimmunization (*prē-im-ū-ni-ZĀ-shun*)	_____	_____
4.	ischemia (*is-KĒ-mē-a*)	_____	_____

Fill in the blanks:

5. Hemorrhage is a profuse flow (-rhage) of _____.

6. Erythroclasis (*er-i-THROK-la-sis*) is the breaking (-clasis) of _____.

7. The term *thrombocythemia* (*throm-bō-sī-THĒ-mē-a*) refers to an increase in the number of _____ in the blood.

8. Leukopoiesis (*lū-kō-poy-Ē-sis*) refers to the production of _____.

9. An immunocyte (*im-ū-nō-SĪT*) is a cell active in _____.

10. A hemocytometer (*hē-mō-sī-TOM-e-ter*) is a device for counting _____.

11. Myelofibrosis (*mi-e-lō-fī-BRO-sis*) is formation of fibrous tissue in _____.

12. Lymphokines (*LIM-fō-kīnz*) are chemicals active in immunity that are produced by _____.

Word building. Write a word for the following definitions:

13. Immature lymphocyte _____

14. Tumor of bone marrow _____

15. Decrease in red blood cells _____

16. Dissolving (-lysis) of a blood clot _____

17. Formation (-poiesis) of bone marrow _____

The suffix -osis added to a root for a type of cell means an increase in that type of cell in the blood. Use this suffix to write a word that means the same as the following:

18. Increase in granulocytes in the blood _____ granulocytosis _____

19. Increase in lymphocytes in the blood _____

20. Increase in red blood cells _____

21. Increase in monocytes in the blood _____

22. Increase in platelets in the blood _____

Table 10·3	Roots for Chemistry		
ROOT	**MEANING**	**EXAMPLE**	**DEFINITION OF EXAMPLE**
azot/o	nitrogenous compounds	azoturia *āz-ō-TŪ-rē-a*	increased nitrogenous compounds in the urine (-uria)
calc/i	calcium (symbol Ca)	calcification *kal-si-fi-KĀ-shun*	deposition of calcium salts
ferr/o, ferr/i	iron (symbol Fe)	ferrous *FER-ous*	pertaining to or containing iron
sider/o	iron	sideroderma *sid-er-ō-DER-ma*	deposition of iron into the skin
kali	potassium (symbol K)	hypokalemia* *hī-per-ka-LĒ-mē-a*	decrease of potassium in the blood
natri	sodium (symbol Na)	natriuresis *nā-trē-ū-RĒ-sis*	excretion of sodium in the urine (ur/o)
ox/y	oxygen (symbol O)	hypoxia *hī-POK-sē-a*	deficiency of oxygen in the tissues

*The i in the root is dropped.

Exercise 10-3

Fill in the blanks:

1. A sideroblast (*SID-er-ō-blast*) is an immature cell containing _____.

2. The term *hyperkalemia* (*hī-per-ka-LĒ-mē-a*) refers to an excess blood concentration of

   _____.

3. The bacterial species *Azotobacter* is named for its ability to metabolize _____.

4. Hypoxemia (*hī-pok-SĒ-mē-a*) is a blood deficiency of _____.

5. Ferritin (*FER-i-tin*) is a compound that contains _____.

6. A calcareous (*kal-KAR-ē-us*) substance contains _____.

Word building. Use the suffix -emia to form words with the following meanings:

7. Presence of potassium in the blood _____

8. Presence of nitrogenous compounds in the blood _____

9. Presence of sodium in the blood _____

10. Presence of calcium in the blood _____

Clinical Aspects of Blood

Anemia

Anemia is defined as an abnormally low amount of hemoglobin in the blood. Anemia may result from too few red blood cells or from cells that are too small (microcytic) or have too little hemoglobin (hypochromic). Key tests in diagnosing anemia are blood counts, mean corpuscular volume (MCV), and mean corpuscular hemoglobin concentration (MCHC). (Reference Box 10-4 describes these and other blood tests. Box 10-5 has information on careers in hematology.)

10

Box 10•4 For Your Reference   *Common Blood Tests*

Test	Abbreviation	Description
red-blood-cell count	RBC	number of red blood cells per μL (microliter) of blood
white-blood-cell count	WBC	number of white blood cells per μL of blood
differential count	Diff	relative percentage of the different types of leukocytes
hematocrit (**Fig. 10–11**)	Ht, Hct, crit	relative percentage of packed red cells in a given volume of blood
packed cell volume	PCV	hematocrit
hemoglobin	Hb, Hgb	amount of hemoglobin in g/dL (100 mL) of blood
mean corpuscular volume	MCV	volume of an average red cell
mean corpuscular hemoglobin	MCH	average weight of hemoglobin in red cells
mean corpuscular hemoglobin concentration	MCHC	average concentration of hemoglobin in red blood cells
erythrocyte sedimentation rate	ESR	rate of settling of erythrocytes per unit of time; used to detect infection or inflammation
complete blood count	CBC	series of tests including cell counts, hematocrit, hemoglobin, and cell volume measurements

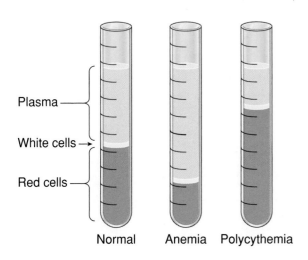

Plasma

White cells

Red cells

Normal   Anemia   Polycythemia

Figure 10-11 Hematocrit. The tube on the left shows a normal hematocrit. The middle tube shows that the percentage of red blood cells is low, indicating anemia. The tube on the right shows an excessively high percentage of red blood cells, as seen in polycythemia.

Box 10·5 Health Professions   *Careers in Hematology*

Hematologists are physicians and other scientists who specialize in the study of blood and blood diseases. In medical practice, hematology is often combined with the study and treatment of blood cancers as the specialty hematology–oncology.

A hematology technician is usually a medical laboratory technician who specializes in blood studies. He or she may work in a clinical laboratory, blood banking, industry, or academic research. The job requires a BS or MS in biological science plus training in laboratory procedures, blood pathology, and testing methods. Hematology technicians perform a full range of blood studies for diagnosis of infections, allergies, anemia, leukemia, and other blood diseases. They also run tests to monitor anticoagulant therapy. They must be able to operate and maintain automated

equipment used to analyze blood. In some cases, they may also draw blood or administer blood transfusions.

A phlebotomist draws blood for testing, transfusions, or research. The blood is often drawn from a vein (venipuncture), but may also be drawn from arteries and by skin puncture. Phlebotomists must be trained in sterile techniques and safety precautions to prevent the spread of infectious diseases. They must take specimens without harming the patient or interfering with medical care and must transport specimens to the proper laboratory. Educational requirements vary among states. Often, in-house training with certification by the National Phlebotomy Association is acceptable. Phlebotomists work in hospitals, laboratories, private physicians' offices, clinics, and blood banks.

The general symptoms of anemia include fatigue, shortness of breath, heart palpitations, pallor, and irritability. There are many different types of anemia, some of which are caused by faulty production of red cells and others by loss or destruction of red cells.

Anemia Due to Impaired Production of Red Cells

➤ **Aplastic anemia** results from bone marrow destruction and affects all blood cells (pancytopenia). It may be caused by drugs, toxins, viruses, radiation, or bone marrow cancer. Aplastic anemia has a high mortality rate but has been treated successfully with bone marrow transplantation.

➤ **Nutritional anemia** may result from a deficiency of vitamin B_{12} or of folic acid, B vitamins needed for RBC development. Most commonly, it is caused by a deficiency of iron, needed to make hemoglobin (Fig. 10-12). Folic acid deficiency commonly appears in those with poor diet, in pregnant and lactating women, and in those who abuse alcohol. Iron-deficiency anemia results from poor diet, poor absorption of iron, or blood loss. Both folic acid deficiency and iron deficiency respond to dietary supplementation.

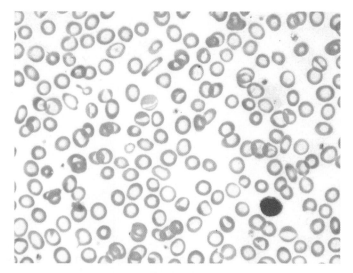

Figure 10-12 Iron-deficiency anemia. Red cells are small (microcytic) and are lacking in hemoglobin (hypochromic).

➤ **Pernicious anemia** is a specific form of B$_{12}$ deficiency. It results from the lack of **intrinsic factor** (IF), a substance produced in the stomach that aids in the absorption of B$_{12}$ from the intestine. Pernicious anemia must be treated with regular injections of B$_{12}$.

➤ In **sideroblastic anemia,** there is adequate iron available, but the iron is not used properly to manufacture hemoglobin. This disorder may be hereditary or acquired, as by exposure to toxins or drugs, or as secondary to another disease. The excess iron precipitates out in immature red cells (normoblasts).

Anemia Due to Loss or Destruction of Red Cells

➤ **Hemorrhagic anemia** results from blood loss. This may be a sudden loss, as from injury, or loss from chronic internal bleeding, as from the digestive tract in cases of ulcers or cancer.

➤ **Thalassemia** is a hereditary disease that appears mostly in Mediterranean populations. It causes production of abnormal hemoglobin and **hemolysis** (destruction) of red cells. Thalassemia is designated as α (alpha) or β (beta), according to the part of the molecule affected. Severe β thalassemia is also called **Cooley anemia.**

➤ In **sickle cell anemia,** a mutation alters the hemoglobin molecule so that it precipitates when it gives up oxygen and distorts the red blood cells into a crescent shape (Fig. 10-13). The altered cells block small blood vessels and deprive tissues of oxygen, an episode termed *sickle cell crisis.* The misshapen cells are also readily destroyed (hemolyzed). The disease predominates in black populations. Genetic carriers of the defect, those with one normal and one abnormal gene, show *sickle cell trait.* They usually have no symptoms, except when oxygen is low, such as at high altitudes. They can, however, pass the defective gene to offspring. Sickle cell anemia, as well as many other genetic diseases, can be diagnosed in carriers and in the fetus before birth.

Reticulocyte counts are useful in diagnosing the causes of anemia. Reticulocytes are immature red blood cells that normally appear as a small percentage of the total erythrocytes. An increase in the number of reticulocytes indicates increased red-cell formation, as in response to hemorrhage or cell destruction. A decrease in reticulocytes indicates a failure in red-cell production, as caused by nutritional deficiency or aplastic anemia (see Box 10-6).

Coagulation Disorders

The most common cause of coagulation problems is a deficiency in the number of circulating platelets, a condition termed **thrombocytopenia.** Possible causes include aplastic anemia, infections, cancer of the bone marrow, and agents that destroy bone marrow, such as x-rays or certain drugs. This disorder results in bleeding into the skin and mucous membranes, variously described as **petechiae** (pinpoint spots), **ecchymoses** (bruises), and **purpura** (purple lesions).

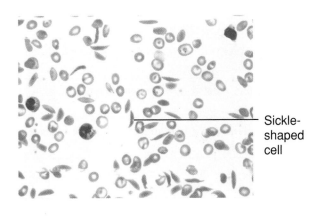

Sickle-shaped cell

Figure 10-13 Sickle cell anemia. A blood smear shows sickled red cells, which take on a crescent shape when they give up oxygen.

Box 10·6 Clinical Perspectives   *Use of Reticulocytes in Diagnosis*

As erythrocytes mature in the red bone marrow, they go through a series of stages in which they lose their nucleus and most other organelles, maximizing the space

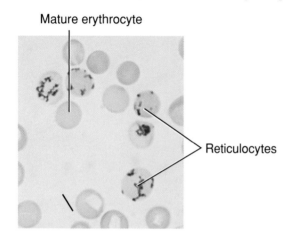

Mature erythrocyte

Reticulocytes

Reticulocytes. Erythrocytes show a network in a late stage of development.

available to hold hemoglobin. In one of the last stages of development, small numbers of ribosomes and some rough endoplasmic reticulum remain in the cell and appear as a network, or reticulum, when stained. Cells at this stage are called reticulocytes. Reticulocytes leave the red bone marrow and enter the bloodstream, where they become fully mature erythrocytes in about 24 to 48 hours. The average number of red cells maturing through the reticulocyte stage at any given time is about 1% to 2%. Changes in these numbers can be used in diagnosing certain blood disorders.

When erythrocytes are lost or destroyed, as from chronic bleeding or some form of hemolytic anemia, red-cell production is "stepped up" to compensate for the loss. Greater numbers of reticulocytes are then released into the blood before reaching full maturity, and counts increase to above normal. On the other hand, a decrease in the number of circulating reticulocytes suggests a problem with red-cell production, as in cases of deficiency anemias or suppression of bone marrow activity.

In **disseminated intravascular coagulation** (DIC) there is widespread clotting in the vessels, which obstructs circulation to the tissues. This is followed by diffuse hemorrhages as clotting factors are removed and the coagulation process is impaired. DIC may result from a variety of causes, including infection, cancer, hemorrhage, injury, and allergy.

Hemophilia is a hereditary deficiency of a specific clotting factor. It is a sex-linked disease that is passed from mother to son. There is bleeding into the tissues, especially into the joints (hemarthrosis). Hemophilia must be treated with transfusions of the necessary clotting factor.

Reference Box 10-7 lists tests done for these and other coagulation disorders.

Box 10·7 For Your Reference   *Coagulation Tests*

Test	Abbreviation	Description
Activated partial thromboplastin time	APTT	Measures time required for clot formation; used to evaluate clotting factors and monitor heparin therapy
Bleeding time	BT	Measures capacity of platelets to stop bleeding after a standard skin incision
Partial thromboplastin time	PTT	Evaluates clotting factors; similar to APTT, but less sensitive
Prothrombin time	PT, Pro Time	Indirectly measures prothrombin; used to monitor anticoagulant therapy; also called Quick test
Thrombin time (thrombin clotting time)	TT (TCT)	Measures how quickly a clot forms

Neoplasms

Leukemia is a neoplasm of white blood cells. The rapidly dividing but incompetent white cells accumulate in the tissues and crowd out the other blood cells. The symptoms of leukemia include anemia, fatigue, easy bleeding, **splenomegaly,** and sometimes hepatomegaly (enlargement of the liver). The causes of leukemia are unknown but may include exposure to radiation or harmful chemicals, hereditary factors, and perhaps viral infection.

The two main categories of leukemia based on origin and the cells involved are:

➤ Myelogenous leukemia, which originates in the bone marrow and involves mainly the granular leukocytes.
➤ Lymphocytic leukemia, which affects B cells and the lymphatic system, causing **lymphadenopathy** (lymph node disease) and adverse effects on the immune system.

Leukemias are further differentiated as acute or chronic based on clinical progress. Acute leukemia is the most common form of cancer in young children. The acute forms are:

➤ Acute myeloblastic (myelogenous) leukemia (AML). The prognosis in AML is poor for both children and adults.
➤ Acute lymphoblastic (lymphocytic) leukemia (ALL). With treatment, the remission rate is high for ALL.

The chronic forms of leukemia are:

➤ Chronic granulocytic leukemia, also called chronic myelogenous leukemia, which affects young to middle-aged adults. Most cases show the **Philadelphia chromosome (Ph),** an inherited anomaly in which part of chromosome 22 shifts to chromosome 9.
➤ Chronic lymphocytic leukemia (CLL), which appears mostly in the elderly and is the most slowly growing form of the disease (Fig. 10-14).

Treatment of leukemia includes chemotherapy, radiation therapy, and bone marrow transplantation. One advance in transplantation is the use of umbilical cord blood to replace blood-forming cells in bone marrow. This blood is more readily available than bone marrow and does not have to match as closely to avoid rejection.

Hodgkin disease is a disease of the lymphatic system that may spread to other tissues. It begins with enlarged but painless lymph nodes in the cervical (neck) region and then progresses to other nodes. A feature of Hodgkin disease is giant cells in the lymph nodes called **Reed–Sternberg cells** (Fig. 10-15). There are fever, night sweats, weight loss, and itching of the skin (pruritus). Persons of any age may be affected, but the disease predominates in young adults and those over age 50. Most cases can be cured with radiation and chemotherapy.

Non-Hodgkin lymphoma (NHL) is also a malignant enlargement of lymph nodes but does not show Reed–Sternberg cells. It is more common than Hodgkin disease and has a higher mortality rate. Cases vary in severity and prognosis. It is most prevalent in the older

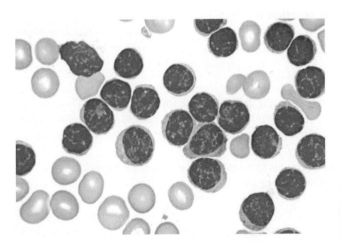

Figure 10-14 Chronic lymphocytic leukemia. A blood smear shows an above normal number of lymphocytes.

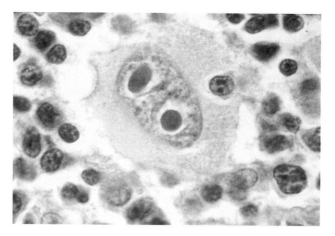

Figure 10-15 Reed–Sternberg cell. These cells are typical of Hodgkin disease.

adult population and in those with AIDS and other forms of immunodeficiency. NHL involves the T or B lymphocytes, and some cases may be related to infection with certain viruses. It requires systemic chemotherapy and, sometimes, bone marrow transplantation.

Multiple myeloma is a cancer of the blood-forming cells in bone marrow, mainly the plasma cells that produce antibodies. The disease causes anemia, bone pain, and weakening of the bones. Patients have a greater susceptibility to infection because of immunodeficiency. Abnormally high levels of calcium and protein in the blood often lead to kidney failure. Multiple myeloma is treated with radiation and chemotherapy, but the prognosis is generally poor.

Clinical Aspects of Immunity

Hypersensitivity

Hypersensitivity is a harmful overreaction of the immune system, commonly known as **allergy**. In cases of allergy, a person is more sensitive to a particular antigen than the average individual. Common **allergens** are pollen, animal dander, dust, and foods, but there are many more. A seasonal allergy to inhaled pollens is commonly called "hay fever." Responses may include itching, redness, or tearing of the eyes (conjunctivitis), skin rash, asthma, runny nose (rhinitis), sneezing, **urticaria** (hives), and **angioedema**, a reaction similar to hives but involving deeper layers of tissue.

An **anaphylactic reaction** is a severe generalized allergic response that can lead rapidly to death as a result of shock and respiratory distress. It must be treated by immediate administration of **epinephrine (adrenaline)** and maintenance of open airways. Oxygen, antihistamines, and corticosteroids may also be given. Common causes of anaphylaxis are drugs, especially penicillin and other antibiotics, vaccines, diagnostic chemicals, foods, and insect venom.

A **delayed hypersensitivity reaction** involves T cells and takes at least 12 hours to develop. A common example is the reaction to contact with plant irritants such as those of poison ivy and poison oak.

Immunodeficiency

The term **immunodeficiency** refers to any failure in the immune system. This may be congenital (present at birth) or acquired and may involve any components of the system. The deficiency may vary in severity but is always evidenced by an increased susceptibility to disease.

AIDS (acquired immunodeficiency syndrome) is acquired by infection with **HIV (human immunodeficiency virus)**, which attacks certain T cells. These cells have a specific surface attachment site, the CD4 receptor, for the virus. HIV is spread by sexual contact, use of contaminated needles, blood transfusions, and passage from an infected mother to a fetus. It leaves the host susceptible to opportunistic infections such as pneumonia caused by the fungus *Pneumocystis jirovicii;* thrush, a fungal infection of the mouth caused by *Candida albicans;* and infection with *Cryptosporidium,* a protozoon that causes cramps and diarrhea. It also predisposes to **Kaposi sarcoma**, a once-rare form of skin cancer. AIDS may also induce autoimmunity or attack the nervous system.

AIDS is diagnosed and monitored by **CD4+ T lymphocyte counts**, a measure of cells with the HIV receptor. A count of less than 200 per μL of blood signifies severe immunodeficiency. HIV antibody levels and direct viral blood counts are also used to track the disease's course. At present there is no vaccine or cure for AIDS, but some drugs can delay its progress.

Autoimmune Diseases

A disorder that results from an immune response to one's own tissues is classified as an **autoimmune disease**. The cause may be a failure in the immune system or a reaction to body cells that have been slightly altered by mutation or disease. The list of diseases that are believed to be caused, at least in part, by autoimmunity is long. Some, such as **systemic lupus erythematosus** (SLE), **systemic sclerosis** (scleroderma), and **Sjögren syndrome**, affect tissues in multiple systems. Others target more specific organs or systems. Examples are pernicious anemia, rheumatoid arthritis, Graves disease (of the thyroid), myasthenia gravis (a muscle disease), fibromyalgia syndrome (a musculoskeletal disorder), rheumatic heart disease, and glomerulonephritis (a kidney disease). These diseases are discussed in more detail in other chapters.

10

TERMINOLOGY Key Terms

DISORDERS

AIDS (acquired immunodeficiency syndrome)	Failure of the immune system caused by infection with HIV (human immunodeficiency virus). The virus infects certain T cells and thus interferes with immunity.
allergen AL-er-jen	A substance that causes an allergic response
allergy AL-er-jē	Hypersensitivity
anaphylactic reaction an-a-fi-LAK-tik	An exaggerated allergic reaction to a foreign substance (root *phylaxis* means . "protection"). It may lead to death caused by circulatory collapse, and respiratory distress if untreated. Also called *anaphylaxis*
anemia a-NĒ-mē-a	A deficiency in the amount of hemoglobin in the blood; may result from blood loss, malnutrition, a hereditary defect, environmental factors, and other causes (see Figs. 10-12 and 10-13)
angioedema an-jē-ō-e-DĒ-ma	A localized edema with large hives (wheals) similar to urticaria but involving deeper layers of the skin and subcutaneous tissue
aplastic anemia ā-PLAS-tik	Anemia caused by bone marrow failure resulting in deficient blood-cell production, especially of red cells; pancytopenia
autoimmune disease aw-tō-i-MŪN	A condition in which the immune system produces antibodies against an individual's own tissues (prefix *auto* means "self")
Cooley anemia	A form of thalassemia (hereditary anemia) in which the B (beta) chain of hemoglobin is abnormal

10

delayed hypersensitivity reaction	An allergic reaction involving T cells that takes at least 12 hours to develop. Examples are various types of contact dermatitis, such as poison ivy or poison oak; the tuberculin reaction (test for TB); and rejections of transplanted tissue.
disseminated intravascular coagulation (DIC)	Widespread formation of clots in the microscopic vessels; may be followed by bleeding caused by depletion of clotting factors
ecchymosis *ek-i-MŌ-sis*	A collection of blood under the skin caused by leakage from small vessels (root *chym* means "juice")
hemolysis *hē-MOL-i-sis*	The rupture of red blood cells and the release of hemoglobin (adjective: hemolytic)
hemophilia *hē-mō-FIL-ē-a*	A hereditary blood disease caused by lack of a clotting factor and resulting in abnormal bleeding
HIV (human immunodeficiency virus)	The virus that causes AIDS; human immunodeficiency virus
Hodgkin disease	A neoplastic disease of unknown cause that involves the lymph nodes, spleen, liver, and other tissues; characterized by the presence of giant Reed-Sternberg cells (see Fig. 10-15)
hypersensitivity	An immunologic reaction to a substance that is harmless to most people; allergy
immunodeficiency *im-ū-nō-dē-FISH-en-sē*	A congenital or acquired failure of the immune system to protect against disease
intrinsic factor	A substance produced in the stomach that aids in the absorption of vitamin B_{12}, necessary for the manufacture of red blood cells. Lack of intrinsic factor causes pernicious anemia.
Kaposi sarcoma *KAP-ō-sē*	Cancerous lesion of the skin and other tissues, seen most often in patients with AIDS
leukemia *lū-KĒ-mē-a*	Malignant overgrowth of immature white blood cells; may be chronic or acute; may affect bone marrow (myelogenous leukemia) or lymphoid tissue (lymphocytic leukemia)
lymphadenopathy *lim-fad-e-NOP-a-thē*	Any disease of the lymph nodes
multiple myeloma *mī-e-LŌ-ma*	A tumor of the blood-forming tissue in bone marrow
non-Hodgkin lymphoma (NHL)	A widespread malignant disease of lymph nodes that involves lymphocytes. It differs from Hodgkin disease in that giant Reed-Sternberg cells are absent.
Philadelphia chromosome (Ph)	An abnormal chromosome found in the cells of most individuals with chronic granulocytic (myelogenous) leukemia

TERMINOLOGY Key Terms

Continued

pernicious anemia *per-NISH-us*	Anemia caused by failure of the stomach to produce intrinsic factor, a substance needed for the absorption of vitamin B_{12}. This vitamin is required for the formation of erythrocytes.
petechiae *pē-TĒ-kē-ē*	Pinpoint, flat, purplish-red spots caused by bleeding within the skin or mucous membrane (singular: petechia)
purpura *PUR-pū-ra*	A condition characterized by hemorrhages into the skin, mucous membranes, internal organs, and other tissues (from Greek word meaning "purple"). Thrombocytopenic purpura is caused by a deficiency of platelets.
sideroblastic anemia *sid-e-rō-BLAS-tik*	Anemia caused by inability to use available iron to manufacture hemoglobin. The excess iron precipitates in normoblasts (developing red blood cells)
Sjögren syndrome *SHŌ-gren*	An autoimmune disease involving dysfunction of the exocrine glands and affecting secretion of tears, saliva, and other body fluids. Deficiency leads to dry mouth, tooth decay, corneal damage, eye infections, and difficulty in swallowing.
sickle cell anemia	A hereditary anemia caused by the presence of abnormal hemoglobin. Red blood cells become sickle-shaped and interfere with normal blood flow to the tissues (see Fig. 10-13). Most common in black populations of West African descent.
splenomegaly *splē-nō-MEG-a-lē*	Enlargement of the spleen
systemic lupus erythematosus *LŪ-pus er-i-thē-ma-TŌ-sus*	Inflammatory disease of connective tissue affecting the skin and multiple organs. Patients are sensitive to light and may have a red butterfly-shaped rash over the nose and cheeks.
systemic sclerosis	A diffuse disease of connective tissue that may involve any system causing inflammation, degeneration, and fibrosis. Also called scleroderma because it causes thickening of the skin.
thalassemia *thal-a-SĒ-mē-a*	A group of hereditary anemias mostly found in populations of Mediterranean descent (the name comes from the Greek word for "sea").
thrombocytopenia *throm-bō-sī-tō-PĒ-nē-a*	A deficiency of thrombocytes (platelets) in the blood
urticaria *ur-ti-KAR-ē-a*	A skin reaction consisting of round, raised eruptions (wheals) with itching; hives

DIAGNOSIS AND TREATMENT

adrenaline *a-DREN-a-lin*	See epinephrine
CD4+ T lymphocyte count	A count of the T cells that have the CD4 receptors for the AIDS virus (HIV). A count of less than 200/μL of blood signifies severe immunodeficiency.

TERMINOLOGY — Key Terms

Continued

epinephrine *ep-i-NEF-rin*	A powerful stimulant produced by the adrenal gland and sympathetic nervous system. Activates the cardiovascular, respiratory, and other systems needed to meet stress. Used as a drug to treat severe allergic reactions and shock. Also called adrenaline.
reticulocyte counts *re-TIK-ū-lō-sīt*	Blood counts of reticulocytes, a type of immature red blood cell; reticulocyte counts are useful in diagnosis to indicate the rate of erythrocyte formation (see Box 10-6)
Reed-Sternberg cells *rēd-SHTERN-berg*	Giant cells that are characteristic of Hodgkin disease. They usually have two large nuclei and are surrounded by a halo (see Fig 10-15).

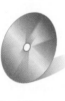

Go to the pronunciation glossary in Chapter 10 on the CD-ROM to hear these words pronounced.

TERMINOLOGY — Supplementary Terms

NORMAL STRUCTURE AND FUNCTION

agglutination *a-glū-ti-NĀ-shun*	The clumping of cells or particles in the presence of specific antibodies
bilirubin *bil-i-RŪ-bin*	A pigment derived from the breakdown of hemoglobin. It is eliminated by the liver in bile.
complement *COM-ple-ment*	A group of plasma enzymes that interacts with antibodies
corpuscle *KOR-pus-l*	A small mass or body. A blood corpuscle is a blood cell.
hemopoietic stem cell *hē-mō-poy-E-tik*	A primitive bone marrow cell that gives rise to all varieties of blood cells
heparin *HEP-a-rin*	A substance found throughout the body that inhibits blood coagulation; an anticoagulant
plasmin *PLAZ-min*	An enzyme that dissolves clots; also called *fibrinolysin*
thrombin *THROM-bin*	The enzyme derived from prothrombin that converts fibrinogen to fibrin

Supplementary Terms

10

SYMPTOMS AND CONDITIONS

agranulocytosis *ā-gran-ū-lō-sī-TŌ-sis*	A condition involving a decrease in the number of granulocytes in the blood; also called *granulocytopenia*
erythrocytosis *e-rith-rō-sī-TŌ-sis*	Increase in the number of red cells in the blood; may be normal, such as to compensate for life at high altitudes, or abnormal, such as in cases of pulmonary or cardiac disease
Fanconi syndrome *fan-KŌ-nē*	Congenital aplastic anemia that appears between birth and 10 years of age; may be hereditary or caused by damage before birth, as by a virus
graft-versus-host reaction (GVHR)	An immunologic reaction of transplanted lymphocytes against tissues of the host; a common complication of bone marrow transplantation.
hairy-cell leukemia	A form of leukemia in which cells have filaments, making them look "hairy"
hematoma *hē-ma-TŌ-ma*	A localized collection of blood, usually clotted, caused by a break in a blood vessel
hemolytic disease of the newborn (HDN)	Disease that results from incompatibility between the blood of a mother and her fetus, usually involving Rh factor. An Rh-negative mother produces antibody to an Rh-positive fetus that, in later pregnancies, will destroy the red cells of an Rh-positive fetus. The problem is usually avoided by treating the mother with antibodies to remove the Rh antigen; erythroblastosis fetalis
hemosiderosis *hē-mō-sid-er-Ō-sis*	A condition involving the deposition of an iron-containing pigment (hemosiderin) mainly in the liver and the spleen. The pigment comes from hemoglobin released from disintegrated red blood cells.
idiopathic thrombocytopenic purpura (ITP)	A clotting disorder caused by destruction of platelets that usually follows a viral illness. Causes petechiae and hemorrhages into the skin and mucous membranes.
infectious mononucleosis *mon-ō-nū-klē-Ō-sis*	An acute infectious disease caused by Epstein–Barr virus (EBV). Characterized by fever, weakness, lymphadenopathy, hepatosplenomegaly, and atypical lymphocytes (resembling monocytes) (Fig. 10-16).
lymphocytosis *lim-fō-sī-TŌ-sis*	An increase in the number of circulating lymphocytes
myelodysplastic syndrome *mī-e-lō-dis-PLAS-tik*	Bone marrow dysfunction resulting in anemia and deficiency of neutrophils and platelets. May develop in time into leukemia; preleukemia
myelofibrosis *mī-e-lō-fī-BRŌ-sis*	Condition in which bone marrow is replaced with fibrous tissue
neutropenia *nū-trō-PĒ-nē-a*	A decrease in the number of neutrophils with increased susceptibility to infection. Causes include drugs, irradiation, and infection. May be a side effect of treatment for malignancy.
pancytopenia *pan-sī-tō-PĒ-nē-a*	A decrease in all cells of the blood, as in aplastic anemia

TERMINOLOGY Supplementary Terms
Continued

polycythemia *pol-ē-sī-THĒ-mē-a*	Any condition in which there is a relative increase in the percent of red blood cells in whole blood. May result from excessive production of red cells because of lack of oxygen, as caused by high altitudes, breathing obstruction, heart failure, or certain forms of poisoning. Apparent polycythemia results from concentration of the blood, as by dehydration.
polycythemia vera *pol-ē-sī-THĒ-mē-a VĒ-ra*	A condition in which overactive bone marrow produces too many red blood cells. These interfere with circulation and promote thrombosis and hemorrhage. Treated by blood removal. Also called *erythremia, Vaquez–Osler disease.*
septicemia *sep-ti-SĒ-mē-a*	Presence of microorganisms in the blood
spherocytic anemia *sfēr-ō-SIT-ik*	Hereditary anemia in which red blood cells are round instead of disk-shaped and rupture (hemolyze) excessively
thrombotic thrombocytopenic purpura (TTP)	An often-fatal disorder in which multiple clots form in blood vessels
von Willebrand disease	A hereditary bleeding disease caused by lack of von Willebrand factor, a substance necessary for blood clotting

DIAGNOSIS (see also Boxes 10–4 and 10–7)

Bence Jones protein	A protein that appears in the urine of patients with multiple myeloma
Coombs test	A test for detection of antibodies to red blood cells such as appear in cases of autoimmune hemolytic anemias
electrophoresis *ē-lek-trō-fo-RĒ-sis*	Separation of particles in a liquid by application of an electrical field; used to separate components of blood.
ELISA	Enzyme-linked immunosorbent assay. A highly sensitive immunologic test used to diagnose HIV infection, hepatitis, and Lyme disease, among others.
monoclonal antibody *mon-ō-KLŌ-nal*	A pure antibody produced in the laboratory; used for diagnosis and treatment
pH	A scale that measures the relative acidity or alkalinity of a solution. Represents the amount of hydrogen ion in the solution.
Schilling test *SHIL-ing*	Test used to determine absorption of vitamin B_{12} by measuring excretion of radioactive B_{12} in the urine. Used to distinguish pernicious from nutritional anemia.
seroconversion *sē-rō-con-VER-zhun*	The appearance of antibodies in the serum in response to a disease or an immunization
Western blot assay	A very sensitive test used to detect small amounts of antibodies in the blood
Wright stain	A commonly used blood stain. Figure 10-2 shows blood cells stained with Wright stain.

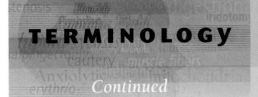

TERMINOLOGY
Supplementary Terms
Continued

TREATMENT

anticoagulant *an-ti-kō-AG-ū-lant*	An agent that prevents or delays blood coagulation
antihistamine *an-ti-HIS-ta-mēn*	A drug that counteracts the effects of histamine and is used to treat allergic reactions
apheresis *af-e-RĒ-sis*	A procedure in which blood is withdrawn, a portion is separated and retained, and the remainder is returned to the donor. Apheresis may be used as a suffix with a root meaning the fraction retained, such as plasmapheresis, leukapheresis.
autologous blood *aw-TOL-ō-gus*	A person's own blood. May be donated in advance of surgery and transfused if needed.
cryoprecipitate *krī-ō-prē-SIP-i-tāt*	A sediment obtained by cooling. The fraction obtained by freezing blood plasma contains clotting factors.
desensitization *dē-sen-si-ti-ZĀ-shun*	Treatment of allergy by small injections of the offending allergen. This causes an increase of antibody to destroy the antigen rapidly on contact.
homologous blood *hō-MOL-ō-gus*	Blood from animals of the same species, such as human blood used for transfusion from one person to another. Blood used for transfusions must be compatible with the blood of the recipient.
immunosuppression *im-ū-nō-sū-PRESH-un*	Depression of the immune response. May be correlated with disease but also may may be induced therapeutically to prevent rejection in cases of tissue transplantation.
protease inhibitor *PRŌ-tē-ās*	An anti-HIV drug that acts by inhibiting an enzyme the virus needs to multiply

 Go to the pronunciation glossary in Chapter 10 on the CD-ROM to hear these words pronounced.

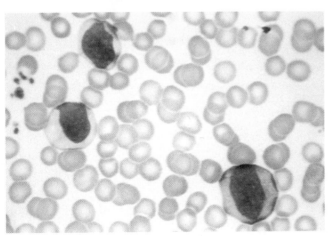

Figure 10-16 Infectious mononucleosis. Atypical lymphocytes characterize this viral disease.

TERMINOLOGY Abbreviations

Ab	Antibody
Ag	Antigen
AIDS	Acquired immunodeficiency syndrome
ALL	Acute lymphoblastic (lymphocytic) leukemia
AML	Acute myeloblastic (myelogenous) leukemia
APTT	Activated partial thromboplastin time
BT	Bleeding time
CBC	Complete blood count
CLL	Chronic lymphocytic leukemia
CML	Chronic myelogenous leukemia
crit	Hematocrit
DIC	Disseminated intravascular coagulation
Diff	Differential count
EBV	Epstein–Barr virus
ELISA	Enzyme-linked immunosorbent assay
EPO	Erythropoietin
ESR	Erythrocyte sedimentation rate
FFP	Fresh frozen plasma
Hb, Hgb	Hemoglobin
Hct, Ht	Hematocrit
HDN	Hemolytic disease of the newborn
HIV	Human immunodeficiency virus
IF	Intrinsic factor
Ig	Immunoglobulin
ITP	Idiopathic thrombocytopenic purpura
lytes	Electrolytes
MCH	Mean corpuscular hemoglobin
MCHC	Mean corpuscular hemoglobin concentration
mcL	Microliter
MCV	Mean corpuscular volume
MDS	Myelodysplastic syndrome
mEq	Milliequivalent
NHL	Non-Hodgkin lymphoma
PCV	Packed cell volume
pH	Scale for measuring hydrogen ion concentration (acidity or alkalinity)
Ph	Philadelphia chromosome
PMN	Polymorphonuclear (neutrophil)
poly	Neutrophil
polymorph	Neutrophil
PT	Pro time; prothrombin time
PTT	Partial thromboplastin time
RBC	Red blood cell; red-blood-cell count
seg	Neutrophil
SLE	Systemic lupus erythematosus
T(C)T	Thrombin (clotting) time
TTP	Thrombotic thrombocytopenic purpura
vWF	von Willebrand factor
WBC	White blood cell; white blood (cell) count

Chapter Review

Labeling Exercise
Blood Cells

Write the name of each numbered part on the corresponding line of the answer sheet.

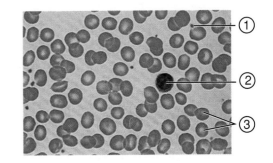

10

Erythrocyte   1._____

Leukocyte   2._____

Platelet   3._____

Leukocytes (white blood cells)

Write the name of each numbered part on the corresponding line of the answer sheet.

Leukocytes (white blood cells)

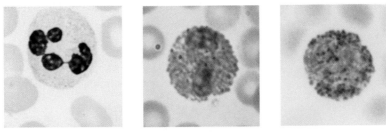

1   2   3

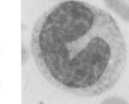

4   5

Basophil   1._____

Eosinophil   2._____

Lymphocyte   3._____

Monocyte   4._____

Neutrophil   5._____

TERMINOLOGY

Match the following terms and write the appropriate letter to the left of each number:

_____	1. myelogenic	**a.** immature bone marrow cell
_____	2. leukopenia	**b.** originating in bone marrow
_____	3. leukemia	**c.** malignant overgrowth of white blood cells
_____	4. myeloblast	**d.** formation of white blood cells
_____	5. leukopoiesis	**e.** deficiency of white blood cells

_____	6. calcidiol	**a.** pertaining to iron
_____	7. hypokalemia	**b.** urinary excretion of nitrogenous compounds
_____	8. ferrous	**c.** hormone involved in the metabolism of calcium
_____	9. siderosis	**d.** decreased potassium in the blood
_____	10. azoturia	**e.** condition involving iron deposits

_____	11. thalassemia	**a.** hives
_____	12. petechiae	**b.** hereditary form of anemia
_____	13. urticaria	**c.** stoppage of blood flow
_____	14. hemophilia	**d.** hereditary clotting disorder
_____	15. hemostasis	**e.** pinpoint spots caused by bleeding into the skin

_____	16. pH	**a.** hematocrit
_____	17. HIV	**b.** scale for measuring acidity or alkalinity
_____	18. CLL	**c.** hormone that stimulates red blood cell formation
_____	19. PCV	**d.** a form of leukemia
_____	20. EPO	**e.** virus that causes an immunodeficiency disease

Supplementary Terms

_____	21. electrophoresis	**a.** separation of blood and use of components
_____	22. heparin	**b.** pigment that comes from hemoglobin
_____	23. apheresis	**c.** anticoagulant
_____	24. ELISA	**d.** method for separating components of a solution
_____	25. bilirubin	**e.** sensitive immunologic test

Fill in the blanks:

26. The engulfing of foreign material by white cells is called _____.

27. The iron-containing pigment in red blood cells that carries oxygen is called _____.

28. A substance that separates into ions in solution is a(n) _____.

29. The cells fragments active in blood clotting are the _____.

30. A substance that induces the formation of antibodies is a(n) _____.

31. A hemocytometer is used to count _____.

32. Oxyhemoglobin is hemoglobin combined with _____.

33. A hematoma is a localized collection of _____.

34. A disorder involving lack of hemoglobin in the blood is _____.

35. A myeloma is a neoplasm that involves the _____.

True–False. Examine the following statements. If the statement is true, write T in the first blank. If the statement is false, write F in the first blank and correct the statement by replacing the <u>underlined</u> word in the second blank.

36. A platelet is also called a <u>lymphocyte</u>.   _____   _____

37. A plasma cell produces <u>antibodies</u>.   _____   _____

38. The liquid that remains after blood coagulates is called <u>serum</u> _____   _____

39. Blood that reacts with both A and B antisera is type <u>AB</u>.   _____   _____

40. A band cell is an immature <u>monocyte</u>.   _____   _____

41. The root natri- pertains to <u>sodium</u>.   _____   _____

The suffixes *-ia, -osis,* and *-hemia* all denote an increase in the type of cell indicated by the word root. Define the following terms:

42. eosinophilia (*ē-ō-sin-ō-FIL-ē-a*) _____

43. *erythrocytosis (e-rith-rō-sī-TŌ-sis)* _____

44. *thrombocythemia (throm-bō-sī-THĒ-mē-a)* _____

45. *neutrophilia (nū-trō-FIL-ē-a)* _____

46. *monocytosis (mon-ō-sī-TŌ-sis)* _____

Word building. Write a word for each of the following:

47. An immature lymphocyte   _____

48. A decrease in the number of platelets (thrombocytes) in the blood _____

49. Formation of white blood cells   _____

50. Presence of pus in the blood   _____

51. Specialist in the study of immunity   _____

52. Profuse flow of blood   _____

Adjectives. Use the ending *-ic* to write the adjective form of the following words:

53. basophil   _____

54. lymphocyte   _____

55. leukemia   _____

56. septicemia   _____

57. hemolysis   _____

58. thrombosis   _____

Define each of the following:

59. myelotoxin _____

60. viremia _____

10

61. neutropenia _____

62. autoimmunity _____

63. hypoxemia _____

Eliminations. In each of the sets below, underline the word that does not fit in with the rest and explain the reason for your choice:

64. fibrin - thrombin - thrombolysis - prothrombin - fibrinogen

_____

65. Diff - Hct - CBC - CD4 - ESR

_____

66. eosinophil - reticulocyte - monocyte - basophil - lymphocyte

_____

67. allergy - hypersensitivity - immunodeficiency - antigen - anaphylaxis

_____

Word analysis. Define the following words, and give the meaning of the word parts in each. Use a dictionary if necessary.

68. Polycythemia (*pol-ē-sī-THĒ-mē-a*) _____

   a. poly _____

   b. cyt/o _____

   c. hem _____

   d. -ia _____

69. Hemochromatosis (*hē-mō-krō-mā-TŌ-sis*) _____

   a. hem/o _____

   b. chromat/o _____

   c. -sis _____

70. Anisocytosis (*an-ī-sō-sī-TŌ-sis*) _____

   a. an- _____

   b. iso- _____

   c. cyt/o _____

   d. -sis _____

71. Myelodysplastic _____

   a. myel/o _____

   b. dys- _____

   c. plast(y) _____

   d. -ic _____

Go to the word exercises in Chapter 10 on the CD-ROM for additional review exercises.

CASE STUDY 10-1: Latex Allergy

M.R., a 36-year-old certified registered nurse anesthetist (CRNA), was diagnosed 7 years ago with latex allergy. She first noticed that contact dermatitis developed when she wore powdered latex gloves. Tachycardia, hypotension, bronchospasm, urticaria, and rhinitis soon developed with contact or proximity to latex in surgery. She had one frightening episode of anaphylaxis. Her allergy is of the type I hypersensitivity, IgE T-cell-mediated latex allergy, which was diagnosed by both a radioallergosorbent test (RAST) and a skin-prick test.

M.R. avoids all contact with any natural rubber latex in her home and at work. She can work only in a pediatric OR because they are latex-free, since many children with congenital disorders are allergic to latex. She wears a medical alert bracelet, uses a bronchodilator inhaler at the first symptom of bronchospasm, and carries a syringe of epinephrine at all times.

CASE STUDY 10-2: Blood Replacement

C.L., a 16-year-old girl, sustained a ruptured liver when she hit a tree while sledding. Emergency surgery was needed to stop the internal bleeding. During surgery, the ruptured segment of the liver was removed and the laceration was sutured with a heavy, absorbable suture on a large smooth needle. Before surgery, her hemoglobin was 10.2 g/dL, but the reading decreased to 7.6 g/dL before hemostasis was attained. Cell salvage, or autotransfusion, was set up. In this procedure, the free blood was suctioned from her abdomen and mixed with an anticoagulant (heparin). The RBCs were washed in a sterile centrifuge with NSS and transfused back to her through tubing fitted with a filter. She also received 6 units of homologous, leukocyte-reduced whole blood, 5 units of fresh frozen plasma, and 2 units of platelets. During the surgery, the CRNA repeatedly tested her Hgb and Hct as well as prothrombin time and partial thromboplastin time to monitor her clotting mechanisms.

C.L. is B-positive. Fortunately, there was enough B-positive blood in the hospital blood bank for her surgery. The lab informed her surgeon that they had 2 units of B-negative and 6 units of O-negative blood, which she could have received safely if she needed more blood during the night. However, her hemoglobin level increased to 12 g/dL, and she was stable during her recovery. She was monitored for DIC and pulmonary emboli.

CASE STUDY 10-3: Myelofibrosis

A.Y., a 52-year-old kindergarten teacher, had myelofibrosis that had been in remission for 25 years. She had seen her hematologist regularly and had had routine blood testing since the age of 27. After several weeks of fatigue, idiopathic joint and muscle aching, weakness, and a frightening episode of syncope, she saw her hematologist for evaluation. Her hemoglobin was 9.0 g/dL and her hematocrit was 29%. Concerned that she was having an exacerbation, her doctor scheduled a bone marrow aspiration, and the results were positive for myelofibrosis.

A.Y. went through a 6-month therapy regimen of iron supplements in the form of ferrous sulfate tablets and received weekly vitamin B_{12} injections. Interferon was given every other week in addition to erythropoiesis therapy, which was unsuccessful. She was treated for presumed aplastic anemia. During treatment, splenomegaly developed, which compromised her abdominal organs and pulmonary function. She continued to lose weight, and her hemoglobin dropped as low as 6.0 g/dL. Weekly transfusions of packed RBCs did not improve her hemoglobin and hematocrit.

After a regimen of high-dose chemotherapy to shrink the fibers in her bone marrow and a splenectomy, A.Y. received a stem-cell transplant. The stem cells were obtained from blood donated by her brother, who was a perfect immunologic match. After a 6-month period of recovery in a protected environment, required because of her immunocompromised state, A.Y. returned home and has been free of disease symptoms for over 1 year.

CASE STUDY QUESTIONS

Multiple choice. Select the best answer and write the letter of your choice to the left of each number:

_____ 1. The natural latex protein in latex gloves may act as a(n):
   a. antibody
   b. allergen
   c. lymphocyte
   d. purpura
   e. immunocyte

_____ 2. Urticaria is commonly called:
   a. rhinitis
   b. dermatitis
   c. hives
   d. ELISA
   e. congenital

_____ 3. The cells involved in a T-cell-mediated allergic response are:
   a. basophils
   b. monocytes
   c. antigen
   d. T lymphocytes
   e. B cells

_____ 4. Anaphylaxis, a life-threatening physiological response, is an extreme form of:
   a. remission
   b. hypersensitivity
   c. hemostasis
   d. exacerbation
   e. homeostasis

_____ 5. The common name for epinephrine is:
   a. heparin
   b. adrenaline
   c. cortisone
   d. apheresis
   e. antihistamine

_____ 6. The removal of part of the liver is called:
   a. partial hepatectomy
   b. hepatomegaly
   c. resection of the liver
   d. a and b
   e. a and c

_____ 7. The unit for hemoglobin measurement (g/dL) means:
   a. grams in decimal point
   b. grains in a decathlon
   c. drops in 50 cc
   d. grams in 100 mL
   e. grains in deciliter

10

_____ 8. Heparin, an anticoagulant, is a drug that:
   a. increases the rate of blood clotting
   b. takes the place of fibrin
   c. supports thrombin
   d. interferes with blood clotting
   e. makes blood thinner than water

_____ 9. The RBCs were washed with NSS. This means: the _____ were washed with _____.
   a. reticulocytes, heparin
   b. red blood cells, nutritional solution
   c. erythrocytes, normal saline solution
   d. reticulocytes, normal simple solution
   e. red blood cells, heparin

_____ 10. Autotransfusion is transfusion of autologous blood, that is, the patient's own blood. Homologous blood is taken from:
   a. another human
   b. synthetic chemicals
   c. plasma with clotting factors
   d. an animal with similar antibodies as humans
   e. IV fluid with electrolytes

_____ 11. Patients who lose a significant amount of blood may lose clotting ability. Effective therapy in such cases would be replacement of:
   a. IV solution with electrolytes
   b. iron supplements
   c. platelets
   d. heparin
   e. packed RBCs

_____ 12. C.L.'s blood type is B-positive. The best blood for her to receive is:
   a. positive
   b. negative
   c. AB-positive
   d. B-negative
   e. B-positive

_____ 13. Myelofibrosis, like aplastic anemia, is a disease in which there is:
   a. overgrowth of RBCs
   b. destruction of the bone marrow
   c. dangerously high hemoglobin and hematocrit
   d. absence of bone marrow
   e. lymphatic tissue in the bone marrow

_____ 14. Erythropoiesis is:
   a. production of blood
   b. production of red cells
   c. production of plasma
   d. destruction of white cells
   e. destruction of platelets

10

_____ 15. The "ferrous" in ferrous sulfate represents:
   a. electrolytes
   b. RBCs
   c. iron
   d. oxygen
   e. B vitamins

_____ 16. Hemoglobin and hematocrit values pertain to:
   a. leukocytes
   b. immune response
   c. granulocytes
   d. red blood cells
   e. fibrinogen

_____ 17. Splenomegaly is:
   a. prolapse of the spleen
   b. movement of the spleen
   c. enlargement of the lymph glands
   d. destruction of the bone marrow
   e. enlargement of the spleen

_____ 18. The stem cells A.Y. received were expected to develop into new:
   a. spleen cells
   b. bone marrow cells
   c. hemoglobin
   d. abdominal organs
   e. cartilage

_____ 19. A.Y.'s health was compromised because the high-dose chemotherapy caused:
   a. immunodeficiency
   b. electrolyte imbalance
   c. anoxia
   d. Rh incompatibility
   e. autoimmunity

Abbreviations. Define the following abbreviations:

20. Ig _____

21. Hgb _____

22. Hct _____

23. FFP _____

24. PT _____

25. PTT _____

26. DIC _____

Blood and Immunity

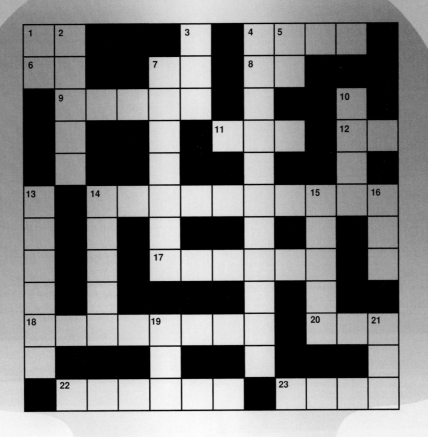

ACROSS

1. Alternative name for antibody (abbreviation)
4. Cold: prefix
6. Chemical symbol for sodium
7. Antibody (abbreviation)
8. Oxygen: root
9. Bone marrow: combining form
11. Oxygen-carrying pigment of red cells (abbreviation)
12. Antigen (abbreviation)
14. The substance that is deficient in cases of anemia
17. Most numerous type of white blood cell: combining form
18. Immature form of red blood cell: combining form
20. Type of widespread coagulation disorder (abbreviation)
22. Name used for a hereditary type of anemia
23. A mineral found in the blood (root)

DOWN

1. Prefix meaning "not"
2. Fraction of the blood that contains antibodies: _____ globulin
3. Common blood type system
4. Blood clotting
5. Prescription (abbreviation)
7. Protein found in the blood
10. Potassium: combining form
13. Iron: combining form
14. Blood: root
15. Fluid that brings oxygen and nutrients to the cells
16. New: prefix
19. Form of lymphocytic leukemia (abbreviation)
21. Comprehensive blood study (abbreviation)

THE RESPIRATORY SYSTEM

11

CHAPTER CONTENTS

OBJECTIVES

After study of this chapter you should be able to:

1. Explain the roles of oxygen and carbon dioxide in the body and describe how each is carried in the blood.
2. Label a diagram of the respiratory tract and briefly explain the function of each part.
3. Describe the mechanism of breathing, including the roles of the diaphragm and phrenic nerve.
4. Identify and use word parts pertaining to the respiratory system.
5. Discuss the major disorders of the respiratory system.
6. Define medical terms related to breathing and diseases of the respiratory system.
7. List and define 10 volumes and capacities commonly used to measure pulmonary function.
8. Interpret abbreviations commonly used with reference to the respiratory system.
9. Analyze several case studies pertaining to diseases that affect respiration.

PRETEST

1. The gas that is supplied to tissues by the respiratory system is _____.

2. The gas that is eliminated by the respiratory system is _____.

3. The air sacs through which gases are exchanged in the lungs are the _____.

4. The tubes that carry air from the trachea into the lungs are the _____.

5. Inflammation of the lungs is called _____.

6. Inflammation of the membranes around the lungs is called _____.

*T*he main function of the respiratory system is to provide **oxygen** to body cells for energy metabolism and to eliminate **carbon dioxide**, a by-product of metabolism. Because these gases must be carried to and from the cells in the blood, the respiratory system works closely with the cardiovascular system to accomplish gas exchange (Fig. 11-1). This activity has two phases:

> ➤ External gas exchange occurs between the outside atmosphere and the blood
> ➤ Internal gas exchange occurs between the blood and the tissues.

External exchange takes place in the lungs, located in the thoracic cavity. The remainder of the respiratory tract consists of a series of passageways that conduct air to and from the lungs. No gas exchange occurs in these regions. Refer to Figure 11-2 as you read the following description of the respiratory tract.

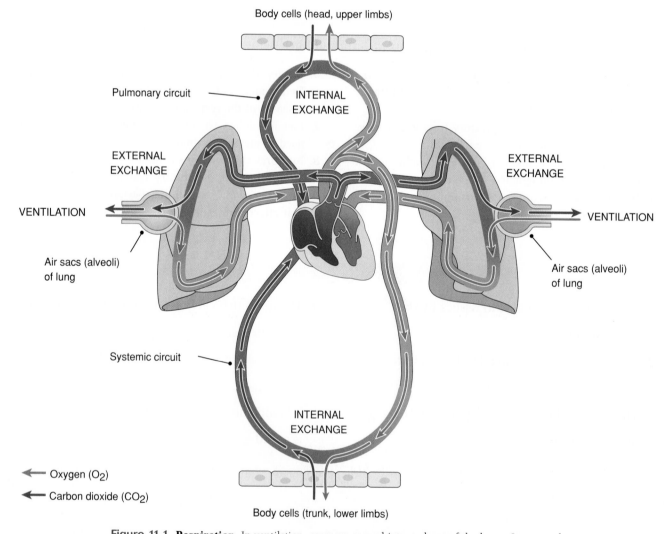

Figure 11-1 Respiration. In ventilation, gases are moved into and out of the lungs. In external exchange, gases move between the air sacs (alveoli) of the lungs and the blood. In internal exchange, gases move between the blood and body cells. The circulation transports gases in the blood.

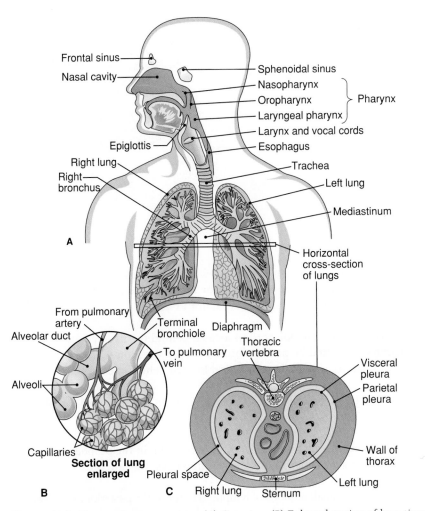

Figure 11-2 The respiratory system. (*A*) Overview. (*B*) Enlarged section of lung tissue showing the relationship between the alveoli (air sacs) and the blood capillaries. (*C*) A transverse section through the lungs.

Upper Respiratory Passageways

The upper respiratory passageways consist of the nose and pharynx (throat). Air can also be exchanged through the mouth, but there are fewer mechanisms for cleansing the air taken in by this route.

The Nose

Air enters through the **nose**, where it is warmed, filtered, and moistened as it passes over the hair-covered mucous membranes of the nasal cavity. Cilia—microscopic hairlike projections from the cells that line the nose—sweep dirt and foreign material toward the throat for elimination. Material that is eliminated from the respiratory tract by coughing or clearing the throat is called **sputum**. Receptors for the sense of smell are located within bony side projections of the nasal cavity called **turbinate bones**, or conchae.

In the bones of the skull and face near the nose are air-filled cavities lined with mucous membranes that drain into the nasal cavity. These chambers lighten the bones and provide resonance for speech production. These cavities are called **sinuses**, and they are named specifically for the bones in which they are located, such as the sphenoid, ethmoid, and maxillary sinuses. Together, because they are near the nose, these cavities are referred to as the paranasal sinuses (see Fig. 11-2).

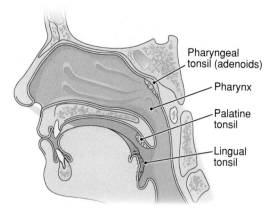

Figure 11-3 The tonsils. All of the tonsils are located in the vicinity of the pharynx (throat).

The Pharynx

Inhaled air passes into the throat, or **pharynx**, where it mixes with air that enters through the mouth and also with food destined for the digestive tract. The pharynx is divided into three regions, which are shown in Figure 11-2:

> ➤ The nasopharynx is the superior portion located behind the nasal cavity.
> ➤ The oropharynx is the middle portion located behind the mouth.
> ➤ The laryngeal pharynx is the inferior portion located behind the larynx.

The tonsils, lymphoid tissue described in Chapter 10, are in the region of the pharynx (Fig. 11-3):

> ➤ The **palatine tonsils** are on either side of the soft palate in the oropharynx.
> ➤ The single pharyngeal tonsil, commonly known as the **adenoids**, is in the nasopharynx.
> ➤ The lingual tonsils are small mounds of lymphoid tissue at the posterior of the tongue.

Opinions on the advisability of removing the tonsils have changed over time, as described in Box 11-1.

Box 11•1 **Clinical Perspectives** *Tonsillectomy: A Procedure Reconsidered*

Tonsillitis, a bacterial infection of the tonsils, is a common childhood illness. In years past, surgical removal of the infected tonsils was a standard procedure, as tonsillectomy was thought to prevent severe infections like strep throat. Because tonsils were thought to have little function in the body, many surgeons removed infected tonsils—even healthy tonsils—in order to prevent tonsillitis later. With the discovery that tonsils play an important immune function, the number of tonsillectomies performed in the United States dropped dramatically, reaching an all-time low in the 1980s.

Today, although many cases of tonsillitis are successfully treated with appropriate antibiotics, tonsillectomy is becoming more frequent; in fact, it is the second most common surgical procedure among American children. Surgery is considered if an infection recurs, or if enlarged tonsils make

swallowing or breathing difficult. Many tonsillectomies are performed in children to treat obstructive sleep apnea, a condition in which the child stops breathing for a few seconds at a time during sleep. Recent studies suggest that tonsillectomy may also be beneficial for children suffering from otitis media (middle ear infection), because bacteria infecting the tonsils may travel to this region of the ear.

Most tonsillectomies are performed by electrocautery, a technique that uses an electrical current to burn the tonsils away from the throat. Now that this operation is becoming more common, surgeons are developing new techniques. For example, coblation tonsillectomy uses radio waves to break down tonsillar tissue. Studies suggest that this procedure results in a faster recovery, fewer complications, and decreased postoperative pain compared with electrocautery.

Lower Respiratory Passageways and Lungs

Air moves from the pharynx into the larynx, commonly called the voice box, because it contains the vocal cords. The larynx is at the top of the trachea, commonly called the windpipe, which conducts air into the bronchial system toward the lungs.

The Larynx

The **larynx** is shaped by nine cartilages, the most prominent of which is the thyroid cartilage at the anterior that forms the "Adam's apple" (Fig. 11-4). The small leaf-shaped cartilage at the top of the larynx is the **epiglottis**. When one swallows, the epiglottis covers the opening of the larynx and helps to prevent food from entering the respiratory tract.

The larynx contains the **vocal cords**, folds of tissue that are important in speech production (Fig. 11-5). Vibrations produced by air passing over the vocal cords form the basis for voice production, although portions of the throat and mouth are needed for proper articulation of speech. The opening between the vocal cords is the **glottis** (the epiglottis is above the glottis).

The Trachea

The **trachea** is a tube reinforced with C-shaped rings of cartilage to prevent its collapse (you can feel these rings if you press your fingers gently against the front of your throat). Cilia in the lining of the trachea move impurities up toward the throat, where they can be eliminated by swallowing or by **expectoration**, coughing them up.

The trachea is contained in a region known as the **mediastinum**, which consists of the space between the lungs together with the organs contained in this space (see Fig. 11-2). In addition to the trachea, the mediastinum contains the heart, esophagus, large vessels, and other tissues.

The Bronchial System

At its lower end, the trachea divides into a right and a left main stem **bronchus**; these enter the lungs. The right bronchus is shorter and wider; it divides into three secondary bronchi in the right lung. The left bronchus divides into two branches that supply the left lung. Further divisions produce an increasing number of smaller tubes that supply air to smaller subdivisions of lung tissue. As the air passageways progress through the lungs, the cartilage in the walls gradually disappears and is replaced by smooth (involuntary) muscle.

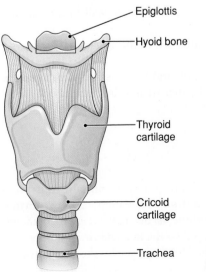

- Epiglottis
- Hyoid bone
- Thyroid cartilage
- Cricoid cartilage
- Trachea

Figure 11-4 **The larynx, anterior view.**

11

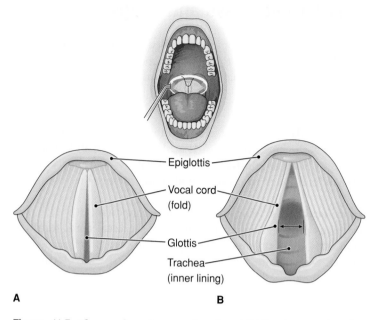

Epiglottis

Vocal cord
(fold)

Glottis

Trachea
(inner lining)

A **B**

Figure 11-5 The vocal cords, superior view. (*A*) The glottis in closed position. (*B*) The glottis in open position.

The smallest of the conducting tubes, the **bronchioles**, carry air into the microscopic air sacs, the **alveoli**, through which gases are exchanged between the lungs and the blood. It is through the ultra-thin walls of the alveoli and their surrounding capillaries that oxygen diffuses into the blood and carbon dioxide diffuses out of the blood for elimination (see Fig. 11-2).

The Lungs

The cone-shaped **lungs** occupy the major portion of the thoracic cavity. The right lung is larger and divided into three lobes. The left lung, which is smaller, to accommodate the heart, is divided into two lobes. The lobes are further subdivided to correspond to divisions of the bronchial network.

A double membrane, the **pleura**, covers the lungs and lines the thoracic cavity (see Fig. 11-2C). The two layers of the pleura are:

> The parietal pleura, the outer layer, which is attached to the wall of the thoracic cavity
> The visceral pleura, the inner layer, which is attached to the surface of the lungs.

The very narrow, fluid-filled space between the two pleural layers is the **pleural space**. The moist pleural membranes slide easily over each other within the chest cavity, allowing the lungs to expand during breathing.

Breathing

Air is moved into and out of the lungs by the process of breathing, technically called **ventilation**. This consists of a steady cycle of **inspiration** (inhalation) and **expiration** (exhalation), separated by a period of rest. Breathing is normally regulated unconsciously by centers in the brainstem. These centers adjust the rate and rhythm of breathing according to changes in the composition of the blood, especially the concentration of carbon dioxide.

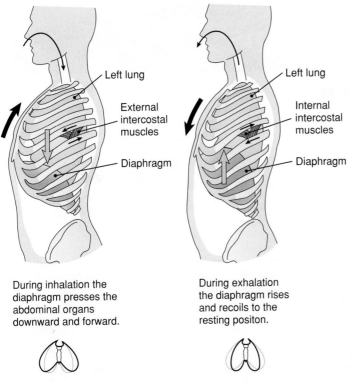

During inhalation the diaphragm presses the abdominal organs downward and forward.

During exhalation the diaphragm rises and recoils to the resting positon.

A. Action of rib cage in inhalation

B. Action of rib cage in exhalation

Figure 11-6 Pulmonary ventilation. (*A*) In inhalation, the diaphragm lowers and the external intercostals elevate the rib cage. (*B*) In exhalation, the diaphragm rises and the internal intercostals draw the ribs downward.

Inspiration

The breathing cycle begins when the **phrenic nerve** stimulates the **diaphragm** to contract and flatten, enlarging the chest cavity considerably. At the same time, external intercostal muscles between the ribs elevate and expand the rib cage. A resulting decrease in pressure within the thorax causes air to be pulled into the lungs (Fig. 11-6). Muscles of the neck and thorax are used in addition for forceful inhalation.

The measure of how easily the lungs expand under pressure is **compliance**. Fluid produced in the lungs, known as **surfactant**, aids in compliance by reducing surface tension within the alveoli.

Expiration

Expiration occurs as the breathing muscles relax and the elastic lungs spring back to their original size. Increased pressure in the smaller thorax forces air out of the lungs. In forceful exhalation, the internal intercostal muscles contract to lower the rib cage, and the abdominal muscles contract, pressing internal organs upward against the diaphragm.

Gas Transport

Oxygen is carried in the blood bound to **hemoglobin** in red blood cells. The oxygen is released to the cells as needed. Carbon dioxide is carried in several ways but is mostly converted to **carbonic acid**. The amount of carbon dioxide that is exhaled is important in regulating the acidity or alkalinity of the blood, based on the amount of carbonic acid that is formed. Dangerous shifts in blood pH can result from exhalation of too much or too little carbon dioxide.

TERMINOLOGY Key Terms

NORMAL STRUCTURE AND FUNCTION

adenoids *AD-e-noyds*	Lymphoid tissue located in the nasopharynx; the pharyngeal tonsils
alveoli *al-VĒ-ō-lī*	The tiny air sacs in the lungs through which gases are exchanged between the atmosphere and the blood in respiration (singular: alveolus). An alveolus, in general, is a small hollow or cavity, and the term is also used to describe the bony socket for a tooth.
bronchiole *BRONG-kē-ōl*	One of the smaller subdivisions of the bronchial tubes (root: *bronchiol*)
bronchus *BRONG-kus*	One of the larger air passageways in the lungs. The bronchi begin as two branches of the trachea and then subdivide within the lungs (plural: bronchi) (root *bronch*).
carbon dioxide (CO$_2$)	A gas produced by energy metabolism in cells and eliminated through the lungs
carbonic acid *kar-BON-ik*	An acid formed by carbon dioxide when it dissolves in water; H$_2$CO$_3$
compliance *kom-PLĪ-ans*	A measure of how easily the lungs expand under pressure. Compliance is reduced in many types of respiratory disorders.
diaphragm *DĪ-a-fram*	The dome-shaped muscle under the lungs that flattens during inspiration (root: *phren/o*)
epiglottis *ep-i-GLOT-is*	A leaf-shaped cartilage that covers the larynx during swallowing to prevent food from entering the trachea
expectoration *ek-spek-to-RĀ-shun*	The act of coughing up material from the respiratory tract; also the material thus released; sputum
expiration *ek-spi-RĀ-shun*	The act of breathing out or expelling air from the lungs; exhalation
glottis *GLOT-is*	The opening between the vocal cords
hemoglobin *HĒ-mō-glō-bin*	The iron-containing pigment in red blood cells that transports oxygen
inspiration *in-spi-RĀ-shun*	The act of drawing air into the lungs; inhalation
larynx *LAR-inks*	The enlarged upper end of the trachea that contains the vocal cords (root: *laryng/o*)
lung	A cone-shaped spongy organ of respiration contained within the thorax (roots: *pneum, pulm*)
mediastinum *mē-dē-as-TĪ-num*	The space between the lungs together with the organs contained in this space
nose *nōz*	The organ of the face used for breathing and for housing receptors for the sense of smell; includes an external portion and an internal nasal cavity (roots: *nas/o, rhin/o*)

TERMINOLOGY   Key Terms

Continued

11

oxygen (O₂) *OK-si-jen*	The gas needed by cells to release energy from food during metabolism
palatine tonsils *PAL-a-tīn*	The paired masses of lymphoid tissue located on either side of the oropharynx; usually meant when the term *tonsils* is used alone
pharynx *FAR-inks*	The throat; a common passageway for food entering the esophagus and air entering the larynx (root: *pharyng/o*)
phrenic nerve *FREN-ik*	The nerve that activates the diaphragm (root: *phrenic/o*)
pleura *PLŪR-a*	A double-layered membrane that lines the thoracic cavity (parietal pleura) and covers the lungs (visceral pleura) (root: *pleur/o*)
pleural space	The thin, fluid-filled space between the two layers of the pleura; pleural cavity
sinus *SĪ-nus*	A cavity or channel; the paranasal sinuses are located near the nose and drain into the nasal cavity.
sputum *SPŪ-tum*	The substance released by coughing or clearing the throat; expectoration. It may contain a variety of material from the respiratory tract.
surfactant *sur-FAK-tant*	A substance that decreases surface tension within the alveoli and eases lung expansion.
trachea *TRĀ-kē-a*	The air passageway that extends from the larynx to the bronchi (root: *trache/o*)
turbinate bones *TUR-bi-nāt*	The bony projections in the nasal cavity that contain receptors for the sense of smell. Also called conchae (KON-kē).
ventilation *ven-ti-LĀ-shun*	The movement of air into and out of the lungs
vocal cords *VŌ-kal*	Membranous folds on either side of the larynx that are important in speech production. Also called vocal folds.

Go to the pronunciation glossary in Chapter 11 on the CD-ROM to hear these words pronounced.

Word Parts Pertaining to the Respiratory System

Table 11·1 Suffixes for Respiration			
SUFFIX	**MEANING**	**EXAMPLE**	**DEFINITION OF EXAMPLE**
-pnea	breathing	orthopnea *or-THOP-nē-a*	breathing difficulty that is relieved by assuming an upright (ortho-) position
-oxia*	level of oxygen	hypoxia *hī-POK-sē-a*	decreased amount of oxygen in the tissues
-capnia*	level of carbon dioxide	hypercapnia *hī-per-KAP-nē-a*	increased carbon dioxide in the tissues
-phonia	voice	dysphonia *dis-FŌ-nē-a*	difficulty in speaking

*When referring to levels of oxygen and carbon dioxide in the blood, the suffix -emia is used, as in hypoxemia, hypercapnemia.

Exercise 11-1

Use the suffix -pnea to build words with the following meanings:

1. lack of breathing   _____ apnea _____

2. slow (brady-) rate of breathing   _____

3. painful or difficult breathing   _____

4. easy, normal breathing   _____

Use the ending -pneic to write the adjective form of the above words:

5. _____ apneic _____

6. _____

7. _____

8. _____

Use the suffixes in Table 11-1 to write a word for each of the following definitions:

9. decreased carbon dioxide in the tissues   _____

10. lack of (an-) oxygen in the tissues   _____

11. normal levels (eu-) of carbon dioxide in the tissues   _____

12. lack of voice   _____

Table 11·2 Roots for the Respiratory Passageways

ROOT	MEANING	EXAMPLE	DEFINITION OF EXAMPLE
nas/o	nose	paranasal *par-a-NĀ-zal*	near the nose
rhin/o	nose	rhinorrhea *rī-NŌ-rē-a*	discharge from the nose
pharyng/o	pharynx	pharyngospasm *fa-RING-gō-spazm*	spasm (sudden contraction) of the pharynx
laryng/o*	larynx	laryngeal *la-RIN-jē-al*	pertaining to the larynx
trache/o	trachea	tracheotome *tra-kē-ō-TŌM*	instrument used to incise the trachea
bronch/o, bronch/i	bronchus	bronchogenic *brong-kō-GEN-ik*	originating in a bronchus
bronchiol	bronchiole	bronchiolectasis *brong-kē-ō-LEK-ta-sis*	dilatation of the bronchioles

*Note addition of e before adjective ending -al.

Exercise 11-2

Write words for the following definitions:

1. plastic repair of the nose _____rhinoplasty_____
2. pertaining to the pharynx (see *larynx* in Table 11-2) _____
3. inflammation of the pharynx _____
4. endoscopic examination of the larynx _____
5. plastic repair of the larynx _____
6. surgical incision of the trachea _____
7. narrowing of a bronchus _____
8. inflammation of the bronchioles _____

Define the following words (note the adjectival endings):

9. intranasal (*in-tra-NĀ-zal*) _____within the nose_____
10. endotracheal (*en-dō-TRĀ-kē-al*) _____
11. nasopharyngeal (*nā-zō-fa-RIN-jē-al*) _____
12. peribronchial (*per-i-BRONG-kē-al*) _____
13. bronchiectasis (*brong-kē-EK-ta-sis*) _____
14. bronchiolar (*brong-KĒ-ō-lar*) _____

Table 11·3 Roots for the Lungs and Breathing

ROOT	MEANING	EXAMPLE	DEFINITION OF EXAMPLE
phren/o	diaphragm	phrenic *FREN-ik*	pertaining to the diaphragm
phrenic/o	phrenic nerve	phrenicotripsy *fren-i-kō-TRIP-sē*	crushing of the phrenic nerve
pleur/o	pleura	pleurodesis *plū-ROD-e-sis*	fusion of the pleura
pulm/o, pulmon/o	lungs	extrapulmonary *EKS-tra-pul-mō-ner-ē*	outside the lungs
pneumon/o	lung	pneumonectomy *nū-mō-NEK-tō-mē*	surgical removal of a lung or lung tissue (pneumectomy and pulmonectomy also used)
pneum/o, pneumat/o	air, gas; also respiration, lung	pneumothorax *nū-mō-THŌ-raks*	presence of air in the thorax (pleural space)
spir/o	breathing	spirometer *spī-ROM-e-ter*	instrument for measuring breathing volumes

Exercise 11-3

Define the following words:

1. pleuralgia *(plū-RAL-jē-a)* _____

2. pleuropulmonary *(plūr-ō-PUL-mō-ner-ē)* _____

3. pneumonitis *(nū-mō-NĪ-tis)* _____

4. pneumoplasty *(NŪ-mō-plas-tē)* _____

5. pulmonology *(pul-mō-NOL-ō-jē)* _____

6. apneumia *(a-NŪ-mē-a)* _____

Write words for the following definitions:

7. within (intra-) the pleura _____

8. above the diaphragm _____

9. surgical puncture of the pleural space _____

10. any disease of the lungs (pneumon/o) _____

11. surgical incision of the phrenic nerve _____

12. record of breathing volumes _____

Clinical Aspects of the Respiratory System

Pulmonary function is affected by conditions that cause resistance to air flow through the respiratory tract or conditions that limit expansion of the chest. These occurrences may be conditions that affect the respiratory system directly, such as infection, injury, allergy, **aspiration** (inhalation) of foreign bodies, or cancer. They also may result from disturbances in other systems, such as in the skeletal, muscular, cardiovascular, or nervous systems.

As noted above, changes in ventilation can affect the blood's pH (acidity or alkalinity). If too much carbon dioxide is exhaled by **hyperventilation**, the blood tends to become too alkaline, a condition termed **alkalosis**. If too little carbon dioxide is exhaled as a result of **hypoventilation**, the blood tends to become too acidic, a condition termed **acidosis**.

Infections

A variety of organisms infect the respiratory system. For your reference, some of these organisms are listed along with the diseases they cause in Box 11-2. Childhood immunizations have dramatically reduced the incidence of some infectious respiratory

Box 11•2 For Your Reference	*Organisms That Infect the Respiratory System*

Organism	Disease
BACTERIA	
Streptococcus pneumoniae *strep-tō-KOK-us nū-MŌ-nē-ē*	Most common cause of pneumonia; streptococcal pneumonia
Haemophilus influenzae *hē-MOF-i-lus in-flū-EN-zē*	Pneumonia, especially in debilitated patients
Klebsiella pneumoniae *kleb-sē-EL-a nū-MŌ-nē-a*	Pneumonia in elderly and debilitated patients
Mycoplasma pneumoniae *mī-kō-PLAZ-ma nū-MŌ-nē-ē*	Mild pneumonia, usually in young adults and children; "walking pneumonia"
Legionella pneumophila *lē-ju-NEL-la nū-MO-fi-la*	Legionellosis (Legionnaire disease); respiratory disease spread through water sources, such as air conditioners, pools, humidifiers
Chlamydia psittaci *kla-MID-ē-a PSI-ta-sē*	Psittacosis (ornithosis); carried by birds
Streptococcus pyogenes *strep-tō-KOK-us pī-OJ-e-nēz*	"Strep throat," scarlet fever
Mycobacterium tuberculosis *mī-kō-bak-TĒR-ē-um tū-ber-kū-LŌ-sis*	Tuberculosis
Bordetella pertussis *bōr-de-TEL-a per-TUS-sis*	Pertussis (whooping cough)
Corynebacterium diphtheriae *kō-RĪ-nē-bak-tēr-ē-um dif-THē-rē-ē*	Diphtheria

Box 11•2 **For Your Reference** *Continued*

VIRUSES

Rhinoviruses *RĪ-nō-vī-rus-es*	Major cause of common cold; also caused by coronaviruses, adenoviruses, and others
Influenzavirus *in-flū-EN-za-vī-rus*	Influenza
Respiratory syncytial virus (RSV) *sin-SISH-al*	Common cause of respiratory disease in infants
SARS coronavirus *kō-RŌ-na-vī-rus*	Severe acute respiratory syndrome; highly infectious disease that appeared in 2003 and spreads from small mammals to humans
Hantavirus *HAN-ta-vī-rus*	Hantavirus pulmonary syndrome (HPS); spread by inhalation of virus released from dried rodent droppings

FUNGI

Histoplasma capsulatum *his-tō-PLAS-ma kap-sū-LĀT-um*	Histoplasmosis; spread by airborne spores
Coccidioides immitis *kok-sid-ē-OY-dēz IM-i-tis*	Coccidioidomycosis (valley fever, San Joaquin fever); found in dry, alkaline soils
Blastomyces dermatitidis *blas-tō-MĪ-sēz der-ma-TIT-i-dis*	Blastomycosis; rare but often fatal fungal disease
Pneumocystis jiroveci (formerly *carinii*) *nū-mō-SIS-tis jir-ō-VE-sē*	Pneumocystis pneumonia (PCP); seen in immunocompromised hosts

diseases, such as **diphtheria** and **pertussis** (the D and P in the DTaP vaccine). Selected infectious diseases are described in greater detail below.

Pneumonia

Pneumonia is caused by many different microorganisms, usually bacteria or viruses. Bacterial agents are most commonly *Streptococcus pneumoniae* and *Klebsiella pneumoniae*. Viral pneumonia is more diffuse and is commonly caused by influenza virus, adenovirus and, in young children, respiratory syncytial virus (RSV). Two forms of pneumonia are (Fig. 11-7):

➤ Bronchopneumonia (bronchial pneumonia), which begins in terminal bronchioles that become clogged with exudate and form consolidated (solidified) patches.
➤ Lobar pneumonia, an acute disease that involves one or more lobes of the lung.

Pneumonia usually can be treated successfully in otherwise healthy people, but in debilitated patients it is a leading cause of death. Immunocompromised patients, such as those with AIDS, are often subject to a form of pneumonia called *Pneumocystis jiroveci* pneumonia (PCP), which is caused by a fungus.

The term *pneumonia* is also applied to lung inflammation caused by noninfectious causes, such as asthma, allergy, or inhalation of irritants. In these cases, however, the more general term **pneumonitis** is often used.

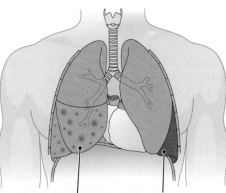

Figure 11-7 Pneumonia. In bronchopneumonia (right lung), patchy areas of consolidation occur. In lobar pneumonia (left lung) an entire lobe is consolidated.

Bronchopneumonia   Lobar pneumonia

Tuberculosis

The incidence of **tuberculosis (TB)** has increased in recent years, along with the increase of AIDS and the appearance of antibiotic resistance in the causative organism, *Mycobacterium tuberculosis* (MTB). (This organism, because of its staining properties, also is referred to as AFB, meaning *acid-fast bacillus*.) The name *tuberculosis* comes from the small lesions, or tubercles, that appear with the infection. The tubercles can liquefy in the center and then rupture to release bacteria into the bloodstream. Generalized TB is known as *miliary tuberculosis* because of the many tubercles that are the size of millet seeds in infected tissue (Fig. 11-8).

The symptoms of TB include fever, weight loss, weakness, cough, and **hemoptysis**, the coughing up of blood-containing sputum, resulting from damage to pulmonary blood vessels. Sputum analysis is used to isolate, stain, and identify infectious organisms. Accumulation of exudate in the alveoli may result in consolidation of lung tissue.

The **tuberculin test** is used to test for tuberculosis infection. The test material, tuberculin, is made from by-products of the tuberculosis organism. PPD (purified protein derivative) is the form of tuberculin commonly used.

BCG vaccine is used worldwide to help to prevent TB; it is not used routinely in the United States because the incidence of TB is relatively low and also because it invalidates the tuberculin test. (The vaccine is named for Calmette and Guérin, discoverers of the avirulent mycobacterium strain it contains.)

Influenza

Influenza ("flu") is a viral disease of the respiratory tract associated with chills, fever, headaches, muscular aches, and coldlike symptoms. It usually resolves in several days, but severe forms of influenza have caused fatal pandemics, most recently in 1918, 1957,

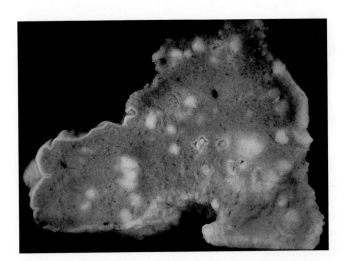

Figure 11-8 Tuberculosis. The cut surface of the lung reveals numerous white nodules in miliary (generalized) tuberculosis.

and 1968. The virus can mutate readily and spread among animals, such as birds or pigs, and humans.

Because influenza viruses change so rapidly, scientists must prepare vaccines against the strains most likely to cause an epidemic in any given year. The virus strains are grouped into categories A–C, with A the most severe and C the least. They are further designated H and N with numbers, such as H3N2, H5N1. The H and N represent surface antigens that the virus uses to infect a host.

Medical personnel combat influenza with vaccines, isolation of infected populations, destruction of infected animals, and antiviral medications.

Common Cold

More than 200 viruses are known to cause the common cold. About one half of these are rhinoviruses, and the others include adenoviruses and coronaviruses. The symptoms, known to all, are sneezing, **acute rhinitis**, which is inflammation of the nasal passageways with copious secretion of watery mucus, tearing of the eyes, and congestion. The infection may spread from the nose and throat to the sinuses, middle ear, and lower respiratory tract.

Cold viruses are mostly spread by airborne virus-filled droplets released by an infected person's coughs and sneezes. Frequent hand washing and not touching one's hands to any part of the face are good preventive measures.

The disorder usually resolves in about a week. Because colds are caused by viruses, antibiotics do not cure them. Rest, fluid intake, symptomatic treatment, and time work best. The many types of cold viruses and their frequent mutation have prevented the development of an effective vaccine.

See Box 11-3 for some history on terminology related to respiratory infections and other disorders.

Emphysema

Emphysema is a chronic disease associated with overexpansion and destruction of the alveoli. Common causes are exposure to cigarette smoke and other forms of pollution as well as chronic infection. Emphysema is the main disorder included under the heading of **chronic obstructive pulmonary disease (COPD)** (also called COLD, chronic obstructive lung disease). Other conditions included in this category are asthma, chronic **bronchitis**, and **bronchiectasis**.

Asthma

Attacks of **asthma** result from narrowing of the bronchial tubes. This constriction, along with edema (swelling) of the bronchial linings, inflammation, and accumulation of mucus, results in wheezing, extreme **dyspnea** (difficulty in breathing), and **cyanosis**.

Box 11•3 Focus on Words   *Don't Breathe a Word*

Some laypersons' terms for respiratory symptoms and conditions are so old-fashioned and quaint that you might see them today only in Victorian novels. Catarrh (ka-TAR) is an old word for an upper respiratory infection with much mucus production. Quinsy (KWIN-zē) referred to a sore throat or tonsillar abscess. Consumption was tuberculosis, and dropsy referred to generalized edema. The grip meant influenza, which we more often abbreviate as "flu."

Some unscientific words are still in use. These include whooping cough for pertussis, croup for laryngeal spasm, cold sore for a herpes lesion, and phlegm for sputum.

Many informal terms are used instead of scientific words by the general public. Health professionals should be familiar with the slang or colloquialisms that are used to describe symptoms so that they can better communicate with their patients.

Asthma is most common in children. Although its causes are uncertain, a main factor is irritation caused by allergy. Heredity may also play a role. Treatment of asthma includes:

- ➤ removal of allergens
- ➤ administration of bronchodilators to widen the airways
- ➤ administration of corticosteroids to reduce inflammation

Pneumoconiosis

Chronic irritation and inflammation caused by inhalation of dust particles is termed **pneumoconiosis**. This is an occupational hazard seen mainly in people involved in the mining and stoneworking industries. Different forms of pneumoconiosis are named for the specific type of dust inhaled: silicosis (silica or quartz), anthracosis (coal dust), asbestosis (asbestos fibers).

Although the term pneumoconiosis is limited to conditions caused by inhalation of inorganic dust, lung irritation may also result from inhalation of organic dusts, such as textile or grain dusts.

Lung Cancer

Lung cancer is the leading cause of cancer-related deaths in both men and women. The incidence of lung cancer has increased steadily over the past 50 years, especially in women. Cigarette smoking is a major risk factor in this as well as other types of cancer. The most common form of lung cancer is squamous carcinoma, originating in the lining of the bronchi (bronchogenic). Lung cancer usually cannot be detected early, and it metastasizes rapidly. The overall survival rate is low.

Methods used to diagnose lung cancer include radiographic studies, computed tomography (CT) scans, and examination of sputum for cancer cells. Physicians can use a **bronchoscope** to examine the airways and to collect tissue samples for study. They may also take samples by surgical or needle biopsies.

Respiratory Distress Syndrome (RDS)

Respiratory distress syndrome of the newborn, also called *hyaline membrane disease*, occurs in premature infants and is the most common cause of death in this group. It results from a lack of surfactant in the lungs, which reduces compliance. **Acute respiratory distress syndrome (ARDS)**, also known as *shock lung*, may result from trauma, allergic reactions, infection, and other causes. It involves edema that can lead to respiratory failure and death if untreated.

Cystic Fibrosis

Cystic fibrosis (CF) is the most common fatal hereditary disease among white children. The flawed gene that causes CF affects glandular secretions by altering chloride transport across cell membranes. Thickening of bronchial secretions leads to infection and other respiratory disorders. Other mucus-secreting glands, sweat glands, and glands of the pancreas are also involved, causing electrolyte imbalance and digestive disturbances.

CF is diagnosed by the increased amounts of sodium and chloride in the sweat. Geneticists also can identify the gene that causes CF by DNA analysis. There is no cure at present for CF. Patients are treated to relieve their symptoms, as by postural drainage, aerosol mists, bronchodilators, antibiotics, and mucolytic agents, which dissolve mucus.

Sudden Infant Death Syndrome (SIDS)

SIDS, also called "crib death", is the unexplained death of a seemingly healthy infant under 1 year of age. Death usually occurs during sleep, leaving no signs of its cause. Neither autopsy nor careful investigation of family history and circumstances of death provides any clues.

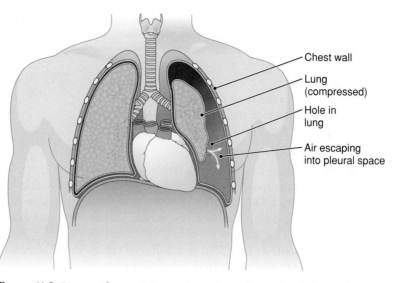

Figure 11-9 Pneumothorax. Injury to lung tissue allows air to leak into the pleural space and put pressure on the lung.

Certain maternal conditions during pregnancy are associated with an increased risk of SIDS, although none is a sure predictor. These include cigarette smoking, age under 20, low weight gain, anemia, illegal drug use, and reproductive or urinary tract infections.

Some practices that have reduced the incidence of SIDS are:

> ➤ Place the baby on its back (supine) for sleep ("back to sleep")
> ➤ Keep the baby in a smoke-free environment
> ➤ Use a firm, flat baby mattress
> ➤ Don't overheat the baby

Pleural Disorders

Pleurisy, also called pleuritis, is an inflammation of the pleura, usually associated with infection. Pain is the common symptom of pleurisy. Because this pain is intensified by breathing or coughing, as the inflamed membranes move, breathing becomes rapid and shallow. Analgesics and anti-inflammatory drugs are used to treat the symptoms of pleurisy.

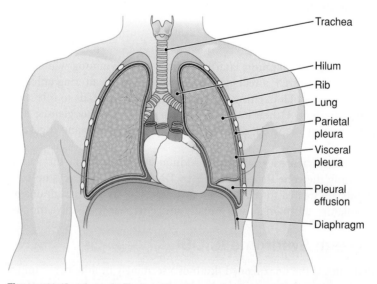

Figure 11-10 Pleural effusion. An abnormal volume of fluid collects in the pleural space.

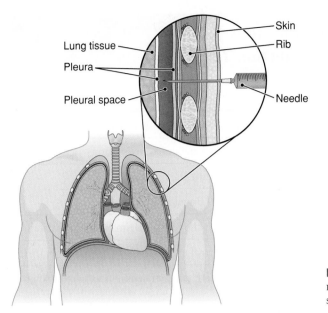

Skin
Rib
Lung tissue
Pleura
Pleural space
Needle

Figure 11-11 Thoracentesis. A needle is inserted into the pleural space.

11

As a result of injury, infection, or weakness in the pleural membrane, substances may accumulate between the layers of the pleura. When air or gas collects in this space, the condition is termed **pneumothorax** (Fig. 11-9). Compression may result in collapse of the lung, termed **atelectasis**.

In **pleural effusion**, other materials accumulate in the pleural space (Fig. 11-10). Depending on the substance involved, these are described as **empyema** (pus), also termed **pyothorax**; **hemothorax** (blood); or **hydrothorax** (fluid). Causes of these conditions include injury, infection, heart failure, and pulmonary embolism. **Thoracentesis**, needle puncture of the chest to remove fluids (Fig. 11-11), or fusion of the pleural membranes (pleurodesis) may be required. A chest tube may be inserted to remove air and fluid from the pleural space.

Diagnosis of Respiratory Disorders

In addition to chest radiographs, CT scans, and magnetic resonance imaging (MRI) scans, methods for diagnosing respiratory disorders include **lung scans**, bronchoscopy, and tests of pleural fluid removed by thoracentesis. **Arterial blood gases (ABGs)** are used to evaluate gas exchange in the lungs by measuring carbon dioxide, oxygen, bicarbonate, and pH in an arterial blood sample. **Pulse oximetry** is routinely used to measure the oxygen saturation of arterial blood by means of a simple apparatus, an oximeter, placed on a thin part of the body, usually the finger or the ear (Fig. 11-12).

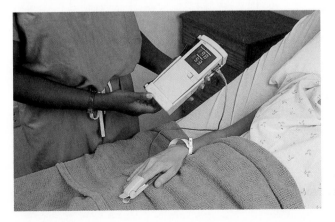

Figure 11-12 Pulse oximetry. The oximeter measures the oxygen saturation of arterial blood.

Box 11·4 For Your Reference — Volumes and Capacities (Sums of Volumes) Used in Pulmonary Function Tests

Volume or Capacity	Definition
tidal volume (TV)	amount of air breathed into or out of the lungs in quiet, relaxed breathing
residual volume (RV)	amount of air that remains in the lungs after maximum exhalation
expiratory reserve volume (ERV)	amount of air that can be exhaled after a normal exhalation
inspiratory reserve volume (IRV)	amount of air that can be inhaled above a normal inspiration
total lung capacity (TLC)	total amount of air that can be contained in the lungs after maximum inhalation
inspiratory capacity (IC)	amount of air that can be inhaled after normal exhalation
vital capacity (VC)	amount of air that can be expelled from the lungs by maximum exhalation after maximum inhalation
functional residual capacity (FRC)	amount of air remaining in the lungs after normal exhalation
forced expiratory volume (FEV)	volume of gas exhaled with maximum force within a given interval of time; the time interval is shown as a subscript, such as FEV_1 (1 second), FEV_3 (3 seconds)
forced vital capacity (FVC)	the volume of gas exhaled as rapidly and completely as possible after a complete inhalation

Pulmonary function tests are used to assess breathing, usually by means of a **spirometer**. They measure the volumes of air that can be moved into or out of the lungs with different degrees of effort. Often used to monitor treatment in cases of allergy, asthma, emphysema, and other respiratory conditions, they are also used to measure progress in cessation of smoking. The main volumes and capacities measured in these tests are summarized in reference Box 11-4 and illustrated in Figure 11-13. A capacity is the sum of two or more volumes.

See Box 11-5 for information on respiratory therapists, who perform many of these tests.

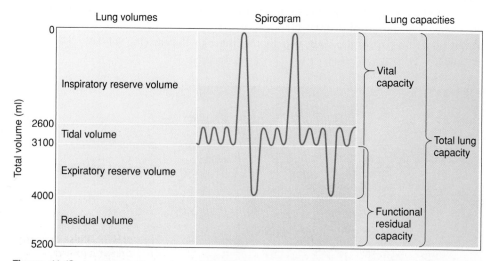

Figure 11-13 A spirogram. A spirometer produces a tracing of lung volumes and capacities (sums of volumes).

| Box 11·5 | Health Professions | *Careers in Respiratory Therapy* |

Respiratory therapists and respiratory therapy technicians specialize in evaluating and treating breathing disorders. Respiratory therapists evaluate the severity of their clients' conditions by taking complete histories and testing respiratory function with specialized equipment. Based on their findings, and in consultation with a physician, therapists design and implement individualized treatment plans, which may include oxygen therapy and chest physiotherapy. They also educate clients on the use of ventilators and other medical devices. Respiratory therapy technicians assist in carrying out evaluations and treatments.

To perform their duties, both types of practitioners need a thorough understanding of anatomy and physiology. Most respiratory therapists in the United States receive their training from an accredited college or university and take a national licensing exam. Respiratory therapists and technicians work in a variety of settings, such as hospitals, nursing care facilities, and private clinics. The American Association for Respiratory Care has information about careers in respiratory therapy.

11

TERMINOLOGY Key Terms

DISORDERS

acidosis *as-i-DŌ-sis*	Abnormal acidity of body fluids. Respiratory acidosis is caused by abnormally high levels of carbon dioxide in the body.
acute respiratory distress syndrome (ARDS)	Pulmonary edema that can lead rapidly to fatal respiratory failure; causes include trauma, aspiration into the lungs, viral pneumonia, and drug reactions; shock lung
acute rhinitis *rī-NĪ-tis*	Inflammation of the nasal mucosa with sneezing, tearing, and profuse secretion of watery mucus, as seen in the common cold
alkalosis *al-ka-LŌ-sis*	Abnormal alkalinity of body fluids. Respiratory alkalosis is caused by abnormally low levels of carbon dioxide in the body.
aspiration *as-pi-RĀ-shun*	The accidental inhalation of food or other foreign material into the lungs. Also means the withdrawal of fluid from a cavity by suction.
asthma *AZ-ma*	A disease characterized by dyspnea and wheezing caused by spasm of the bronchial tubes or swelling of their mucous membranes
atelectasis *at-e-LEK-ta-sis*	Incomplete expansion of a lung or part of a lung; lung collapse. May be present at birth (as in respiratory distress syndrome) or be caused by bronchial obstruction or compression of lung tissue (prefix *atel/o* means "imperfect").
bronchiectasis *brong-kē-EK-ta-sis*	Chronic dilatation of a bronchus or bronchi
bronchitis *brong-KĪ-tis*	Inflammation of a bronchus
chronic obstructive pulmonary disease (COPD)	Any of a group of chronic, progressive, and debilitating respiratory diseases, which includes emphysema, asthma, bronchitis, and bronchiectasis
cyanosis *sī-a-NŌ-sis*	Bluish discoloration of the skin caused by lack of oxygen in the blood (adjective, cyanotic) (see Fig. 3-4)

TERMINOLOGY Key Terms

Continued

cystic fibrosis (CF) *SIS-tik fi-BRō-sis*	An inherited disease that affects the pancreas, respiratory system, and sweat glands. Characterized by mucus accumulation in the bronchi causing obstruction and leading to infection.
diphtheria *dif-THĒR-ī-a*	Acute infectious disease, usually limited to the upper respiratory tract, characterized by the formation of a surface pseudomembrane composed of cells and coagulated material
dyspnea *dysp-NĒ-a*	Difficult or labored breathing, sometimes with pain; "air hunger"
emphysema *em-fi-SĒ-ma*	A chronic pulmonary disease characterized by enlargement and destruction of the alveoli
empyema *em-pī-Ē-ma*	Accumulation of pus in a body cavity, especially the pleural space; pyothorax
hemoptysis *hē-MOP-ti-sis*	The spitting of blood from the mouth or respiratory tract (*ptysis* means "spitting")
hemothorax *hē-mō-THOR-aks*	Presence of blood in the pleural space
hydrothorax *hī-drō-THOR-aks*	Presence of fluid in the pleural space
hyperventilation *hī-per-ven-ti-LĀ-shun*	Increased rate and depth of breathing; increase in the amount of air entering the alveoli
hypoventilation *hī-pō-ven-ti-LĀ-shun*	Decreased rate and depth of breathing; decrease in the amount of air entering the alveoli
influenza *in-flū-EN-za*	An acute, contagious respiratory infection causing fever, chills, headache, and muscle pain; "flu"
pertussis *per-TUS-is*	An acute, infectious disease characterized by a cough ending in a whooping inspiration; whooping cough
pleural effusion *PLŪR-al e-FŪ-zhun*	Accumulation of fluid in the pleural space. The fluid may contain blood (hemothorax) or pus (pyothorax or empyema).
pleurisy *PLŪR-i-sē*	Inflammation of the pleura; pleuritis. A symptom of pleurisy is sharp pain on breathing.
pneumoconiosis *nū-mō-kō-nē-Ō-sis*	Disease of the respiratory tract caused by inhalation of dust particles. Named more specifically by the type of dust inhaled, such as silicosis, anthracosis, asbestosis.
pneumonia *nū-Mō-nē-a*	Inflammation of the lungs generally caused by infection. May involve the bronchioles and alveoli (bronchopneumonia) or one or more lobes of the lung (lobar pneumonia).
pneumonitis *nū-mō-NĪ-tis*	Inflammation of the lungs; may follow infection or be caused by asthma, allergy, or inhalation of irritants

TERMINOLOGY Key Terms

Continued

pneumothorax *nū-mō-THOR-aks*	Accumulation of air or gas in the pleural space. May result from injury or disease or may be produced artificially to collapse a lung.
pyothorax *pī-ō-THOR-aks*	Accumulation of pus in the pleural space; empyema
respiratory distress syndrome (RDS)	A respiratory disorder that affects premature infants born without enough surfactant in the lungs. It is treated with respiratory support and administration of surfactant.
sudden infant death syndrome (SIDS)	The sudden and unexplained death of an apparently healthy infant; crib death
tuberculosis *tū-ber-kū-LŌ-sis*	An infectious disease caused by the tubercle bacillus, *Mycobacterium tuberculosis*. Often involves the lungs but may involve other parts of the body as well. Miliary (*MIL-ē-ar-ē*) tuberculosis is an acute generalized form of the disease with formation of minute tubercles that resemble millet seeds

DIAGNOSIS

arterial blood gases (ABGs)	The concentrations of gases, specifically oxygen and carbon dioxide, in arterial blood. Reported as the partial pressure (P) of the gas in arterial (a) blood, such as PaO_2 or $PaCO_2$. These measurements are important in measuring acid-base balance.
bronchoscope *BRONG-kō-skōp*	An endoscope used to examine the tracheobronchial passageways. Also allows access for biopsy of tissue to removal of a foreign object (see Fig. 7-7).
lung scan	Study based on the accumulation of radioactive isotope in lung tissue. A *ventilation scan* measures ventilation after inhalation of radioactive material. A *perfusion scan* measures blood supply to the lungs after injection of radioactive material. Also called a pulmonary scintiscan.
pulse oximetry *ok-SIM-e-trē*	Determination of the oxygen saturation of arterial blood by means of a photoelectric apparatus (oximeter), usually placed on the finger or the ear; reported as SpO_2 in percent (see Fig. 11-12).
pulmonary function tests	Tests done to assess breathing, usually by spirometry
spirometer *spī-ROM-e-ter*	An apparatus used to measure breathing volumes and capacities; record of test is a spirogram (see Fig. 11-13)
thoracentesis *thor-a-sen-Tē-sis*	Surgical puncture of the chest for removal of air or fluids, such as may accumulate after surgery or as a result of injury, infection, or cardiovascular problems. Also called thoracocentesis (see Fig. 11-11).
tuberculin test *tū-BER-kū-lin*	A skin test for tuberculosis. Tuberculin, the test material made from products of the tuberculosis organism, is injected below the skin or inoculated with a four-pronged device (tine test).

Go to the pronunciation glossary in Chapter 11 on the CD-ROM to hear these words pronounced.

TERMINOLOGY Supplementary Terms

NORMAL STRUCTURE AND FUNCTION

carina *ka-RĪ-na*	A projection of the lowest tracheal cartilage that forms a ridge between the two bronchi. Used as a landmark for endoscopy. Any ridge or ridgelike structure (from a Latin word that means "keel").
hilum *HĪ-lum*	An anatomical depression in an organ where vessels and nerves enter
nares *NĀ-rēz*	The external openings of the nose; the nostrils (singular, naris)
nasal septum	The partition that divides the nasal cavity into two parts (root *sept/o* means "septum")

SYMPTOMS AND CONDITIONS

anoxia *an-OK-sē-a*	Lack or absence of oxygen in the tissues; often used incorrectly to mean hypoxia
asphyxia *as-FIK-sē-a*	Condition caused by inadequate intake of oxygen; suffocation (literally "lack of pulse")
Biot respirations *bē-Ō*	Deep, fast breathing interrupted by sudden pauses; seen in spinal meningitis and other disorders of the central nervous system
bronchospasm *BRONG-kō-spazm*	Narrowing of the bronchi caused by smooth muscle spasms; common in cases of asthma and bronchitis
Cheyne-Stokes respiration *chān-stōks*	A repeating cycle of gradually increased and then decreased respiration followed by a period of apnea; caused by depression of the breathing centers in the brain stem; seen in cases of coma and in terminally ill patients
cor pulmonale *kor pul-mō-NĀ-lē*	Enlargement of the heart's right ventricle caused by disease of the lungs or pulmonary blood vessels
coryza *kō-RĪ-za*	Acute inflammation of the nasal passages with profuse nasal discharge; acute rhinitis
croup *krūp*	A childhood disease usually caused by a viral infection that involves inflammation and obstruction of the upper airway. Croup is characterized by a barking cough, difficulty breathing, and laryngeal spasm.
deviated septum	A shifted nasal septum; may require surgical correction
epiglottitis *ep-i-glo-TĪ-tis*	Inflammation of the epiglottis that may lead to obstruction of the upper airway. Commonly seen in cases of croup (also spelled *epiglottiditis*).
epistaxis *ep-i-STAK-sis*	Hemorrhage from the nose; nosebleed (Greek -*staxis* means "dripping")
fremitus *FREM-i-tus*	A vibration, especially as felt through the chest wall on palpation

TERMINOLOGY *Continued*

Supplementary Terms

Kussmaul respiration *KOOS-mawl*	Rapid and deep gasping respiration without pause; characteristic of severe acidosis
pleural friction rub	A sound heard on auscultation that is produced by the rubbing together of the two pleural layers; a common sign of pleurisy
rales *rahlz*	Abnormal chest sounds heard when air enters small airways or alveoli containing fluid; usually heard during inspiration (sing. rale [*rahl*]). Also called crackles.
rhonchi *RONG-kī*	Abnormal chest sounds produced in airways with accumulated fluids; more noticeable during expiration (singular, rhonchus)
stridor *STRĪ-dor*	A harsh, high-pitched sound caused by obstruction of an upper air passageway
tussis *TUS-is*	A cough. An antitussive drug is one that relieves or prevents coughing.
wheeze	A whistling or sighing sound caused by narrowing of a respiratory passageway

DISORDERS

byssinosis *bis-i-NŌ-sis*	Obstructive airway disease caused by reaction to the dust in unprocessed plant fibers
sleep apnea *AP-nē-a*	Intermittent periods of breathing cessation during sleep. Central sleep apnea arises from failure of the brain stem to stimulate breathing. Obstructive sleep apnea results from airway obstruction during deep sleep, as from obesity or enlarged tonsils.
small cell carcinoma	A highly malignant type of bronchial tumor involving small, undifferentiated cells; "oat cell" carcinoma

DIAGNOSIS

Mantoux test *man-TOO*	A test for tuberculosis in which PPD (tuberculin) is injected into the skin. The test does not differentiate active from inactive cases.
mediastinoscopy *mē-dē-as-ti-NOS-kō-pē*	Examination of the mediastinum by means of an endoscope inserted through an incision above the sternum
plethysmograph *ple-THIZ-mō-graf*	An instrument that measures changes in gas volume and pressure during respiration
pneumotachometer *nū-mō-tak-OM-e-ter*	A device for measuring air flow
thoracoscopy *thor-a-KOS-kō-pē*	Examination of the pleural cavity through an endoscope; pleuroscopy

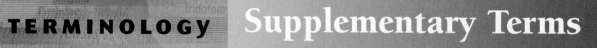

tine test	A test for tuberculosis in which PPD (tuberculin) is introduced into the skin with a multi-pronged device. The test does not differentiate active from inactive cases.

TREATMENT

aerosol therapy	Treatment by inhalation of a drug or water in spray form
continuous positive airway pressure (CPAP)	Use of a mechanical respirator to maintain pressure throughout the respiratory cycle in a patient who is breathing spontaneously
extubation	Removal of a previously inserted tube
intermittent positive pressure breathing (IPPB)	Use of a ventilator to inflate the lungs at intervals under positive pressure during inhalation
intermittent positive pressure ventilation (IPPV)	Use of a mechanical ventilator to force air into the lungs while allowing for passive exhalation
nasal cannula KAN-ū-la	A two-pronged plastic device inserted into the nostrils for delivery of oxygen (Fig. 11-14)
orthopneic position or-thop-NĒ-ik	An upright or semiupright position that aids breathing
positive end-expiratory pressure (PEEP)	Use of a mechanical ventilator to increase the volume of gas in the lungs at the end of exhalation, thus improving gas exchange
postural drainage POS-tū-ral	Use of body position to drain secretions from the lungs by gravity. The patient is placed so that secretions will move passively into the larger airways for elimination.
thoracic gas volume (TGV, V_{TG})	The volume of gas in the thoracic cavity calculated from measurements made with a body plethysmograph

SURGERY

adenoidectomy ad-e-noyd-EK-tō-mē	Surgical removal of the adenoids
intubation in-tū-BĀ-shun	Insertion of a tube into a hollow organ, such as into the larynx or trachea for entrance of air (Fig. 11-15). Patients may be intubated during surgery for administration of anesthesia or to maintain an airway. Endotracheal intubation may be used as an emergency measure when airways are blocked.
lobectomy lō-BEK-tō-mē	Surgical removal of a lobe of the lung or of another organ
pneumoplasty NŪ-mō-plas-tē	Plastic surgery of the lung. In reduction pneumoplasty, nonfunctional portions of the lung are removed, as in cases of advanced emphysema.

TERMINOLOGY
Continued

Supplementary Terms

tracheotomy
trā-kē-OT-ō-mē

Incision of the trachea through the neck, usually to establish an airway in cases of tracheal obstruction

tracheostomy
trā-kē-OS-tō-mē

Surgical creation of an opening into the trachea to form an airway or to prepare for the insertion of a tube for ventilation (Fig. 11-16), also the opening thus created

DRUGS

antihistamine
an-ti-HIS-ta-mēn

Agent that prevents responses mediated by histamine, such as allergic and inflammatory reactions

antitussive
an-ti-TUS-iv

Drug that prevents or relieves coughing

asthma maintenance drug

Agent used to prevent asthma attacks and for chronic treatment of asthma

bronchodilator
brong-kō-DĪ -lā-tor

Drug that relieves bronchial spasm and widens the bronchi

corticosteroid
kor-ti-kō-STĒR-oyd

Hormone from the adrenal cortex; used to reduce inflammation

decongestant
dē-kon-JES-tant

Agent that reduces congestion or swelling

expectorant
ek-SPEK-tō-rant

Agent that aids in removal of bronchopulmonary secretions

isoniazid (INH)
ī-sō-NĪ -a-zid

Drug used to treat tuberculosis

mucolytic
mū-kō-LIT-ik

Agent that loosens mucus to aid in its removal

Go to the pronunciation glossary in Chapter 11 on the CD-ROM to hear these words pronounced.

11

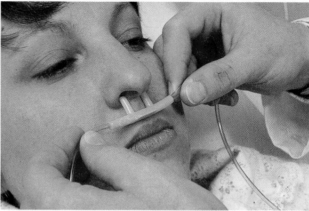

Figure 11-14 **A nasal cannula.**

Intranasal intubation

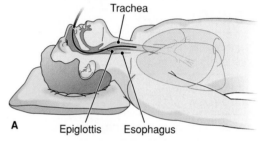

Trachea

A   Epiglottis   Esophagus

Oral intubation

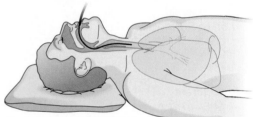

Figure 11-15 **Endotracheal intubation.**
(*A*) Nasal endotracheal catheter in proper position. (*B*) Oral endotracheal intubation.

B

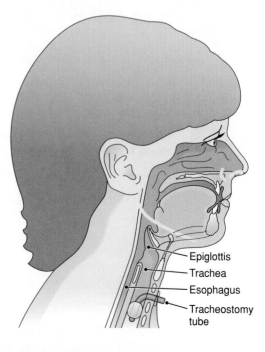

Epiglottis

Trachea

Esophagus

Tracheostomy tube

Figure 11-16 **A tracheostomy tube in place.**

TERMINOLOGY Abbreviations

ABG(s)	Arterial blood gas(es)
AFB	Acid-fast bacillus (usually *Mycobacterium tuberculosis*)
ARDS	Acute respiratory distress syndrome; shock lung
ARF	Acute respiratory failure
BCG	Bacillus Calmette-Guérin (tuberculosis vaccine)
BS	Breath sounds
C	Compliance
CF	Cystic fibrosis
CO_2	Carbon dioxide
COLD	Chronic obstructive lung disease
COPD	Chronic obstructive pulmonary disease
CPAP	Continuous positive airway pressure
CXR	Chest radiograph, chest x-ray
DTaP	Diphtheris, tetanus, acellular pertussis (vaccine)
ERV	Expiratory reserve volume
FEV	Forced expiratory volume
FRC	Functional residual capacity
FVC	Forced vital capacity
HPS	*Hantavirus* pulmonary syndrome
IC	Inspiratory capacity
INH	Isoniazid
IPPB	Intermittent positive pressure breathing
IPPV	Intermittent positive pressure ventilation
IRV	Inspiratory reserve volume
LLL	Left lower lobe (of lung)
LUL	Left upper lobe (of lung)
MEFR	Maximal expiratory flow rate
MMFR	Maximum midexpiratory flow rate
O_2	Oxygen
Pa_{CO_2}	Arterial partial pressure of carbon dioxide
Pa_{O_2}	Arterial partial pressure of oxygen
PCP	*Pneumocystis* pneumonia
PEEP	Positive end-expiratory pressure
PEFR	Peak expiratory flow rate
PFT	Pulmonary function test(s)
PIP	Peak inspiratory pressure
PND	Paroxysmal nocturnal dyspnea
PPD	Purified protein derivative (tuberculin)
R	Respiration
RDS	Respiratory distress syndrome
RLL	Right lower lobe (of lung)
RML	Right middle lobe (of lung)
RSV	Respiratory syncytial virus
RUL	Right upper lobe (of lung)
RV	Residual volume
SARS	Severe acute respiratory syndrome
SIDS	Sudden infant death syndrome
SpO_2	Oxygen percent saturation
T & A	Tonsils and adenoids; tonsillectomy and adenoidectomy
TB	Tuberculosis
TGV	Thoracic gas volume
TLC	Total lung capacity
TV	Tidal volume
URI	Upper respiratory infection
VC	Vital capacity
V_{TG}	Thoracic gas volume

11

CHAPTER REVIEW

LABELING EXERCISE
The Respiratory System

Write the name of each numbered part on the corresponding line of the answer sheet.

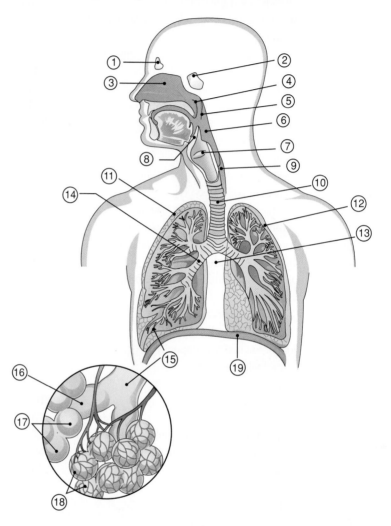

Alveolar duct	1.	_____
Alveoli	2.	_____
Capillaries	3.	_____
Diaphragm	4.	_____
Epiglottis	5.	_____
Esophagus	6.	_____
Frontal sinus	7.	_____
Laryngeal pharynx	8.	_____
Larynx and vocal cords	9.	_____

Left lung

10. _____

Mediastinum

11. _____

Nasal cavity

12. _____

Nasopharynx

13. _____

Oropharynx

14. _____

Right bronchus

15. _____

Right lung

16. _____

Sphenoidal sinus

17. _____

Terminal bronchiole

18. _____

Trachea

19. _____

11

TERMINOLOGY

Match the following terms and write the appropriate letter to the left of each number:

_____ 1. pneumoconiosis
_____ 2. hyperpnea
_____ 3. sputum
_____ 4. surfactant
_____ 5. aspiration

a. accidental inhalation of foreign material into the lungs
b. increased rate and depth of breathing
c. substance that reduces surface tension
d. respiratory disease caused by dust inhalation
e. expectoration

_____ 6. hypercapnemia
_____ 7. emphysema
_____ 8. atelectasis
_____ 9. compliance
_____ 10. pertussis

a. pulmonary disease with destruction of alveoli
b. increased carbon dioxide in the blood
c. a measure of how easily the lungs expand
d. whooping cough
e. incomplete expansion of lung tissue

_____ 11. PCP
_____ 12. INH
_____ 13. RSV
_____ 14. RDS
_____ 15. CF

a. virus that causes respiratory disease in young children
b. respiratory condition seen most often in newborns
c. hereditary disease that affects respiration
d. pneumonia seen in compromised patients
e. drug used to treat tuberculosis

Supplementary Terms

_____	**16.** hilum	**a.** suffocation
_____	**17.** rhonchi	**b.** nosebleed
_____	**18.** asphyxia	**c.** anatomical depression in an organ
_____	**19.** expectorant	**d.** abnormal chest sounds
_____	**20.** epistaxis	**e.** agent that helps remove bronchial secretions
_____	**21.** croup	**a.** irregular respiration seen in terminally ill patients
_____	**22.** Cheyne-Stokes	**b.** device used to measure air flow
_____	**23.** fremitus	**c.** high pitches sound caused by obstruction
_____	**24.** pneumotachometer	**d.** childhood disease with barking cough
_____	**25.** stridor	**e.** vibration felt through the chest wall

11

Fill in the blanks:

26. The gas produced in the tissues and exhaled in respiration is _____.

27. The phrenic nerve activates the _____.

28. The turbinate bones contain receptors for the sense of _____.

29. The double membrane that covers the lungs and lines the thoracic cavity is the

_____.

30. The small air sacs in the lungs through which gases are exchanged between the atmosphere and the blood are the

_____.

31. The trachea divides into the right and left main stem _____.

32. A pneumotropic virus is one that invades the _____.

33. The term *acid-fast bacillus* (AFB) is commonly applied to the organism that causes

_____.

34. In orthopnea, breathing difficulty is relieved by assuming a position that is _____.

Supplementary Terms

35. The amount of air moved into or out of the lungs in quiet breathing is the _____.

36. An antitussive agent prevents _____.

37. A mucolytic agent dissolves _____.

38. The partition between the two portions of the nasal cavity is the nasal _____.

39. Intermittent periods of not breathing during sleep is termed sleep _____.

40. The amount of air that remains in the lungs after maximal exhalation is the

_____.

True-False. Examine the following statements. If the statement is true, write T in the first blank. If the statement is false, write F in the first blank and correct the statement by replacing the <u>underlined</u> word in the second blank.

41. The diaphragm flattens during <u>inhalation</u>. _____ _____

42. The pharynx is the <u>throat</u>. _____ _____

43. The vocal cords are located in the <u>pharynx</u>.   _____ _____

44. The right lung has <u>two</u> lobes.   _____ _____

45. The opening between the vocal cords is the <u>glottis</u>.   _____ _____

46. The adenoids are in the <u>nasopharynx</u>.   _____ _____

Word building. Write words for the following definitions:

47. incision of the phrenic nerve   _____

48. hernia of the pleura   _____

49. inflammation of the throat   _____

50. inflammation of the bronchioles   _____

51. creation of an opening into the trachea   _____

The word *thorax* (chest) is used as an ending in compound words that mean the accumulation of substances in the pleural space. Define the following terms:

52. pneumothorax _____ accumulation of air or gas in the pleural space _____

53. hemothorax _____

54. pyothorax _____

55. hydrothorax _____

Define the following words:

56. pleurodynia _____

57. hypoxia _____

58. pneumonopathy _____

59. bradypnea _____

60. bronchiectasis _____

61. intrapulmonary _____

62. rhinoplasty _____

63. pharyngoxerosis _____

Identify and define the root in the following words:

	Root	Meaning of Root
64. respiration	_____	_____
65. pulmonologist	_____	_____
66. empyema	_____	_____
67. subphrenic	_____	_____
68. pneumatic	_____	_____

Opposites. Write a word that means the opposite of the following:

69. hypocapnia   _____

70. inspiration   _____

71. tachypnea   _____

72. intubation   _____

Adjectives. Write the adjective form of the following words:

73. alveolus _____

74. larynx _____

75. pleura _____

76. nose _____

77. trachea _____

78. bronchus _____

Plurals. Write the plural form of the following words:

79. naris _____

80. pleura _____

81. alveolus _____

82. concha _____

83. bronchus _____

Eliminations. In each of the sets below, underline the word that does not fit in with the rest and explain the reason for your choice:

84. turbinates – septum – nares – mediastinum – conchae

_____

85. sinus – thyroid cartilage – epiglottis – cricoid cartilage – vocal cords

_____

86. diphtheria – tuberculosis – asthma – common cold – influenza

_____

87. RUL – URI – LUL – LLL – RML

_____

Word analysis. Define the following words and give the meaning of the word parts in each. Use a dictionary if necessary.

88. atelectasis (*at-e-LEK-ta-sis*) _____

    a. atel/o- _____

    b. -ectasis _____

89. pneumatocardia (*nū-ma-tō-KAR-dē-a*) _____

    a. pneumato _____

    b. cardi _____

    c. -ia _____

Go to the word exercises in Chapter 11 on the CD-ROM for additional review exercises.

CASE STUDIES

CASE STUDY 11-1: Preoperative Testing in a Patient With Asthma

A.D., 15 years old, was seen in the preadmission testing unit in preparation for her elective spinal surgery. She has a history of mild asthma since age 4, with at least one attack per week. In an acute attack, she will have mild dyspnea, diffuse wheezing, yet an adequate air exchange that responds to bronchodilators. She was sent to pulmonary health services for a consult with a specialist and pulmonary function studies to clear her for surgery. The anesthesiologist reviewed the pulmonologist's report.

Her prebronchodilator spirometry showed a mild reduction in vital capacity but with a moderate to severe decrease in FEV_1 and FEV_1/FVC ratio. After bronchodilator administration, there was a mild but insignificant improvement in FEV_1. The postbronchodilator FEV_1 was 55% of predicted and was considered moderately abnormal. The flow volume loops and spirographic curves were consistent with airflow obstruction.

CASE STUDY 11-2: Giant Cell Sarcoma of the Lung

L.E., a 68-year-old man, was admitted to the pulmonary unit with chest pain on inspiration, dyspnea, and diaphoresis. He had smoked 1-1/2 packs of cigarettes per day for 52 years and had quit 3 months ago. L.E. was retired from the advertising industry and admitted to occasional alcohol use. He was treated for primary giant cell sarcoma of the left lung 3 years ago with a lobectomy of the left lung followed by radiation and chemotherapy.

Physical examination was unremarkable except for a thoracotomy scar in the left hemithorax, decreased breath sounds, and dullness to percussion of the left base. There was no hemoptysis. Radionucleotide bone scan showed increased activity in the left upper posterior hemithorax. Chest and upper abdomen CT scan showed findings compatible with recurrent sarcoma of the left hemithorax. Abnormal mediastinal nodes were evident. Thoracentesis was attempted but did not yield fluid. L.E. was scheduled for a left thoracoscopy, mediastinoscopy, and biopsy.

CASE STUDY 11-3: Terminal Dyspnea

N.A., a 76-year-old woman, was in the ICU in the terminal stage of multisystem organ failure. She had been admitted to the hospital for bacterial pneumonia, which had not resolved with antibiotic therapy. She had a 20-year history of COPD. She was not conscious and was unable to breathe on her own. Her ABGs were abnormal, and she was diagnosed with refractory ARDS. The decision was made to support her breathing with endotracheal intubation and mechanical ventilation. After 1 week and several unsuccessful attempts to wean her from the ventilator, the pulmonologist suggested a permanent tracheostomy and family consideration of continuing or withdrawing life support. Her physiologic status met the criteria of remote or no chance for recovery.

N.A.'s family discussed her condition and decided not to pursue aggressive life-sustaining therapies. N.A. was assigned DNR status. After the written orders were read and signed by the family, the endotracheal tube, feeding tube, pulse oximeter, and ECG electrodes were removed and a morphine IV drip was started with prn boluses ordered to promote comfort and relieve pain and other symptoms of dying. The family sat with N.A. for many hours while her breaths became shallow with Cheyne-Stokes respirations. She died surrounded by her family with the hospital chaplain.

CASE STUDY QUESTIONS

Multiple choice. Select the best answer and write the letter of your choice to the left of each number:

_____ 1. The root *spir/o*, as in *spirometry*, means:
   a. turbulence
   b. breathing

    c. twisted
    d. air quality
    e. saturation

_____ 2. The root *pulmon*, as in *pulmonary*, means:
    a. chest
    b. air
    c. lung
    d. breath sound
    e. blood vessel

_____ 3. Hemoptysis is:
    a. drooping eyelids
    b. discoloration of skin
    c. blue nail beds
    d. spitting of blood
    e. acute leukemia

_____ 4. Dyspnea could NOT be described as:
    a. difficulty breathing
    b. eupnea
    c. air hunger
    d. orthopnea
    e. Cheyne-Stokes respirations

_____ 5. Pulse oximetry is used to measure:
    a. forced expiratory volume
    b. tidal volume
    c. end-tidal CO_2
    d. oxygen saturation of blood
    e. positive end-expiratory pressure

_____ 6. An endotracheal tube is placed:
    a. under the trachea
    b. beyond the carina
    c. within the bronchus
    d. around the airway
    e. within the trachea

Write words from the case histories with the following meanings:

7. Whistling breath sounds due to narrowing of the breathing passageways _____

8. A drug that enlarges the lumen of the bronchi _____

9. Removal of a lobe _____

10. Profuse sweating _____

11. Surgical incision of the chest _____

12. Endoscopic examination of the chest cavity _____

13. Half of the chest _____

14. Endoscopic examination of the space between the lungs _____

15. Movement of air into and out of the lungs _____

Abbreviations. Define the following abbreviations:

16. COPD _____

17. FVC _____

18. ABG _____

19. ARDS _____

20. DNR _____

11

The Respiratory System

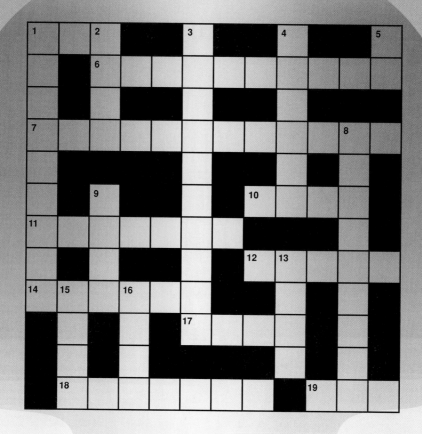

ACROSS

1. Drug used to treat tuberculosis (abbreviation)
6. Portion of the throat behind the mouth
7. Instrument used to examine the larynx
10. Blood: combining form
11. RDS may appear in a newborn, also called a(n)
12. Rapid: prefix
14. Respiratory disease involving constriction of the bronchial tubes
17. An organ of respiration
18. Abnormal chest sounds
19. Chest radiograph (abbreviation)

DOWN

1. Infectious disease of the respiratory tract
2. The abbreviation qh means every _____
3. Pertaining to the cartilage above the larynx
4. The tube between the throat and the bronchi: root
5. Diagnosis (abbreviation)
8. Accumulation of pus in the pleural space
9. After, behind: prefix
13. Vessel: root
15. Breathing: root
16. Under, below, decreased: prefix

CHAPTER TWELVE

THE DIGESTIVE SYSTEM

OBJECTIVES

After study of this chapter you should be able to:

1. Explain the function of the digestive system.
2. Label a diagram of the digestive tract, and describe the function of each part.
3. Label a diagram of the accessory organs, and explain the role of each in digestion.
4. Identify and use the roots pertaining to the digestive system.
5. Describe the major disorders of the digestive system.
6. Define medical terms used in reference to the digestive system.
7. Interpret abbreviations used in referring to the gastrointestinal system.
8. Analyze case studies concerning gastroenterology.

PRETEST

1. The organ that carries food from the pharynx to the stomach is the _____ .

2. The word root for the stomach is _____ .

3. The main portion of the large intestine is the _____ .

4. The word root *enter/o* refers to the _____ .

5. The process of moving digested nutrients from the intestine into the circulation is called _____ .

6. The organ that secretes bile is the _____ .

7. Cholecystitis is inflammation of the _____ .

The function of the digestive system is to prepare food for intake by body cells. Nutrients must be broken down by mechanical and chemical means into molecules that are small enough to be absorbed into the circulation. Within cells, the nutrients are used for energy and for rebuilding vital cell components. (Box 12-1 has information on dieticians and nutritionists, who help people to obtain proper nutrients.)

Digestion takes place in the digestive tract proper, which extends from the mouth to the anus (Fig. 12-1). **Peristalsis,** wavelike contractions of the organ walls, moves food through the digestive tract and also moves undigested waste material out of the body. Also contributing to the digestive process are several accessory organs that release secretions into the digestive tract.

Box 12•1 Health Professions | *Dietitians and Nutritionists*

Dietitians and nutritionists specialize in planning and supervising food programs for institutions such as hospitals, schools, and nursing-care facilities. They assess their clients' nutritional needs and design individualized meal plans. Dietitians and nutritionists also work in community settings, educating the public about disease prevention through healthy eating. Increased public awareness about food and nutrition has also led to new opportunities in the food manufacturing industry. To perform their duties, dietitians and nutritionists need a thorough understanding of anatomy and physiology. Most dietitians and nutritionists in the United States receive their training from a college or university and take a licensing exam.

Job prospects for dietitians and nutritionists are good. As the American population ages, the need for nutritional planning in hospital and nursing-care settings is expected to rise. In addition, many people now place an emphasis on healthy eating and may consult nutritionists privately. The American Dietetic Association has information about these careers.

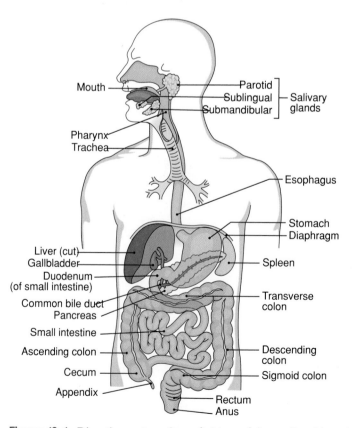

Figure 12-1 Digestive system. Some divisions of the small and large intestine are shown. The accessory organs are the salivary glands, liver, gallbladder, and pancreas. The trachea, diaphragm, and spleen are shown for reference.

Box 12•2 For Your Reference — *Organs of the Digestive Tract*

Organ	Digestive Actions
Mouth	Used to bite and chew food. Mixes food with saliva, which contains salivary amylase, an enzyme that begins the digestion of starch. Shapes food into small portions, which the tongue pushes into the pharynx.
Pharynx	Swallows food by reflex action and moves it into the esophagus
Esophagus	Moves food into the stomach by peristalsis
Stomach	Stores food; churns to mix food with water and digestive juices. Secretes protein-digesting hydrochloric acid (HCl) and the enzyme pepsin.
Small intestine	Secretes enzymes. Receives secretions from the accessory organs, which digest and neutralize food. Site of most digestion and absorption of nutrients into the circulation.
Large intestine	Forms, stores, and eliminates undigested waste material

The Digestive Tract

The digestive tract, also known as the alimentary canal or gastrointestinal (GI) tract, is essentially a long tube modified into separate organs with special functions. Reference Box 12-2 summarizes the activities of the digestive organs described below.

The Mouth to the Stomach

Digestion begins in the **mouth** (Fig. 12-2), also called the oral cavity. Here food is chewed into small bits by the teeth. There are 32 teeth in a complete adult set, including incisors and canines to bite food and molars for grinding. The structural features of a molar tooth and its surrounding tissue are shown in Figure 12-3. The **palate** is the roof of the mouth; the anterior portion (hard palate) is formed by bone and the posterior part (soft palate) is made of soft tissue. The fleshy **uvula**, used in speech production, hangs from the soft palate.

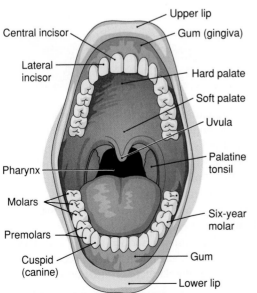

Figure 12-2 The mouth. The teeth, pharynx, tonsils, and other structures in the oral cavity are shown.

Central incisor
Lateral incisor
Pharynx
Molars
Premolars
Cuspid (canine)
Upper lip
Gum (gingiva)
Hard palate
Soft palate
Uvula
Palatine tonsil
Six-year molar
Gum
Lower lip

12

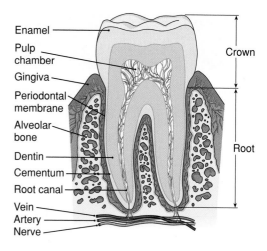

Figure 12-3 A molar tooth. The bony socket, gums, blood vessels, and nerve supply are shown, as well as portions of the tooth.

In the process of chewing, or **mastication**, the tongue, lips, cheeks, and palate also help to break up the food and mix it with **saliva**, a secretion that moistens the food and begins the digestion of starch. The salivary glands (see Fig. 12-1) secrete saliva into the mouth and are considered to be accessory organs of digestion.

Portions of moistened food are moved toward the **pharynx** (throat), where swallowing reflexes push it into the **esophagus**. Peristalsis moves the food through the esophagus and into the **stomach**. At its distal end, where it joins the stomach, the esophagus has muscle tissue that contracts to keep stomach contents from refluxing. This **lower esophageal sphincter** (LES) is also called the "cardiac sphincter" because it lies above the stomach's cardia, the region around its upper opening.

In the stomach, food is further broken down as it is churned and mixed with secretions containing the enzyme pepsin and powerful hydrochloric acid (HCl), both of which break down proteins. The partially digested food then passes through the lower portion of the stomach, the **pylorus**, into the **intestine**.

The Small Intestine

Food leaving the stomach enters the **duodenum**, the first portion of the **small intestine**. As the food continues through the **jejunum** and **ileum**, the remaining sections of the small intestine, digestion is completed (see Box 12-3). The digestive substances active in

---

Box 12•3 Focus on Words   *Homonyms*

Homonyms are words that sound alike but have different meanings. One must know the context in which they are used in order to understand the intended meaning. For example, the ilium is the upper portion of the pelvis, but the ileum is the last portion of the small intestine. Different adjectives are preferred for each, iliac for the first and ileal for the second.

The word *meiosis* refers to the type of cell division that halves the chromosomes to form the gametes, but miosis means abnormal contraction of the pupil. Both words come from the Greek word that means a decrease.

Similar-sounding names lead to some funny misspellings. The large bone of the upper arm is the humerus, but this bone is often written as humorous. The vagus nerve (cranial nerve X) is named with a root that means "wander," as in the words vague and vagabond, because this nerve branches to many of the internal organs. Students often write the name as if it had some relation to the famous gambling city in Nevada.

Homonyms may have a more serious side as well. Drug names may sound or look so similar that clinicians confuse them, leading to some dangerous situations.

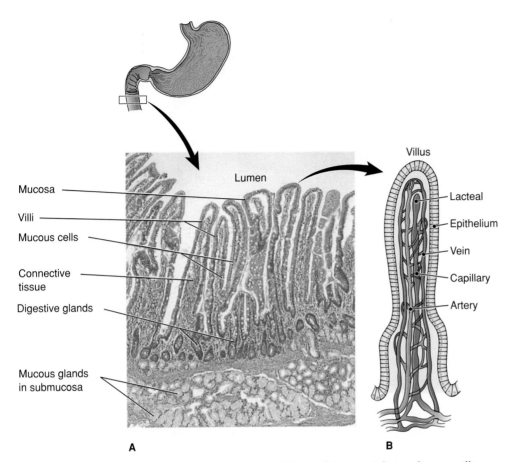

Figure 12-4 Intestinal villi. (*A*) Microscopic view of the small intestine's lining showing villi and glands that secrete mucus and digestive juices. The lumen is the central opening. (*B*) A villus of the small intestine. Each villus has blood vessels and a lacteal (lymphatic capillary) for nutrient absorption.

the small intestine include enzymes from the intestine itself and products from accessory organs that secrete into the duodenum.

The digested nutrients, as well as water, minerals, and vitamins, are absorbed into the circulation, aided by small projections in the lining of the small intestine called **villi** (Fig. 12-4). Each villus has blood capillaries to absorb nutrients into the bloodstream and lymphatic capillaries, or **lacteals,** to absorb small molecules of digested fats into the lymph. These fats join the blood when the lymph flows into the bloodstream near the heart.

The Large Intestine

Any food that has not been digested, along with water and digestive juices, passes into the **large intestine**. This part of the digestive tract begins in the lower right region of the abdomen with a small pouch, the **cecum,** to which the **appendix** is attached. (The appendix does not aid in digestion, but contains lymphatic tissue and may function in immunity.) The large intestine continues as the **colon,** a name that is often used to mean the large intestine because the colon constitutes such a large portion of that organ. The colon travels upward along the right side of the abdomen as the ascending colon, crosses below the stomach as the transverse colon, then continues down the left side of the abdomen as the descending colon. As food is pushed through the colon, water is reabsorbed and stool or **feces** is formed. This waste material passes into the S-shaped **sigmoid colon** and is stored in the **rectum** until eliminated through the **anus.**

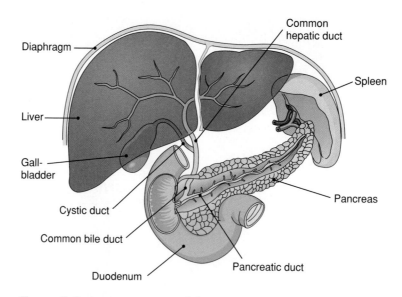

Figure 12-5 Accessory organs of digestion. The organs and ducts are shown. The diaphragm and spleen are shown for reference.

The Accessory Organs

The salivary glands, which secrete into the mouth, are the first accessory organs to act on food. They secrete an enzyme (salivary amylase) that begins the digestion of starch. The remainder of the accessory organs are in the abdomen and secrete into the duodenum (Fig. 12-5). The **liver** is a large gland with many functions. A major part of its activity is to process blood brought to it by a special circulatory pathway called the **hepatic portal system**. The liver's role in digestion is the secretion of **bile**, which emulsifies fats (breaks them down into smaller units). The **gallbladder** stores bile until it is needed in digestion. The common hepatic duct from the liver and the cystic duct from the gallbladder merge to form the **common bile duct**, which empties into the duodenum.

The **pancreas** produces a mixture of digestive enzymes that is delivered into the duodenum through the pancreatic duct. It also secretes large amounts of bicarbonate, which neutralizes the strong stomach acid. Reference Box 12-4 summarizes the functions of the accessory organs.

Box 12•4 For Your Reference	*The Accessory Organs*

Organ	Digestive Actions
Salivary glands	Secrete saliva, which moistens food and contains salivary amylase, an enzyme that begins the digestion of starch
Liver	Secretes bile salts that break down (emulsify) fats.
Gallbladder	Stores bile and releases it into the digestive tract when needed
Pancreas	Secretes a variety of digestive enzymes. Also secretes bicarbonate to neutralize stomach acid and water to dilute food.

TERMINOLOGY Key Terms

NORMAL STRUCTURE AND FUNCTION

anus Ā-nus	The distal opening of the digestive tract (root: *an/o*)
appendix a-PEN-diks	An appendage; usually means the narrow tube of lymphatic tissue attached to the cecum, the vermiform (wormlike) appendix
bile bīl	The fluid secreted by the liver that emulsified fats and aids in their absorption (roots: *chol/e, bili*)
cecum SĒ-kum	A blind pouch at the beginning of the large intestine (root: cec/o)
colon KŌ-lon	The major portion of the large intestine; extends from the cecum to the rectum and is formed by ascending, transverse, and descending portions (root: *col/o, colon/o*)
common bile duct	The duct that carries bile into the duodenum; formed by the union of the cystic duct and the common hepatic duct (root: *choledoch/o*)
duodenum dū-ō-DĒ-num	The first portion of the small intestine (root: *duoden/o*)
esophagus ē-SOF-a-gus	The muscular tube that carries food from the pharynx to the stomach.
feces FĒ-sēz	The waste material eliminated from the intestine (adjective: fecal); stool
gallbladder	A sac on the undersurface of the liver that stores bile (root: *cholecyst/o*)
hepatic portal system	A special pathway of the circulation that brings blood directly from the abdominal organs to the liver for processing (also called simply the *portal system*). The vessel that enters the liver is the hepatic portal vein (portal vein).
ileum IL-ē-um	The terminal portion of the small intestine (root: *ile/o*)
intestine in-TES-tin	The portion of the digestive tract between the stomach and the anus. It consists of the small intestine and large intestine. It functions in digestion, absorption, and elimination of waste (root *enter/o*). The bowel (*BOW-el*)
jejunum je-JŪ-num	The middle portion of the small intestine (root: *jejun/o*)
lacteal lak-TĒL	A lymphatic capillary in a villus of the small intestine. Lacteals absorb digested fats into the lymph.
large intestine in-TES-tin	The terminal portion of the digestive tract, consisting of the cecum, colon, rectum, and anus. It stores and eliminates undigested waste material (feces).
liver LIV-er	The large gland in the upper right part of the abdomen. In addition to many other functions, it secretes bile needed for digestion and absorption of fats (root: *hepat/o*).
lower esophageal sphincter (LES) ē-sof-a-JĒ-al SFINK-ter	Muscle tissue at the distal end of the esophagus (gastroesophageal junction) that prevents stomach contents from refluxing into the esophagus. Also called the cardiac sphincter

12

TERMINOLOGY Key Terms

Continued

mastication *mas-ti-KĀ-shun*	Chewing
mouth	The oral cavity; contains the tongue and teeth. Used to take in and chew food, mix it with saliva, and move it toward the throat to be swallowed.
palate *PAL-at*	The roof of the mouth; the partition between the mouth and nasal cavity; consists of an anterior portion formed by bone, the hard palate, and a posterior portion formed of tissue, the soft palate (root: *palat/o*)
pancreas *PAN-krē-as*	A large, elongated gland behind the stomach. It produces hormones that regulate sugar metabolism and also produces digestive enzymes (root: *pancreat/o*).
peristalsis *per-i-STAL-sis*	Wavelike contractions of an organ's walls
pharynx *FAR-inks*	The throat; a common passageway for food entering the esophagus and air entering the larynx (root: *pharyng/o*)
pylorus *pī-LOR-us*	The stomach's distal opening into the duodenum. The opening is controlled by a ring of muscle, the pyloric sphincter (root: *pylor/o*).
rectum *REK-tum*	The distal portion of the large intestine. It stores and eliminates undigested waste (root: *rect/o, proct/o*).
saliva *sa-LĪ-va*	The clear secretion released into the mouth that moistens food and contains an enzyme that digests starch. It is produced by three pairs of glands: the parotid, submandibular, and sublingual glands (see Fig. 12-1) (root: *sial/o*).
sigmoid colon	Distal s-shaped portion of the large intestine located between the descending colon and the rectum.
small intestine *in-TES-tin*	The portion of the intestine between the stomach and the large intestine; comprised of the duodenum, jejunum, and ileum. Accessory organs secrete into the small intestine, and almost all digestion and absorption occur there.
stomach *STUM-ak*	A muscular saclike organ below the diaphragm that stores food and secretes juices that digest proteins (root: *gastr/o*)
uvula *Ū-vū-la*	The fleshy mass that hangs from the soft palate; aids in speech production (literally "little grape") (root: *uvul/o*)
villi *VIL-ī*	Tiny projections in the lining of the small intestine that absorb digested foods into the circulation (singular: *villus*)

Go to the pronunciation glossary in Chapter 12 on the CD-ROM to hear these words pronounced.

Roots Pertaining to Digestion

Table 12·1	Roots for the Mouth		
ROOT	**MEANING**	**EXAMPLE**	**DEFINITION OF EXAMPLE**
bucc/o	cheek	buccoversion *buk-kō-VER-zhun*	turning toward the cheek
dent/o, dent/i	tooth, teeth	edentulous *ē-DEN-tū-lus*	without teeth
odont/o	tooth, teeth	periodontics *per-ē-ō-DON-tiks*	dental specialty that deals with the study and treatment of the tissues around the teeth
gingiv/o	gum (gingiva)	gingivectomy *jin-ji-VEK-tō-mē*	excision of gum tissue
gloss/o	tongue	glossoplegia *glos-ō-PLĒ-jē-a*	paralysis (-plegia) of the tongue
lingu/o	tongue	orolingual *or-ō-LING-gwal*	pertaining to the mouth and tongue
gnath/o	jaw	prognathous *PROG-na-thus*	having a projecting jaw
labi/o	lip	labium *LĀ-bē-um*	lip or liplike structure
or/o	mouth	circumoral *sir-kum-OR-al*	around the mouth
stoma, stomat/o	mouth	xerostomia *zē-rō-STŌ-mē-a*	dryness (xero-) of the mouth
palat/o	palate	palatine *PAL-a-tīn*	pertaining to the palate (also palatal)
sial/o	saliva, salivary gland, salivary duct	sialogram *sī-AL-ō-gram*	radiograph of the salivary glands and ducts
uvul/o	uvula	uvulotome *Ū-vū-lō-tōm*	instrument (-tome) for incising the uvula

Exercise 12-1

Use the adjective suffix -al to write a word that has the same meaning as the following:

1. pertaining to the mouth   _____ oral _____

2. pertaining to the teeth   _____

3. pertaining to the gums   _____

4. pertaining to the tongue   _____

5. pertaining to the cheek   _____

6. pertaining to the lip   _____

Fill in the blanks:

7. Micrognathia (*mī-krō-NĀ-thē-a*) is excessive smallness of the _____.

8. Hemiglossal (*hem-ī-GLOS-al*) means pertaining to one half of the _____.

9. Stomatoplasty (*STŌ-ma-tō-plas-tē*) is any plastic repair of the _____.

10. The oropharynx is the part of the pharynx that is located behind the _____.

11. A sialolith (*sī-AL-ō-lith*) is a stone formed in a _____ gland or duct.

12. A dentifrice (*DEN-ti-fris*) is an agent used to clean the _____.

13. An orthodontist (*or-thō-DON-itst*) specializes in straightening (ortho-) of the _____.

Define the following words:

14. sublingual (*sub-LING-gwal*) _____

15. palatorrhaphy (*pal-at-OR-a-fē*) _____

16. gingivitis (*jin-ji-VĪ-tis*) _____

17. labiodental (*lā-bē-ō-DEN-tal*) _____

18. hypoglossal (*hī-pō-GLOS-al*) _____

19. extrabuccal (*eks-tra-BUK-al*) _____

20. uvuloptosis (*ū-vū-lop-TŌ-sis*) _____

Table 12•2 Roots for the Digestive Tract (Except the Mouth)

ROOT	MEANING	EXAMPLE	DEFINITION OF EXAMPLE
esophag/o	esophagus	esophageal* ē-sof-a-JĒ-al	pertaining to the esophagus
gastr/o	stomach	gastroparesis gas-trō-pa-RĒ-sis	partial paralysis (paresis) of the stomach
pylor/o	pylorus	pyloroplasty pī-LOR-ō-plas-tē	plastic repair of the pylorus
enter/o	intestine	dysentery DIS-en-ter-ē	infectious disease of the intestine
duoden/o	duodenum	duodenostomy dū-ō-de-NOS-tō-mē	surgical creation of an opening into the duodenum
jejun/o	jejunum	jejunectomy je-jū-NEK-ō-mē	excision of the jejunum
ile/o	ileum	ileitis il-ē-Ī-tis	inflammation of the ileum
cec/o	cecum	cecoptosis sē-kop-TŌ-sis	downward displacement of the cecum
col/o, colon/o	colon	coloclysis kō-lō-KLĪ-sis	irrigation (-clysis) of the colon

Table 12·2	Continued		
sigmoid/o	sigmoid colon	sigmoidoscope *sig-MOY-dō-skōp*	an endoscope for examining the sigmoid colon
rect/o	rectum	rectocele *REK-tō-sēl*	hernia of the rectum
proct/o	rectum	proctopexy *PROK-tō-pek-sē*	surgical fixation of the rectum
an/o	anus	perianal *per-ē-Ā-nal*	around the anus

*Note addition of e before –al.

12

Exercise 12-2

Use the adjective suffix -ic to write a word for the following definitions:

1. pertaining to the stomach _____ gastric _____

2. pertaining to the intestine _____

3. pertaining to the pylorus _____

4. pertaining to the colon _____

Use the adjective suffix -al to write a word for the following definitions:

5. pertaining to the duodenum _____ duodenal _____

6. pertaining to the jejunum _____

7. pertaining to the ileum _____

8. pertaining to the cecum _____

9. pertaining to the anus _____

Write a word for the following definitions:

10. study of the stomach and intestines _____

11. inflammation of the esophagus _____

12. surgical fixation of the stomach _____

13. downward displacement of the pylorus _____

14. excision of the ileum _____

15. endoscopic examination of the duodenum _____

16. surgical creation of an opening into the jejunum _____

17. Pertaining to the anus and rectum _____

Use the root col/o to write a word for the following definitions:

18. surgical creation of an opening into the colon _____

19. surgical fixation of the colon _____

20. inflammation of the colon _____

21. surgical puncture of the colon _____

Use the root colon/o to write a word for the following definitions:

22. any disease of the colon _____

23. endoscopic examination of the colon _____

Two organs of the digestive tract or even two parts of the same organ may be surgically connected by a passage (anastomosis) after removal of damaged tissue. Such a procedure is named for the connected organs plus the ending -stomy. Use two roots plus the suffix -stomy to write a word for the following definitions:

24. surgical creation of a passage between the esophagus and stomach _____ esophagogastrostomy _____

25. surgical creation of a passage between the stomach and intestine _____

26. surgical creation of a passage between the stomach and the jejunum _____

27. surgical creation of a passage between the duodenum and the ileum _____

28. surgical creation of a passage between the sigmoid colon and the rectum (proct/o) _____

Table 12•3 Roots for the Accessory Organs

ROOT	MEANING	EXAMPLE	DEFINITION OF EXAMPLE
hepat/o	liver	hepatocyte *HEP-a-tō-sīt*	a liver cell
bili	bile	biliary *BIL-ē-ar-ē*	pertaining to the bile or bile ducts
chol/e, chol/o	bile, gall	cholestasis *kō-lē-STĀ-sis*	stoppage of bile flow
cholecyst/o	gallbladder	cholecystogram *kō-lē-SIS-tō-gram*	radiograph of the gallbladder
cholangi/o	bile duct	cholangioma *kō-lan-jē-Ō-ma*	cancer of the bile ducts
choledoch/o	common bile duct	choledochal *kō-LED-o-kal*	pertaining to the common bile duct
pancreat/o	pancreas	pancreatotropic *pan-krē-at-ō-TROP-ik*	acting on the pancreas

Exercise 12-3

Use the suffix -ic to write a word for the following definitions:

1. pertaining to the liver _____

2. pertaining to the gallbladder _____

3. pertaining to the pancreas _____

Use the suffix -graphy to write a word for the following definitions:

4. radiographic study of the liver _____

5. radiographic study of the gallbladder _____

6. radiographic study of the bile ducts _____

7. radiographic study of the pancreas _____

Use the suffix -lithiasis to write a word for the following definitions:

8. condition of having a stone in the common bile duct _____

9. condition of having a stone in the pancreas _____

Fill in the blanks:

10. Hepatomegaly (*hep-a-tō-MEG-a-lē*) is enlargement of the _____.

11. A cholelith (*KŌ-lē-lith*) is a(n) _____.

12. The word biligenesis (*bil-i-JEN-e-sis*) means the formation of _____.

13. Choledochotomy (*kō-led-o-KOT-o-mē*) is incision of the _____.

14. Inflammation of the liver is called _____.

15. Pancreatolysis (*pan-krē-a-TOL-i-sis*) is dissolving of the _____.

16. Cholangitis (*kō-lan-JĪ-tis*) is inflammation of a(n) _____.

17. Cholecystorrhaphy (*kō-lē-sis-TOR-a-fē*) is suture of the _____.

Clinical Aspects of the Digestive System

Digestive Tract

Infection

A variety of organisms can infect the gastrointestinal tract, from viruses and bacteria to protozoa and worms. Some produce short-lived upsets with **gastroenteritis**, **nausea**, **diarrhea**, and **emesis** (vomiting). Others, such as typhoid, cholera, and dysentery, are more serious, even fatal.

Appendicitis results from infection of the appendix, often secondary to its obstruction. Surgery is necessary to avoid rupture and **peritonitis**, infection of the peritoneal cavity.

Ulcers

An ulcer is a lesion of the skin or a mucous membrane marked by inflammation and tissue damage. Ulcers caused by the damaging action of gastric, or peptic, juices on the lining of the GI tract are termed **peptic ulcers**. Most peptic ulcers appear in the first portion of the duodenum. The origins of such ulcers are not completely known, although infection with a bacterium, *Helicobacter pylori,* has been identified as a major cause. Heredity and stress may be factors, as well as chronic inflammation and exposure to damaging drugs, such as aspirin and other NSAIDs, or to irritants in food and drink.

Current ulcer treatment includes the administration of antibiotics to eliminate *H. pylori* infection and use of drugs that inhibit gastric acid secretion. Ulcers may lead to hemorrhage or to perforation of the digestive tract wall.

Ulcers can be diagnosed by **endoscopy** (Fig. 12-6, Box 12-5) and by radiographic study of the GI tract using a contrast medium, usually barium sulfate. A **barium study** can reveal a variety of GI disorders in addition to ulcers, including tumors and obstruc-

12

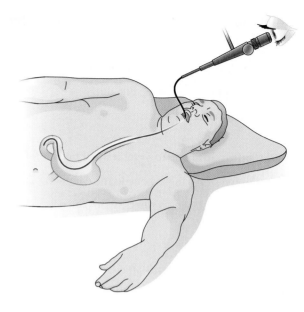

Figure 12-6 Endoscopy. A patient undergoing gastroscopy is shown.

tions. A barium swallow is used for study of the pharynx and esophagus; an upper GI series examines the esophagus, stomach, and small intestine.

Cancer

The most common sites for GI tract cancer are the colon and rectum. Together these colorectal cancers rank among the most frequent causes of cancer deaths in the United States in both men and women. A diet low in fiber and calcium and high in fat is a major risk factor in colorectal cancer. Heredity is also a factor, as is chronic inflammation of the colon (colitis). **Polyps** (growths) in the intestine often become cancerous and should be removed. Polyps can be identified and even removed by endoscopy.

One sign of colorectal cancer is bleeding into the intestine, which can be detected by testing the stool for blood. Because this blood may be present in very small amounts, it is described as **occult** ("hidden") **blood**. Colorectal cancers are staged according to **Dukes' classification**, ranging from A to C according to severity.

Examiners can observe the interior of the intestine with various endoscopes named for the specific area in which they are used, such as proctoscope (rectum), sigmoidoscope (sigmoid colon), colonoscope (colon) (Fig. 12-7).

Box 12•5 Clinical Perspectives   *Endoscopy*

Modern medicine has made great strides toward looking into the body without resorting to surgery. The endoscope, an instrument that is inserted through a body opening or small incision, has allowed the noninvasive examination of passageways, hollow organs, and body cavities. The first endoscopes were rigid lighted telescopes that could be inserted only a short distance into the body. Today, physicians can navigate the twists and turns of the digestive tract using long fiberoptic endoscopes composed of flexible, light-transmitting bundles of glass or plastic.

Physicians can detect structural abnormalities, ulcers, inflammation, and tumors in the GI tract endoscopically.

In addition, they use endoscopes to remove fluid samples or tissue biopsy specimens. Some surgery can even be done with an endoscope, such as polyp removal from the colon or sphincter expansion. Endoscopy can also be used to examine and operate on joints (arthroscopy), the bladder (cystoscopy), respiratory passages (bronchoscopy), and the abdominal cavity (laparoscopy).

Capsular endoscopy, a recent technological advance, has made examination of the GI tract even easier. It uses a pill-sized camera that a patient can swallow! As the camera moves through the digestive tract, it transmits video images to a data recorder worn on the patient's belt.

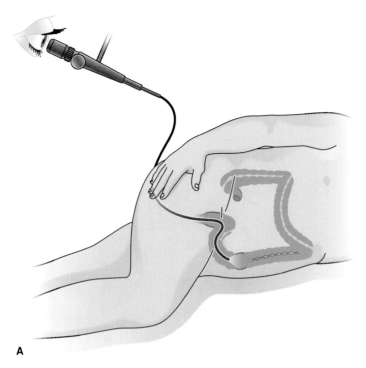

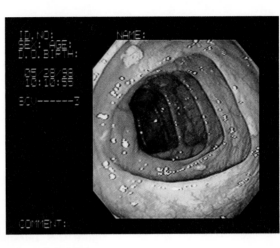

A **B**

Figure 12-7 Colonoscopy. (*A*) Sigmoidoscopy. The flexible fiberoptic endoscope is advanced past the proximal sigmoid colon and then into the descending colon. (*B*) Endoscopic image of the cecum, the first portion of the large intestine.

In some cases of cancer, and for other reasons as well, it may be necessary to surgically remove a portion of the GI tract and create a **stoma** (opening) on the abdominal wall for elimination of waste. Such **ostomy** surgery (Fig. 12-8) is named for the organ involved, such as ileostomy (ileum) or colostomy (colon). When an **anastomosis** (connection) is formed between two organs of the tract, both organs are included in naming, such as gastroduodenostomy (stomach and duodenum) or coloproctostomy (colon and rectum).

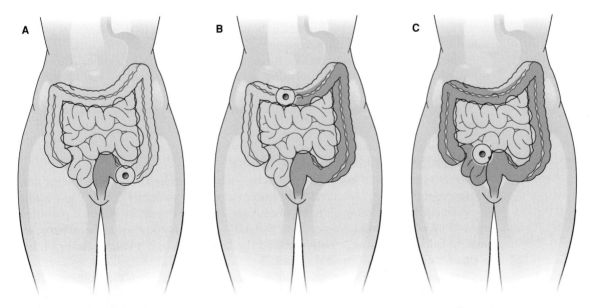

A **B** **C**

Figure 12-8 Ostomy surgery. Various locations are shown. The shaded portions represent the bowel sections that have been removed or are inactive. (*A*) Sigmoid colostomy. (*B*) Transverse colostomy. (*C*) Ileostomy.

12

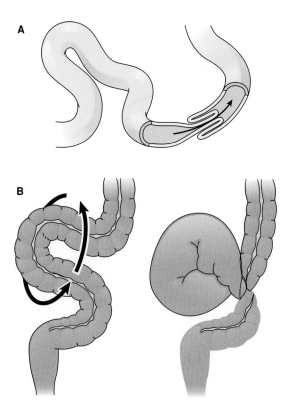

Figure 12-9 Intestinal obstruction.
(*A*) Intussusception. (*B*) Volvulus, showing counterclockwise twist.

Obstructions

A hernia is the protrusion of an organ through an abnormal opening. The most common type is an inguinal hernia, described in Chapter 14 (see Fig. 14-7). In a **hiatal hernia**, part of the stomach moves upward into the chest cavity through the space (hiatus) in the diaphragm where the esophagus passes through (see Fig. 6-7). Often this condition produces no symptoms, but it may result in chest pain, **dysphagia** (difficulty in swallowing), or reflux (backflow) of stomach contents into the esophagus.

In **pyloric stenosis**, the opening between the stomach and small intestine is too narrow. This usually occurs in infants, and in boys more often than in girls. A sign of pyloric stenosis is projectile vomiting. Surgery may be needed to correct it.

Other types of obstruction include **intussusception** (Fig. 12-9), slipping of a part of the intestine into a part below it; **volvulus**, twisting of the intestine (see Fig. 12-9B); and **ileus**, intestinal obstruction often caused by lack of peristalsis.

Hemorrhoids are varicose veins in the rectum associated with pain, bleeding, and, in some cases, prolapse of the rectum.

Gastroesophageal Reflux Disease (GERD)

GERD refers to reflux of gastric juices into the esophagus caused by weakness at the gastroesophageal junction, specifically the lower esophageal sphincter (LES). These acidic secretions irritate the lining of the esophagus and even the throat and mouth if propelled upward by **regurgitation**. A symptom of GERD commonly known as **heartburn**, an upward-radiating burning sensation behind the sternum, does not involve the heart, but is experienced in the area near the heart.

Symptoms of GERD are more likely to occur after meals when the stomach is full, when one is lying or bending down, and with hiatal hernia, obesity, and pregnancy. Treatment includes weight reduction if needed, elevating the head of the bed 4 to 6 inches, avoidance of irritating foods, and drugs to reduce secretion of stomach acid. Surgery to repair an incompetent LES might be needed.

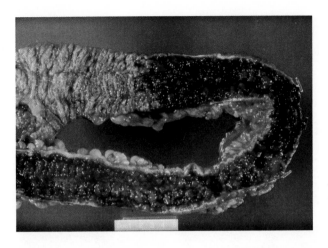

Figure 12-10 Ulcerative colitis. Prominent erythema and ulceration of the colon begin in the ascending colon and are most severe in the rectosigmoid area.

12

Inflammatory Intestinal Disease

Two similar diseases are included under the heading of inflammatory bowel disease (IBD):

➤ **Crohn disease** is a chronic inflammation of intestinal wall segments, usually in the ileum and colon, causing pain, diarrhea, abscess, and often formation of an abnormal passageway, or **fistula**.

➤ **Ulcerative colitis** involves a continuous inflammation of the colon lining that begins in the rectum and extends proximally (Fig. 12-10)

Both forms of IBD occur mainly in adolescents and young adults and show a hereditary pattern. They originate with an abnormal immunologic response, perhaps to the normal flora of the intestine, along with autoimmunity. Treatment is with antiinflammatory agents, immunosuppressants, and frequently surgery to remove damaged portions of the colon.

Celiac disease is characterized by the inability to absorb foods containing gluten, a protein found in wheat and some other grains. It affects the upper part of the small intestine and originates with an excess immune response to gluten. Inflammation of the mucosa reduces the intestinal villi and interferes with absorption. Celiac disease is treated with a gluten-free diet.

Diverticulitis most commonly affects the colon. Diverticula are small pouches in the wall of the intestine. If these pouches are present in large numbers the condition is termed **diverticulosis**, which has been attributed to a diet low in fiber. Collection of waste and bacteria in these sacs leads to diverticulitis, which is accompanied by pain and sometimes bleeding. Diverticula can be seen by radiographic studies of the lower GI tract using barium as a contrast medium, a so-called barium enema (Fig. 12-11). Although there is no cure, diverticulitis is treated with diet, stool softeners, and drugs to reduce motility (antispasmodics).

Accessory Organs

Hepatitis

In the United States and other industrialized countries, **hepatitis** is most often caused by viral infection. More than six types of hepatitis virus have now been identified. Vaccines are available for hepatitis A and hepatitis B.

➤ Hepatitis A virus (HAV) is the most common hepatitis virus. It is spread by fecal–oral contamination, often by food handlers, and in crowded, unsanitary conditions. It may also be acquired by eating contaminated food, especially seafood.

➤ Hepatitis B virus (HBV) is spread by blood and other body fluids. It may be transmitted sexually, by sharing needles used for injection, and by close interpersonal contact. Infected individuals may become carriers of the disease. Most patients recover, but the disease may be serious, even fatal, and may lead to liver cancer.

12

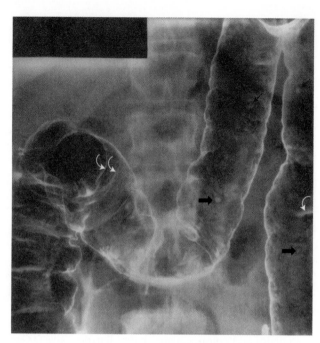

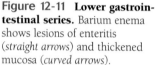

Figure 12-11 Lower gastrointestinal series. Barium enema shows lesions of enteritis (*straight arrows*) and thickened mucosa (*curved arrows*).

> ➤ Hepatitis C is spread through blood and blood products or by close contact with an infected person.
> ➤ Hepatitis D, the delta virus, is highly pathogenic but infects only those already infected with hepatitis B.
> ➤ Hepatitis E, like HAV, is spread by contaminated food and water. It has caused epidemics in Asia, Africa, and Mexico.
> ➤ Hepatitis G is believed to be spread through contact with blood of an infected person.

The name *hepatitis* simply means "inflammation of the liver," but this disease also causes necrosis (death) of liver cells. Hepatitis also may be caused by other infections and by drugs and toxins. Liver-function tests performed on blood serum are important in diagnosis.

Jaundice, or **icterus**, is a symptom of hepatitis and other diseases of the liver and biliary system (Fig. 12-12). It appears as yellowness of the skin, whites of the eyes, and mucous membranes caused by the presence of bile pigments, mainly **bilirubin**, in the blood.

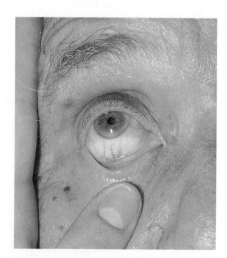

Figure 12-12 Jaundice. Yellowish discoloration due to bile pigments in the blood is seen in the eye.

Cirrhosis

Cirrhosis is a chronic liver disease characterized by **hepatomegaly**, edema, **ascites** (fluid in the abdomen), and jaundice. Progression of the disease leads to internal bleeding, and brain damage caused by changes in the blood's composition. One complication of cirrhosis is **portal hypertension**, increased pressure in the hepatic portal system, which is the vascular network that carries blood from the abdominal organs to the liver. Portal hypertension causes **splenomegaly** and the formation of varices (varicose veins) in the distal portion of the esophagus with possible hemorrhage. The main cause of cirrhosis is the excess consumption of alcohol.

Gallstones

Cholelithiasis refers to the presence of stones in the gallbladder or bile ducts, which is usually associated with **cholecystitis**, inflammation of the gallbladder. Cholelithiasis is characterized by **biliary colic** (pain) in the right upper quadrant (RUQ), nausea, and vomiting.

Most gallstones are composed of cholesterol, an ingredient of bile. They form more commonly in women than in men, and are promoted by conditions that increase estrogen, as this hormone raises the cholesterol in bile. These predisposing conditions include pregnancy, use of oral contraceptives, and obesity. Oddly, the rapid weight loss that follows stomach reduction surgery to treat morbid obesity commonly leads to gallstones because of changes in bile production and cholesterol precipitation in the bile. Drugs may dissolve gallstones, but often the cure is removal of the gallbladder in a **cholecystectomy**. This procedure was originally performed through a major abdominal incision, but now the gallbladder is almost always removed laparoscopically through a small incision in the abdomen. Following removal of the gallbladder, bile flows directly into the duodenum through the common bile duct.

Ultrasonography, radiography, and magnetic resonance imaging (MRI) are used for the diagnosis of gallstones (Fig. 12-13). **Endoscopic retrograde cholangiopancreatography (ERCP)** (Fig. 12-14) is a technique for viewing the pancreatic and bile ducts and for performing certain techniques to relieve obstructions. Contrast medium is injected into the biliary system from the duodenum and radiographs are taken.

Pancreatitis

Pancreatitis, or inflammation of the pancreas, may result from alcohol abuse, drug toxicity, bile obstruction, infections, and other causes. Blood tests in acute pancreatitis show increased levels of the enzymes amylase and lipase. Glucose and bilirubin levels may also be elevated. Often the disease subsides with only treatment of the symptoms.

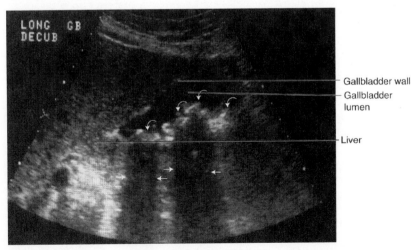

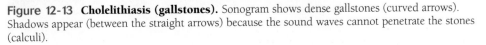

Figure 12-13 Cholelithiasis (gallstones). Sonogram shows dense gallstones (curved arrows). Shadows appear (between the straight arrows) because the sound waves cannot penetrate the stones (calculi).

12

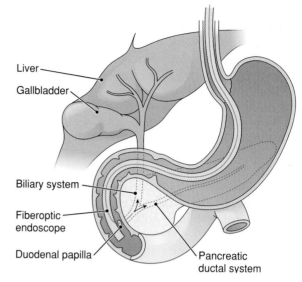

Figure 12-14 Endoscopic retrograde cholangiopancreatography (ERCP). A contrast medium is injected into the pancreatic and bile ducts in preparation for radiography.

Liver
Gallbladder
Biliary system
Fiberoptic endoscope
Duodenal papilla
Pancreatic ductal system

TERMINOLOGY   Key Terms

DISORDERS

appendicitis *a-pen-di-SĪ-tis*	Inflammation of the appendix
Ascites *a-SĪ-tēz*	Accumulation of fluid in the abdominal cavity; a form of edema. May be caused by heart disease, lymphatic or venous obstruction, cirrhosis, or changes in plasma composition.
biliary colic *BIL-ē-ar-ē KOL-ik*	Acute abdominal pain caused by gallstones in the bile ducts
bilirubin *bil-i-RŪ-bin*	A pigment released in the breakdown of hemoglobin from red blood cells; mainly excreted by the liver in bile
celiac disease *SĒ-lē-ak*	Inability to absorb foods containing gluten, a protein found in wheat and some other grains; caused by an excess immune response to gluten
cholecystitis *kō-lē-sis-TĪ-tis*	Inflammation of the gallbladder
cholelithiasis *kō-lē-li-THĪ-a-sis*	The condition of having stones in the gallbladder; also used to refer to stones in the common bile duct
cirrhosis *sir-RŌ-sis*	Chronic liver disease with degeneration of liver tissue
Crohn disease *krōn*	A chronic inflammatory disease of the gastrointestinal tract usually involving the ileum and colon
diarrhea *dī-a-RĒ-a*	The frequent passage of watery bowel movements
diverticulitis *dī-ver-tik-ū-LĪ-tis*	Inflammation of diverticula (small pouches) in the wall of the digestive tract, especially in the colon

TERMINOLOGY   Key Terms

Continued

diverticulosis dī-ver-tik-ū-LŌ-sis	The presence of diverticula, especially in the colon
dysphagia dis-FĀ-jē-a	Difficulty in swallowing
emesis EM-e-sis	Vomiting
fistula FIS-tū-la	An abnormal passageway between two organs or from an organ to the body surface, such as between the rectum and anus (anorectal fistula)
gastroenteritis gas-trō-en-ter-Ī-tis	Inflammation of the stomach and intestine
gastroesophageal reflux disease (GERD) gas-trō-ē-sof-a-JĒ-al	Condition caused by reflux of gastric juices into the esophagus resulting in heartburn, regurgitation, inflammation, and possible damage to the esophagus; caused by weakness of the lower esophageal sphincter (LES)
heartburn HART-burn	A warm or burning sensation felt behind the sternum and radiating upward. Commonly associated with gastroesophageal reflux. Medical name is pyrosis (*pyr/o* means "heat")
hemorrhoids HEM-ō-roydz	Varicose veins in the rectum associated with pain, bleeding, and sometimes prolapse of the rectum
hepatitis hep-a-TĪ-tis	Inflammation of the liver; commonly caused by a viral infection
hepatomegaly hep-a-tō-MEG-a-lē	Enlargement of the liver
hiatal hernia hī-Ā-tal	A protrusion of the stomach through the opening (hiatus) in the diaphragm through which the esophagus passes (see Fig. 6-7)
icterus IK-ter-us	Jaundice
ileus IL-ē-us	Intestinal obstruction. May be caused by lack of peristalsis (adynamic, paralytic ileus) or by contraction (dynamic ileus). Intestinal matter and gas may be relieved by passage of a tube for drainage.
intussusception in-tu-su-SEP-shun	Slipping of one part of the intestine into another part below it. Occurs mainly in male infants in the ileocecal region (see Fig. 12-9A). May be fatal if untreated for more than 1 day.
jaundice JAWN-dis	A yellowish color of the skin, mucous membranes, and whites of the eye caused by bile pigments in the blood (from French jaune meaning "yellow"). The main pigment is bilirubin, a by-product of the breakdown of red blood cells. (See Fig 12-12.)
nausea NAW-zha	An unpleasant sensation in the upper abdomen that often precedes vomiting. Typically occurs in digestive upset, motion sickness, and sometimes early pregnancy

12

TERMINOLOGY   Key Terms
Continued

occult blood *o-KULT*	Blood present in such small amounts that it can be detected only microscopically or chemically; in the feces, a sign of intestinal bleeding (*occult* means "hidden")
pancreatitis *pan-krē-a-TĪ-tis*	Inflammation of the pancreas
peptic ulcer *PEP-tik UL-ser*	A lesion in the mucous membrane of the esophagus, stomach, or duodenum caused by the action of gastric juice
peritonitis *per-i-tō-NĪ-tis*	Inflammation of the peritoneum, the membrane that lines the abdominal cavity and covers the abdominal organs. May result from perforation of an ulcer, rupture of the appendix, or infection of the reproductive tract, among other causes.
polyp *POL-ip*	A tumor that grows on a stalk and bleeds easily
portal hypertension	An abnormal increase in pressure in the hepatic portal system. May be caused by cirrhosis, infection, thrombosis, or tumors.
pyloric stenosis *pī-LOR-ik*	Narrowing of the opening between the stomach and the duodenum; pylorostenosis
regurgitation *rē-gur-ji-TĀ-shun*	A backward flowing, such as the backflow of undigested food
splenomegaly *splē-nō-MEG-a-lē*	Enlargement of the spleen
ulcerative colitis *UL-ser-a-tiv kō-LĪ-tis*	Chronic ulceration of the rectum and colon; the cause is unknown, but may involve autoimmunity
volvulus *VOL-vū-lus*	Twisting of the intestine resulting in obstruction. Usually involves the sigmoid colon and occurs most often in children and in the elderly. May be caused by congenital malformation, a foreign body, or adhesion. Failure to treat immediately may result in death (see Fig. 12-9B).

DIAGNOSIS AND TREATMENT

anastomosis *a-nas-to-MŌ-sis*	A passage or communication between two vessels or organs. May be normal or pathologic, or may be created surgically.
barium study	Use of barium sulfate as a liquid contrast medium for fluoroscopic or radiographic study of the digestive tract. Can show obstruction, tumors, ulcers, hiatal hernia, and motility disorders, among other things.
cholecystectomy *kō-lē-sis-TEK-tō-mē*	Surgical removal of the gallbladder
Dukes classification	A system for staging colorectal cancer based on degree of penetration of the bowel wall and lymph node involvement; severity is graded from A to C

TERMINOLOGY Key Terms

Continued

12

endoscopy *en-DOS-kō-pē*	Use of a fiberoptic endoscope for direct visual examination. GI studies include esophagogastroduodenoscopy, proctosigmoidoscopy (rectum and distal colon), and colonoscopy (all regions of the colon) (see Figs. 12-6 and 12-7).
ERCP	Endoscopic retrograde cholangiopancreatography; a technique for viewing the pancreatic and bile ducts and for performing certain techniques to relieve obstructions. Contrast medium is injected into the biliary system from the duodenum and radiographs are taken (see Fig. 12-14).
ostomy *OS-tō-mē*	An opening into the body; generally refers to an opening created for elimination of body waste. Also refers to the operation done to create such an opening (see stoma).
stoma *STŌ-ma*	A surgically created opening to the body surface or between two organs (literally "mouth") (see Fig. 12-8)

Go to the pronunciation glossary in Chapter 12 on the CD-ROM to hear these words pronounced.

TERMINOLOGY Supplementary Terms

NORMAL STRUCTURE AND FUNCTION

bolus *BŌ-lus*	A mass, such as the rounded mass of food that is swallowed
cardia *KAR-dē-a*	The part of the stomach near the esophagus, named for its closeness to the heart
chyme *kīm*	The semiliquid partially digested food that moves from the stomach into the small intestine
defecation *def-e-KĀ-shun*	The evacuation of feces from the rectum
deglutition *deg-lū-TISH-un*	Swallowing
duodenal bulb	The part of the duodenum near the pylorus; the first bend (flexure) of the duodenum

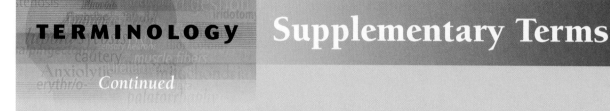

TERMINOLOGY *Continued*

Supplementary Terms

duodenal papilla	The raised area where the common bile duct and pancreatic duct enter the duodenum (see Fig. 12-14); papilla of Vater (FA-ter)
greater omentum *ō-MEN-tum*	A fold of the peritoneum that extends from the stomach over the abdominal organs
hepatic flexure	The right bend of the colon, forming the junction between the ascending colon and the transverse colon (see Fig. 12-1)
ileocecal valve *il-ē-ō-SĒ-kal*	A valvelike structure between the ileum of the small intestine and the cecum of the large intestine
mesentery *MES-en-ter-ē*	The portion of the peritoneum that folds over and supports the intestine
mesocolon *mes-ō-KŌ-lon*	The portion of the peritoneum that folds over and supports the colon
papilla of Vater	See duodenal papilla
peritoneum *per-i-tō-NĒ-um*	The serous membrane that lines the abdominal cavity and supports the abdominal organs
rugae *Rū-jē*	The large folds in the lining of the stomach seen when the stomach is empty
sphincter of Oddi *OD-ē*	The ring of muscle at the opening of the common bile duct into the duodenum
splenic flexure	The left bend of the colon, forming the junction between the transverse colon and the descending colon (see Fig. 12-1)

DISORDERS

achalasia *ak-a-LĀ-zē-a*	Failure of a smooth muscle to relax, especially the lower esophageal sphincter, so that food is retained in the esophagus
achlorhydria *ā-klor-HĪ-drē-a*	Lack of hydrochloric acid in the stomach; opposite is hyperchlorhydria
anorexia *an-ō-REK-sē-a*	Loss of appetite. Anorexia nervosa is a psychologically induced refusal or inability to eat (adjectives: anorectic, anorexic).
aphagia *a-FĀ-jē-a*	Refusal or inability to eat; inability to swallow or difficulty in swallowing
aphthous ulcer *AF-thus*	A small ulcer in the mucous membrane of the mouth
Barrett syndrome	Lower esophageal ulcer resulting from chronic esophagitis, often with constriction caused by mucosal changes; may be premalignant. Also called Barrett esophagus.

Supplementary Terms

bruxism *BRUK-sizm*	Clenching and grinding of the teeth, usually during sleep
bulimia *bū-LIM-ē-a*	Excessive, insatiable appetite. A disorder characterized by overeating followed by induced vomiting, diarrhea, or fasting.
cachexia *ka-KEK-sē-a*	Profound ill health, malnutrition, and wasting
caries *KAR-ēz*	Tooth decay
celiac disease *SĒ-lē-ak*	A disease characterized by the inability to absorb foods containing gluten
cheilosis *kī-LŌ-sis*	Cracking at the corners of the mouth, often caused by B vitamin deficiency (root cheil/o means "lip")
cholestasis *kō-lē-STA-sis*	Stoppage of bile flow
constipation *con-sti-PĀ-shun*	Infrequency or difficulty in defecation and the passage of hard, dry feces
dyspepsia *dis-PEP-sē-a*	Poor or painful digestion
eructation *e-ruk-TĀ-shun*	Belching
familial adenomatous polyposis (FAP)	A heredity condition in which multiple polyps form in the colon and rectum, predisposing to colorectal cancer
flatulence *FLAT-ū-lens*	Condition of having gas or air in the GI tract
flatus *FLĀ-tus*	Gas or air in the gastrointestinal tract; gas or air expelled through the anus
hematemesis *hē-ma-TEM-e-sis*	Vomiting of blood
irritable bowel syndrome (IBS)	A chronic stress-related disease characterized by diarrhea, constipation, and pain associated with rhythmic contractions of the intestine. Mucous colitis; spastic colon.
megacolon *meg-a-KŌ-lon*	An extremely dilated colon. Usually congenital but may occur in acute ulcerative colitis.
melena *MEL-ē-na*	Black tarry feces resulting from blood in the intestines. Common in newborns. May also be a sign of gastrointestinal bleeding.
obstipation *ob-sti-PĀ-shun*	Extreme constipation

12

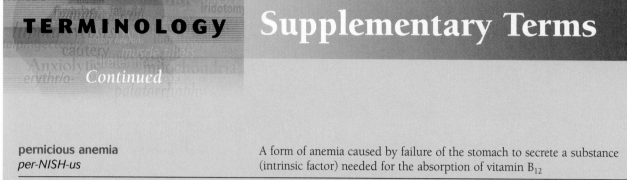

pernicious anemia *per-NISH-us*	A form of anemia caused by failure of the stomach to secrete a substance (intrinsic factor) needed for the absorption of vitamin B_{12}
pilonidal cyst *pī-lō-NĪ-dal*	A dermal cyst in the region of the sacrum, usually at the top of the cleft between the buttocks. May become infected and begin to drain.

DIAGNOSIS AND TREATMENT

appendectomy *ap-en-DEK-tō-mē*	Surgical removal of the appendix
bariatrics *bar-ē-AT-riks*	The branch of medicine concerned with prevention and control of obesity and associated diseases (from Greek baros, meaning "weight")
Billroth operations	Gastrectomy with anastomosis of the stomach to the duodenum (Billroth I) or to the jejunum (Billroth II) (Fig. 12-15)
gastric bypass surgery	Division of the stomach and anastomosis of its upper part to the small intestine (jejunum) to reduce nutrient absorption; used to treat morbid obesity (Fig. 12-16). Other surgical methods are used for this purpose, including partition of the stomach with rows of staples (gastric stapling).
gavage *ga-VAHZH*	Process of feeding through a nasogastric tube into the stomach
lavage *la-VAJ*	Washing out of a cavity; irrigation
manometry *man-OM-e-trē*	Measurement of pressure; pertaining to the GI tract, measurement of pressure in the portal system as a sign of obstruction
Murphy sign	Inability to take a deep breath when fingers are pressed firmly below the right arch of the ribs (below the liver). Signifies gallbladder disease.
nasogastric (NG) tube	Tube that is passed through the nose into the stomach (Fig. 12-17). May be used for emptying the stomach, administering medication, giving liquids, or sampling stomach contents.
parenteral hyperalimentation *pa-REN-ter-al*	Complete intravenous feeding for one who cannot take in food. Total parenteral nutrition (TPN).
percutaneous endoscopic gastrostomy (PEG) tube	Tube inserted into the stomach for long-term feeding (Fig. 12-18)
vagotomy *vā-GOT-ō-mē*	Interruption of impulses from the vagus nerve to reduce stomach secretions in the treatment of gastric ulcer. Originally done surgically but may also be done with drugs.

DRUGS

antacid *ant-AS-id*	Agent that counteracts acidity, usually gastric acidity

TERMINOLOGY

Continued

Supplementary Terms

12

antidiarrheal *an-ti-di-a-RĒ-al*	Treats or prevents diarrhea by reducing intestinal motility or absorbing irritants and soothing the intestinal lining
antiemetic *an-tē-e-MET-ik*	Agent that relieves or prevents nausea and vomiting
antiflatulent *an-ti-FLAT-ū-lent*	Agent that prevents or relieves flatulence
antispasmodic *an-ti-spas-MOD-ik*	Agent that relieves spasm, usually of smooth muscle
emetic *e-MET-ik*	An agent that causes vomiting
histamine H₂ antagonist	Drug that decreases secretion of stomach acid by interfering with the action of histamine at H_2 receptors. Used to treat ulcers and other gastrointestinal problems. H_2-receptor-blocking agent.
laxative *LAK-sa-tiv*	Promotes elimination from the large intestine. Types include stimulants, substances that retain water (hyperosmotics), stool softeners, and bulk-forming agents.
proton-pump inhibitor (PPI)	Agent that inhibits secretion of stomach acid by blocking the transport of hydrogen ions (protons) into the stomach.

Go to the pronunciation glossary in Chapter 12 on the CD-ROM to hear these words pronounced.

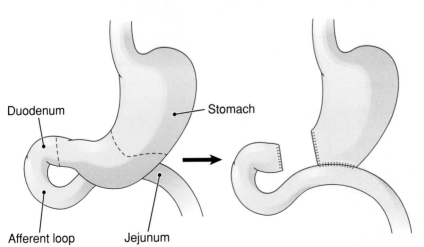

Figure 12-15 Gastrojejunostomy (Billroth II operation). The dotted lines show the portion removed.

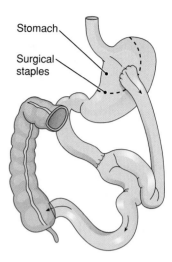

Figure 12-16 Gastric bypass. For treatment of morbid obesity, a small pouch is created in the stomach to limit food intake. The pouch is attached to the jejunum in a gastrojejunostomy to bypass the stomach and reduce nutrient absorption.

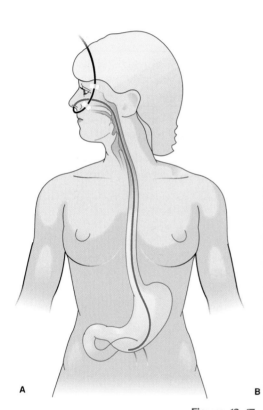

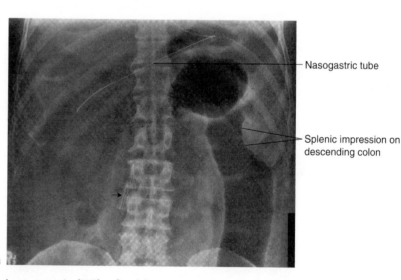

Figure 12-17 A nasogastric (NG) tube. (*A*) Diagram showing an NG tube in place. (*B*) Abdominal radiograph showing an NG tube. The filter (*arrow*) shown in the inferior vena cava is meant to trap emboli that might originate in the lower extremities and pelvis.

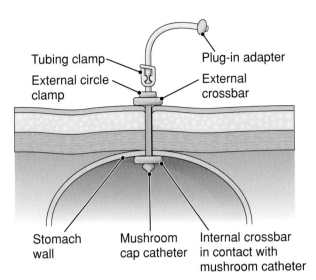

Tubing clamp

External circle clamp

Plug-in adapter

External crossbar

Stomach wall

Mushroom cap catheter

Internal crossbar in contact with mushroom catheter

Figure 12-18 Percutaneous endoscopic gastrostomy (PEG) tube. The tube is shown in place in the stomach.

12

TERMINOLOGY Abbreviations

BE	Barium enema (for radiographic study of the colon)	**HEV**	Hepatitis E virus
BM	Bowel movement	**HCl**	Hydrochloric acid
CBD	Common bile duct	**IBD**	Inflammatory bowel disease
ERCP	Endoscopic retrograde cholangiopancreatography	**IBS**	Irritable bowel syndrome
		LES	Lower esophageal sphincter
FAP	Familial adenomatous polyposis	**NG**	Nasogastric (tube)
GERD	Gastroesophageal reflux disease	**N & V**	Nausea and vomiting
GI	Gastrointestinal	**N/V/D**	Nausea, vomiting, and diarrhea
HAV	Hepatitis A virus	**PONV**	Postoperative nausea and vomiting
HBV	Hepatitis B virus	**PPI**	Proton-pump inhibitor
HCV	Hepatitis C virus	**TPN**	Total parenteral nutrition
HDV	Hepatitis D virus	**UGI**	Upper gastrointestinal (radiograph series)

12

CHAPTER REVIEW

LABELING EXERCISE
The Digestive System

Write the name of each numbered part on the corresponding line of the answer sheet.

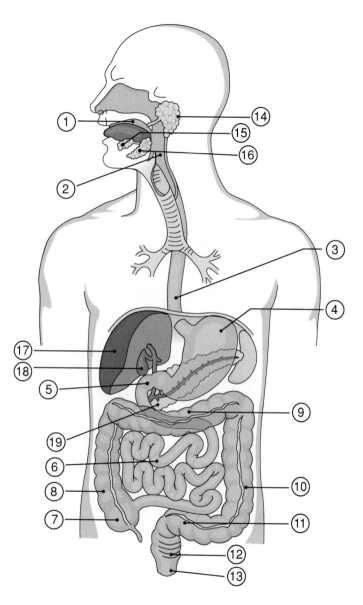

Anus	1._____
Ascending colon	2._____
Cecum	3._____
Descending colon	4._____
Duodenum (of small intestine)	5._____
Esophagus	6._____

Gallbladder   7._____

Liver   8._____

Mouth   9._____

Pancreas   10._____

Parotid salivary glands   11._____

Pharynx   12._____

Rectum   13._____

Sigmoid colon   14._____

Small intestine   15._____

Stomach   16._____

Sublingual salivary glands   17._____

Submandibular salivary glands   18._____

Transverse colon   19._____

Accessory Organs of Digestion

Write the name of each numbered part on the corresponding line of the answer sheet.

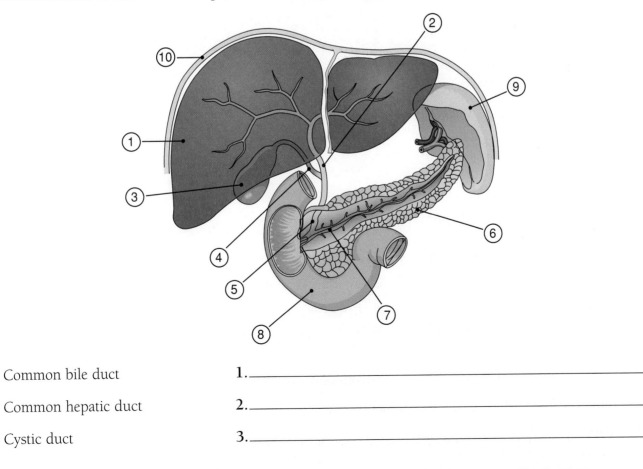

Common bile duct   1._____

Common hepatic duct   2._____

Cystic duct   3._____

Diaphragm   4._____

Duodenum   5._____

Gallbladder   6._____

Liver   7._____

Pancreas   8._____

Pancreatic duct   9._____

12 Spleen   10._____

TERMINOLOGY

Match the following terms and write the appropriate letter to the left of each number:

_____ 1. agnathia   **a.** hypoglossal

_____ 2. sublingual   **b.** pertaining to the lip

_____ 3. labial   **c.** substance that induces vomiting

_____ 4. emetic   **d.** jaundice

_____ 5. icterus   **e.** absence of the jaw

_____ 6. choledochal   **a.** any disease of the intestine

_____ 7. cirrhosis   **b.** pertaining to the common bile duct

_____ 8. cholangiectasis   **c.** crushing of a biliary calculus

_____ 9. enteropathy   **d.** dilatation of a bile duct

_____ 10. cholelithotripsy   **e.** a type of liver disease

_____ 11. cecopexy   **a.** dropping of the cecum

_____ 12. colocentesis   **b.** surgical repair of the rectum

_____ 13. proctocele   **c.** surgical fixation of the cecum

_____ 14. cecoptosis   **d.** surgical puncture of the colon

_____ 15. proctorrhaphy   **e.** hernia of the rectum

Supplementary Terms

_____ 16. peritoneum   **a.** part of the stomach near the esophagus

_____ 17. cardia   **b.** chewing

_____ 18. deglutition   **c.** serous membrane in the abdomen

_____ 19. bolus   **d.** swallowing

_____ 20. mastication   **e.** a mass, as of food

_____ 21. gavage   **a.** inability to eat

_____ 22. caries   **b.** partially digested food

_____ 23. aphagia   **c.** malnutrition and wasting

_____ 24. cachexia   d. feeding through a tube

_____ 25. chyme   e. tooth decay

Fill in the blanks:

26. The palatine tonsils are located on either side of the _____

27. Dentin is the main substance of the _____

28. Glossorrhaphy is suture of the _____

29. From its name you might guess that the buccinator muscle is in the _____

30. An enterovirus is a virus that infects the _____

31. The blind pouch at the beginning of the colon is the _____

32. The anticoagulant heparin is found throughout the body, but it is named for its presence in the

   _____

33. The substance cholesterol is named for its chemical composition (sterol) and for its presence in

   _____

34. The hepatic portal system carries blood to the _____

35. The organ that stores bile is the _____

Eliminations. In each of the sets below, underline the word that does not fit in with the rest and explain the reason for your choice:

36. gingival – pylorus – palate – uvula – incisor

   _____

37. spleen – cecum – colon – rectum – anus

   _____

38. pancreas – gallbladder – liver – villi – salivary glands

   _____

39. diarrhea – emesis – nausea – regurgitation – peristalsis

   _____

True–False. Examine the following statements. If the statement is true, write T in the first blank. If the statement is false, write F in the first blank and correct the statement by replacing the underlined word in the second blank.

40. The epigastrium is the region of the abdomen <u>below</u> the stomach.   _____ _____

41. The middle portion of the small intestine is the <u>duodenum</u>.   _____ _____

42. Polysialia is the excess secretion of <u>bile</u>.   _____ _____

43. The cystic duct carries bile to and from the <u>gallbladder</u>.

44. The appendix is attached to the <u>cecum</u>.   _____ _____

45. The common hepatic duct and the cystic duct merge to form the <u>common bile duct</u>.   _____ _____

Word building. Write a word for the following definitions:

46. a dentist who specializes in treating the tissues around the teeth   _____

47. surgical excision of the stomach   _____

48. surgical repair of the palate   _____

49. narrowing of the pylorus   _____

50. inflammation of the pancreas _____

51. pertaining to the ileum and cecum _____

52. hernia of the rectum _____

53. medical specialist who treats diseases of the stomach and intestine _____

54. surgical creation of an opening into the colon _____

55. surgical creation of a passage between the stomach and the duodenum _____

56. inflammation of the ileum _____

57. within (intra-) the liver _____

Plurals. Write the plural form of the following words:

58. diverticulum _____

59. gingiva _____

60. calculus _____

61. anastomosis _____

Write the meaning of the following abbreviations:

62. TPN _____

63. GERD _____

64. GI _____

65. HCl _____

66. PEG (tube) _____

67. HAV _____

Word analysis. Define each of the following words, and give the meaning of the word parts in each. Use a dictionary if necessary.

68. myenteric (*mī-en-TER-ik*) _____

    a. my/o _____

    b. enter/o _____

    c. -ic _____

69. cholescintigraphy (*kō-lē-sin-TIG-ra-fē*) _____

    a. chole _____

    b. scinti _____ spark (radiation) _____

    c. -graphy _____

70. parenteral (*pa-REN-ter-al*) _____

    a. par(a) _____

    b. enter/o _____

    c. -al _____

Go to the word exercises in Chapter 12 on the CD-ROM for additional review exercises.

CASE STUDIES

CASE STUDY 12-1: Cholecystectomy

G.L., a 42-year-old obese Caucasian woman, entered the hospital with nausea and vomiting, flatulence and eructation, a fever of 100.5°F, and continuous right upper quadrant and subscapular pain. Examination on admission showed rebound tenderness in the RUQ with a positive Murphy sign. Her skin, nails, and conjunctivae were yellowish, and she reported frequent clay-colored stools. Her leukocyte count was 16,000. An ERCP and ultrasound of the abdomen suggested many small stones in her gallbladder and possibly the common bile duct. Her diagnosis was cholecystitis with cholelithiasis.

A laparoscopic cholecystectomy was attempted, with an intraoperative cholangiogram and common bile duct exploration. Because of G.L.'s size and some unexpected bleeding, visualization was difficult and the procedure was converted to an open approach. Small stones and granular sludge were irrigated from her common duct, and the gallbladder was removed. She had a T-tube inserted into the duct for bile drainage; this tube was removed on the second postoperative day. An NG tube in place before and during the surgery was also removed on day 2. She was discharged on the fifth postoperative day with a prescription for prn pain medication and a low-fat diet.

CASE STUDY 12-2: Surgical Pathology Report

Gross Description: The specimen is received in formalin labeled "ruptured duodenal diverticula" and consists of enteric tissue measuring approximately 6.3 × 2.8 × 0.7 cm. The serosal surface is markedly dull in appearance and fibrotic. The mucosal surface is hemorrhagic. Representative sections are taken for microscopic examination.

Microscopic Description: Sectioned slide shows segments of duodenal tissues with areas of gangrenous change in the bowel wall, and acute and chronic inflammatory infiltrates. There are chronic and focal acute-inflammatory-cell infiltrates with hemorrhage in the mesenteric fatty tissue. There are areas of acute inflammatory exudates noted in the fatty tissue. Histopathologic changes are consistent with ruptured duodenal diverticula.

CASE STUDY 12-3: Colonoscopy with Biopsy

S.M., a 24-year-old man, had a recent history of lower abdominal pain with frequent loose mucoid stools. He described symptoms of occasional dysphagia, dyspepsia, nausea, and aphthous ulcers of his tongue and buccal mucosa. A previous barium enema examination showed some irregularities in the sigmoid and rectal segments of his large bowel. Stool samples for culture, ova, and parasites were negative. His tentative diagnosis was irritable bowel syndrome.

He followed a lactose-free, low-residue diet and took Imodium to reduce intestinal motility. His gastroenterologist recommended a colonoscopy. After a 2-day regimen of a soft-to-clear-liquid diet, laxatives, and an enema the morning of the procedure, he reported to the endoscopy unit. He was transported to the procedure room. ECG electrodes, a pulse oximeter sensor, and a blood pressure cuff were applied for monitoring, and an IV was inserted in S.M.'s right arm. An IV bolus of Demerol and a bolus of Versed were given, and S.M. was positioned on his left side. The colonoscope was gently inserted through the anal sphincter and advanced proximally. S.M. was instructed to take a deep breath when the scope approached the splenic flexure and the hepatic flexure to facilitate comfortable passage.

The physician was able to advance past the ileocecal valve, examining the entire length of the colon. Ulcerated granulomatous lesions were seen throughout the colon, with a concentration in the sigmoid segment. Many biopsy specimens were taken. The mucosa of the distal ileum was normal. Pathology examination of the biopsy samples was expected to establish a diagnosis of IBD.

CASE STUDY QUESTIONS

Multiple choice. Select the best answer and write the letter of your choice to the left of each number:

_____ 1. Flatulence and eructation represent:
   a. regurgitation of chyme
   b. distention of the esophagus
   c. passage of gas or air from the GI tract
   d. muscular movement of the alimentary tract
   e. sounds heard only by abdominal auscultation

_____ 2. The Murphy sign is tested for:
   a. under the ribs on the left
   b. near the spleen
   c. in the lower right abdomen
   d. under the ribs on the right
   e. in the lower left abdomen

_____ 3. The NG tube is inserted through the _____ and terminates in the _____:
   a. nose/stomach
   b. nostril/gallbladder
   c. glottis/nephron
   d. anus/cecum
   e. Nissen/glottis

_____ 4. Enteric tissue is found in the:
   a. gallbladder
   b. stomach
   c. esophagus
   d. liver
   e. intestine

_____ 5. The mucosal surface of a digestive organ is the:
   a. outer surface
   b. medulla
   c. cortex
   d. inner surface
   e. central opening

_____ 6. Diverticula are:
   a. small pouches in the wall of the colon
   b. communications between two organs
   c. ducts in the liver
   d. intestinal obstructions
   e. polyps in the intestine

_____ 7. Dysphagia and dyspepsia are difficulty or pain with:
   a. chewing and intestinal motility
   b. speaking and motility
   c. swallowing and digestion
   d. breathing and absorption
   e. swallowing and nutrition

_____ 8. The buccal mucosa is in the:
  a. nostril, medial side
  b. mouth, inside of the cheek
  c. greater curvature of the stomach
  d. lesser curvature near the duodenum
  e. base of the tongue

_____ 9. A gastroenterologist is a physician who specializes in study of:
  a. respiration and pathology
  b. mouth and teeth
  c. stomach, intestines, and related structures
  d. musculoskeletal system
  e. nutritional and weight loss diets

_____ 10. The splenic and hepatic flexures are bends in the colon near the:
  a. liver and splanchnic vein
  b. common bile duct and biliary tree
  c. spleen and appendix
  d. spleen and liver
  e. mesenteric vessels and liver

_____ 11. Intestinal motility refers to:
  a. chewing
  b. peristalsis
  c. absorption
  d. antiemetics
  e. ascites

_____ 12. A colonoscopy is:
  a. a radiograph of the small intestine
  b. an endoscopic study of the esophagus
  c. an upper endoscopy with biopsy
  d. a type of barium enema
  e. an endoscopic examination of the large bowel

_____ 13. The ileocecal valve is:
  a. part of a colonoscope
  b. at the distal ileum
  c. in the pylorus
  d. at the proximal ileum
  e. near the liver

Write the meaning of each of the following abbreviations:

14. ERCP _____

15. RUQ _____

16. NG _____

17. IBD _____

CASE STUDIES

Give the word or words in the case studies with each of the following meanings:

18. pertaining to the first part of the small intestine _____

19. pertaining to the membrane that supports the intestine _____

20. localized _____

21. fluid that escapes from blood vessels as a result of inflammation _____

22. hidden or microscopic blood _____

23. jaundice _____

24. drug that treats nausea and vomiting _____

25. presence of stones in the gallbladder _____

26. endoscopic surgery of the gallbladder _____

27. inflammation of the gallbladder _____

28. radiographic study of the gallbladder and biliary system _____

29. ring of muscle that regulates the distal opening of the colon _____

30. surgical excision of tissue for pathology examination _____

Digestion

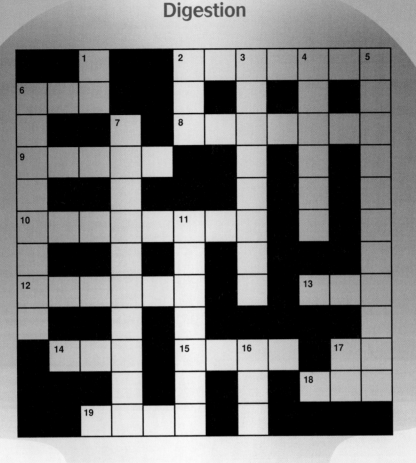

ACROSS

2. Pertaining to the jaw
6. Major portion of the large intestine: root
8. Mouth: combining form
9. Tooth: combining form
10. Small appendage to the cecum
12. Stomach: combining form
13. Inflammatory condition of the bowel (abbreviation)
14. Parenteral hyperalimentation (abbreviation)
15. Technique for viewing the accessory ducts (abbreviation)
17. Two, twice: prefix
18. Blind pouch at the beginning of the large intestine: root
19. Last portion of the small intestine: combining form

DOWN

1. 1/1000 of 1 liter (abbreviation)
2. Results in flatulence
3. Loss of appetite
4. Pertaining to the opening in the diaphragm that the esophagus passes through
5. Pertaining to the gallbladder
6. Bile duct: root
7. Enteric
11. First portion of the small intestine: combining form
16. Duct that carries bile into the intestine (abbreviation)
17. Down, without, removal: prefix

CHAPTER THIRTEEN

THE URINARY SYSTEM

CHAPTER CONTENTS

OBJECTIVES

After study of this chapter you should be able to:

1. Label a diagram of the urinary tract and follow the flow of urine through the body.
2. Label diagrams of the kidney and the urinary bladder.
3. Identify the portions of the nephron, and explain how each functions in urine formation.
4. Explain the relationship between the kidney and the blood circulation.
5. Identify and use the roots pertaining to the urinary system.
6. Describe the major disorders of the urinary system.
7. Define medical terms commonly used in reference to the urinary system.
8. Interpret abbreviations used in reference to the urinary system.
9. Analyze several case studies pertaining to urinary disorders.

PRETEST

1. The organs that form urine are the

   _____.

2. The tube that carries urine out of the body is the

   _____.

3. The hormone erythropoietin stimulates

   production of _____.

4. Micturition is the scientific term for

   _____.

5. With reference to the urinary system, the root

   cyst/o means _____.

6. Glomerulonephritis is inflammation of the

   _____.

7. Separation of substances by passage through a

   membrane is termed _____.

*T*he urinary system excretes metabolic waste. In forming and eliminating urine, it also regulates the composition, volume, and acid–base balance (pH) of body fluids. The system is thus of critical importance in maintaining homeostasis, the state of internal balance. As shown in Figure 13-1, the urinary system consists of:

> Two kidneys, the organs that form urine
> Two ureters, which transport urine from the kidneys to the bladder
> The urinary bladder, which stores and eliminates urine
> The urethra, which carries urine out of the body

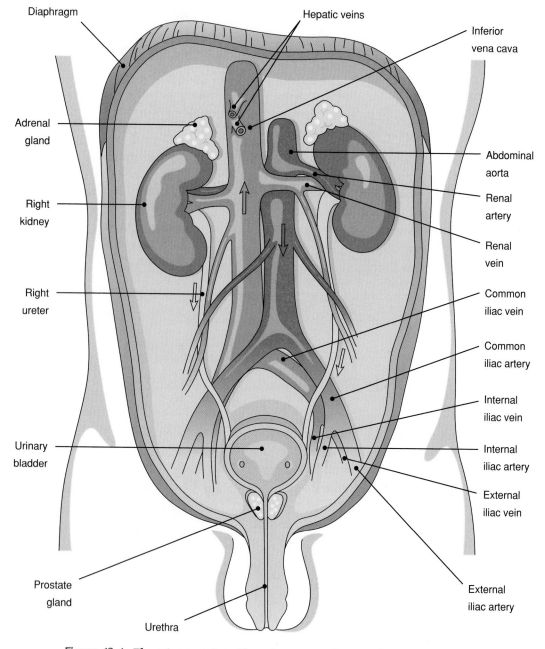

Figure 13-1 The urinary system. The male system is shown, with associated and nearby blood vessels.

The Kidneys

The kidneys are the organs that form urine from substances filtered out of the blood. In addition to metabolic wastes, urine contains water and ions, so its formation is important in regulating the blood's volume and composition. In addition, the kidneys produce two substances that act on the circulatory system:

➤ **Erythropoietin (EPO)**, a hormone that stimulates red-blood-cell production in the bone marrow
➤ **Renin**, an enzyme that functions to raise blood pressure. It does so by activating a blood component called **angiotensin**, which causes constriction of the blood vessels. The drugs known as ACE inhibitors (angiotensin-converting-enzyme inhibitors) lower blood pressure by interfering with the production of angiotensin.

Location and Structure of the Kidneys

The **kidneys** are located behind the peritoneum in the lumbar region. On the top of each kidney rests an adrenal gland. The kidney is encased in a capsule of fibrous connective tissue overlaid with fat. An outermost layer of connective tissue supports the kidney and anchors it to the body wall.

If you look inside the kidney (Fig. 13-2), you will see that it has an outer region, the **renal cortex**, and an inner region, the **renal medulla** (See Box 13-1). The medulla is divided into triangular sections, the **renal pyramids**. These pyramids have a lined appearance because they are made up of the loops and collecting tubules of the nephrons, the kidney's functional units. Each collecting tubule empties into a urine-collecting area called a **calyx** (from the Latin word meaning "cup"). Several of the smaller minor calices merge to form a major calyx. The major calices then unite to form the **renal pelvis**, the upper funnel-shaped portion of the ureter.

The Nephrons

The tiny working units of the kidneys are the **nephrons** (Fig. 13-3). These microscopic structures are basically a single tubule coiled and folded into various shapes. At the beginning of the tubule is the cup-shaped **glomerular** (Bowman) **capsule**, which is part of the nephron's blood-filtering device. The tubule then folds into the proximal convoluted

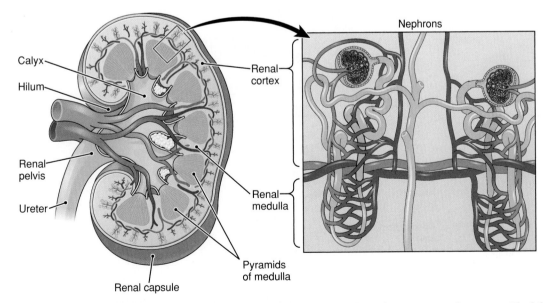

Figure 13-2 The kidney. (*Left*) A longitudinal section through the kidney shows its internal structure. The hilum is the point where blood vessels and ducts connect with the kidney. (*Right*) An enlarged diagram of nephrons. Each kidney contains more than 1 million nephrons.

Box 13•1 Focus on Words — *Words That Serve Double Duty*

Some words appear in more than one body system to represent different structures. The medulla of the kidney is the inner portion of the organ. Other organs, such as the adrenal gland, ovary, and lymph nodes, may also be divided into a central medulla and outer cortex. But *medulla* means "marrow," and this term is also applied to the bone marrow, to the spinal cord, and to the part of the brain that connects with the spinal cord, the medulla oblongata.

A ventricle is a chamber. There are ventricles in the brain and in the heart. The word *fundus* means the back part or base of an organ. The uterus has a fundus, the upper rounded portion farthest from the cervix, as does the stomach. The fundus of the eye, examined for signs of diabetes and glaucoma, is the innermost layer, where the retina is located. A macula is a spot. There is a macula in the eye, which is the point of sharpest vision. There is also a macula in the ear, which contains receptors for equilibrium.

In interpreting medical terminology, it is often important to know the context in which a word is used.

tubule, straightens out to form the loop of Henle, coils again into the distal convoluted tubule, and then finally straightens out to form a collecting duct.

Blood Supply to the Kidney

Blood enters the kidney through a renal artery, a short branch of the abdominal aorta. This vessel subdivides into smaller vessels as it branches throughout the kidney tissue,

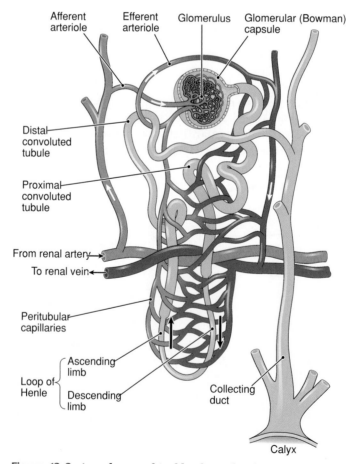

Figure 13-3 A nephron and its blood supply. The nephron regulates the proportion of water, waste, and other materials in urine according to the body's constantly changing needs. A nephron consists of a glomerular capsule, convoluted tubules, the loop of Henle, and a collecting duct. Blood filtration occurs through the glomerulus in the glomerular capsule. Materials that enter the nephron can be returned to the blood through the surrounding peritubular capillaries.

until finally blood is brought into the glomerular (Bowman) capsule and circulated through a cluster of capillaries, called a **glomerulus**, within the capsule.

Blood leaves the kidney by a series of vessels that finally merge to form the renal vein, which empties into the inferior vena cava.

Urine Formation

As blood flows through the glomerulus, blood pressure forces materials through the glomerular wall and through the wall of the glomerular capsule into the nephron. The fluid that enters the nephron, the **glomerular filtrate**, consists mainly of water, electrolytes, soluble wastes, nutrients, and toxins. The main waste material is **urea**, the nitrogenous (nitrogen-containing) by-product of protein metabolism. The filtrate should not contain any cells or proteins, such as albumin.

The waste material and the toxins must be eliminated, but most of the water, electrolytes, and nutrients must be returned to the blood or we would rapidly starve and dehydrate. This return process, termed **tubular reabsorption**, occurs through the peritubular capillaries that surround the nephron.

As the filtrate flows through the nephron, other processes further regulate its composition and pH. The concentration of the filtrate is also adjusted under the effects of the pituitary hormone **antidiuretic hormone (ADH)**. Finally, the filtrate, now called **urine**, flows into the collecting tubules to be eliminated.

Transport and Removal of Urine

Urine is drained from the renal pelvis and carried by the **ureter** on the left and right sides to the **urinary bladder** (Fig. 13-4), where it is stored. The bladder expands upward as it fills, leaving a triangle at its base unstretched. This triangle, the **trigone**, is marked by the ureteral openings and the urethral opening below (see Fig. 13-4). The trigone's stability prevents urine from refluxing back up into the ureters.

Fullness stimulates a reflex contraction of the bladder muscle and expulsion of urine through the **urethra**. The female urethra is short (4 cm [1.5 in.]) and carries only urine. The male urethra is longer (20 cm [8 in.]) and carries both urine and semen.

The voiding (release) of urine, technically called **micturition** or **urination**, is regulated by two sphincters (circular muscles) that surround the urethra. The superior muscle, the internal urethral sphincter, is around the entrance to the urethra and functions involuntarily; the inferior muscle, the external urethral sphincter, is under conscious control.

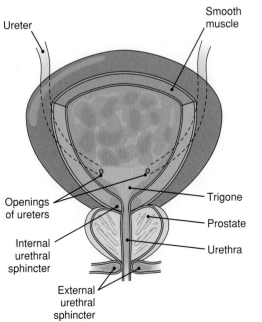

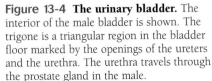

Figure 13-4 The urinary bladder. The interior of the male bladder is shown. The trigone is a triangular region in the bladder floor marked by the openings of the ureters and the urethra. The urethra travels through the prostate gland in the male.

TERMINOLOGY   Key Terms

NORMAL STRUCTURE AND FUNCTION

antidiuretic hormone (ADH)
an-ti-dī-ū-RET-ik

A hormone released from the pituitary gland that causes water reabsorption in the kidneys, thus concentrating the urine

angiotensin
an-jē-ō-TEN-sin

A substance that increases blood pressure; activated in the blood by renin, an enzyme produced by the kidneys

calyx
KĀ-liks

A cuplike cavity in the pelvis of the kidney; also calix (plural: calices) (root: *cali, calic*)

erythropoietin (EPO)
e-rith-rō-POY-e-tin

A hormone produced by the kidneys that stimulates red-blood-cell production in the bone marrow

glomerular capsule
glō-MER-ū-lar KAP-sūl

The cup-shaped structure at the beginning of the nephron that surrounds the glomerulus and receives material filtered out of the blood; Bowman (*BŌ-man*) capsule

glomerular filtrate
glō-MER-ū-lar FIL-trāt

The fluid and dissolved materials that filter out of the blood and enter the nephron through the glomerular capsule

glomerulus
glō-MER-ū-lus

The cluster of capillaries within the glomerular capsule (plural: glomeruli) (root: *glomerul/o*)

kidney
KID-nē

An organ of excretion (root: *ren/o, nephr/o*); the two kidneys filter the blood and form urine, which contains metabolic waste products and other substances as needed to regulate the water and electrolyte balance and the pH of body fluids

micturition
mik-tū-RISH-un

The voiding of urine; urination

nephron
NEF-ron

A microscopic functional unit of the kidney; working with blood vessels, the nephron filters the blood and balances the composition of urine

renal cortex
RĒ-nal KOR-tex

The outer portion of the kidney; contains portions of the nephrons

renal medulla
me-DUL-la

The inner portion of the kidney; contains portions of the nephrons and ducts that transport urine toward the renal pelvis

renal pelvis
PEL-vis

The expanded upper end of the ureter that receives urine from the kidney; Greek root *pyel/o* means "basin"

renal pyramid
PIR-a-mid

A triangular structure in the medulla of the kidney; composed of the loops and collecting ducts of the nephrons

renin
RĒ-nin

An enzyme produced by the kidneys that activates angiotensin in the blood

trigone
TRĪ-gōn

A triangle at the base of the bladder formed by the openings of the two ureters and the urethra (see Fig. 13-4)

tubular reabsorption
TŪB-ū-lar rē-ab-SORP-shun

The return of substances from the glomerular filtrate to the blood through the peritubular capillaries

urea
ū-RĒ-a

The main nitrogenous (nitrogen-containing) waste product in the urine

TERMINOLOGY Key Terms

Continued

ureter Ū-rē-ter	The tube that carries urine from the kidney to the bladder (root: *ureter/o*)
urethra ū-RĒ-thra	The tube that carries urine from the bladder to the outside of the body (root: *urethr/o*)
urinary bladder ū-ri-NAR-ē BLAD-der	The organ that stores and eliminates urine excreted by the kidneys (root: *cyst/o, vesic/o*)
urination ū-ri-NĀ-shun	The voiding of urine; micturition
urine Ū-rin	The fluid excreted by the kidneys. It consists of water, electrolytes, urea, other metabolic wastes, and pigments. A variety of other substances may appear in urine in cases of disease (root: *ur/o*).

Go to the pronunciation glossary in Chapter 13 on the CD-ROM to hear these words pronounced.

Roots Pertaining to the Urinary System

Table 13•1	Roots for the Kidney		
ROOT	**MEANING**	**EXAMPLE**	**DEFINITION OF EXAMPLE**
ren/o	kidney	prerenal prē-RĒ-nal	before or in front of the kidney
nephr/o	kidney	nephrosis nef-RŌ-sis	any noninflammatory disease condition of the kidney
glomerul/o	glomerulus	juxtaglomerular juks-ta-glō-MER-ū-lar	near the glomerulus
pyel/o	renal pelvis	pyelectasis pī-e-LEK-ta-sis	dilatation of the renal pelvis
cali/o, calic/o	calyx	calicectomy kal-i-SEK-tō-mē	excision of a renal calyx

Exercise 13-1

Use the root ren/o to write a word for the following:

1. behind (post-) the kidney   _____ postrenal _____

2. within (intra-) the kidney   _____

3. above (supra-) the kidney   _____

4. around the kidneys   _____

Use the root nephr/o to write a word for the following:

5. surgical removal of the kidney   _____

6. study of the kidney   _____

7. softening of the kidney   _____

8. poisonous or toxic to the kidney   _____

9. any disease of the kidney   _____

Use the appropriate root to write a word for the following:

10. inflammation of a glomerulus   _____

11. dilatation of a renal calyx   _____

12. radiograph of the renal pelvis   _____

13. plastic repair of the renal pelvis   _____

14. radiographic study (-graphy) of the   _____

15. hardening of a glomerulus   _____

16. inflammation of the renal pelvis and kidney   _____

Table 13·2   Roots for the Urinary Tract (Except the Kidney)

ROOT	MEANING	EXAMPLE	DEFINITION OF EXAMPLE
ur/o	urine, urinary tract	urosepsis ū-rō-SEP-sis	generalized infection that originates in the urinary tract
urin/o	urine	nocturia nok-TŪ-rē-a	urination during the night (noct/i)
ureter/o	ureter	ureterostenosis ū-rē-ter-ō-ste-NŌ-sis	narrowing of the ureter
cyst/o	urinary bladder	cystocele SIS-tō-sel	hernia of the bladder
vesic/o	urinary bladder	supravesical sū-pra-VES-i-kal	superior to the urinary bladder
urethr/o	urethra	urethrotome ū-RĒ-thrō-tōm	instrument for incising the urethra

Exercise 13-2

*Use the root **ur/o** to write a word for the following:*

1. study of the urinary tract   _____

2. radiography of the urinary tract   _____

3. a urinary calculus (stone)   _____

4. presence of urinary waste products in the blood (-emia)   _____

*The root **ur/o-** is used in the suffix **-uria**, which means "condition of urine or of urination." Use **-uria** to write a word for the following:*

5. lack of urine   _____anuria_____

6. painful or difficult urination   _____

7. formation of excess (poly-) urine   _____

8. presence of cells in the urine   _____

9. presence of blood (hemat/o) in the urine   _____

*The suffix **-uresis** means "urination." Use **-uresis** to write a word for the following:*

10. increased excretion of urine   _____diuresis_____

11. lack of urination   _____

12. excretion of sodium (natri-) in the urine   _____

13. excretion of potassium (kali-) in the urine   _____

*The adjective ending for the above words is **-uretic**, as in **diuretic** (pertaining to diuresis) and **natriuretic** (pertaining to the excretion of sodium in the urine).*

Use the appropriate root to write a word for the following:

14. endoscopic examination of the urethra   _____

15. a ureteral calculus   _____

16. surgical creation of an opening in the ureter   _____

17. surgical fixation of the urethra   _____

*Use the root **cyst/o** to write a word for the following:*

18. inflammation of the urinary bladder   _____

19. surgical fixation of the urinary bladder   _____

20. an instrument for examining the inside of the bladder   _____

21. incision of the bladder   _____

*Use the root **vesic/o** to write a word for the following:*

22. within (intra-) the bladder   _____

23. pertaining to the urethra and bladder   _____

Define the following terms:

24. transurethral (*trans-ū-RĒ-thral*) _____

25. ureterotomy (*ū-rē-ter-OT-ō-mē*) _____

26. cystalgia (*sis-TAL-jē-a*) _____

27. uropoiesis (*ū-rō-poy-Ē-sis*) _____

Clinical Aspects of the Urinary System

Infections

Organisms that infect the urinary tract generally enter through the urethra and ascend toward the bladder, producing **cystitis**. Untreated, the infection can ascend even further into the urinary tract. The infecting organisms are usually colon bacteria carried in feces, particularly *Escherichia coli*. Although urinary tract infections (UTIs) do occur in men, they appear more commonly in women because the female urethra is shorter than the male urethra and the opening is closer to the anus. Poor toilet habits and **urinary stasis** are contributing factors. In the hospital, UTIs may result from procedures involving the urinary system, especially **catheterization**, in which a tube is inserted into the bladder to withdraw urine (Fig. 13-5). Less frequently, UTIs originate in the blood and descend through the urinary system.

An infection that involves the kidney and renal pelvis is termed **pyelonephritis**. As in cystitis, signs of this condition include **dysuria**, painful or difficult urination, and the presence of bacteria and pus in the urine, **bacteriuria** and **pyuria**, respectively.

Urethritis is inflammation of the urethra, generally associated with sexually transmitted infections such as gonorrhea and chlamydial infections (see Chapter 14).

Glomerulonephritis

Although the name simply means inflammation of the glomeruli and kidney, **glomerulonephritis** is a specific disorder that follows an immunologic reaction. It is usually a response to infection in another system, commonly a streptococcal infection of the respiratory tract or a skin infection. It may also accompany autoimmune diseases such as lupus erythematosus. The symptoms are hypertension, edema, and **oliguria**, the passage of small amounts of urine. This urine is highly concentrated. Because of damage to kidney tissue, blood and proteins escape into the nephrons, causing **hematuria**, blood in the urine, and **proteinuria**, protein in the urine. Blood cells may also form into small molds of the kidney tubule, called **casts**, which can be found in the urine.

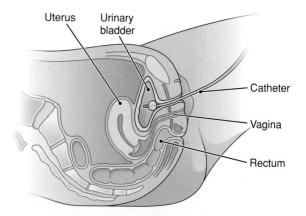

Figure 13-5 An indwelling (Foley) catheter. The catheter is shown in place in the female bladder.

Most patients recover fully from glomerulonephritis, but in some cases, especially among the elderly, the disorder may lead to chronic renal failure (CRF) or end-stage renal disease (ESRD). In such cases, urea and other nitrogen-containing compounds accumulate in the blood, a condition termed **uremia**. These compounds affect the central nervous system, causing irritability, loss of appetite, stupor, and other symptoms. There is also electrolyte imbalance and **acidosis**.

Nephrotic Syndrome

Glomerulonephritis is one cause of **nephrotic syndrome**, a disease in which the glomeruli become overly permeable and allow the loss of proteins. Other possible causes of nephrotic syndrome are renal vein thrombosis, diabetes, systemic lupus erythematosus, toxins, or any other condition that damages the glomeruli.

Nephrotic syndrome is marked by proteinuria and **hypoproteinemia**, low blood protein. The low plasma protein level affects capillary exchange and results in edema. There is also an increase in blood lipids, as the liver compensates for lost protein by releasing lipoproteins.

Acute Renal Failure

Injury, shock, exposure to toxins, infections, and other renal disorders may cause damage to the nephrons, resulting in acute renal failure (ARF). There is rapid loss of kidney function with oliguria and accumulation of nitrogenous wastes in the blood. Failure of the kidneys to eliminate potassium leads to **hyperkalemia**, along with other electrolyte imbalances and acidosis (see Box 13-2). When destruction (necrosis) of kidney tubules is involved, the condition may be referred to as acute tubular necrosis (ATN).

Renal failure may lead to a need for kidney **dialysis** or, ultimately, **renal transplantation**. Dialysis refers to the movement of substances across a semipermeable membrane; it is a method used for removing harmful or unnecessary substances from the body when the kidneys are impaired or have been removed (Fig. 13-6). Two approaches are used:

> ➤ In **hemodialysis**, blood is cleansed by passage over a membrane surrounded by fluid (dialysate) that draws out unwanted substances. Most people on hemodialysis are treated for 4 hours 3 times a week in a dialysis center. Some patients are able to use simpler machines at home for daily dialysis. Box 13-3 has information on careers in hemodialysis treatment.

Box 13•2 Clinical Perspectives — *Sodium and Potassium: Causes and Consequences of Imbalance*

The concentrations of sodium and potassium in body fluids are important measures of water and electrolyte balance. An excess of sodium in body fluids is termed **hypernatremia**, taken from the Latin name for sodium, *natrium*. This condition accompanies dehydration and severe vomiting and may cause hypertension, edema, convulsions, and coma. **Hyponatremia**, a deficiency of sodium in body fluids, can come from water intoxication (overhydration), heart failure, kidney failure, cirrhosis of the liver, pH imbalance, or endocrine disorders. It can cause muscle weakness, hypotension, confusion, shock, convulsions, and coma.

The term **hyperkalemia** is taken from the Latin name for potassium, *kalium*. It refers to excess potassium in body fluids, which may result from kidney failure, dehydration, and other causes. Its signs and symptoms include nausea, vomiting, muscular weakness, and severe cardiac arrhythmias. **Hypokalemia**, or low potassium in body fluids, may result from taking diuretics, which cause potassium to be lost along with water. It may also result from pH imbalance or secretion of too much aldosterone from the adrenal cortex, resulting in potassium excretion. Hypokalemia causes muscle fatigue, paralysis, confusion, hypoventilation, and cardiac arrhythmias.

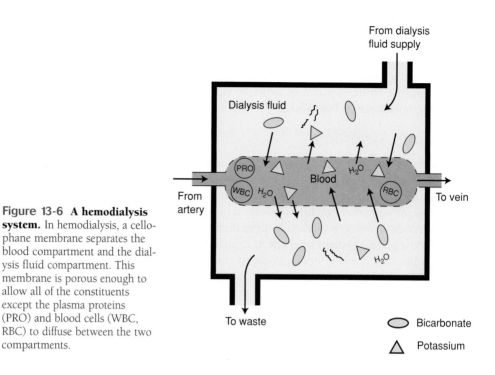

Figure 13-6 A hemodialysis system. In hemodialysis, a cellophane membrane separates the blood compartment and the dialysis fluid compartment. This membrane is porous enough to allow all of the constituents except the plasma proteins (PRO) and blood cells (WBC, RBC) to diffuse between the two compartments.

> ➤ In **peritoneal dialysis**, fluid is introduced into the peritoneal cavity. The fluid, along with waste products, is periodically withdrawn and replaced (Fig. 13-7). Fluid may be exchanged at intervals throughout the day in continuous ambulatory peritoneal dialysis (CAPD) or during the night in continuous cyclic peritoneal dialysis (CCPD).

Urinary Stones

Urinary lithiasis (condition of having stones) may be related to infection, irritation, diet, or hormone imbalances that lead to an increased level of calcium in the blood. Most urinary calculi (stones) are made up of calcium salts, but they may be composed of other materials as well. Causes of stone formation include dehydration, infection, abnormal pH

Box 13•3 **Health Professions**   *Hemodialysis Technician*

A hemodialysis technician, also called a renal technician or a nephrology technician, specializes in the safe and effective delivery of renal dialysis therapy to patients suffering from kidney failure. Before treatment begins, the technician prepares the dialysis solutions and ensures that the dialysis machine is clean, sterile, and in proper working order. The technician measures and records the patient's weight, temperature, and vital signs, inserts a catheter into the patient's arm, and connects the dialysis machine to it. During dialysis, the technician monitors the patient for adverse reactions and guards against any equipment malfunction. After the treatment is completed, the technician again measures and records the patient's

weight, temperature, and vital signs. To perform these duties, hemodialysis technicians need a thorough understanding of anatomy and physiology. Most technicians in the United States receive their training from a college or technical school, and many states require that the technician be certified.

Hemodialysis technicians work in a variety of settings, such as hospitals, clinics, and patients' homes. As populations age, the incidence of kidney disease is expected to rise, as will the need for hemodialysis. The National Association of Nephrology Technicians has more information on this career.

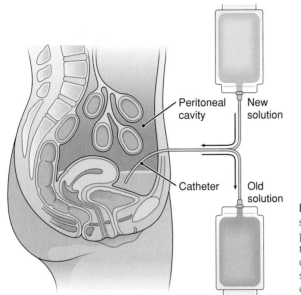

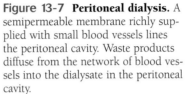

Figure 13-7 Peritoneal dialysis. A semipermeable membrane richly supplied with small blood vessels lines the peritoneal cavity. Waste products diffuse from the network of blood vessels into the dialysate in the peritoneal cavity.

13

of urine, urinary stasis, and metabolic imbalances. The stones generally form in the kidney and may move to the bladder (Fig. 13-8). This results in great pain, termed **renal colic**, and obstruction that can promote infection and cause **hydronephrosis** (collection of urine in the renal pelvis) (Fig. 13-9).

Because they are radiopaque, stones can usually be seen on simple radiographs of the abdomen. Stones may dissolve and pass out of the body on their own. If not, they may be removed surgically, in a **lithotomy**, or by using an endoscope. External shock waves are used to crush stones in the urinary tract in a procedure called extracorporeal (outside the body) shock-wave **lithotripsy** (crushing of stones).

Cancer

Carcinoma of the bladder has been linked to occupational exposure to chemicals, parasitic infections, and cigarette smoking. A key symptom is sudden, painless hematuria.

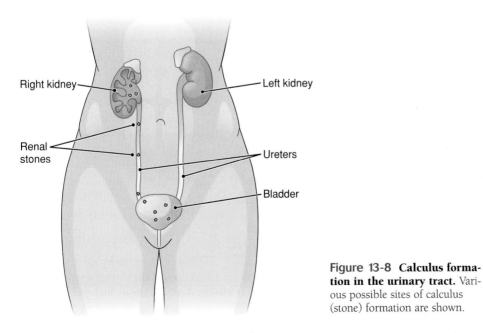

Figure 13-8 Calculus formation in the urinary tract. Various possible sites of calculus (stone) formation are shown.

13

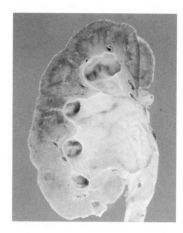

Figure 13-9 Hydronephrosis. Urinary tract obstruction has led to dilation of the ureters, pelves, and calices.

Often the cancer can be seen by viewing the lining of the bladder with a **cystoscope** (Fig. 13-10). This instrument can also be used to biopsy tissue for study.

If treatment is not effective in permanently removing the tumor, a **cystectomy** (removal of the bladder) may be necessary. In this case, the ureters must be vented elsewhere, such as directly to the surface of the body through the ileum in an **ileal conduit** (Fig. 13-11), or to some other portion of the intestine.

Cancer may also involve the kidney and renal pelvis. Additional means for diagnosing cancer and other disorders of the urinary tract include ultrasound, computed tomography scans, and radiographic studies such as **intravenous urography** (Fig. 13-12), also called **intravenous pyelography**, and **retrograde pyelography**.

Urinalysis

Urinalysis (UA) is a simple and widely used method for diagnosing urinary tract disorders. It may also reveal disturbances in other systems when abnormal by-products are eliminated in the urine. In a routine urinalysis, the urine is grossly examined for color and turbidity (a sign that bacteria are present); **specific gravity** (a measure of concentration) and pH are recorded; tests are performed for chemical components such as glucose, ketones, and hemoglobin; and the urine is examined microscopically for cells, crystals, and casts. In more detailed tests, drugs, enzymes, hormones, and other metabolites may be analyzed and bacterial cultures may be performed.

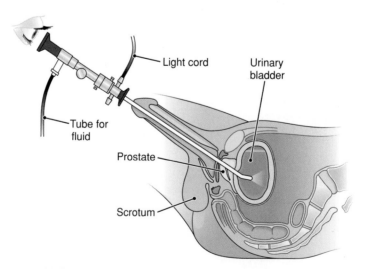

Figure 13-10 Cystoscopy. A lighted cystoscope is introduced through the urethra into the bladder of a male subject. Sterile fluid is used to inflate the bladder. Cystoscopes are used to examine the bladder, remove specimens for biopsy, and remove tumors.

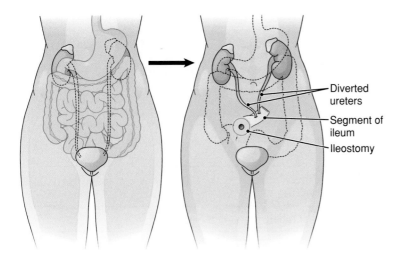

Figure 13-11 **Ileal conduit.** In this surgery, the ureters are vented to the body surface through the ileum when the bladder is removed or nonfunctional.

13

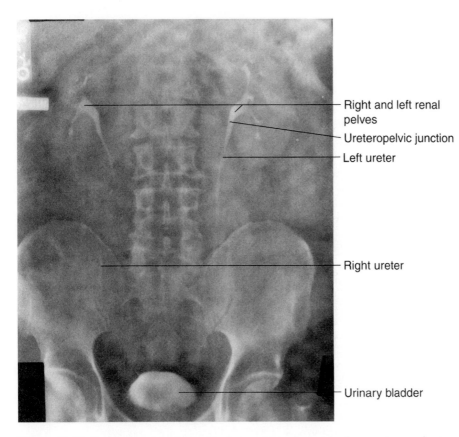

Figure 13-12 **Intravenous urogram.** The image shows the renal pelves, ureters, and urinary bladder.

TERMINOLOGY Key Terms

DISORDERS

acidosis *as-i-DŌ-sis*	Excessive acidity of body fluids
bacteriuria *bak-tē-rē-Ū-rē-a*	Presence of bacteria in the urine
cast	A solid mold of a renal tubule found in the urine
cystitis *sis-TĪ-tis*	Inflammation of the urinary bladder, usually as a result of infection
dysuria *dis-Ū-rē-a*	Painful or difficult urination
glomerulonephritis *glō-mer-ū-lō-nef-RĪ-tis*	Inflammation of the kidney primarily involving the glomeruli. The acute form usually occurs after an infection elsewhere in the body; the chronic form varies in cause and usually leads to renal failure.
hematuria *hē-mat-Ū-rē-a*	Presence of blood in the urine
hydronephrosis *hī-drō-nef-RŌ-sis*	Collection of urine in the renal pelvis caused by obstruction; causes distention and atrophy of renal tissue. Also called nephrohydrosis or nephydrosis (see Fig. 13-9)
hypokalemia *hī-pō-ka-LĒ-mē-a*	Deficiency of potassium in the blood
hyponatremia *hī-pō-na-TRĒ-mē-a*	Deficiency of sodium in the blood
hypoproteinemia *hī-pō-prō-tē-NĒ-mē-a*	Decreased amount of protein in the blood; may result from protein loss caused by kidney damage
hyperkalemia	Excess amount of potassium in the blood
hypernatremia	Excess amount of sodium in the blood
nephrotic syndrome *nef-ROT-ik*	Condition that results from glomerular damage leading to loss of protein in the urine (proteinuria). There is low plasma protein (hypoproteinemia), edema, and increased blood lipids as the liver releases lipoproteins. Also called nephrosis.
oliguria *ol-ig-Ū-rē-a*	Elimination of small amounts of urine
proteinuria *prō-tē-NŪ-rē-ā*	Presence of protein, mainly albumin, in the urine
pyelonephritis *pī-e-lō-ne-FRĪ-tis*	Inflammation of the renal pelvis and kidney, usually as a result of infection
pyuria *pī-Ū-rē-a*	Presence of pus in the urine
renal colic *KOL-ik*	Radiating pain in the region of the kidney associated with the passage of a stone

TERMINOLOGY Key Terms

Continued

uremia *ū-RĒ-mē-a*	Presence in the blood of toxic levels of nitrogen-containing substances, mainly urea, as a result of renal insufficiency
urethritis *ū-rē-THRĪ-tis*	Inflammation of the urethra, usually as a result of infection
urinary stasis *STĀ-sis*	Stoppage of urine flow; urinary stagnation

DIAGNOSIS AND TREATMENT

catheterization *kath-e-ter-i-ZĀ-shun*	Introduction of a tube into a passage, such as through the urethra into the bladder for withdrawal of urine (see Fig. 13-5)
cystoscope *SIS-tō-skōp*	An instrument for examining the inside of the urinary bladder. Also used for removing foreign objects, for surgery, and for other forms of treatment.
dialysis *dī-AL-i-sis*	Separation of substances by passage through a semipermeable membrane. Dialysis is used to rid the body of unwanted substances when the kidneys are impaired or missing. The two forms of dialysis are hemodialysis and peritoneal dialysis.
hemodialysis *hē-mō-dī-AL-i-sis*	Removal of unwanted substances from the blood by passage through a semipermeable membrane (see Fig. 13-6)
intravenous pyelography (IVP) *pī-e-LOG-ra-fē*	Intravenous urography (see Fig. 13-12)
intravenous urography (IVU) *ū-ROG-ra-fē*	Radiographic visualization of the urinary tract after intravenous administration of a contrast medium that is excreted in the urine; also called excretory urography or intravenous pyelography, although the latter is less accurate because the procedure shows more than just the renal pelvis
lithotripsy *LITH-ō-trip-sē*	Crushing of a stone
peritoneal dialysis *per-i-tō-NĒ-al dī-AL-i-sis*	Removal of unwanted substances from the body by introduction of a dialyzing fluid into the peritoneal cavity followed by removal of the fluid (see Fig. 13-7)
retrograde pyelography *RET-rō-grād pī-e-LOG-ra-fē*	Pyelography in which the contrast medium is injected into the kidneys from below, by way of the ureters
specific gravity (SG)	The weight of a substance compared with the weight of an equal volume of water. The specific gravity of normal urine ranges from 1.015 to 1.025. This value may increase or decrease in disease.
urinalysis *ū-ri-NAL-i-sis*	Laboratory study of the urine. Physical and chemical properties and microscopic appearance are included.

TERMINOLOGY Key Terms

Continued

SURGERY

cystectomy *sis-TEK-tō-mē*	Surgical removal of all or part of the urinary bladder
ileal conduit *IL-ē-al KON-dū-it*	Diversion of urine by connection of the ureters to an isolated segment of the ileum. One end of the segment is sealed, and the other drains through an opening in the abdominal wall (see Fig. 13-11). A procedure used when the bladder is removed or nonfunctional. Also called ileal bladder.
lithotomy *lith-OT-ō-mē*	Incision of an organ to remove a stone (calculus)
renal transplantation	Surgical implantation of a donor kidney into a patient

Go to the pronunciation glossary in Chapter 13 on the CD-ROM to hear these words pronounced.

TERMINOLOGY Supplementary Terms

NORMAL STRUCTURE AND FUNCTION

aldosterone *al-DOS-ter-ōn*	A hormone secreted by the adrenal gland that regulates electrolyte excretion by the kidneys
clearance	The volume of plasma that can be cleared of a substance by the kidneys per unit of time; renal plasma clearance
creatinine *krē-AT-in-in*	A nitrogen-containing by-product of muscle metabolism. An increase in blood creatinine is a sign of renal failure.
detrusor muscle *dē-TRŪ-sor*	The muscle in the bladder wall
diuresis *dī-ū-RĒ-sis*	Increased excretion of urine

TERMINOLOGY

Continued

Supplementary Terms

glomerular filtration rate (GFR)	The amount of filtrate formed per minute by the nephrons of both kidneys
maximal transport capacity (Tm)	The maximum rate at which a given substance can be transported across the renal tubule; tubular maximum
renal corpuscle *KOR-pus-l*	The glomerular capsule and the glomerulus considered as a unit; the filtration device of the kidney

SYMPTOMS AND CONDITIONS

anuresis *an-ū-RĒ-sis*	Lack of urination
anuria *an-Ū-rē-a*	Lack of urine formation
azotemia *az-ō-TĒ-mē-a*	Presence of an increased amount of nitrogenous waste, especially urea, in the blood
azoturia *az-ō-TŪ-rē-a*	Presence of an increased amount of nitrogen-containing compounds, especially urea, in the urine
cystocele *SIS-tō-sēl*	Herniation of the bladder into the vagina (see Fig. 15-11); vesicocele
dehydration *dē-hī-DRĀ-shun*	Excessive loss of body fluids
diabetes insipidus *dī-a-BĒ-tēz in-SIP-id-us*	A condition caused by inadequate production of antidiuretic hormone, resulting in excessive excretion of dilute urine and extreme thirst
enuresis *en-ū-RĒ-sis*	Involuntary urination, usually at night; bed-wetting
epispadias *ep-i-SPĀ-dē-as*	A congenital condition in which the urethra opens on the dorsal surface of the penis as a groove or cleft; anaspadias
glycosuria *glī-kō-SŪ-rē-a*	Presence of glucose in the urine, as in cases of diabetes mellitus
horseshoe kidney	A congenital union of the lower poles of the kidneys, resulting in a horseshoe-shaped organ (Fig. 13-13)
hydroureter *hī-drō-ū-RĒ-ter*	Distention of the ureter with urine caused by obstruction
hypospadias *hī-pō-SPĀ-dē-as*	A congenital condition in which the urethra opens on the undersurface of the penis or into the vagina (Fig. 13-14)
hypovolemia *hī-pō-vō-LĒ-mē-a*	A decrease in blood volume

13

TERMINOLOGY *Continued*

Supplementary Terms

incontinence *in-KON-tin-ens*	Inability to retain urine. Incontinence may originate with a neurologic disorder, trauma to the spinal cord, weakness of the pelvic muscles, urinary retention, or impaired bladder function. Term also applies to inability to retain semen or feces.
neurogenic bladder *nū-rō-JEN-ik*	Any bladder dysfunction that results from a central nervous system lesion
nocturia *nok-TŪ-rē-a*	Excessive urination at night (*noct/o* means "night")
pitting edema	Edema in which the skin, when pressed firmly with the finger, will maintain the depression produced (see Fig. 9-21)
polycystic kidney disease *pol-ē-SIS-tik*	A hereditary condition in which the kidneys are enlarged and contain many cysts (Fig. 13-15)
polydipsia *pol-ē-DIP-sē-a*	Excessive thirst
polyuria *pol-ē-Ū-rē-a*	Elimination of large amounts of urine, as in diabetes mellitus
retention of urine	Accumulation of urine in the bladder because of an inability to urinate
staghorn calculus	A kidney stone that fills the renal pelvis and calices to give a "staghorn" appearance (Fig. 13-16)
ureterocele *ū-RĒ-ter-ō-sēl*	A cystlike dilation of the ureter near its opening into the bladder. Usually results from a congenital narrowing of the ureteral opening (Fig. 13-17).
urinary frequency	A need to urinate often without an increase in average output
urinary urgency	Sudden need to urinate
water intoxication *in-tok-si-KĀ-shun*	Excess intake or retention of water with decrease in sodium concentration. May result from excess drinking, excess ADH, or replacement of a large amount of body fluid with pure water. Causes an imbalance in the cellular environment, with edema and other disturbances.
Wilms tumor	A malignant tumor of the kidney that usually appears in children before the age of 5 years

DIAGNOSIS

anion gap *AN-ī-on*	A measure of electrolyte imbalance
blood urea nitrogen (BUN)	Nitrogen in the blood in the form of urea. An increase in BUN indicates an increase in nitrogenous waste products in the blood and renal failure.
clean-catch specimen	A urine sample obtained after thorough cleansing of the urethral opening and collected in midstream to minimize the chance of contamination

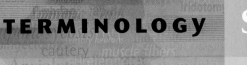

TERMINOLOGY

Continued

Supplementary Terms

cystometrography *sis-tō-me-TROG-ra-fē*	A study of bladder function in which the bladder is filled with fluid or air and the pressure exerted by the bladder muscle at varying degrees of filling is measured. The tracing recorded is a cystometrogram.
protein electrophoresis (PEP)	Laboratory study of the proteins in urine; used to diagnose multiple myeloma, systemic lupus erythematosus, and lymphoid tumor
urinometer *ū-ri-NOM-e-ter*	Device for measuring the specific gravity of urine

TREATMENT

diuretic *dī-ū-RET-ik*	A substance that increases the excretion of urine; pertaining to diuresis
indwelling Foley catheter	A urinary tract catheter with a balloon at one end that prevents the catheter from leaving the bladder (see Fig. 13-5)
lithotrite *LITH-ō-trīt*	Instrument for crushing a bladder stone

Go to the pronunciation glossary in Chapter 13 on the CD-ROM to hear these words pronounced.

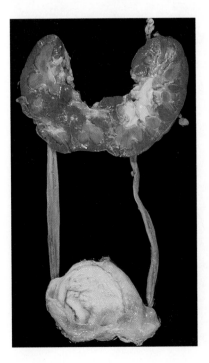

Figure 13-13 Horseshoe kidney. The photograph shows the kidneys fused at the poles.

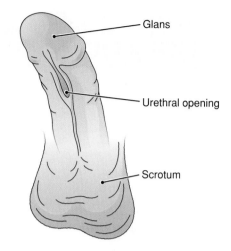

Glans

Urethral opening

Scrotum

Figure 13-14 Hypospadias. The urethra is shown opening on the ventral surface of the penis.

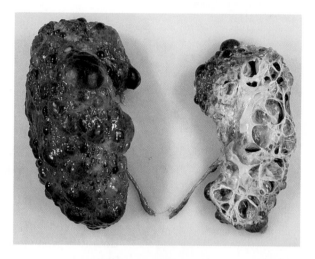

Figure 13-15 Adult polycystic disease. The kidney is enlarged and the active tissue is almost entirely replaced by cysts of varying size. (*Left*) Surface view. (*Right*) Longitudinal section.

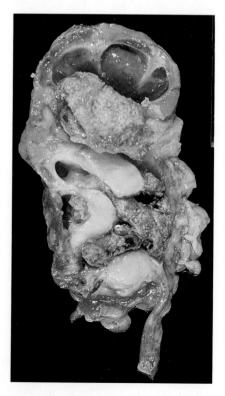

Figure 13-16 Staghorn calculus. The kidney shows hydronephrosis and stones that are casts of the dilated calices.

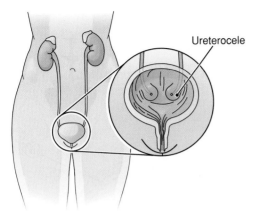

Figure 13-17 Ureterocele. The ureter bulges into the bladder. The resulting obstruction causes urine to reflux into the ureter (hydroureter) and renal pelvis (hydronephrosis).

13

TERMINOLOGY Abbreviations

ADH	Antidiuretic hormone
ARF	Acute renal failure
ATN	Acute tubular necrosis
BUN	Blood urea nitrogen
CAPD	Continuous ambulatory peritoneal dialysis
CCPD	Continuous cyclic peritoneal dialysis
CMG	Cystometrography; cystometrogram
CRF	Chronic renal failure
EPO	Erythropoietin
ESRD	End-stage renal disease
ESWL	Extracorporeal shock-wave lithotripsy
GFR	Glomerular filtration rate

GU	Genitourinary
IVP	Intravenous pyelography
IVU	Intravenous urography
K	Potassium
KUB	Kidney–ureter–bladder (radiography)
Na	Sodium
PEP	Protein electrophoresis
SG	Specific gravity
Tm	Maximal transport capacity
UA	Urinalysis
UTI	Urinary tract infection

13

CHAPTER REVIEW

LABELING EXERCISE
Urinary System

Write the name of each numbered part on the corresponding line of the answer sheet.

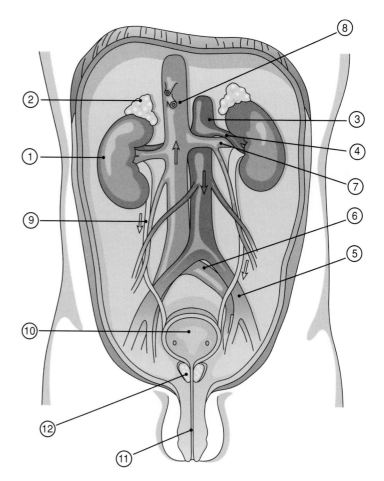

Abdominal aorta	1. _____
Adrenal gland	2. _____
Common iliac artery	3. _____
Common iliac vein	4. _____
Inferior vena cava	5. _____
Prostate gland	6. _____
Renal artery	7. _____
Renal vein	8. _____
Right kidney	9. _____

Right ureter   10. _____

Urethra   11. _____

Urinary bladder   12. _____

The Kidney

Write the name of each numbered part on the corresponding line of the answer sheet.

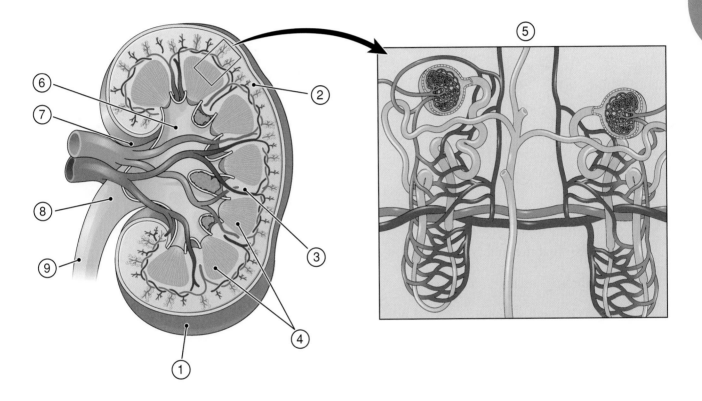

Calyx   1. _____

Hilum   2. _____

Nephrons   3. _____

Pyramids of medulla   4. _____

Renal capsule   5. _____

Renal medulla   6. _____

Renal pelvis   7. _____

Renal cortex   8. _____

Ureter   9. _____

The Urinary Bladder

Write the name of each numbered part on the corresponding line of the answer sheet.

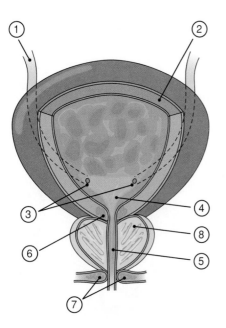

External urethral sphincter	1. _____
Internal urethral sphincter	2. _____
Openings of ureters	3. _____
Prostate	4. _____
Smooth muscle	5. _____
Trigone	6. _____
Ureter	7. _____
Urethra	8. _____

TERMINOLOGY

Match the following terms and write the appropriate letter to the left of each number:

_____	1. pyuria	**a.**	abnormal color of urine
_____	2. oliguria	**b.**	pus in the urine
_____	3. chromaturia	**c.**	elimination of small amounts of urine

_____ 4. albuminuria   d. excessive urination during the night

_____ 5. nocturia   e. proteinuria

_____ 6. uropenia   a. absence of a bladder

_____ 7. catheterization   b. stagnation, as of urine

_____ 8. stasis   c. deficiency of urine

_____ 9. acystia   d. enzyme that increases blood pressure

_____ 10. renin   e. introduction of a tube

Supplementary Terms

_____ 11. aldosterone   a. bed-wetting

_____ 12. anuresis   b. presence of glucose in the urine

_____ 13. azoturia   c. presence of nitrogenous waste in the urine

_____ 14. glycosuria   d. hormone that regulates electrolytes

_____ 15. enuresis   e. lack of urination

_____ 16. creatinine   a. excessive thirst

_____ 17. diabetes insipidus b. a nitrogenous by-product of metabolism

_____ 18. epispadias   c. inability to retain urine

_____ 19. incontinence   d. congenital misplacement of the ureteral opening

_____ 20. polydipsia   e. condition caused by lack of ADH

Fill in the blanks:

21. A microscopic working unit of the kidney is called a(n) _____.

22. The cluster of capillaries within the glomerular capsule is the _____.

23. Micturition is the scientific term for _____.

24. Laboratory study of the urine is a(n) _____.

25. The main nitrogenous waste product in urine is _____.

26. A solid mold of the renal tubule found in the urine is a(n) _____.

True-False. Examine the following statements. If the statement is true, write T in the first blank. If the statement is false, write F in the first blank and correct the statement by replacing the <u>underlined</u> word in the second blank.

27. Pyelitis is inflammation of the <u>renal pelvis</u>.   _____   _____

28. A reniform structure is shaped like the <u>bladder.</u>   _____   _____

29. The adjective *vesical* refers to the <u>bladder.</u>   _____   _____

30. The inner portion of the kidney is the <u>cortex.</u>   _____   _____

31. The tube that carries urine out of the body is the <u>ureter.</u>   _____   _____

32. EPO stimulates the production of <u>red blood cells.</u>   _____   _____

33. A lithotomy is an incision to remove a <u>calculus.</u>   _____   _____

34. Kaliuresis refers to the excretion of <u>sodium</u> in the urine.   _____   _____

Define the following words:

35. prerenal (*prē-RĒ-nal*) _____

36. dysuria (*dis-Ū-rē-a*) _____

37. nephrotropic (*nef-rō-TROP-ik*) _____

38. juxtaglomerular (*juks-ta-glō-MER-ū-lar*) _____

39. caliceal (*kal-i-SĒ-al*) (note addition of e) _____

40. urethrostenosis (*ū-rē-thrō-ste-NŌ-sis*) _____

Word building. Write a word for the following definitions:

41. any disease of the kidney (nephr/o) _____

42. radiograph of the bladder (cyst/o) and urethra _____

43. excision of the bladder (cyst/o) _____

44. softening of a kidney (nephr/o) _____

45. inflammation of the renal pelvis and the kidney _____

46. plastic repair of a ureter and renal pelvis _____

47. surgical creation of an opening between a ureter and the sigmoid colon _____

48. dilatation of the renal pelvis and calices _____

Eliminations. In each of the sets below, underline the word that does not fit in with the rest and explain the reason for your choice:

49. capsule — trigone — pyramid — nephron — cortex

_____

50. loop of Henle — distal convoluted tubule — glomerular capsule — prostate — proximal convoluted tubule

_____

51. ileal conduit — hydronephrosis — dialysis — cystoscopy — lithotripsy

_____

Opposites. Write a word that means the opposite of the following:

52. hydration _____

53. hypovolemia _____

54. diuretic _____

55. hypernatremia _____

56. uresis _____

Adjectives. Write the adjective form of the following:

57. vesica (bladder) _____

58. urology _____

59. uremia _____

60. diuresis _____

61. nephrosis _____

62. ureter _____

63. urethra _____

Plurals. Write the plural form of the following:

64. glomerulus _____

65. calyx _____

66. pelvis _____

Write the meaning of the following abbreviations:

67. IVP _____

68. ADH _____

69. EPO _____

70. IVU _____

71. Na _____

72. GFR _____

73. UA _____

Word analysis. Define the following words, and give the meaning of the word parts in each. Use a dictionary if necessary.

74. cystometrography (*sis-tō-me-TROG-ra-fē*) _____

    a. cyst/o _____

    b. metr/o _____

    c. -graphy _____

75. ureteroneocystostomy (*ū-rē-ter-ō-nē-ō-sis-TOS-tō-mē*) _____

    a. ureter/o _____

    b. neo- _____

    c. cyst/o _____

    d. -stomy _____

Go to the word exercises in Chapter 13 on the CD-ROM for additional review exercises.

13

CASE STUDY 13-1: Renal Calculi

A.A., a 48-year-old woman, was admitted to the inpatient unit from the ER with severe right flank pain unresponsive to analgesics. Her pain did not decrease with administration of 100 mg of IV meperidine. She had a 3-month history of chronic UTI. Six months ago she had been prescribed calcium supplements for low bone density. Her gynecologist warned her that calcium could be a problem for people who are "stone-formers." A.A. was unaware that she might be at risk. An IV urogram showed a right staghorn calculus. The diagnosis was further confirmed by a renal ultrasound. A renal flow scan showed normal perfusion and no obstruction. Kidney function was 37% on the right and 63% on the left. The pain became intermittent, and A.A. had no hematuria, dysuria, frequency, urgency, or nocturia. Urinalysis revealed no albumin, glucose, bacteria, or blood; there was evidence of cells, crystals, and casts.

A.A. was transferred to surgery for a cystoscopic ureteral laser lithotripsy, insertion of a right retrograde ureteral catheter, and right percutaneous nephrolithotomy. A ureteral calculus was fragmented with a pulsed-dye laser. Most of the staghorn was removed from the renal pelvis with no remaining stone in the renal calices. She was discharged 2 days later and ordered to strain her urine for the next week for evidence of stones.

CASE STUDY 13-2: End-Stage Renal Disease

M.C., a 20-year-old part-time college student, has had chronic glomerulonephritis since age 7. He has been treated at home with CAPD for the past 16 months as he awaits kidney transplantation. His doctor advised him to go immediately to the ER when he reported chest pain, shortness of breath, and oliguria. On admission, M.C. was placed on oxygen and given a panel of blood tests and an ECG to rule out an acute cardiac episode. His hemoglobin was 8.2 and his hematocrit was 26%. He had bilateral lung rales. ABGs were: pH, 7.0; $PaCO_2$, 28; PaO_2, 50; HCO_3, 21. His BUN, serum creatinine, and BUN/creatinine ratio were abnormally high. His ECG and liver enzyme studies were normal. His admission diagnosis was ESRD, fluid overload, and metabolic acidosis. He was typed and crossed for blood; tested for HIV, hepatitis B antigen, and sexually transmitted disease; and sent to hemodialysis. A bed was reserved for him on the transplant unit.

CASE STUDY 13-3: Setup for Cystoscopy

Renovations had been completed recently in the new surgical suite, and J.O., a surgical technologist, set up the two new adjoining "cysto" rooms. Each room had a new cystoscopy bed with padded knee crutches for lithotomy position, a drainage drawer for irrigation solution collection, and radiology capability. The instrument storage carts were stocked with rigid and flexible cystoscopes, sheaths with obturators, and resectoscopes with assorted fulgurating loops, connectors, guide wires, laser fibers, and fiberoptic light cords. Sterile storage closets held assorted urethral and ureteral catheters, irrigation tubing and syringes, collection bags, biopsy needles and forceps, basic soft-tissue instruments, and dressing supplies.

An electrosurgery machine was placed in each room. Cysto no. 1 had the CMG machine and urinometer. Cysto no. 2 had a Nd:YAG (neodymium:yttrium-aluminum-garnet) and a liquid tunable pulsed-dye laser machine. Each room had a machine to collect and decontaminate the liquid waste, instead of the former floor drains.

The substerile room between Cysto no. 1 and no. 2 had a steam sterilizer, a peracetic acid processor/sterilizer, and glutaraldehyde soaking pans under a ventilation hood to high-level-disinfect the instruments between cases. A warming closet contained blankets and sterile PSS, H_2O, and glycine for bladder irrigation during the procedures. J.O. wished there was room left for an ESWL system.

CASE STUDIES

CASE STUDY QUESTIONS

Multiple choice. Select the best answer and write the letter of your choice to the left of each number:

_____ 1. The term *perfusion* means:
   a. size
   b. shape
   c. passage of fluid
   d. surrounding tissue
   e. metabolism

_____ 2. M.C.'s chronic glomerulonephritis means that he has had:
   a. long-term kidney stones
   b. an acute bout of kidney infection
   c. short-term bladder inflammation
   d. a long-term kidney infection
   e. dysuria for 13 years

_____ 3. Renal dialysis can be performed by shunting venous blood through a dialysis machine and returning the blood to the patient's arterial system. This procedure is called:
   a. hemodialysis
   b. arteriovenous transplant
   c. CAPD
   d. phlebotomy
   e. glomerular filtration rate

_____ 4. A surgical endoscope that can enter and visualize the bladder is a(n) _____, whereas a scope that cuts tissue is called a(n) _____.
   a. cystoscope, resectoscope
   b. resectoscope, fulgurating loop
   c. urinometer, obturator with sheath
   d. cystoscope, scissorscope
   e. urethrascope, ureteralscope

_____ 5. A transurethral approach for examination or surgery always begins with inserting a catheter or scope:
   a. through the ureter
   b. alongside of the urethra
   c. between the ureters
   d. through the urethra
   e. below the perineum

Write a term from the case studies with the following meanings:

6. intravenous injection of contrast dye and radiographic study of the urinary tract

_____

7. production of a reduced amount of urine _____

8. getting up to go to the bathroom at night _____

9. crushing a stone in the ureter with a laser _____

10. kidney replacement _____

11. surgical incision for removal of a stone _____

13

CASE STUDIES

Abbreviations. Define the following abbreviations:

12. UTI _____

13. CAPD _____

14. BUN _____

15. ESRD _____

16. HIV _____

17. CMG _____

18. PSS _____

19. ESWL _____

13

Urinary System

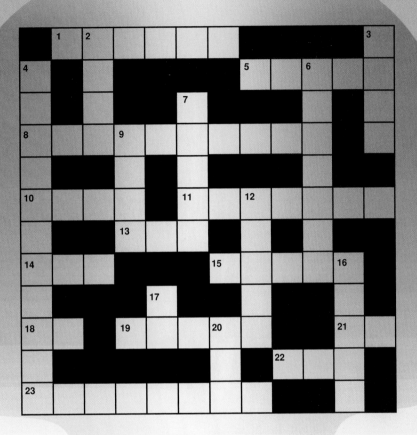

13

ACROSS

1. Tube that carries urine from the kidney to the bladder
5. Water; fluid: combining form
8. Cluster of capillaries in the glomerular capsule
10. Few; scant: prefix
11. Microscopic functional unit of the kidney
13. Drug that reduces blood pressure, _____ inhibitor
14. Hormone that stimulates red-cell production: abbreviation
15. Pertaining to the kidney
18. Measure of the weight of a substance as compared to water: abbreviation
19. Urinary bladder: combining form
21. Maximum amount of a substance that can be reabsorbed: abbreviation
22. Pituitary hormone that regulates water reabsorption: abbreviation
23. Excessive urination at night

DOWN

2. Kidney: combining form
3. Organism often involved in urinary tract infections, E. _____
4. Substance produced in response to renin that increases blood pressure
6. Painful or difficult urination
7. The fluid excreted by the kidneys
9. Large or abnormally large: prefix
12. Renal pelvis: combining form
16. Calculus (stone): combining form
17. Pus: root
20. Three: prefix

CHAPTER FOURTEEN

THE MALE REPRODUCTIVE SYSTEM

14

CHAPTER CONTENTS

OBJECTIVES

After study of this chapter you should be able to:

1. Label a diagram of the male reproductive tract and describe the function of each part.
2. Describe the contents and functions of semen.
3. Identify and use roots pertaining to the male reproductive system.
4. Describe the main disorders of the male reproductive system.
5. Interpret abbreviations used in referring to the reproductive system.
6. Analyze several case studies concerning the male reproductive system.

PRETEST

1. The male germ cell, or gamete, is the _____.

2. Gametes develop in a gonad, which in males is called the _____.

3. The main male sex hormone is _____.

4. The secretion that transports gametes in males is _____.

5. The gland below the bladder in males is the _____.

6. Protrusion of an organ or tissue through an abnormal body opening is a(n) _____.

7. Orchitis is inflammation of the _____.

T he function of the **gonads** (sex glands) in both males and females is to produce the reproductive cells, the **gametes,** and to produce hormones. The gametes are generated by **meiosis,** a process of cell division that halves the chromosome number from 46 to 23. When male and female gametes unite in fertilization, the original chromosome number is restored.

The sex hormones aid in the manufacture of the gametes, function in pregnancy and lactation, and also produce the secondary sex characteristics such as the typical size, shape, body hair, and voice that we associate with the male and female genders.

The reproductive tract develops in close association with the urinary tract. In females, the two systems become completely separate, whereas the male reproductive and urinary tracts share a common passage, the urethra. Thus, the two systems are referred to together as the genitourinary (GU) or urogenital (UG) tract, and urologists are called on to treat disorders of the male reproductive system as well as those of the urinary system.

The Testes

The male germ cells, the **spermatozoa** (sperm cells), are produced in the paired **testes** (singular: testis) that are suspended outside of the body in the **scrotum** (Fig. 14-1). Although the testes develop in the abdominal cavity, they normally descend through the **inguinal canal** into the scrotum before birth or shortly thereafter (Fig. 14-2).

From the start of sexual maturation, or **puberty**, spermatozoa form continuously within the testes in coiled seminiferous tubules (Fig. 14-3). Their development requires

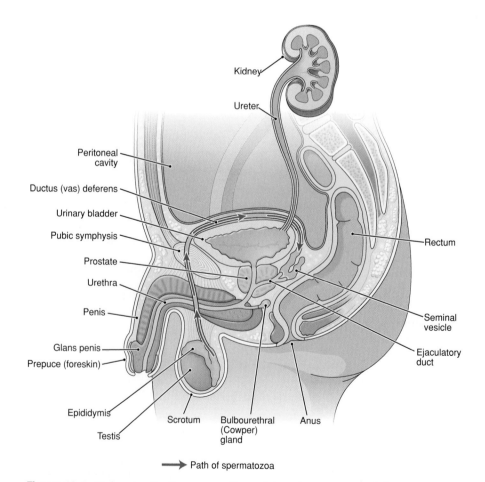

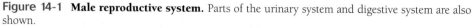

Figure 14-1 Male reproductive system. Parts of the urinary system and digestive system are also shown.

14

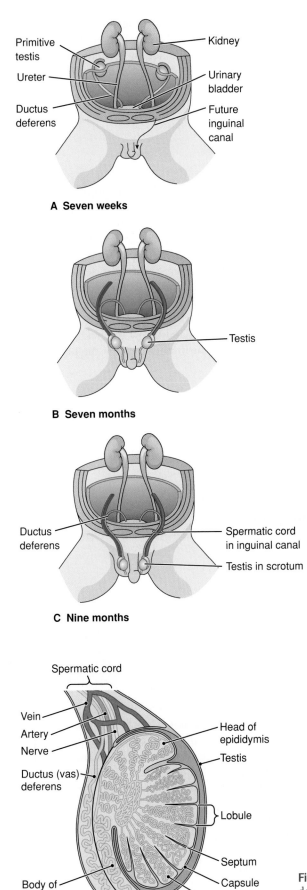

A Seven weeks

B Seven months

C Nine months

Figure 14-2 Descent of the testes. Drawings show formation of the inguinal canals and descent of the testes at three different times during fetal development. (*A*) At seven weeks, the testis is in the dorsal abdominal wall. (*B*) At seven months, the testis is passing through the inguinal canal. (*C*) At nine months, the testis is in the scrotum, suspended by the spermatic cord.

Figure 14-3 The testis. Spermatozoa develop in the seminiferous tubules in the lobules of the testis. The epididymis and spermatic cord are also shown.

the aid of special **Sertoli cells** and male sex hormones, or **androgens**, mainly **testosterone**. These hormones are manufactured in **interstitial cells** located between the tubules. In both males and females, the gonads are stimulated by **follicle-stimulating hormone (FSH)** and **luteinizing hormone (LH)**, released from the anterior **pituitary gland** beneath the brain. These hormones are chemically the same in males and females, although they are named for their actions in female reproduction.

Transport of Spermatozoa

After their manufacture, sperm cells are stored in a much-coiled tube on the surface of each testis, the **epididymis** (see Figs. 14-1 and 14-3). Here they remain until **ejaculation** propels them into a series of ducts that lead out of the body. The first of these is the **ductus (vas) deferens**, which is contained in the **spermatic cord** along with nerves and blood vessels that supply the testis (see Figs. 14-2 and 14-3). The spermatic cord ascends through the inguinal canal into the abdominal cavity, where the ductus deferens leaves the cord and travels behind the bladder. (See Box 14-1, which discusses how alternative names can be a challenge to learning medical terminology.)

A short continuation of the ductus deferens, the **ejaculatory duct**, delivers spermatozoa to the **urethra** as it passes through the prostate gland below the bladder. Finally, the cells, now mixed with other secretions, travel in the urethra through the **penis** to be released (see Fig. 14-1).

The Penis

The penile urethra transports both urine and semen. The penis is the male organ of sexual intercourse, or **coitus**. It is composed of three segments of spongy tissue, which become engorged with blood to produce an **erection**, a stiffening of the penis. As shown in Figure 14-4, the two corpora cavernosa are lateral bodies; the corpus spongiosum, through which the urethra travels, is in the center. The corpus spongiosum enlarges at the tip to form the **glans penis**, which is covered by loose skin—the **prepuce**, or foreskin. Surgery to remove the foreskin is **circumcision**. This may be performed for medical reasons, but is most often performed electively in male infants for reasons of hygiene, cultural preferences, or religion.

Box 14•1 **Focus on Words** *Which Is It?*

Some of the work of learning medical terminology is made more difficult by the fact that many structures and processes are known by two or even more names. This duplication may occur because different names have been assigned at different times or places or because the name is in a state of transition to another name and the new one has not been universally accepted.

The tube that leads from the testis to the urethra in males was originally called the vas deferens, *vas* being a general term for *vessel*. To distinguish this tube from a blood vessel, efforts have been made to change the name to ductus deferens. The original name has lingered, however,

because the surgical procedure used to sterilize a man is still called a vasectomy and not a "ductusectomy."

Similar inconsistencies appear in other systems. Dorsal is also posterior; ventral could be anterior. Human growth hormone is also called somatotropin. ADH, a hormone that increases blood pressure, is also known as vasopressin.

In the nervous system, the little swellings at the ends of axons that contain neurotransmitters are variously called end-feet, end-bulbs, terminal knobs, terminal feet, and even more. In the woman, the tube that carries the ovum from the ovary to the uterus is referred to as the oviduct, or maybe the Fallopian tube . . . or the uterine tube . . . or . . .

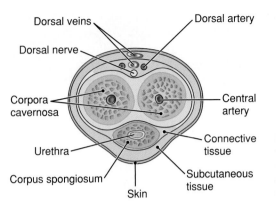

Figure 14-4 The penis. This cross section shows the erectile bodies of the penis (corpora cavernosa and corpus spongiosum), the centrally located urethra, as well as blood vessels and a nerve.

14

Formation of Semen

Semen is the thick, whitish fluid that transports spermatozoa. It contains, in addition to sperm cells, secretions from three types of accessory glands (see Fig. 14-1). Following the sequence of sperm transport, these are:

1. The paired **seminal vesicles**, which release their secretions into the ejaculatory duct on each side.
2. The **prostate gland**, which secretes into the first part of the urethra beneath the bladder. As men age, enlargement of the prostate gland may compress the urethra and cause urinary problems.
3. The two **bulbourethral** (Cowper) **glands**, which secrete into the urethra just below the prostate gland.

Together these glands produce a slightly alkaline mixture that nourishes and transports the sperm cells and also protects them by neutralizing the acidity of the female vaginal tract.

TERMINOLOGY Key Terms

NORMAL STRUCTURE AND FUNCTION

androgen *AN-drō-jen*	Any hormone that produces male characteristics; root *andr/o* means "male"
bulbourethral gland *bul-bō-ū-RĒ-thral*	A small gland beside the urethra below the prostate that secretes part of the seminal fluid. Also called Cowper gland.
circumcision *ser-kum-SI-zhun*	Surgical removal of the end of the prepuce (foreskin)
coitus *KŌ-i-tus*	Sexual intercourse
ductus deferenz *DUK-tus DEF-er-enz*	The duct that conveys spermatozoa from the epididymis to the ejaculatory duct. Also called vas deferens.

TERMINOLOGY
Key Terms

Continued

ejaculation ē-jak-ū-LĀ-shun	Ejection of semen from the male urethra
ejaculatory duct ē-JAK-ū-la-tōr-ē	The duct formed by union of the ductus deferens and the duct of the seminal vesicle; it carries spermatozoa and seminal fluid into the urethra
epididymis ep-i-DID-i-mis	A coiled tube on the surface of the testis that stores sperm until ejaculation (root: *epididym/o*)
erection ē-REK-shun	The stiffening or hardening of the penis or the clitoris, usually because of sexual excitement
follicle-stimulating hormone (FSH)	A hormone secreted by the anterior pituitary that acts on the gonads. In the male, FSH stimulates development of sperm cells.
gamete GAM-ēt	A mature reproductive cell, the spermatozoon in the male and the ovum in the female
glans penis glanz PĒ-nis	The bulbous end of the penis
gonad GŌ-nad	A sex gland; testis or ovary
inguinal canal ING-gwin-al	The channel through which the testis descends into the scrotum in the male
interstitial cells in-ter-STISH-al	Cells located between the seminiferous tubules of the testes that produce hormones, mainly testosterone. Also called cells of Leydig (LĪ-dig).
luteinizing hormone (LH) LŪ-tē-in-ī-zing	A hormone secreted by the anterior pituitary that acts on the gonads
meiosis mī-Ō-sis	The type of cell division that forms the gametes; it results in cells with 23 chromosomes, half the number found in other body cells (from the Greek word *meiosis* meaning "diminution")
penis PĒ-nis	The male organ of copulation and urination (adjective: penile)
pituitary gland pi-TŪ-i-tar-ē	An endocrine gland at the base of the brain
prepuce PRĒ-pūs	The fold of skin over the glans penis; the foreskin
prostate gland PROS-tāt	A gland that surrounds the urethra below the bladder in males and contributes secretions to the semen (root: *prostat/o*)
puberty PŪ-ber-tē	Period during which the ability for sexual reproduction is attained and secondary sex characteristics begin to develop
scrotum SKRŌ-tum	A double pouch that contains the testes (root: *osche/o*)

TERMINOLOGY   Key Terms

Continued

semen	The thick secretion that transports spermatozoa (root: *semin, sperm/i, spermat/o*)
seminal vesicle *SEM-i-nal VES-i-kl*	A saclike gland behind the bladder that contributes secretions to the semen (root: *vesicul/o*)
Sertoli cells *ser-TŌ-lē*	Cells in the seminiferous tubules that aid in the development of spermatozoa; sustentacular (*sus-ten-TAK-ū-lar*) cells
spermatic cord *sper-MAT-ik*	Cord attached to the testis that contains the ductus deferens, blood vessels, and nerves enclosed within a fibrous sheath (see Fig. 14-3)
spermatozoa *sper-ma-tō-ZŌ-a*	Mature male sex cells (singular, spermatozoon) (root: *sperm/i, spermat/o*)
testis *TES-tis*	The male reproductive gland (plural: testes; root: *test/o*); also called testicle
testosterone *tes-TOS-ter-ōn*	The main male sex hormone
urethra *ū-RĒ-thra*	The duct that carries urine out of the body and also transports semen in the male
vas deferens *DEF-er-enz*	The duct that conveys spermatozoa from the epididymis to the ejaculatory duct. Also called ductus deferens.

Go to the pronunciation glossary in Chapter 14 on the CD-ROM to hear these words pronounced.

Roots Pertaining to Male Reproduction

Table 14·1	Roots Pertaining to Male Reproduction		
ROOT	**MEANING**	**EXAMPLE**	**DEFINITION OF EXAMPLE**
test/o	testis, testicle	testosterone *tes-TOS-te-rōn*	hormone produced in the testis
orchi/o, orchid/o	testis	anorchism *an-OR-kizm*	absence of a testis
osche/o	scrotum	oscheal *OS-kē-al*	pertaining to the scrotum

Table 14·1	Continued		
semin	semen	inseminate *in-SEM-i-nāt*	to introduce semen into a vagina
sperm/i, spermat/o	semen, spermatozoa	polyspermia *pol-ē-SPER-mē-a*	secretion of excess semen
epididym/o	epididymis	epididymotomy *ep-i-did-i-MOT-ō-mē*	incision of the epididymis
vas/o	vas deferens, ductus deferens; also vessel	vasostomy *vas-OS-tō-mē*	surgical creation of an opening in the ductus deferens
vesicul/o	seminal vesicle	vesiculogram *ve-SIK-ū-lō-gram*	radiograph of a seminal vesicle
prostat/o	prostate	prostatometer *pros-ta-TOM-e-ter*	instrument for measuring the prostate

Exercise 14-1

Define the following words:

1. testopathy (*tes-TOP-a-thē*) _____

2. prostatodynia (*pros-ta-tō-DIN-ē-a*) _____

3. oscheoplasty (*os-kē-ō-PLAS-tē*) _____

4. epididymectomy (*ep-i-did-i-MEK-tō-mē*) _____

5. orchialgia (*or-kē-AL-jē-a*) _____

6. seminal (*SEM-i-nal*) _____

7. orchiepididymitis (*or-kē-ep-i-did-i-MĪ-tis*) _____

Use the root orchi/o to write a word that means the same as the following. Each is also written with the root orchid/o.

8. incision of a testis _____

9. plastic repair of a testis _____

10. surgical fixation of a testis _____

Use the root spermat/o to write a word that means the same as the following:

11. formation (-genesis) of spermatozoa _____

12. a sperm-forming cell _____

13. excessive discharge (-rhea) of semen _____

14. destruction (-lysis) of sperm _____

15. condition of having sperm in the urine (-uria) _____

The ending -spermia means "condition of sperm or semen." Add a prefix to -spermia to form a word that means the same as the following:

16. lack of semen _____

17. presence of blood in the semen _____

Exercise 14-1

18. presence of pus in the semen   _____

19. deficiency of (olig/o) semen   _____

Write a word that means the same as the following:

20. excision of the vas deferens   _____

21. inflammation of a seminal vesicle   _____

22. excision of the prostate gland   _____

23. tumor of the scrotum   _____

24. radiographic study of a seminal vesicle   _____

25. suture of the vas deferens   _____

26. inflammation of the epididymis   _____

Clinical Aspects of the Male Reproductive System

Infection

Most infections of the male reproductive tract are **sexually transmitted infections (STIs)**, listed in Box 14-2 . The most common STI in the United States is caused by the bacterium *Chlamydia trachomatis*, which mainly causes **urethritis** in males. This same organism also causes lymphogranuloma venereum, an STI associated with lymphadenopathy, which occurs most commonly in tropical regions. Both forms of these chlamydial infections respond to treatment with antibiotics.

Box 14•2 **For Your Reference** *Sexually Transmitted Infections*

Disease	Organism	Description
BACTERIAL		
chlamydial infection	*Chlamydia trachomatis* types D to K	Ascending infection of reproductive and urinary tracts. May spread to pelvis in women, causing pelvic inflammatory disease (PID).
lymphogranuloma venereum	*Chlamydia trachomatis* type L	General infection with swelling of inguinal lymph nodes; scarring of genital tissue
gonorrhea	*Neisseria gonorrhoeae;* gonococcus (GC)	Inflammation of reproductive and urinary tracts. Urethritis in men. Vaginal discharge and inflammation of the cervix (cervicitis) in women, leading to pelvic inflammatory disease (PID). Possible systemic infection. May spread to newborns. Treated with antibiotics.
bacterial vaginosis	*Gardnerella vaginalis*	Vaginal infection with foul-smelling discharge
syphilis	*Treponema pallidum* (a spirochete)	Primary stage: chancre (lesion); secondary stage: systemic infection and syphilitic warts; tertiary stage: degeneration of other systems. Cause of spontaneous abortions, stillbirths, and fetal deformities. Treated with antibiotics.

14

Box 14•2 **For Your Reference** *Continued*

VIRAL

acquired immunodeficiency syndrome (AIDS)	human immunodeficiency virus (HIV)	An often fatal disease that infects T cells of the immune system, weakening the host and leading to other diseases
genital herpes	herpes simplex virus (HSV)	Painful genital lesions. In women, may be a risk factor in cervical carcinoma. Often fatal infections of newborns. No cure at present.
hepatitis B	hepatitis B virus (HBV)	Causes liver inflammation, which may be acute or may develop into a chronic carrier state. Linked to liver cancer.
condyloma acuminatum (genital warts)	human papillomavirus (HPV)	Benign genital warts. In women, predisposes to cervical dysplasia and carcinoma.

PROTOZOAL

trichomoniasis	*Trichomonas vaginalis*	Vaginitis. Green, frothy discharge with itching; pain on intercourse (dyspareunia); and painful urination (dysuria).

Gonorrhea is caused by *Neisseria gonorrhoeae,* the gonococcus (GC). Infection usually centers in the urethra, causing urethritis with burning, a purulent discharge, and dysuria. Untreated, the disease can spread through the reproductive system. Gonorrhea is treated with antibiotics, but there has been rapid development of resistance to these drugs by gonococci.

Another common STI is herpes infection, caused by a virus. Other STIs are discussed in Chapter 15.

Mumps is a non-sexually transmitted viral disease that can infect the testes and lead to sterility. Other microorganisms can infect the reproductive tract as well, causing urethritis, **prostatitis**, **orchitis**, or **epididymitis**.

Benign Prostatic Hyperplasia

As men age, the prostate gland commonly enlarges, a condition known as **benign prostatic hyperplasia (BPH)**. Although not cancerous, this overgrown tissue can press on the urethra near the bladder and interfere with urination. Urinary retention, infection, and other complications may follow if an obstruction is not corrected.

Medications to relax smooth muscle in the prostate and bladder neck are used to treat the symptoms of BPH. Alpha-adrenergic blocking agents interfere with sympathetic nervous stimulation in these regions to improve urinary flow rate. One example is tamsulosin (Flomax). Because testosterone stimulates enlargement of the prostate, drugs that interfere with prostatic testosterone activity may slow progress of the disorder. One example is finasteride (Proscar). An herbal remedy that seems to act in this same manner is an extract of the berries of the saw palmetto, a low-growing palm tree. Saw palmetto has been found to delay the need for surgery in some cases of BPH.

In advanced cases of BPH, removal of the prostate, or **prostatectomy**, may be required. When this is performed through the urethra, the procedure is called a transurethral resection of the prostate (TURP) (Fig. 14-5A). The prostate may also be cut in a transurethral incision of the prostate (TUIP) to reduce pressure on the urethra (Fig. 14-5B). Other forms

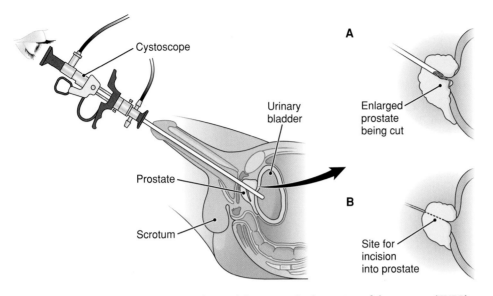

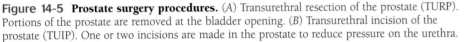

Figure 14-5 Prostate surgery procedures. (*A*) Transurethral resection of the prostate (TURP). Portions of the prostate are removed at the bladder opening. (*B*) Transurethral incision of the prostate (TUIP). One or two incisions are made in the prostate to reduce pressure on the urethra.

of energy, such as a laser beam or heat, have also been used to destroy prostatic tissue. BPH is diagnosed by digital rectal examination (DRE) or imaging studies.

Cancer

Cancer of the Prostate

Cancer of the prostate is the most common malignancy in men in the United States. Only lung cancer and colon cancer cause more cancer-related deaths in men who are past middle age. In cases of prostatic cancer, a protein produced by prostate cells increases in the blood. This prostate-specific antigen (PSA) is used, along with palpation and digital rectal examinations, to screen for prostate cancer and to assess the results of treatment.

The TNM system for staging prostate cancer includes the following categories:

> ➤ T_1: tumor not palpable by rectal examination; detected by biopsy or abnormal PSA
> ➤ T_2: tumor palpable and confined to the prostate
> ➤ T_3: tumor has spread locally beyond the prostate
> ➤ M: distant metastases

Methods of treatment include surgery (prostatectomy); radiation; inhibition of male hormones (androgens), which stimulate prostatic growth; and chemotherapy. Radiation is usually delivered by implantation of radioactive seeds. Another approach is termed "watchful waiting" or deferred therapy, which consists of monitoring without therapy. Choice of this option is based on a man's age and tumor invasiveness, and the probability that an untreated tumor will result in harm to a patient during his lifetime.

Testicular Cancer

Cancer of the testis represents less than 1% of cancer in adult males. It usually appears between the ages of 25 and 45 years and shows no sign of genetic inheritance. This cancer typically originates in germ cells and can spread to abdominal lymph nodes. More than half of testicular tumors release markers that can be detected in the blood. Treatment may include removal of the testis (orchiectomy), radiation, and chemotherapy.

Cryptorchidism

It is fairly common that one or both testes will fail to descend into the scrotum by the time of birth (Fig. 14-6). This condition is termed **cryptorchidism**, literally hidden

14

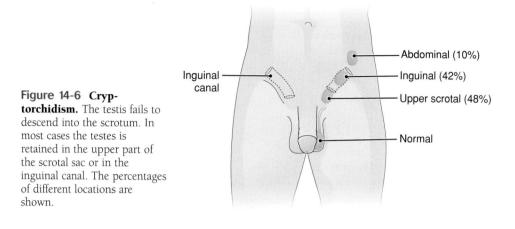

Figure 14-6 Cryptorchidism. The testis fails to descend into the scrotum. In most cases the testes is retained in the upper part of the scrotal sac or in the inguinal canal. The percentages of different locations are shown.

(crypt/o) testis (orchid/o). The condition usually corrects itself within the first year of life. If not, it must be corrected surgically to avoid sterility and an increased risk of cancer.

Infertility

An inability or a diminished ability to reproduce is termed **infertility**. Its causes may be hereditary, hormonal, disease-related, or the result of exposure to chemical or physical agents. The most common causes of infertility are STIs. A total inability to produce offspring may be termed **sterility**. Men may be voluntarily sterilized by cutting and sealing the vas deferens on both sides in a **vasectomy** (see Fig. 15-5).

Erectile Dysfunction
Erectile dysfunction, also called **impotence**, is the male lack of ability to perform intercourse because of failure to initiate or maintain an erection until ejaculation. About 10 to 20% of such cases are psychogenic—that is, caused by emotional factors, such as stress, depression, or emotional trauma. More often, erectile dysfunction has a physical cause, which may be:

> ➤ A vascular disorder, such as arteriosclerosis, varicose veins, or damage caused by diabetes
> ➤ A neurologic problem, as caused by a tumor, trauma, the effects of diabetes, or damage caused by radiation or surgery
> ➤ A side effect of a drug, such as an antihypertensive agent, anti-ulcer medication, or an appetite suppressant

Drugs that are used to treat erectile dysfunction work by dilating arteries in the penis to increase blood flow to that organ. Nondrug approaches include corrective surgery, vacuum pumps to draw blood into the penis, penile injections to dilate blood vessels, and penile prostheses. Box 14-3 has more information on erectile dysfunction.

Inguinal Hernia

The inguinal canal, through which the testis descends, may represent a weakness in the abdominal wall that can lead to a hernia. In the most common form of **inguinal hernia** (Fig. 14-7), an abdominal organ, usually the intestine, enters the inguinal canal and may extend into the scrotum. This is an indirect, or external, inguinal hernia. In a direct, or internal, inguinal hernia, the organ protrudes through the abdominal wall into the scrotum. If blood supply to the organ is cut off, the hernia is said to be *strangulated*. Surgery to correct a hernia is a **herniorrhaphy**.

Approximately 25 million American men and their partners are affected by **erectile dysfunction (ED)**, the inability to achieve an erection. Although ED is more common in men over the age of 65, it can occur at any age and can have many causes.

Erection results from an interaction between the autonomic nervous system and penile blood vessels. Sexual arousal stimulates parasympathetic nerves in the penis to release a compound called nitric oxide (NO). This substance activates an enzyme in vascular smooth muscle that promotes vasodilation, increasing blood flow into the penis and causing erection. Physical factors that cause ED prevent these physiological changes.

Drugs that target the physiologic mechanisms of erection are helping men who suffer from ED. These include sildenafil (trade name, Viagra), vardenafil (Levitra), and tadalafil (Cialis). These drugs prevent the breakdown of vasodilators, thus prolonging the effects of NO. Although effective in about 80% of ED cases, these drugs can cause some relatively minor side effects, including headache, nasal congestion, stomach upset, and blue-tinged vision. They should never be used by men who are taking nitrate drugs to treat angina. Because nitrates elevate NO levels, taking them with drugs for ED and prolonging the effects of NO can cause life-threatening hypotension. They are also contraindicated in men with low blood pressure and heart failure.

14

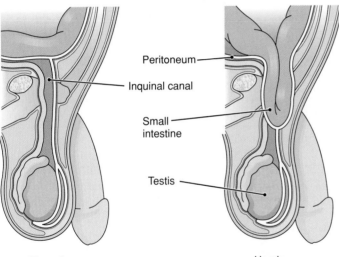

Peritoneum
Inquinal canal
Small intestine
Testis

Normal   Hernia

Figure 14-7 Inguinal hernia. Weakness in the abdominal wall allows the intestine or other abdominal contents to protrude into the inguinal canal. The hernial sac is a continuation of the peritoneum.

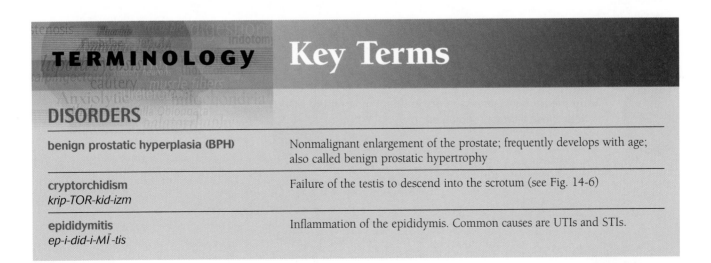

TERMINOLOGY   **Key Terms**

DISORDERS

benign prostatic hyperplasia (BPH)	Nonmalignant enlargement of the prostate; frequently develops with age; also called benign prostatic hypertrophy
cryptorchidism *krip-TOR-kid-izm*	Failure of the testis to descend into the scrotum (see Fig. 14-6)
epididymitis *ep-i-did-i-MĪ-tis*	Inflammation of the epididymis. Common causes are UTIs and STIs.

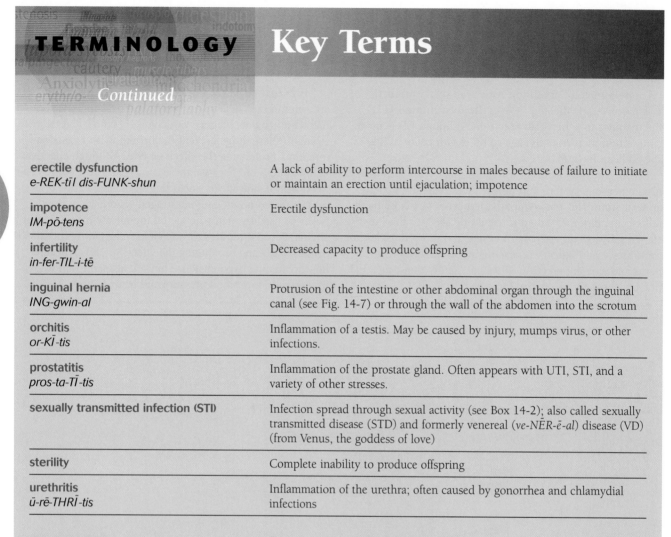

TERMINOLOGY *Continued*

Key Terms

erectile dysfunction *e-REK-tĭl dis-FUNK-shun*	A lack of ability to perform intercourse in males because of failure to initiate or maintain an erection until ejaculation; impotence
impotence *IM-pō-tens*	Erectile dysfunction
infertility *in-fer-TIL-i-tē*	Decreased capacity to produce offspring
inguinal hernia *ING-gwin-al*	Protrusion of the intestine or other abdominal organ through the inguinal canal (see Fig. 14-7) or through the wall of the abdomen into the scrotum
orchitis *or-KĪ-tis*	Inflammation of a testis. May be caused by injury, mumps virus, or other infections.
prostatitis *pros-ta-TĪ-tis*	Inflammation of the prostate gland. Often appears with UTI, STI, and a variety of other stresses.
sexually transmitted infection (STI)	Infection spread through sexual activity (see Box 14-2); also called sexually transmitted disease (STD) and formerly venereal (*ve-NĒR-ē-al*) disease (VD) (from Venus, the goddess of love)
sterility	Complete inability to produce offspring
urethritis *ū-rē-THRĪ-tis*	Inflammation of the urethra; often caused by gonorrhea and chlamydial infections

SURGERY

herniorrhaphy *her-nē-OR-a-fē*	Surgical repair of a hernia
prostatectomy *pros-ta-TEK-tō-mē*	Surgical removal of the prostate
vasectomy *va-SEK-tō-mē*	Excision of the vas deferens. Usually done bilaterally to produce sterility (see Fig. 15-5). May be accomplished through the urethra (transurethral resection).

Go to the pronunciation glossary in Chapter 14 on the CD-ROM
to hear these words pronounced.

TERMINOLOGY Supplementary Terms

NORMAL STRUCTURE AND FUNCTION

emission ē-MISH-un	The discharge of semen
genitalia jen-i-TĀL-ē-a	The organs concerned with reproduction, divided into internal and external components
insemination in-sem-i-NĀ-shun	Introduction of semen into a woman's vagina
orgasm OR-gazm	A state of physical and emotional excitement, especially that which occurs at the climax of sexual intercourse
phallus FAL-us	The penis

DISORDERS

balanitis bal-a-NĪ-tis	Inflammation of the glans penis and mucous membrane beneath it (root *balan/o* means "glans penis")
bladder neck obstruction (BNO)	Blockage of urine flow at the outlet of the bladder. The common cause is benign prostatic hyperplasia.
hydrocele HĪ-drō-sēl	The accumulation of fluid in a saclike cavity, especially within the covering of the testis or spermatic cord (Fig. 14-8)
phimosis fī-MŌ-sis	Narrowing of the opening of the prepuce so that the foreskin cannot be pushed back over the glans penis
priapism PRĪ-a-pizm	Abnormal, painful, continuous erection of the penis, as may be caused by drugs or specific damage to the spinal cord
seminoma sem-i-NŌ-ma	A tumor of the testis
spermatocele SPER-ma-tō-sēl	An epididymal cyst containing spermatozoa (see Fig. 14-8)
varicocele VAR-i-kō-sēl	Enlargement of the veins of the spermatic cord (see Fig. 14-8)

DIAGNOSIS AND TREATMENT

brachytherapy brak-ē-THER-a-pē	Radiation therapy by placement of encapsulated radiation sources, such as seeds, directly into a tumor or nearby tissue (from Greek *brachy-*, meaning "short")
castration kas-TRĀ-shun	Surgical removal of the testes or ovaries. Hormones and drugs can inhibit the gonads, to produce functional castration.

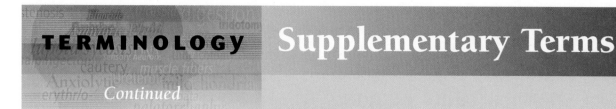

TERMINOLOGY

Supplementary Terms

Continued

Gleason tumor grade *GLĒ-son*	A system for assessing the severity of cancerous changes in the prostate; reported as a Gleason score.
Whitmore-Jewett staging *WIT-mōr-JEW-et*	A method for staging prostatic tumors; and alternate to TNM staging

Go to the pronunciation glossary in Chapter 14 on the CD-ROM to hear these words pronounced.

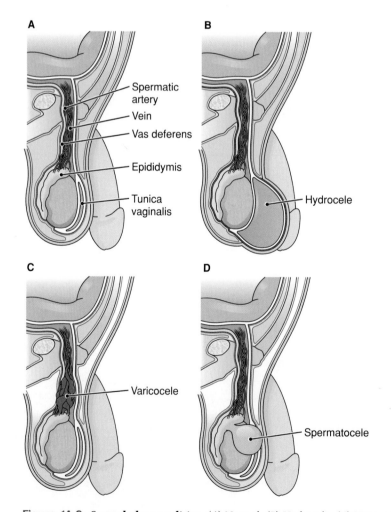

Figure 14-8 Scrotal abnormalities. (*A*) Normal. (*B*) Hydrocele. (*C*) Varicocele. (*D*) Spermatocele.

TERMINOLOGY Abbreviations

AIDS	Acquired immunodeficiency syndrome	**STD**	Sexually transmitted disease
BNO	Bladder neck obstruction	**STI**	Sexually transmitted infection
BPH	Benign prostatic hyperplasia (hypertrophy)	**TPUR**	Transperineal urethral resection
DRE	Digital rectal examination	**TSE**	Testicular self-examination
FSH	Follicle-stimulating hormone	**TUIP**	Transurethral incision of prostate
GC	Gonococcus	**TURP**	Transurethral resection of prostate
GU	Genitourinary	**UG**	Urogenital
HBV	Hepatitis B virus	**UTI**	Urinary tract infection
HIV	Human immunodeficiency virus	**VD**	Venereal disease (sexually transmitted infection)
HSV	Herpes simplex virus		
LH	Luteinizing hormone	**VDRL**	Venereal Disease Research Laboratory (test for syphilis)
NGU	Nongonococcal urethritis		
PSA	Prostate-specific antigen		

14

CHAPTER REVIEW

LABELING EXERCISE
Male Reproductive System

Write the name of each numbered part on the corresponding line of the answer sheet.

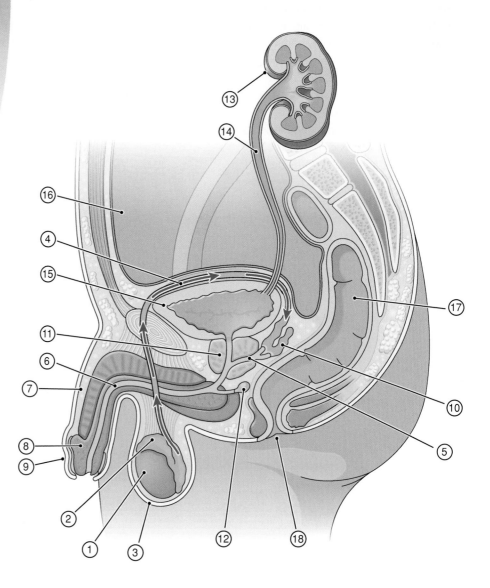

anus	1. _____
bulbourethral (Cowper) gland	2. _____
ductus (vas) deferens	3. _____
ejaculatory duct	4. _____
epididymis	5. _____
glans penis	6. _____

14

kidney   7. _____

penis   8. _____

peritoneal cavity   9. _____

prepuce (foreskin)   10. _____

prostate   11. _____

rectum   12. _____

scrotum   13. _____

seminal vesicle   14. _____

testis   15. _____

ureter   16. _____

urethra   17. _____

urinary bladder   18. _____

14

TERMINOLOGY

Match the following terms and write the appropriate letter to the left of each number:

_____ 1. gonad   **a.** a reproductive cell

_____ 2. glans   **b.** surgical removal of the foreskin

_____ 3. gamete   **c.** gland located below the bladder in males

_____ 4. circumcision   **d.** end of the penis

_____ 5. prostate   **e.** sex gland

_____ 6. meiosis   **a.** excision of the ductus deferens

_____ 7. coitus   **b.** erectile dysfunction

_____ 8. impotence   **c.** overgrowth of tissue

_____ 9. vasectomy   **d.** cell division that forms the gametes

_____ 10. hyperplasia   **e.** sexual intercourse

Supplementary Terms

_____ 11. priapism   **a.** accumulation of fluid in a saclike cavity

_____ 12. insemination   **b.** prolonged erection of the penis

_____ 13. hydrocele   **c.** tumor of the testis

_____ 14. phimosis   **d.** narrowing of the foreskin opening

_____ 15. seminoma   **e.** introduction of semen into a woman's vagina

_____ 16. castration   **a.** epididymal cyst

_____ 17. balanitis   **b.** a form of radiation treatment

_____ 18. brachytherapy   **c.** discharge of semen

_____ 19. emission   **d.** removal of the testes

_____ 20. spermatocele   **e.** inflammation of the glans penis

Fill in the blanks:

21. The male gonad is the _____.

22. The sac that holds the testis is the _____.

23. The thick fluid that transports spermatozoa is _____.

24. The main male sex hormone is _____.

25. The channel through which the testis descends is the _____.

26. The coiled tube that stores sperm cells on the surface of the testis is the _____.

True–False. Examine the following statements. If the statement is true, write T in the first blank. If the statement is false, write F in the first blank and correct the statement by replacing the underlined word in the second blank.

27. Any male sex hormone is an <u>androgen.</u>   _____   _____

28. The adjective *oscheal* refers to the <u>seminal vesicle.</u>   _____   _____

29. The spirochete *Treponema pallidum* causes <u>syphilis.</u>   _____   _____

30. Herpes simplex is a <u>virus.</u>   _____   _____

31. The <u>ureter</u> carries both urine and semen in males.   _____   _____

32. FSH and LH are produced by the <u>pituitary gland.</u>   _____   _____

Define the following terms:

33. vasorrhaphy (*vas-OR-a-fē*) _____

34. anorchism (*an-OR-kizm*) _____

35. oscheoma (*os-kē-Ō-ma*) _____

36. vesiculotomy (*ve-sik-ū-LOT-ō-mē*) _____

37. prostatometer (*pros-ta-TOM-e-ter*) _____

38. hemospermia (*hē-mō-SPER-mē-a*) _____

Word building. Write a word for the following definitions:

39. inflammation of a seminal vesicle   _____

40. surgical incision of the prostate   _____

41. stone in the scrotum   _____

42. surgical fixation of the testis   _____

43. plastic repair of the scrotum   _____

44. surgical creation of an opening between two parts of a cut ductus deferens (done to reverse a vasectomy)   _____

Eliminations. In each of the sets below, underline the word that does not fit in with the rest and explain the reason for your choice:

45. bulbourethral gland – prostate – testis – spermatic cord – seminal vesicle

_____

46. FSH – semen – testosterone – androgen – LH

_____

47. condyloma acuminatum – AIDS – hernia – trichomoniasis – herpes

_____

Adjectives. Write the adjective form of the following words:

48. semen _____

49. prostate _____

50. penis _____

51. urethra _____

52. scrotum _____

Write the meaning of the following abbreviations:

53. STI _____

54. TUIP _____

55. GC _____

56. PSA _____

57. GU _____

58. DRE _____

Word analysis. Define the following words, and give the meaning of the word parts in each. Use a dictionary if necessary.

59. cryptorchidism (*krip-TOR-kid-izm*) _____

    a. crypt- _____

    b. orchid/o _____

    c. -ism _____

60. vasovesiculitis (*vas-ō-ve-sik-ū-LĪ-tis*) _____

    a. vas/o _____

    b. vesicul/o _____

    c. -itis _____

14

Go to the word exercises in Chapter 14 on the CD-ROM for additional review exercises.

CASE STUDY 14–1: Herniorrhaphy and Vasectomy

E.D., a 48-year-old married dock worker with three children, had inguinal bulging and pain on exertion when he lifted heavy objects. An occupational health service advised a surgical referral. The surgeon diagnosed E.D. with bilateral direct inguinal hernias and suggested that he not delay surgery, although he was not at high risk for a strangulated hernia. E.D. asked the surgeon if he could also be sterilized at the same time. He was scheduled for bilateral inguinal herniorrhaphy and elective vasectomy.

During the herniorrhaphy procedure an oblique incision was made in each groin. The incision continued through the muscle layers by either resecting or splitting the muscle fibers. The spermatic vessels and vas deferens were identified, separated, and gently retracted. The spermatic cord was examined for an indirect hernia. Repair began with suturing the defect in the rectus abdominis muscles, transverse fascia, cremaster muscle, external oblique aponeurosis, and Scarpa fascia with heavy-gauge synthetic nonabsorbable suture material.

The vasectomy began with the identification of the vas deferens through the scrotal skin. An incision was made, and the vas was gently dissected and retracted through the opening. Each vas was clamped with a small hemostat, and a 1-cm length was resected. Both cut ends were coagulated with electrosurgery and tied independently with a fine-gauge absorbable suture material. The testicles were examined, and the scrotal incision was closed with an absorbable suture material.

CASE STUDY 14–2: Benign Prostatic Hyperplasia with TURP

C.S., a 62-year-old businessman, saw a urologist because of decreased force of urine stream and ejaculation, hesitancy, and sensation of incomplete bladder emptying. He stated that he had taken prostate-health herbal supplements without any real benefit for 2 years before making the appointment. He reported no dysuria, hematuria, or flank pain. He had no history of UTI, epididymitis, prostatitis, renal disease, or renal calculi. Rectal examination revealed a 50-g prostate with slight firmness in the right prostatic lobe. Bladder ultrasound showed no intravesical lesions or prostate protrusion into the bladder base. C.S. was diagnosed with benign prostatic hyperplasia with bladder neck obstruction and was scheduled for a TURP.

CASE STUDY 14–3: Circumcision

S.G., a 12-year-old Jewish Russian immigrant, was preparing for his bar mitzvah. He had not been circumcised on the eighth day after his birth, as is Jewish tradition, because he had been unable to practice his religion within the former soviet system. On recommendation of his rabbi, his family brought him to a urologist for referral and surgery. On examination, the phallus and meatus were normal and without lesions. S.G. had no signs of discharge, phimosis, or balanitis. Surgery for an adult circumcision was scheduled along with the attendance of a mohel, a Jewish ritual circumciser.

S.G. was positioned in the supine position after administration of general anesthesia. His penis and scrotum were prepped with an antimicrobial solution and draped in sterile sheets. The surgeon and mohel scrubbed in and donned sterile gowns and gloves. The mohel chanted several prayers in Hebrew before and after making the first small cut below the foreskin, enough to draw blood. The urologist completed the resection of the redundant foreskin and approximated the circumferential incisions with fine-gauge absorbable suture material. After the incision was dressed with petrolatum gauze, and S.G. recovered enough to be returned to his room, the mohel met with him and his family to continue the sacred rite with prayer and ceremonial wine.

CASE STUDY QUESTIONS

Multiple choice. Select the best answer and write the letter of your choice to the left of each number:

_____ 1. The term for male sterilization surgery is:
   a. herniorrhaphy
   b. circumcision
   c. vagotomy
   d. vasectomy
   e. vasovasotomy

_____ 2. An oblique surgical incision follows what direction?
   a. slanted or angled
   b. superior to inferior
   c. lateral
   d. circumferential
   e. elliptical

_____ 3. When the ends of the vas were coagulated with electrosurgery, they were:
   a. probed
   b. dilated
   c. sealed
   d. sutured
   e. clamped

_____ 4. A urologist is a physician who treats health and disease conditions of the:
   a. male reproductive system
   b. urinary system
   c. digestive system
   d. a and b
   e. b and c

_____ 5. A person with painful, blood-tinged, scanty urination would be described as having:
   a. hematocrit, dyspnea, and oliguria
   b. dystonia, hematuria, and oliguria
   c. dysuria, hematuria, and oliguria
   d. oliguria, hematogenesis, and dystonia
   e. dyspnea, hematuria, and polyuria

_____ 6. Another name for the foreskin is the:
   a. prepuce
   b. phimosis
   c. phallus
   d. glans
   e. balan

_____ 7. The circumferential incisions followed a direction:
   a. inferior to the scrotum
   b. suprapubic and transverse
   c. around the penis
   d. lateral to the prostate
   e. medial to the inguinal canal

CASE STUDIES

14

Write a term from the case studies with the following meanings:

8. surgical repair of a weak abdominal muscle in the groin area on both sides _____

9. entrapment of a loop of bowel in a hernia _____

10. inflammation of the prostate gland _____

11. within the urinary bladder _____

12. inflammation of the glans penis _____

13. narrowing of the distal opening of the foreskin _____

Abbreviations. Define the following abbreviations:

14. BPH _____

15. TURP _____

16. BNO _____

17. UTI _____

Male Reproductive System

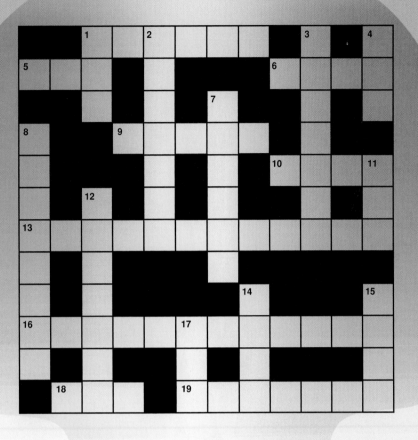

ACROSS

1. The male gonad
5. Abnormal, painful, difficult: prefix
6. Pertaining to condition of urine: suffix
9. A reproductive organ
10. Stone or calculus: root
13. Male gamete or sex cell
16. Main male sex hormone
18. Protein associated with prostate cancer: abbreviation
19. Semen or spermatozoa: root

DOWN

1. Self-examination of the testis: abbreviation
2. Sac that holds the testis
3. Testis: combining form
4. Ductus deferens: root
7. A reproductive or germ cell
8. Gland that contributes to semen
11. High blood pressure: abbreviation
12. Type of cell division that forms the gametes
14. Hernia or localized dilation: suffix
15. Male reproductive gland: root
17. Condition of: suffix

CHAPTER FIFTEEN

THE FEMALE REPRODUCTIVE SYSTEM; PREGNANCY AND BIRTH

OBJECTIVES

After study of this chapter you should be able to:

1. Label a diagram of the female reproductive tract and describe the function of each part.
2. Describe the structure and function of the mammary glands.
3. Outline the events in the menstrual cycle.
4. Describe the main disorders of the female reproductive system.
5. Outline the major events that occur in the first 2 months after fertilization.
6. Describe the structure and function of the placenta.
7. Describe the three stages of childbirth.
8. List the hormonal and nervous controls over lactation.
9. Identify and use roots pertaining to the female reproductive system, pregnancy, and birth.
10. Interpret abbreviations used in referring to reproduction.
11. Analyze several case studies concerning the female reproductive system, pregnancy, and birth.

PRETEST

1. The female gonad is the _____.
2. The two ovarian hormones are _____ and _____.
3. Use of artificial methods to prevent fertilization is termed _____.
4. During the first two months of growth, the developing offspring is called a(n) _____.
5. The structure that nourishes the developing fetus is the _____.
6. Production of milk is technically called _____.
7. The root *gyn/o* means _____.
8. The roots *metr/o* and *hyster/o* mean _____.
9. Any disorder present at birth is described as _____.

Unlike the continuous gametogenesis in males, formation of the female gamete is cyclic, with an egg released midway in the menstrual cycle. Each month, the uterus is prepared to receive a fertilized egg. If fertilization occurs, the developing offspring is nourished and protected by the placenta and surrounding fluids until birth. If the released egg is not fertilized, the lining of the uterus is sloughed off in menstruation.

The Female Reproductive System

The Ovaries

The female gonads are the paired **ovaries** (singular: ovary) that are held by ligaments in the pelvic cavity on either side of the uterus (Fig. 15-1). It is within the ovaries that the female gametes, the eggs or **ova** (singular: ovum), develop. Every month several ova ripen, each within a cluster of cells called a **graafian follicle**. At the time of ovulation, usually only one ovum is released from an ovary and the remainder of the ripening ova degenerate. The follicle remains behind and continues to function for about 2 weeks if there is no fertilization of the ovum and for about 2 months if the ovum is fertilized.

The Oviducts, Uterus, and Vagina

After ovulation, the ovum travels into an **oviduct** (also called the **fallopian tube** or uterine tube), one of the two tubes attached to the upper lateral portions of the uterus (see Fig. 15-1). These tubes arch above the ovaries and have fingerlike projections called **fimbriae** that sweep the released ovum into the oviduct. If fertilization occurs, it usually takes place in the oviduct.

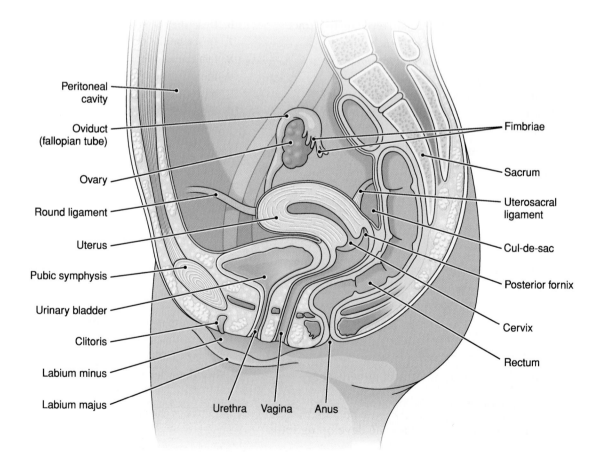

Figure 15-1 Female reproductive system. The system is seen in sagittal section along with some adjacent structures.

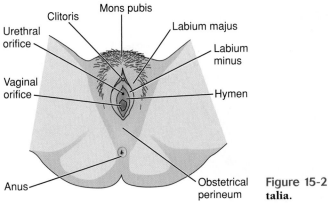

Figure 15-2 **The external female genitalia.**

The **uterus** is the organ that nourishes the developing offspring. It is pear-shaped, with an upper rounded fundus, a triangular cavity, and a lower narrow **cervix** that projects into the vagina. The recess around the cervix in the superior vagina is the **fornix**. At the posterior cervix, the peritoneum dips downward to form a blind pouch, or **cul-de-sac** (from French, meaning "bottom of the bag"), the lowest point of the peritoneal cavity.

The innermost layer of the uterine wall, the **endometrium**, has a rich blood supply. It receives the fertilized ovum and becomes part of the placenta during pregnancy. The endometrium is shed during the menstrual period if no fertilization occurs. The muscle layer of the uterine wall is the **myometrium**.

The **vagina** is a muscular tube that receives the penis during intercourse, functions as a birth canal, and transports the menstrual flow out of the body (see Fig. 15-1).

The External Genital Organs

All of the external female genitalia together are called the **vulva** (Fig. 15-2). This includes the large outer **labia majora** and small inner **labia minora** that enclose the openings of the vagina and the urethra. The **clitoris**, anterior to the urethral opening, is similar in origin to the penis and responds to sexual stimulation.

In both males and females, the region between the thighs, from the external genital organs to the anus, is the **perineum**. During childbirth, an incision may be made between the vagina and the anus to facilitate birth and prevent the tearing of tissue, a procedure called an *episiotomy*. (This procedure is actually a perineotomy, as the root *episi/o* means "vulva.")

The Mammary Glands

The **mammary glands**, or breasts, are composed mainly of glandular tissue and fat (Fig. 15-3). Their purpose is to provide nourishment for the newborn. The milk secreted by the glands is carried in ducts to the nipple.

The Menstrual Cycle

Reproductive activity in the female normally begins during puberty with **menarche**, the first menstrual period. Each month, the menstrual cycle is controlled, like reproductive activity in the male, by hormones from the anterior pituitary gland.

Follicle-stimulating hormone (FSH) begins the cycle by causing the ovum to ripen in the graafian follicle (Fig. 15-4). The follicle secretes **estrogen**, a hormone that starts development of the endometrium in preparation for the fertilized egg.

A second pituitary hormone, **luteinizing hormone (LH)**, triggers **ovulation** and conversion of the follicle to the **corpus luteum**. This structure, left behind in the ovary,

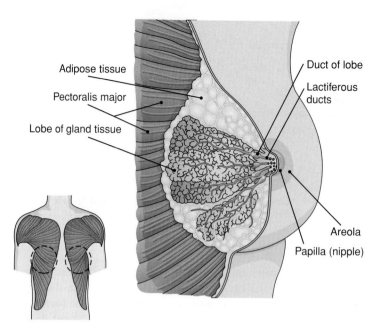

Figure 15-3 **Section of the breast.**

secretes **progesterone** and estrogen, which further the growth of the endometrium. If no fertilization occurs, hormone levels decline, and the endometrium sloughs off in the process of **menstruation**.

The average menstrual cycle lasts 28 days, with the first day of menstruation taken as day 1 and ovulation occurring on about day 14. Throughout the cycle, estrogen and progesterone feed back to the pituitary to regulate the production of FSH and LH. Hormonal methods of birth control act by supplying estrogen and progesterone, which inhibit the pituitary and prevent ovulation, while not interfering with menstruation.

Figure 15-4 shows changes occurring simultaneously in the ovary and uterus during the course of one menstrual cycle under the effects of pituitary and ovarian hormones.

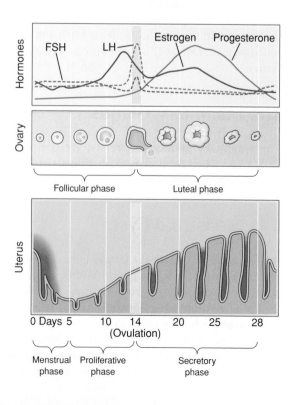
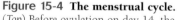

Figure 15-4 **The menstrual cycle.** (*Top*) Before ovulation on day 14, the follicle is ripening in the ovary; after ovulation, the follicle becomes the corpus luteum. (*Bottom*) Changes in the endometrium of the uterus during the menstrual cycle.

Menopause

Menopause is the cessation of monthly menstrual cycles. This generally occurs between the ages of 45 and 55 years. Levels of reproductive hormones decline, and egg cells in the ovaries gradually degenerate. Some women experience unpleasant symptoms, such as hot flashes, headaches, insomnia, mood swings, and urinary problems. There is also some atrophy of the reproductive tract, with vaginal dryness. Most importantly, the decline in estrogen levels is associated with weakening of the bones (osteoporosis).

Hormone-replacement therapy (HRT) has been used to alleviate menopausal symptoms. This treatment usually consists of the administration of estrogen in combination with progestin, a synthetic progesterone given to minimize the risk of endometrial cancer. Replacement hormones reduce bone loss associated with aging. Concerns about the safety of HRT, however, have caused reconsideration of this therapy beyond the early postmenopausal years. Studies with the most widely used form of HRT showed an increased risk of endometrial cancer, breast cancer, heart disease, and blood clots with extended use. Additional studies are ongoing.

Aside from HRT, antidepressants and vitamin E may help to relieve symptoms; locally applied estrogen and moisturizers relieve vaginal dryness. Nonhormonal drugs that increase bone density are also available if needed. As always, exercise and a balanced diet with adequate calcium are important in maintaining health throughout life.

Contraception

Contraception is the use of artificial methods to prevent fertilization of the ovum or its implantation in the uterus. Temporary methods of birth control function to:

> ➤ Block sperm penetration of the uterus (e.g. condom, diaphragm)
> ➤ Prevent implantation of the fertilized egg (e.g. intrauterine device, or IUD)
> ➤ Prevent ovulation (e.g. hormones). Hormonal methods differ in dosage and route of delivery, such as oral intake (the "birth control pill"), injection, skin patch, vaginal ring.

The so-called morning after pill is intended for emergency contraception. It considerably reduces the chance of pregnancy if taken within 72 hours after unprotected sexual intercourse. One such product, Plan B, consists of two doses of progestin taken 12 hours apart.

Surgical sterilization provides the most effective and usually permanent contraception. In males, this procedure is a vasectomy; in females, surgical sterilization is a **tubal ligation**, in which the fallopian tubes are cut and tied on both sides (Fig. 15-5). The preferred

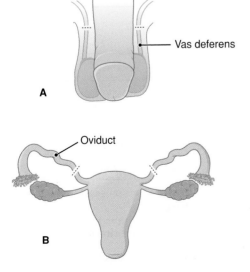

A

Vas deferens

B

Oviduct

Figure 15-5 Sterilization. (*A*) Vasectomy. (*B*) Tubal ligation.

15

15

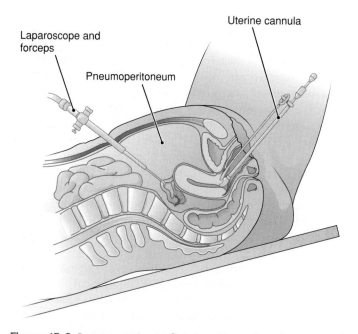

Laparoscope and forceps

Pneumoperitoneum

Uterine cannula

Figure 15-6 Laparoscopic sterilization. The peritoneal cavity is inflated (pneumoperitoneum) and the oviducts are cut laparoscopically through a small incision.

method for performing this surgery is through the abdominal wall with the use of a laparoscope (Fig. 15-6).

RU486 (mifepristone) is more widely used for birth control in other countries than in the United States. It terminates an early pregnancy by blocking progesterone and causing the endometrium to break down. Technically, it is an abortion-causing agent (abortifacient), not a contraceptive.

Box 15-1 describes the main methods of contraception currently in use. Each has advantages and disadvantages over other methods, but they are listed roughly in order of decreasing effectiveness.

Box 15•1 **For Your Reference** *Main Methods of Birth Control Currently in Use*

Method	Description
SURGICAL	
Vasectomy/tubal ligation	Cutting and tying of tubes carrying gametes
HORMONAL	
Birth control pills	Estrogen and progestin or progestin alone taken orally to prevent ovulation
Birth control shot	Injection of synthetic progesterone every 3 months to prevent ovulation
Birth control patch	Adhesive patch placed on body that administers estrogen and progestin through the skin; left on for 3 weeks and removed for a fourth week
Birth control ring	Flexible ring inserted into vagina that releases hormones internally; left in place for 3 weeks and removed for a fourth week.

Box 15•1 For Your Reference *Continued*

BARRIER

Male condom	Sheath that fits over erect penis and prevents release of semen
Diaphragm (with spermicide)	Rubber cap that fits over cervix and prevents entrance of sperm
Contraceptive sponge (with spermicide)	Soft, disposable foam disk containing spermicide, which is moistened with water and inserted into vagina
Intrauterine device (IUD)	Metal or plastic device inserted into uterus through vagina; prevents fertilization and implantation by release of copper or birth control hormones

OTHER

Spermicide	Chemicals used to kill sperm; best when used in combination with a barrier method
Fertility awareness	Abstinence during fertile part of cycle as determined by menstrual history, basal body temperature, or quality of cervical mucus

15

TERMINOLOGY Key Terms

Female Reproductive System

NORMAL STRUCTURE AND FUNCTION

cervix SER-viks	Neck. Usually means the lower narrow portion (neck) of the uterus; cervix uteri (*U-ter-ī*) (*root cervic/o*)
clitoris KLIT-o-ris	A small erectile body anterior to the urethral opening that is similar in origin to the penis (root: *clitor/o, clitorid/o*)
contraception kon-tra-SEP-shun	The prevention of pregnancy
corpus luteum KOR-pus LŪ-tē-um	The small yellow structure that develops from the graafian follicle after ovulation and secretes progesterone and estrogen
cul-de-sac kul-di-SAK	A blind pouch, such as the recess between the rectum and the uterus; the rectouterine pouch or pouch of Douglas (see Fig. 15-1)
endometrium en-dō-MĒ-trē-um	The inner lining of the uterus
estrogen ES-trō-jen	A group of hormones that produce female characteristics and prepare the uterus for the fertilized egg. The most active of these is estradiol.
fallopian tube fa-LŌ-pē-an	A tube extending from the upper lateral portion of the uterus that carries the ovum to the uterus. Also called oviduct or uterine tube (root: *salping/o*).
fimbriae FIM-brē-ē	The long fingerlike extensions of the oviduct that wave to capture the released ovum (see Fig. 15-1) (singular: *fimbria*)

TERMINOLOGY

Key Terms

Continued

follicle-stimulating hormone (FSH)	A hormone secreted by the anterior pituitary that acts on the gonads. In the female, it stimulates ripening of the ova in the ovary.
fornix *FOR-niks*	An archlike space, such as the space between the uppermost wall of the vagina and the cervix (see Fig. 15-1); from Latin meaning "arch"
graafian follicle *GRAF-ē-an*	The cluster of cells in which the ovum ripens in the ovary. Also called ovarian follicle.
labia majora *LĀ-bē-a ma-JOR-a*	The two large folds of skin that form the sides of the vulva (root *labi/o* means "lip") (singular: *labium majus*)
labia minora *LĀ-bē-a mī-NOR-a*	The two small folds of skin within the labia majora (singular: *labium minus*)
luteinizing hormone (LH) *LŪ-tē-in-ī-zing*	A hormone secreted by the anterior pituitary that acts on the gonads. In the female, it stimulates ovulation and formation of the corpus luteum.
mammary gland *MAM-a-rē*	A specialized gland capable of secreting milk in the female; the breast (root: *mamm/o, mast/o*)
menarche *men-AR-kē*	The first menstrual period, which normally occurs during puberty
menopause *MEN-ō-pawz*	Cessation of menstrual cycles in the female
menstruation *men-strū-Ā-shun*	The cyclic discharge of blood and mucosal tissues from the lining of the nonpregnant uterus (root: *men/o, mens*); menstrual period, menses (*MEN-sēz*)
myometrium *mī-ō-MĒ-trē-um*	The muscular wall of the uterus
ovary *Ō-va-rē*	A female gonad (root: *ovari/o, oophor/o*)
oviduct *Ō-vi-dukt*	A tube extending from the upper lateral portion of the uterus that carries the ovum to the uterus. Also called fallopian or uterine tube (root: *salping/o*).
ovulation *ov-ū-LĀ-shun*	The release of a mature ovum from the ovary (from *ovule*, meaning "little egg")
ova *Ō-va*	The female gamete or reproductive cell (singular: *ovum*) (root: *oo, ov/o*)
perineum *per-i-NĒ-um*	The region between the thighs from the external genitals to the anus (root: *perine/o*)
progesterone *prō-JES-ter-ōn*	A hormone produced by the corpus luteum and the placenta that maintains the endometrium for pregnancy
tubal ligation *lī-GĀ-shun*	Surgical constriction of the oviducts to produce sterilization (see Figs. 15-5 and 15-6)
uterus *Ū-ter-us*	The organ that receives the fertilized egg and maintains the developing offspring during pregnancy (root: *uter/o, metr, hyster/o*) See Box 15-2

TERMINOLOGY   Key Terms

Continued

vagina va-JĪ-na	The muscular tube between the cervix and the vulva (root: *vagin/o, colp/o*)
vulva VUL-va	The external female genital organs (root: *vulv/o, episi/o*)

15

Go to the pronunciation glossary in Chapter 15 on the CD-ROM
to hear these words pronounced.

Box 15•2 **Focus on Words**   *Crazy Ideas*

Most women would be shocked and surprised to learn the origin of the root hyster/o, used for the uterus. It comes from the same root as the words hysterical and hysterics and was based on the very old belief that the womb was the source of mental disturbances in women.

A similar history lies at the origin of the word hypochondriac, a term for someone who has imaginary illnesses. The hypochondriac regions are in the upper portions of the abdomen, an area that the ancients believed was the seat of mental disorders.

Roots Pertaining to the Female Reproductive System

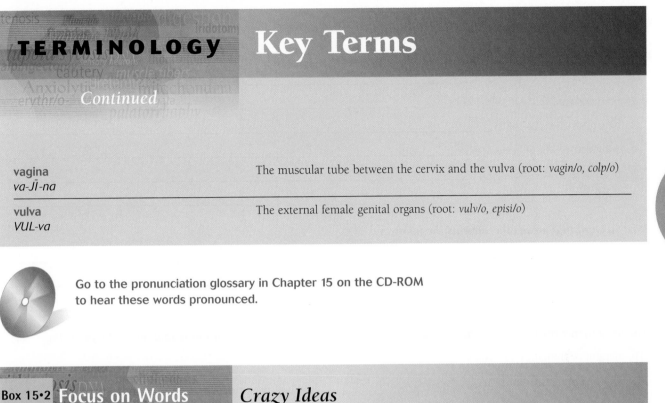

Table 15•1 Roots for Female Reproduction and the Ovaries

ROOT	MEANING	EXAMPLE	DEFINITION OF EXAMPLE
gyn/o, gynec/o*	woman	gynecology gī-ne-KOL-ō-jē	study of women's diseases
men/o, mens	month, menstruation	intermenstrual in-ter-MEN-strū-al	between menstrual periods
oo	ovum, egg cell	oocyte Ō-ō-sīt	cell that gives rise to an ovum
ov/o, ovul/o	ovum, egg cell	ovulatory OV-ū-la-tōr-ē	pertaining to ovulation
ovari/o	ovary	ovariopexy ō-var-ē-ō-PEK-sē	surgical fixation of an ovary
oophor/o	ovary	oophorectomy ō-of-ō-REK-tō-mē	excision of an ovary

This root may also be pronounced with a soft g, as in jin-e-KOL-ō-jē.

Exercise 15-1

Define the following words:

1. gynecopathy (*ji-ne-KOP-a-thē*) _____

2. premenstrual (*prē-MEN-strū-al*) _____

3. oogenesis (*ō-ō-JEN-e-sis*) _____

4. anovulatory (*an-OV-ū-la-tō-rē*) _____

5. ovarian (*ō-VAR-ē-an*) _____

6. oophoritis (*ō-of-ō-RĪ-tis*) _____

Write a word that means the same as the following:

7. a physician who specializes in the study of diseases of women _____

8. after ovulation _____

9. profuse bleeding (-rhagia) at the time of menstruation _____

The word menorrhea means "menstruation." Add a prefix to menorrhea to form words that mean the following:

10. painful or difficult menstruation _____

11. absence of menstruation _____

12. scanty menstrual flow _____

Use the root ovari/o to write words that mean the following:

13. surgical puncture of an ovary _____

14. hernia of an ovary _____

15. rupture of an ovary _____

Use the root oophor/o to write words that mean the following:

16. incision of an ovary _____

17. malignant tumor of the ovary _____

Table 15·2 Roots for the Oviducts, Uterus, and Vagina

ROOT	MEANING	EXAMPLE	DEFINITION OF EXAMPLE
salping/o	oviduct, tube	salpingoplasty *sal-PING-ō-plas-tē*	plastic repair of an oviduct
uter/o	uterus	intrauterine *in-tra-Ū-ter-in*	within the uterus
metr/o, metr/i	uterus	metrorrhea *mē-trō-RĒ-a*	abnormal uterine discharge
hyster/o	uterus	hysterotomy *his-ter-OT-ō-mē*	incision of the uterus
cervic/o	cervix, neck	endocervical *en-dō-SER-vi-kal*	pertaining to the lining of the cervix

Table 15·2	Continued		
vagin/o	vagina	vaginometer *vaj-i-NOM-e-ter*	instrument for measuring the vagina
colp/o	vagina	colpostenosis *kol-pō-sten-Ō-sis*	narrowing of the vagina

Exercise 15-2

Define the following terms:

1. salpingectomy (*sal-pin-JEK-tō-mē*) _____

2. hysteroscopy (*his-ter-OS-kō-pē*) _____

3. metromalacia (*mē-trō-ma-LĀ-shē-a*) _____

4. uterovesical (*ū-ter-ō-VES-i-kal*) _____

5. intracervical (*in-tra-SER-vi-kal*) _____

6. vaginoplasty (*vaj-i-nō-PLAS-tē*) _____

7. colpodynia (*kol-pō-DIN-ē-a*) _____

Write words for the following:

8. surgical fixation of an oviduct _____

9. radiographic study of the oviduct _____

*The root **salping/o** is taken from the word **salpinx**, which means "tube." Add a prefix to **salpinx** to write a word for the following:*

10. Presence of pus in an oviduct _____

11. Collection of fluid in an oviduct _____

*Note how the roots **salping/o** and **oophor/o** are combined to form **salpingo-oophoritis** (inflammation of an oviduct and ovary). Write a word with the following meaning:*

12. surgical removal of an oviduct and ovary _____

Use the roots indicated to write a word that means the same as the following:

13. pertaining to the uterus (uter/o) _____

14. radiograph of the uterus (hyster/o) and oviducts _____

15. surgical fixation of the uterus (hyster/o) _____

16. prolapse of the uterus (metr/o) _____

17. narrowing of the uterus (metr/o) _____

18. through the cervix _____

19. inflammation of the vagina (vagin/o) _____

20. hernia of the vagina (colp/o) _____

15

Table 15•3	Roots for the Female Accessory Structures		
ROOT	**MEANING**	**EXAMPLE**	**DEFINITION OF EXAMPLE**
vulv/o	vulva	vulvar *VUL-var*	pertaining to the vulva
episi/o	vulva	episiotomy *e-piz-ē-OT-ō-mē*	incision of the vulva
perine/o	perineum	perineal *per-i-NĒ-al*	pertaining to the perineum
clitor/o, clitorid/o	clitoris	clitorectomy *klī-tō-REK-tō-mē*	excision of the clitoris
mamm/o	breast, mammary gland	mammoplasty *mam-ō-PLAS-tē*	plastic surgery of the breast
mast/o	breast, mammary gland	amastia *a-MAS-tē-a*	absence of the breasts

Exercise 15-3

Write a word that means the same as the following:

1. any disease of the vulva (vulv/o) _____

2. suture of the vulva (episi/o) _____

3. pertaining to the vagina (vagin/o) and perineum _____

4. inflammation of the clitoris _____

5. radiograph of the breast (mamm/o) _____

6. inflammation of the breast (mast/o) _____

7. excision of the breast _____

Clinical Aspects of Female Reproduction

Infection

The major organisms that cause sexually transmitted infections in both men and women are given in Box 14-2.

Genital herpes is a presently incurable viral infection that affects over 25% of adults in the United States. Once infection occurs, the virus lives in the nervous system, causing intermittent outbreaks that may include genital sores, itching, burning, and urinary problems. The virus is easily spread to sexual partners even if there are no active signs of the disease. Pregnant women can pass the virus to their babies during delivery, resulting in possible disabilities and even death. Some basic hygiene measures and condom use can reduce viral spread.

A fungus that infects the vulva and vagina is *Candida albicans*, causing **candidiasis**. **Vaginitis** is inflammation of the vagina that produces a thick, white, cheesy discharge and causes itching; pregnancy, diabetes mellitus, and use of antibiotics, steroids, or birth control pills predispose to this infection. If the infection is recurrent, the patient's partner should be treated to prevent reinfections. Antifungal agents (mycostatics) are used in treatment.

Pelvic inflammatory disease (PID) is the spread of infection from the reproductive organs into the pelvic cavity. It is most often caused by the gonorrhea organism or by chlamydia, although bacteria normally living in the reproductive tract may also be responsible when conditions allow. PID is a serious disorder that may result in septicemia or shock. Inflammation of the oviducts, called **salpingitis**, may close off these tubes and cause infertility.

Fibroids

A **fibroid** is a benign smooth-muscle tumor usually occurring in the wall of the uterus (the myometrium) (Fig. 15-7). This type of growth, technically called a **leiomyoma**, is one of the most common uterine disorders, but it usually causes no symptoms and requires no treatment. Fibroids may, however, cause heavy menstrual bleeding (menorrhagia), and rectal or bladder pressure. Treatments include:

➤ Suppression of hormones that stimulate fibroid growth
➤ Surgical removal of the fibroids (myomectomy)
➤ Surgical removal of the uterus (hysterectomy)
➤ Uterine artery embolization (UAE), a new method that has reduced the need for hysterectomies. A specially trained radiologist uses a catheter to inject particles into uterine arteries, blocking blood supply to the fibroid and causing it to shrink.

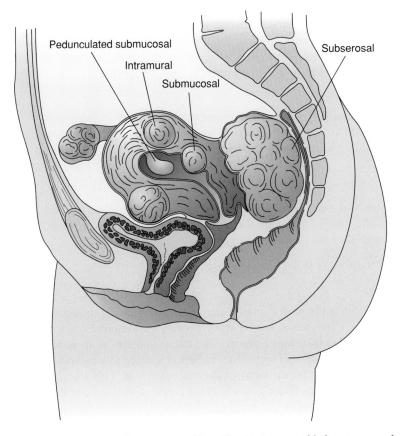

Figure 15-7 Uterine leiomyomas (fibroids). Various possible locations are shown. They may be within the uterine wall (intramural), below the mucous membrane (submucosal), on a stalk (pedunculated), or below the outer serous membrane (subserosal). One tumor is shown compressing the urinary bladder and another the rectum.

Endometriosis

Growth of endometrial tissue outside the uterus is termed **endometriosis**. Commonly the ovaries, oviducts, peritoneum, and other pelvic organs are involved. Stimulated by normal hormones, the endometrial tissue causes inflammation, fibrosis, and adhesions in surrounding areas. The results may be pain, **dysmenorrhea** (painful or difficult menstruation), and infertility. Laparoscopy is used to diagnose endometriosis and also to remove the abnormal tissue.

Menstrual Disorders

Menstrual abnormalities include flow that is too scanty (oligomenorrhea) or too heavy (menorrhagia) and the absence of monthly periods (amenorrhea). Dysmenorrhea, when it occurs, usually begins at the start of menstruation and lasts 1 to 2 days. Together these disorders are classified as dysfunctional uterine bleeding (DUB). These responses may be caused by hormone imbalances, systemic disorders, or uterine problems. They are most common in adolescence or near menopause. At other times they are often related to life changes and emotional upset.

Premenstrual syndrome (PMS) describes symptoms that appear during the second half of the menstrual cycle and includes emotional changes, fatigue, bloating, headaches, and appetite changes. Possible causes of PMS have been under study. Symptoms may be relieved by hormone therapy, antidepressants, or antianxiety medications. Exercise, dietary control, rest, and relaxation strategies may also be helpful. Avoidance of caffeine and vitamin E supplements may relieve breast tenderness; one should also drink adequate water and limit salt intake.

Polycystic Ovarian Syndrome

Polycystic ovarian syndrome (PCOS) is discussed here because the symptoms of this disorder first described were enlarged ovaries with multiple cysts. These signs are not always present in PCOS, although the ovaries do show abnormalities. PCOS is an endocrine disorder involving increased androgen and estrogen secretion that interferes with normal secretion of pituitary FSH and LH. Some effects include:

> ➤ anovulation and infertility
> ➤ scant or absent menses (oligomenorrhea or amenorrhea)
> ➤ Excessive growth of hair (hirsutism), caused by excess androgen (male hormone)
> ➤ resistance to insulin, a hormone that lowers blood sugar, resulting in symptoms of diabetes mellitus
> ➤ obesity

PCOS is treated with hormones to regulate hormonal imbalance, drugs to increase responsiveness to insulin, weight reduction (estrogen is produced in adipose tissue), and sometimes partial removal of the ovaries.

Cancer of the Female Reproductive Tract

Endometrial Cancer

Cancer of the endometrium is the most common cancer of the female reproductive tract. Women at risk should have biopsies taken regularly because endometrial cancer is not always detected by **Pap (Papanicolaou) smear**. Treatment consists of **hysterectomy** (removal of the uterus) (Fig. 15-8) and sometimes radiation therapy. A small percentage of cases occur after overgrowth (hyperplasia) of the endometrium. This tissue can be removed by **dilation and curettage (D&C)**, in which the cervix is widened and the lining of the uterus is scraped with a curette.

Cervical Cancer

Almost all patients with cancer of the cervix have been infected with human papillomavirus (HPV), a virus that causes genital warts. Incidence also is related to high sexual activity and other sexually transmitted viral infections, such as herpes.

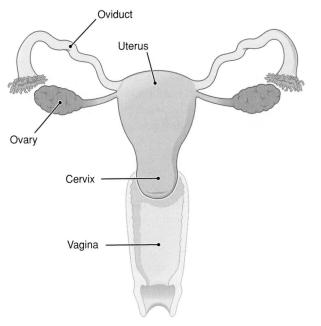

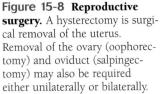

Figure 15-8 Reproductive surgery. A hysterectomy is surgical removal of the uterus. Removal of the ovary (oophorectomy) and oviduct (salpingectomy) may also be required either unilaterally or bilaterally.

In the 1940s and 1950s, the synthetic steroid DES (diethylstilbestrol) was given to prevent miscarriages. A small percentage of daughters born to women treated with this drug have shown an increased risk for cancer of the cervix and vagina. These women need to be examined regularly.

Cervical carcinoma is often preceded by abnormal growth (dysplasia) of the epithelial cells lining the cervix. Growth is graded as CIN I, II, or III, depending on the depth of tissue involved. CIN stands for cervical intraepithelial neoplasia. Diagnosis of cervical cancer is by a Pap smear, examination with a **colposcope**, and biopsy. In a **cone biopsy** (Fig. 15-9), a cone-shaped piece of tissue is removed from the lining of the cervix for study. Often in the procedure, all of the abnormal cells are removed as well.

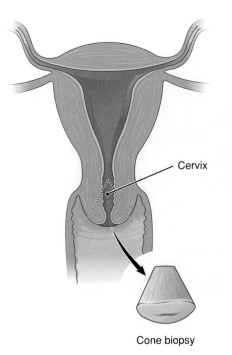

Figure 15-9 Cone biopsy of the uterine cervix.

Ovarian Cancer

Cancer of the ovary has a high mortality rate because it usually causes no distinct early symptoms and there is no accurate routine screening test yet available. Women may overlook the vague possible signs of ovarian cancer, such as bloating, change in bowel habits, backache, urinary changes, abnormal bleeding, weight loss, and fatigue. Often by the time of diagnosis, the tumor has invaded the pelvis and abdomen. Removal of the ovaries (**oophorectomy**) and oviducts (**salpingectomy**) along with the uterus is required (see Fig. 15-7), in addition to chemotherapy and radiation therapy.

Breast Cancer

Carcinoma of the breast is second only to lung cancer in causing cancer-related deaths among women in the United States. This cancer metastasizes readily through the lymph nodes and blood to other sites such as the lung, liver, bones, and ovaries.

Diagnosis

Palpation is a simple first step in breast cancer diagnosis. Regular breast self-examination (BSE) is of utmost importance, because most breast cancers are discovered by women themselves.

Mammography, which provides two-dimensional x-ray images of the breast, is still the standard diagnostic procedure for breast cancer (Fig. 15-10). After the age of 40, women should have mammograms yearly. In digital mammography, x-ray images are stored on computers instead of on film. These images can be manipulated electronically to aid interpretation. They are more easily stored and retrieved or sent to other medical facilities.

Ultrasound and MRI studies are adjuncts to mammography. Ultrasound can show whether a lump seen on mammography is simply a benign cyst. MRI with a contrast medium can show abnormal blood vessel formation signifying a tumor.

Any suspicious breast tissue must be biopsied by needle aspiration or surgical excision for further study. In a **stereotactic biopsy**, a physician uses a computer-guided imaging system to locate suspicious tissue and remove samples with a needle. This method is less invasive than surgical biopsy.

Treatment

Treatment of breast cancer is usually some form of **mastectomy**, or removal of breast tissue:

> ➤ In a radical mastectomy, the entire breast is removed. Underlying muscle and axillary lymph nodes (in the armpit) also are removed.

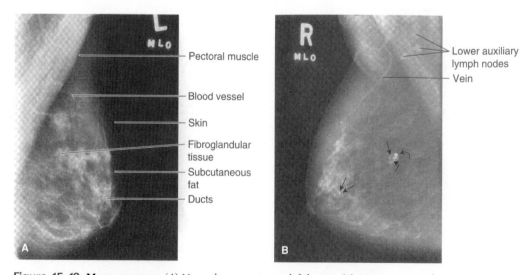

Figure 15-10 Mammograms. (*A*) Normal mammogram, left breast. (*B*) Mammogram of right breast showing lesions (*arrows*). In mammograms, fat tissue appears gray; breast tissue, calcium deposits, and benign or cancerous tumors appear white.

➤ In a modified radical mastectomy, the breast and lymph nodes are removed, but muscles are left in place.

➤ In a segmental mastectomy, or "lumpectomy," just the tumor itself is removed. When the tumor is small and surgery is followed by additional treatment, this procedure gives survival rates as high as those with more radical surgeries.

Surgeons can assess the extent of tumor spread and conserve lymphatic tissue using a **sentinel-node biopsy**. A dye or radioactive tracer identifies the first lymph nodes that receive lymph from a tumor. Study of possible tumor spread to these "sentinel nodes" guides further treatment.

Often after breast surgery a patient receives chemotherapy and/or radiation therapy. It is now possible in some cases to deliver radiation to just the tumor area (brachytherapy) instead of irradiating the whole breast. A radiation source is delivered through catheters or implanted in the breast tissue for a short time.

Progress in breast cancer treatment involves genetic studies and tumor analysis that allows therapy more specific to each particular case. About 8% of these cancers are linked to a defective gene (*BRCA1* or *BRCA2*) that is transmitted within families. Women with these genetic predispositions can be screened more carefully or treated prophylactically.

Some types of specific drug treatments for breast cancer, which may be given in combination, are:

➤ Drugs that block estrogen production or block estrogen receptors in breast tissue if a tumor responds to this hormone

➤ Drugs that inhibit tumor growth factors

➤ Drugs that inhibit growth of blood vessels that supply the tumor (antiangiogenesis agents)

These and other anticancer drugs are described in more detail in the list of supplementary terms.

TERMINOLOGY Key Terms

Female Reproductive System

DISORDERS

candidiasis *kan-di-DĪ-a-sis*	Infection with the fungus *Candida,* a common cause of vaginitis
dysmenorrhea *DIS-men-ō-rē-a*	Painful or difficult menstruation. A common disorder that may be caused by infection, use of an intrauterine device, endometriosis, overproduction of prostaglandins, or other factors.
endometriosis *en-dō-mē-trē-Ō-sis*	Growth of endometrial tissue outside the uterus, usually in the pelvic cavity
fibroid *FĪ-broyd*	Benign tumor of smooth muscle (see leiomyoma)
leiomyoma *lī-ō-mī-Ō-ma*	Benign tumor of smooth muscle, usually in the uterine wall (myometrium). In the uterus, may cause bleeding and pressure on the bladder or rectum. Also called fibroid or myoma. (See Figure 15-7.)

TERMINOLOGY Key Terms
Continued

pelvic inflammatory disease (PID)	Condition caused by the spread of infection from the reproductive tract into the pelvic cavity. Commonly caused by sexually transmitted gonorrhea and chlamydial infections.
salpingitis *sal-pin-JĪ-tis*	Inflammation of the oviduct; typically caused by urinary tract infection or sexually transmitted infection. Chronic salpingitis may lead to infertility or ectopic pregnancy (development of the fertilized egg outside of the uterus).
vaginitis *vaj-i-NĪ-tis*	Inflammation of the vagina

DIAGNOSIS AND TREATMENT

colposcope *KOL-pō-skōp*	Instrument for examining the vagina and cervix
cone biopsy	Removal of a cone of tissue from the lining of the cervix for cytologic examination; also called conization (see Fig. 15-9)
dilation and curettage (D&C) *kū-re-TAJ*	Procedure in which the cervix is dilated (widened) and the lining of the uterus is scraped with a curette
hysterectomy *his-ter-EK-tō-mē*	Surgical removal of the uterus. Most commonly done because of tumors. Often the oviducts and ovaries are removed as well (see Fig. 15-8).
mammography *mam-OG-ra-fē*	Radiographic study of the breast for the detection of breast cancer
mastectomy *mas-TEK-tō-mē*	Excision of the breast to eliminate malignancy
oophorectomy *ō-of-ō-REK-tō-mē*	Excision of an ovary (see Fig. 15-8)
Pap smear	Study of cells collected from the cervix and vagina for early detection of cancer. Also called Papanicolaou smear or Pap test.
salpingectomy *sal-pin-JEK-tō-mē*	Surgical removal of the oviduct (see Fig. 15-8)
sentinel-node biopsy *SEN-ti-nel*	Biopsy of the first lymph nodes to receive drainage from a tumor; used to determine spread of cancer in planning treatment.
stereotactic biopsy *ster-ē-ō-TAK-tik*	Needle biopsy using a computer-guided imaging system to locate suspicious tissue and remove samples for study

Go to the pronunciation glossary in Chapter 15 on the CD-ROM to hear these words pronounced.

TERMINOLOGY Supplementary Terms

Female Reproductive System

NORMAL STRUCTURE AND FUNCTION

adnexa *ad-NEK-sa*	Appendages, such as the adnexa uteri—the ovaries, oviducts, and uterine ligaments
areola *a-RĒ-ō-la*	A pigmented ring, such as the dark area around the nipple of the breast
greater vestibular gland	A small mucus-secreting gland on the side of the vestibule (see below) near the vaginal opening. Also called Bartholin (*BAR-tō-lin*) gland (see Fig. 15-12).
hymen *HĪ-men*	A fold of mucous membrane that partially covers the entrance of the vagina
mons pubis *monz PŪ-bis*	The rounded, fleshy elevation in front of the pubic joint that is covered with hair after puberty
oocyte *Ō-ō-sīt*	An immature ovum
perimenopause *per-i-MEN-ō-pawz*	The period immediately before and after menopause; begins at the time of irregular menstrual cycles and ends 1 year after the last menstrual period; averages 3 to 4 years
vestibule *VES-ti-būl*	The space between the labia minora that contains the openings of the urethra, vagina, and ducts of the greater vestibular glands

DISORDERS

cystocele *SIS-tō-sēl*	Herniation of the urinary bladder into the wall of the vagina (Fig. 15-11)
dyspareunia *dis-par-Ū-nē-a*	Pain during sexual intercourse
fibrocystic disease of the breast *fī-brō-SIS-tik*	A condition in which there are palpable lumps in the breasts, usually associated with pain and tenderness. These lumps or "thickenings" change with the menstrual cycle and must be distinguished from malignant tumors by diagnostic methods.
hirsutism *HIR-sū-tizm*	Excess growth of hair
leukorrhea *lū-kō-RĒ-a*	White or yellowish discharge from the vagina. Infection and other disorders may change the amount, color, or odor of the discharge.
microcalcification *mī-krō-kal-si-fi-KĀ-shun*	Small deposit of calcium that appears as a white spot on mammograms. Most microcalcifications are harmless, but some might indicate breast cancer.
prolapse of the uterus	Downward displacement of the uterus with the cervix sometimes protruding from the vagina

TERMINOLOGY Supplementary Terms
Continued

rectocele	Herniation of the rectum into the wall of the vagina; also called proctocele
REK-tō-sēl	(see Fig. 15-11)

DIAGNOSIS AND TREATMENT

episiorrhaphy	Suture of the vulva or suture of the perineum cut in an episiotomy (incision
e-pis-ē-OR-a-fē	to ease childbirth)

laparoscopy	Endoscopic examination of the abdomen; may include surgical procedures,
lap-a-ROS-kō-pē	such as tubal ligation (see Fig. 15-5)

myomectomy	Surgical removal of a uterine leiomyoma (fibroid, myoma)
mī-ō-MEK-tō-mē	

speculum	An instrument used to enlarge the opening of a passage or cavity to allow
SPEK-ū-lum	examination

teletherapy	Delivery of radiation to a tumor from an external beam source, as compared
tel-e-THER-a-pē	to implantation of radioactive material (brachytherapy) or systemic
	administration of radionuclide

DRUGS

aromatase inhibitor (AI)	Agent that inhibits estrogen production; used for postmenopausal treatment
a-RŌ-ma-tās	of breast cancers that respond to estrogen. Examples are exemestane
	(Aromasin), anastrozole (Arimidex), letrozole (Femara).

bisphosphonate	Agent used to prevent and treat osteoporosis; increases bone mass by
bis-FOS-fō-nāt	decreasing bone turnover. Examples are alendronate (Fosamax) and
	risedronate (Actonel).

HER2 inhibitor	Drug used to treat breast cancers that show excess receptors (HER2) for
	human epidermal growth factor. Example is trastuzumab (Herceptin).

paclitaxel	Antineoplastic agent derived from yew trees used mainly in treatment of
pak-li-TAKS-el	breast and ovarian cancer; Taxol

selective estrogen receptor modulator	Drug that acts on estrogen receptors. Tamoxifen (Nolvodex) is used to
(SERM)	prevent and treat estrogen-sensitive breast cancer; Raloxifene (Avista) is
	used to prevent bone loss after menopause.

Go to the pronunciation glossary in Chapter 15 on the CD-ROM
to hear these words pronounced.

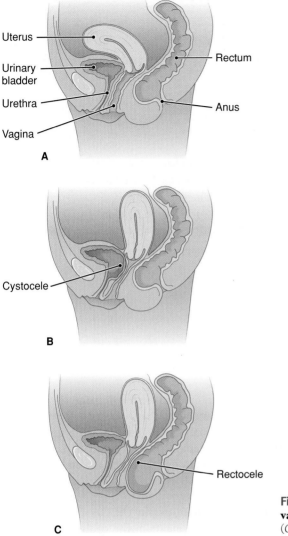

Uterus

Urinary bladder

Urethra

Vagina

Rectum

Anus

A

Cystocele

B

Rectocele

C

Figure 15-11 Herniation into the vagina. (*A*) Normal. (*B*) Cystocele. (*C*) Rectocele.

15

TERMINOLOGY Abbreviations

Female Reproductive System

AI	Aromatase inhibitor		**DES**	Diethylstilbestrol
BRCA1	Breast cancer gene 1		**DUB**	Dysfunctional uterine bleeding
BRCA2	Breast cancer gene 2		**FSH**	Follicle-stimulating hormone
BSE	Breast self-examination		**GC**	Gonococcus (cause of gonorrhea)
BSO	Bilateral salpingo-oophorectomy		**GYN**	Gynecology
BV	Bacterial vaginosis		**HPV**	Human papillomavirus
CIN	Cervical intraepithelial neoplasia		**HRT**	Hormone-replacement therapy
D&C	Dilation and curettage		**IUD**	Intrauterine device

TERMINOLOGY   Abbreviations

Continued

LH	Luteinizing hormone	**STI**	Sexually transmitted infection
NGU	Nongonococcal urethritis	**TAH**	Total abdominal hysterectomy
PCOS	Polycystic ovarian syndrome	**TSS**	Toxic shock syndrome
PID	Pelvic inflammatory disease	**UAE**	uterine artery embolization
PMS	Premenstrual syndrome	**VD**	Venereal disease (sexually transmitted
SERM	Selective estrogen receptor modulator		disease)
STD	Sexually transmitted disease		

Pregnancy and Birth

Fertilization and Early Development

Penetration of an ovulated egg cell by a spermatozoon results in **fertilization** (Fig. 15-12). This union normally occurs in the oviduct. The nuclei of the sperm and egg cells fuse, restoring the chromosome number to 46 and forming a **zygote**. As the zygote travels through the oviduct toward the uterus, it divides rapidly. Within 6 to 7 days, the fertilized egg reaches the uterus and implants into the endometrium, and the **embryo** begins to develop.

During the first 8 weeks of growth, all of the major body systems are established. Embryonic tissue produces **human chorionic gonadotropin (hCG)**, a hormone that keeps the corpus luteum functional in the ovary to maintain the endometrium. (The presence of hCG in urine is the basis for the most commonly used tests for pregnancy.) After 2 months, placental hormones take over this function and the corpus luteum degenerates. At this time the embryo becomes a **fetus** (Fig. 15-13).

The Placenta

During development, the fetus is nourished by the **placenta**, an organ formed from the outermost layer of the embryo, the **chorion**, and the innermost layer of the uterus, the endometrium (Fig. 15-14). Here, exchanges take place between the bloodstreams of the mother and the fetus through fetal capillaries.

The **umbilical cord** contains the blood vessels that link the fetus to the placenta. Fetal blood is carried to the placenta in two umbilical arteries. While traveling through the placenta, the blood picks up nutrients and oxygen and gives up carbon dioxide and metabolic waste. Replenished blood is carried from the placenta to the fetus in a single umbilical vein.

Although the bloodstreams of the mother and the fetus do not mix, and all exchanges take place through capillaries, some materials do manage to get through the placenta in both directions. For example, some viruses, such as HIV and rubella, as well as drugs, alcohol, and other harmful substances are known to pass from the mother to the fetus; fetal proteins can enter the mother's blood and cause immunologic reactions.

During **gestation** (the period of development), the fetus is cushioned and protected by fluid contained in the **amniotic sac** (amnion) (Fig. 15-15), commonly called the bag of waters. This sac ruptures at birth.

15

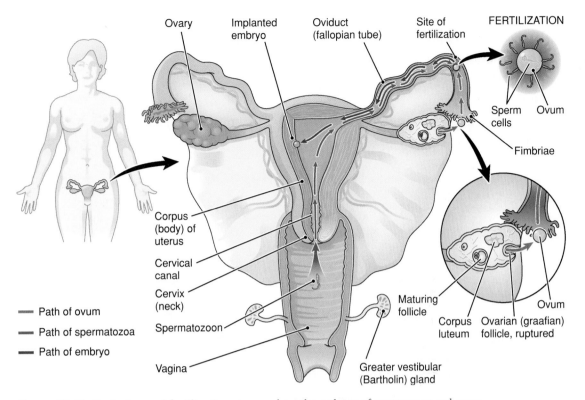

Figure 15-12 Ovulation and fertilization. Arrows show the pathway of spermatozoa and ovum. Fertilization occurs in the oviduct, after which the zygote implants in the uterine lining.

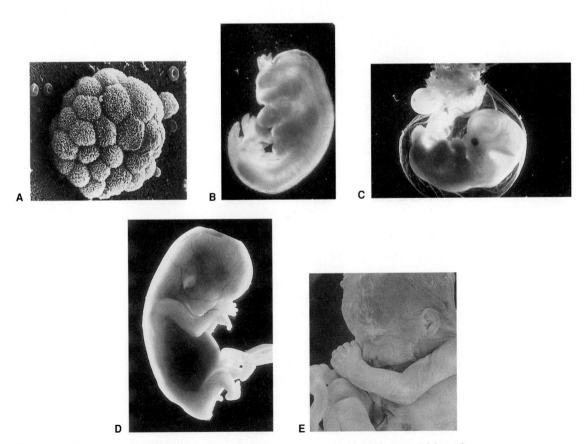

Figure 15-13 Human development. Human embryos and an early fetus are shown. (*A*) Implantation in the uterus 7 to 8 days after conception. (*B*) Embryo at 32 days. (*C*) At 37 days. (*D*) At 41 days. (*E*) Fetus at 12 to 15 weeks.

15

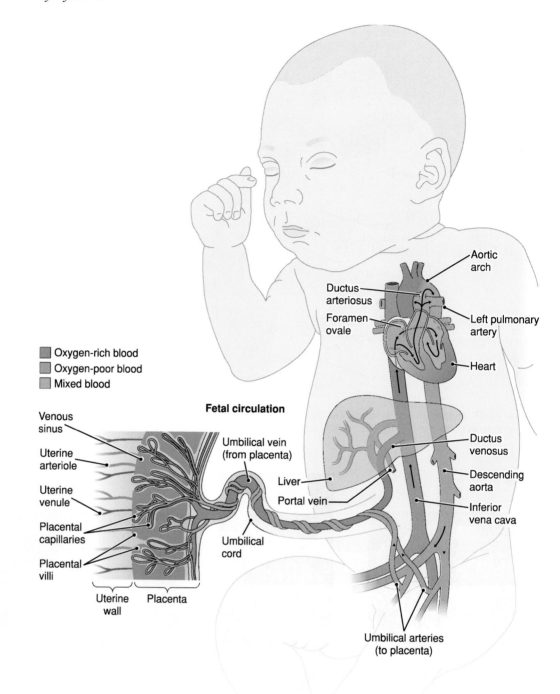

Figure 15-14 **Fetal circulation.** A section of the placenta is also shown. Colors show relative oxygen content of blood.

Fetal Circulation

The fetus has several adaptations that serve to bypass the lungs, which are not needed to oxygenate the blood. When blood coming from the placenta enters the right atrium, the **foramen ovale**, a small hole in the septum between the atria, allows some of the blood to go directly into the left atrium, thus bypassing the pulmonary artery. Further, blood pumped out of the right ventricle can shunt directly into the aorta through a short vessel, the **ductus arteriosus**, which connects the pulmonary artery with the descending aorta (see Fig. 15-14). Both of these passages close off at birth when the pulmonary circuit is established. Their failure to close taxes the heart and may require medical attention.

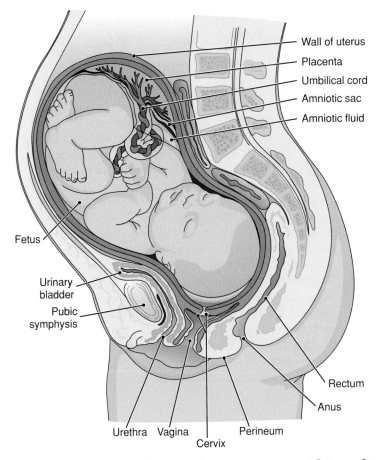

Wall of uterus
Placenta
Umbilical cord
Amniotic sac
Amniotic fluid

Fetus

Urinary
bladder
Pubic
symphysis

Rectum

Anus

Urethra   Vagina   Perineum
              Cervix

Figure 15-15 Midsagittal section of a pregnant uterus with intact fetus.

Childbirth

The length of pregnancy, from fertilization of the ovum to birth, is about 38 weeks, or 266 days. In practice, it is calculated as approximately 280 days or 40 weeks from the first day of the last menstrual period (LMP). For study purposes, pregnancy is divided into 3-month periods (trimesters), during which defined changes can be observed in the fetus.

Childbirth, or **parturition**, occurs in three stages:

1. onset of regular uterine contractions and dilation of the cervix
2. expulsion of the fetus
3. delivery of the placenta and fetal membranes

The third stage of childbirth is followed by contraction of the uterus and control of bleeding. The factors that start labor are not completely understood, but it is clear that the hormone **oxytocin** from the posterior pituitary gland and other hormones called **prostaglandins** are involved. Box 15-3 has career information on midwives and other birth assistants.

The term **gravida** refers to a pregnant woman. The term **para** refers to a woman who has given birth. This means the production of a viable infant (500 g or more or over 20 weeks' gestation) regardless of whether the infant is alive at birth or whether the birth is single or multiple. Prefixes are added to both terms to indicate the number of pregnancies or births, such as:

> nulli-   none
> primi-   one
> secundi-   two
> tri- or terti- three

Box 15•3 Health Professions | *Nurse-Midwives and Other Birth Assistants*

A midwife is someone, not a physician and traditionally a woman, who assists women in childbirth. The term literally means "with woman," and the practice is termed midwifery (mid-WĪF-rē or mid-WIF-er-ē). A certified nurse-midwife (CNM) is a graduate nurse who takes special training in midwifery leading to a certificate or masters degree. CNMs assist women in labor, delivery, and postpartum care as well as routine gynecologic care. The practice is legal throughout the United States, but states vary in requirements and restrictions. In most, CNMs have some prescription-writing privileges and insurance reimbursement for their services is mandated. Most CNMs work in hospitals, but they may also work in private practice, birth centers, and homes, usually in cooperation with an obstetrician.

A certified midwife (CM) can enter specialized training with a high-school diploma. Education in social sciences, health sciences, and nursing practices leads to a certificate

or degree in midwifery. A CM may assist alone at a birth, but is trained to detect complications and obtain medical assistance if needed. They are licensed by states, which may require prior examination of the mother by a physician or qualified nurse and supervision by an obstetrician. States also may place limitations on the cases they can handle based on medical conditions.

A birth assistant is someone who works with families during pregnancy, through labor, and after delivery. Birth assistants may help with early labor at home, give care between home and the hospital, and provide continuity and support throughout the hospital stay. A "doula" may or may not assist at a birth, but helps a mother and her family for some time after the birth. The name comes from Greek and refers to the most important female servant in the household, who probably assisted the lady of the house in childbearing. Both doulas and birth assistants have professional associations that set standards for training and certification.

> ➤ quadri-   four
> ➤ multi-   two or more

Alternatively, a number can be added after the term to indicate events, such as gravida 1, para 3, etc.

Lactation

The secretion of milk from the breasts, called **lactation**, is started by the hormone prolactin from the anterior pituitary gland, as well as hormones from the placenta. The baby's suckling then stimulates the release of milk. The pituitary hormone oxytocin is needed for this release or "letdown" of milk. For the first few days after delivery, only **colostrum** is produced. This has a slightly different composition than milk, but like the milk, it has protective antibodies.

TERMINOLOGY Key Terms

Pregnancy and Birth

NORMAL STRUCTURE AND FUNCTION

amniotic sac am-nē-OT-ik	The membranous sac filled with fluid that holds the fetus; also called amnion (root: *amnio*)
chorion KOR-ē-on	The outermost layer of the embryo that, with the endometrium, forms the placenta (adjective: chorionic)
colostrum kō-LOS-trum	Breast fluid that is secreted in the first few days after giving birth, before milk is produced

Key Terms

15

ductus arteriosus *DUK-tus ar-tēr-ē-Ō-sus*	A fetal blood vessel that connects the pulmonary artery with the descending aorta, thus allowing blood to bypass the lungs
embryo *EM-brē-ō*	The stage in development between the zygote and the fetus, extending from the second through the eighth week of growth in the uterus (adjective: embryonic; root: *embry/o*)
fertilization *fer-ti-li-ZĀ-shun*	The union of an ovum and a spermatozoon
fetus *FĒ-tus*	The developing child in the uterus from the third month to birth (adjective: fetal; root: *fet/o*)
foramen ovale *fō-RĀ-men ō-VĀ-lē*	A small hole in the septum between the atria in the fetal heart that allows blood to pass directly from the right to the left side of the heart
gestation *jes-TĀ-shun*	The period of development from conception to birth
gravida *GRAV-i-da*	Pregnant woman
human chorionic gonadotropin (hCG) *kor-ē-ON-ik GŌ-na-dō-trō-pin*	A hormone secreted by the embryo early in pregnancy that maintains the corpus luteum so that it will continue to secrete hormones
lactation *lak-TĀ-shun*	The secretion of milk from the mammary glands
oxytocin *ok-sē-TŌ-sin*	A pituitary hormone that stimulates contractions of the uterus. It also stimulates release ("letdown") of milk from the breasts.
para	Woman who has produced a viable infant. Multiple births are considered as single pregnancies.
parturition *par-tū-RI-shun*	Childbirth (root: *nat/i*); labor (root: *toc/o*)
placenta *pla-SEN-ta*	The organ, composed of fetal and maternal tissues, that nourishes and maintains the developing fetus
prostaglandins *PROS-ta-glan-dinz*	A group of hormones with varied effects, including the stimulation of uterine contractions
umbilical cord *um-BIL-i-kal*	The structure that connects the fetus to the placenta. It contains vessels that carry blood between the mother and the fetus.
zygote *ZĪ-gōt*	The fertilized ovum

Go to the pronunciation glossary in Chapter 15 on the CD-ROM to hear these words pronounced.

Table 15·4 Roots Pertaining to Pregnancy and Birth

ROOT	MEANING	EXAMPLE	DEFINITION OF EXAMPLE
amnio	amnion, amniotic sac	diamniotic dī-am-nē-OT-ik	showing two amniotic sacs
embry/o	embryo	embryonic em-brē-ON-ik	pertaining to the embryo
fet/o	fetus	fetometry fē-TOM-e-trē	measurement of a fetus
toc/o	labor	dystocia dis-TŌ-sē-ā	difficult labor
nat/i	birth	neonate NĒ-ō-nāt	newborn
lact/o	milk	lactose LAK-tōs	sugar (-ose) found in milk
galact/o	milk	galactogogue ga-LAK-tō-gog	agent that promotes (-agogue) the flow of milk
gravida	pregnant woman	nulligravida nul-i-GRAV-i-da	woman who has never (nulli-) been pregnant
para	woman who has given birth	multipara mul-TIP-a-ra	woman who has given birth two or more times

Exercise 15-4

Define the following words:

1. embryogenesis (*em-brē-ō-JEN-e-sis*) _____

2. prenatal (*prē-NĀ-tal*) _____

3. neonatal (*nē-ō-NĀ-tal*) _____

4. monoamniotic (*mon-ō-am-nē-OT-ik*) _____

5. fetoscopy (*fē-TOS-kō-pē*) _____

6. hyperlactation (*hī-per-lak-TĀ-shun*) _____

7. agalactia (*ā-ga-LAK-shē-a*) _____

Use the appropriate roots to write words for the following:

8. incision of the amnion (to induce labor)   _____

9. rupture of the amniotic sac   _____

10. cell (-cyte) found in amniotic fluid   _____

11. study of an embryo   _____

12. instrument for endoscopic examination of the fetus   _____

13. any disease of an embryo   _____

14. study of the newborn   _____

15. after birth   _____

16. woman who is pregnant for the first time   _____

17. woman who has been pregnant two or more times   _____

18. woman who has never given birth   _____

19. woman who has given birth to one child   _____

Use the suffix -tocia, *meaning "condition of labor," to write words for the following:*

20. dry labor   _____

21. slow labor   _____

Use the root galact/o *to write words for the following:*

22. cystic enlargement (-cele) of a milk duct   _____

23. discharge of milk   _____

15

Clinical Aspects of Pregnancy and Birth

Infertility

About 10 to 15% of couples who want children are unable to conceive or to sustain a pregnancy. Some of the possible causes of infertility are discussed in Chapter 14 and in this section. In men, these causes include low sperm count, low sperm motility, blockage of the ducts that transport the sperm cells, and erectile dysfunction. In women they include:

> ➤ lack of ovulation
> ➤ blockage in the oviducts, as caused by infection or excess growth of tissue
> ➤ uterine problems, such as tumors or abnormal growth of endometrial tissue
> ➤ cervical scarring or infection
> ➤ excess vaginal acidity that harms spermatozoa, or antibodies to sperm cells
> ➤ drugs, including temporary or permanent infertility following cessation of birth control pills

Box 15-4 describes some clinical approaches to helping infertile couples have children when all other diagnostic and therapeutic methods have failed.

Ectopic Pregnancy

Development of a fertilized egg outside of its normal position in the uterine cavity is termed an **ectopic pregnancy** (Fig. 15-16). Although it may occur elsewhere in the abdominal cavity, an ectopic pregnancy usually occurs in the oviduct, resulting in a tubal pregnancy. Salpingitis, endometriosis, and PID may lead to ectopic pregnancy by blocking passage of the ovum into the uterus. Continued growth will rupture the oviduct, causing dangerous hemorrhage. Symptoms of ectopic pregnancy are pain, tenderness, swelling, and shock. Diagnosis is by measurement of the hormone hCG and ultrasonography, confirmed by laparoscopic examination. Prompt surgery is required, sometimes including removal of the tube.

Pregnancy-Induced Hypertension

Pregnancy-induced hypertension (PIH), also referred to as preeclampsia or toxemia of pregnancy, is a state of hypertension during pregnancy in association with oliguria,

Box 15•4 Clinical Perspectives *Assisted Reproductive Technology: The "Art" of Conception*

At least 1 in 10 American couples is affected by infertility. Assisted reproductive technologies such as in vitro fertilization (IVF), gamete intrafallopian transfer (GIFT), and zygote intrafallopian transfer (ZIFT) can help these couples have children.

In vitro fertilization refers to fertilization of an egg outside the mother's body in a laboratory dish, and it is often used when a woman's fallopian tubes are blocked or when a man has a low sperm count. The woman participating in IVF is given hormones to cause ovulation of several eggs. These are then withdrawn with a needle and fertilized with the father's sperm. After a few divisions, some of the fertilized eggs are placed in the uterus, thus bypassing the fallopian tubes. Additional fertilized eggs can be frozen to repeat the procedure in case of failure or for later pregnancies.

GIFT can be used when the woman has at least one normal fallopian tube and the man has an adequate sperm count. As in IVF, the woman is given hormones to cause ovulation of several eggs, which are collected. Then, the eggs and the father's sperm are placed into the fallopian tube using a catheter. Thus, in GIFT, fertilization occurs inside the woman, not in a laboratory dish.

ZIFT is a combination of IVF and GIFT. Fertilization takes place in a laboratory dish, and then the zygote is placed into the fallopian tube.

Because of a lack of guidelines or restrictions in the United States in the field of assisted reproductive technology, some problems have arisen. These issues concern the use of stored embryos and gametes, use of embryos without consent, and improper screening for disease among donors. In addition, the implantation of more than one fertilized egg has resulted in a high incidence of multiple births, even up to seven or eight offspring in a single pregnancy, a situation that imperils the survival and health of the babies.

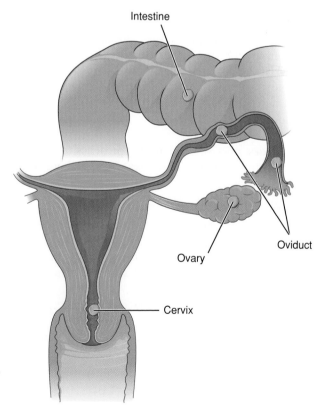

Figure 15-16 Ectopic pregnancy. Possible sites where a fertilized ovum might develop outside the body of the uterus.

proteinuria, and edema. The cause is a hormone imbalance that results in constriction of blood vessels. If untreated, PIH may lead to **eclampsia**, with seizures, coma, and possibly death.

Abortion

For a variety of reasons, a pregnancy may terminate before the fetus is capable of surviving outside the uterus. An **abortion** is loss of an embryo or fetus before the 20th week of pregnancy or before a weight of 500 g (1.1 lb). When this occurs spontaneously, it is commonly referred to as a miscarriage. Most spontaneous abortions occur within the first 3 months of pregnancy. Causes include poor maternal health, hormone imbalance, incompetence (weakness) of the cervix, immune reactions, tumors, and most commonly, fetal abnormalities. If all gestational tissues are not eliminated, the abortion is described as incomplete, and a physician must remove the remaining tissue.

An induced abortion is the intentional termination of a pregnancy. A common method for inducing an abortion is **dilatation and evacuation (D&E)**, in which the cervix is dilated and the fetal tissue is removed by suction.

Rh Incompatibility

Incompatibility between the blood of a mother and her fetus is a problem in certain pregnancies. If a mother lacks the Rh blood antigen (see Chapter 10) and her baby is positive for that factor (inherited from the father), the mother's body may make Rh antibodies as her baby's blood crosses the placenta during pregnancy or enters the mother's bloodstream during childbirth. In a subsequent pregnancy with an Rh-positive fetus, the antibodies may enter the fetus and destroy its red cells. **Hemolytic disease of the newborn (HDN)** is prevented by giving the mother preformed antibodies to the Rh factor during pregnancy and shortly after delivery to remove these proteins from her blood.

Placental Abnormalities

If the placenta attaches near or over the cervix instead of in the upper portion of the uterus, the condition is termed **placenta previa**. This disorder may cause bleeding in the later stages of pregnancy. If bleeding is heavy, it may be necessary to terminate the pregnancy.

Placental abruption (abruptio placentae) describes premature separation of the placenta from its point of attachment. The separation causes hemorrhage, which if extensive, may result in fetal or maternal death or a need to end the pregnancy. Causative factors include injury, maternal hypertension, and advanced maternal age.

Mastitis

Inflammation of the breast, or **mastitis**, may occur at any time but usually occurs in the early weeks of breastfeeding. It is commonly caused by staphylococcus or streptococcus bacteria that enter through cracks in the nipple. The breast becomes red, swollen, and tender, and the patient may experience chills, fever, and general discomfort.

Congenital Disorders

Congenital disorders are those present at birth (birth defects). They fall into two categories:

➤ developmental disorders that occur during growth of the fetus
➤ hereditary (familial) disorders that can be passed from parents to children through the germ cells.

Genetic disorders are caused by a **mutation** (change) in the genes or chromosomes of the cells. They may involve changes in the number or structure of the chromosomes or changes in single or multiple genes. The appearance and severity of genetic disorders may also involve abnormal genes interacting with environmental factors. Examples are the diseases that "run in families," such as diabetes mellitus, heart disease, hypertension, and certain forms of cancer. Box 15-5 describes some of the most common genetic disorders.

A **carrier** of a genetic disorder is an individual who has a genetic defect that does not appear but that can be passed to offspring. Laboratory tests can identify carriers of some genetic disorders.

15

Box 15•5 For Your Reference *Genetic Disorders**

Disease	Cause	Description
albinism	recessive gene mutation	lack of pigmentation
cystic fibrosis	recessive gene mutation	affects respiratory system, pancreas, and sweat glands; most common hereditary disease in white populations (see Chapter 11)
Down syndrome	extra chromosome 21	slanted eyes, short stature, mental retardation, and others (Fig. 15-17); incidence increases with increasing maternal age; trisomy 21
fragile X chromosome	defect in an X (sex-determining) chromosome	reduced intellectual abilities, autism, hyperactivity; enlarged head and ears; passed from mothers to sons with the X chromosome
hemophilia hē-mō-FIL-ē-a	recessive gene mutation on the X chromosome	bleeding disease inherited from mothers with the X chromosome and usually appearing in sons
Huntington disease	dominant gene mutation	altered metabolism destroys specific nerve cells; appears in adulthood and is fatal within about 10 years; causes motor and mental disorders
Klinefelter syndrome	extra X chromosome	lack of sexual development, lowered intelligence
Marfan syndrome	dominant gene mutation	disease of connective tissue with weakness of the aorta
neurofibromatosis nū-rō-fī-brō-ma-TŌ-sis	dominant gene mutation	multiple skin tumors containing nerve tissue
phenylketonuria (PKU) fen-il-kē-tō-NŪ-rē-a	recessive gene mutation	lack of enzyme to metabolize an amino acid; neurologic signs, mental retardation, lack of pigment; tested for at birth; special diet can prevent retardation
sickle cell anemia	recessive gene mutation	abnormally shaped red cells block blood vessels; mainly affects black populations
Tay–Sachs disease	recessive gene mutation	an enzyme deficiency causes lipid to accumulate in nerve cells and other tissues; causes death in early childhood; carried in Jewish populations in eastern Europe
Turner syndrome	single X chromosome	sexual immaturity, short stature, possible lowered intelligence

*A dominant gene is one for a trait that always appears if the gene is present; that is, it will affect the offspring even if inherited from only one parent. A recessive gene is one for a trait that will appear only if the gene is inherited from both parents.

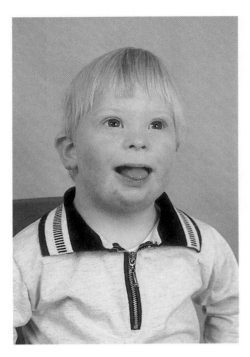

Figure 15-17 Child with Down syndrome (trisomy 21). The typical facial features are visible in this photo.

Teratogens are factors that cause malformations in the developing fetus. These include infections—such as **rubella** (German measles), herpes simplex, and syphilis—alcohol, drugs, chemicals, and radiation. The fetus is most susceptible to teratogenic effects during the first 3 months of pregnancy.

Examples of developmental disorders are **atresia** (absence or closure of a normal body opening), **anencephaly** (absence of a brain), **cleft lip**, **cleft palate**, and congenital heart disease. **Spina bifida** is incomplete closure of the spine, through which the spinal cord and its membranes may project (Fig. 15-18). This usually occurs in the lumbar region. If there is no herniation of tissue, the condition is spina bifida occulta. Protrusion of the meninges through the opening is a meningocele; in a myelomeningocele, both the spinal cord and membranes herniate through the defect, as seen in Figure 15-18D and Figure 15-19. Note that folic acid, a B vitamin, can prevent embryonic spinal malformations, known as neural-tube defects. This vitamin is found in vegetables,

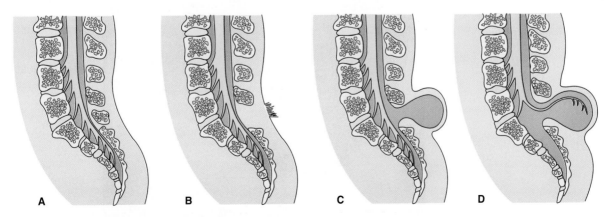

Figure 15-18 Spinal defects. (A) Normal spinal cord. (B) Spina bifida occulta. (C) Meningocele. (D) Myelomeningocele.

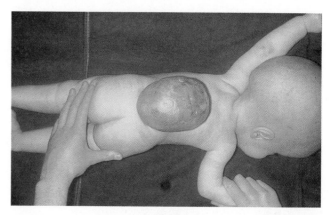

Figure 15-19 A myelomeningocele.

liver, legumes and seeds, but it is now added to some commercial foods, including cereals and breads, to provide young women with this vitamin early on in case they become pregnant.

Diagnosis of Congenital Disorders

Many congenital disorders can now be detected before birth. **Ultrasonography** (Fig. 15-20), in addition to its use for monitoring pregnancies and determining fetal sex, can also reveal certain fetal abnormalities. In **amniocentesis** (Fig. 15-21), a sample is withdrawn from the amniotic cavity with a needle. The fluid obtained is analyzed for chemical abnormalities. The cells are grown in the laboratory and tested for biochemical disorders. A **karyotype** is prepared to study the genetic material (see Fig. 4-10).

In **chorionic villus sampling (CVS)**, small amounts of the membrane around the fetus are obtained through the cervix for analysis. This can be done at 8 to 10 weeks of pregnancy, in comparison with 14 to 16 weeks for amniocentesis.

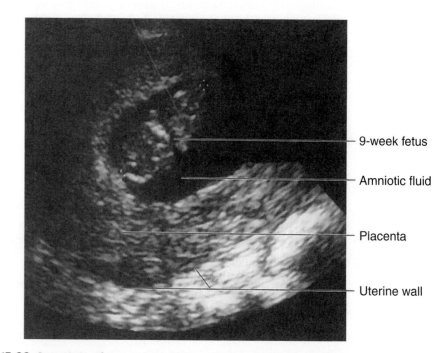

— 9-week fetus

— Amniotic fluid

— Placenta

— Uterine wall

Figure 15-20 Sonogram. This transvaginal sonogram shows a 9-week-old fetus.

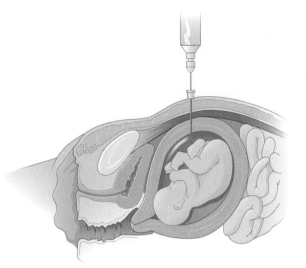

Figure 15-21 Amniocentesis. A sample is removed from the amniotic sac. Cells and fluid are tested for fetal abnormalities.

TERMINOLOGY   Key Terms

Pregnancy and Birth

DISORDERS

abortion *a-BOR-shun*	Termination of a pregnancy before the fetus is capable of surviving outside the uterus, usually at 20 wk or 500 g. May be spontaneous or induced. A spontaneous abortion is commonly called a miscarriage.
anencephaly *an-en-SEF-a-lē*	Congenital absence of a brain
atresia *a-TRĒ-zē-a*	Congenital absence or closure of a normal body opening
carrier	An individual who has an unexpressed genetic defect that can be passed to his or her children
cleft lip	A congenital separation of the upper lip
cleft palate	A congenital split in the roof of the mouth
congenital disorder *kon-GEN-i-tal*	A disorder that is present at birth. May be developmental or hereditary (familial).
eclampsia *e-KLAMP-sē-a*	Convulsions and coma occurring during pregnancy or after delivery and associated with the conditions of pregnancy-induced hypertension (see below) (adjective: eclamptic)
ectopic pregnancy *ek-TOP-ik*	Development of the fertilized ovum outside the body of the uterus. Usually occurs in the oviduct (tubal pregnancy) but may occur in other parts of the reproductive tract or abdominal cavity (see Fig. 15-16).

TERMINOLOGY Key Terms

Continued

hemolytic disease of the newborn (HDN)	Disease that results from Rh incompatibility between the blood of a mother and her fetus. An Rh-negative mother produces antibody to Rh-positive fetal red cells that enter her circulation. These antibodies can destroy Rh-positive fetal red cells in a later pregnancy unless the mother is treated with antibodies to remove the Rh antigen. Formerly called erythroblastosis fetalis.
mastitis *mas-TĪ-tis*	Inflammation of the breast, usually associated with the early weeks of breastfeeding
mutation *mū-TĀ-shun*	A change in the genetic material of the cell. Most mutations are harmful. If the change appears in the sex cells, it can be passed to future generations.
placental abruption *ab-RUP-shun*	Premature separation of the placenta; abruptio placentae
placenta previa *PRĒ-vē-a*	A placenta that is attached in the lower portion of the uterus instead of the upper portion, as is normal. May result in hemorrhage late in pregnancy.
pregnancy-induced hypertension (PIH)	A toxic condition of late pregnancy associated with hypertension, edema, and proteinuria that, if untreated, may lead to eclampsia. Also called preeclampsia (*prē-e-KLAMP-sē-a*) and toxemia of pregnancy.
rubella *rū-BEL-la*	German measles. The virus can cross the placenta and cause fetal abnormalities, such as eye defects, deafness, heart abnormalities, and mental retardation. The virus is most damaging during the first trimester.
spina bifida *SPĪ-na BIF-i-da*	A congenital defect in the closure of the spinal column through which the spinal cord and its membranes may project (see Figs. 15-18 and 15-19)
teratogen *ter-AT-ō-jen*	A factor that causes developmental abnormalities in the fetus (adjective: teratogenic); root *terat/o* means "malformed fetus"

DIAGNOSIS AND TREATMENT

amniocentesis *am-nē-ō-sen-TĒ-sis*	Transabdominal puncture of the amniotic sac to remove amniotic fluid for testing. Tests on the cells and fluid obtained can reveal congenital abnormalities, blood incompatibility, and sex of the fetus (see Fig. 15-21).
chorionic villus sampling (CVS)	Removal of chorionic cells through the cervix for prenatal testing. Can be done earlier in pregnancy than amniocentesis.
dilatation and evacuation (D&E)	Widening of the cervix and removal of conception products by suction
karyotype *KAR-ē-ō-tīp*	A picture of the chromosomes of a cell arranged in order of decreasing size; can reveal abnormalities in the chromosomes themselves or in their number or arrangement (root *kary/o* means "nucleus") (see Fig. 4-10)
ultrasonography	The use of high-frequency sound waves to produce a photograph of an organ or tissue (see Fig. 15-20). Used in obstetrics to diagnose pregnancy, multiple births, and abnormalities and also to study and measure the fetus. The picture obtained is a sonogram or ultrasonogram.

Go to the pronunciation glossary in Chapter 15 on the CD-ROM to hear these words pronounced.

TERMINOLOGY Supplementary Terms

Pregnancy and Birth

NORMAL STRUCTURE AND FUNCTION

afterbirth	The placenta and membranes delivered after birth of a child
antepartum *an-tē-PAR-tum*	Before childbirth, with reference to the mother
Braxton–Hicks contractions	Light uterine contractions that occur during pregnancy and increase in frequency and intensity during the third trimester. They strengthen the uterus for delivery.
chloasma *klō-AZ-ma*	Brownish pigmentation that appears on the face during pregnancy; melasma
fontanel *fon-tan-EL*	A membrane-covered space between cranial bones in the fetus that later becomes ossified; a soft spot. Also spelled fontanelle.
intrapartum *in-tra-PAR-tum*	Occurring during childbirth
linea nigra *LIN-ē-a NĪ-gra*	A dark line on the abdomen from the umbilicus to the pubic region that may appear late in pregnancy
lochia *LŌ-kē-a*	The mixture of blood, mucus, and tissue discharged from the uterus after childbirth
meconium *me-KŌ-nē-um*	The first feces of the newborn
peripartum *per-i-PAR-tum*	Occurring during the end of pregnancy or the first few months after delivery, with reference to the mother
postpartum	After childbirth, with reference to the mother
premature	Describing an infant born before the organ systems are fully developed; immature
preterm	Occurring before the 37th week of gestation; describing an infant born before the 37th week of gestation
puerperium *pū-er-PĒR-ē-um*	The first 42 days after childbirth, during which the mother's reproductive organs usually return to normal (root: *puer* means "child")
striae atrophicae *STRĪ-ē a-TRŌ-fi-kē*	Pinkish or gray lines that appear where skin has been stretched, as in pregnancy; stretch marks, striae gravidarum
umbilicus *um-bi-LĪ-kus*	The scar in the middle of the abdomen that marks the attachment point of the umbilical cord to the fetus; the navel
vernix caseosa *VER-niks kā-sē-Ō-sa*	The cheeselike deposit that covers and protects the fetus (literally "cheesy varnish")

15

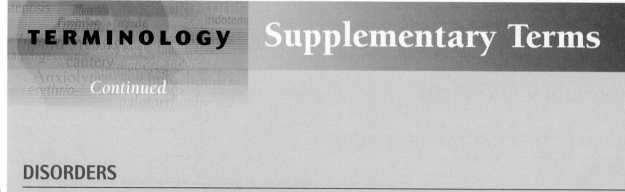

Supplementary Terms

15

DISORDERS

cephalopelvic disproportion *sef-a-lō-PEL-vik*	The condition in which the head of the fetus is larger than the pelvic outlet; also called fetopelvic disproportion
choriocarcinoma *kor-ē-ō-kar-si-NŌ-ma*	A rare malignant neoplasm composed of placental tissue
galactorrhea *ga-lak-tō-RĒ-a*	Excessive secretion of milk or continuation of milk production after breastfeeding has ceased. Often results from excess prolactin secretion and may signal a pituitary tumor.
hydatidiform mole *hī-da-TID-i-form*	A benign overgrowth of placental tissue. The placenta dilates and resembles grapelike cysts. The neoplasm may invade the wall of the uterus, causing rupture. Also called hydatid mole.
hydramnios *hī-DRAM-nē-os*	An excess of amniotic fluid; also called polyhydramnios
oligohydramnios *ol-i-gō-hī-DRAM-nē-os*	A deficiency of amniotic fluid
patent ductus arteriosus (PDA) *PĀ-tent*	Persistence of the ductus arteriosus after birth so that blood continues to shunt from the pulmonary artery to the aorta
puerperal infection *pū-ER-per-al*	Infection of the genital tract after delivery

DIAGNOSIS AND TREATMENT

abortifacient *a-bor-ti-FĀ-shent*	Agent that induces abortion
alpha-fetoprotein (AFP)	A fetal protein that may be elevated in amniotic fluid and maternal serum in cases of certain fetal disorders
Apgar score	A system of rating an infant's physical condition immediately after birth. Five features are rated as 0, 1, or 2 at 1 minute and 5 minutes after delivery, and sometimes thereafter. The maximum possible score at each interval is 10. Infants with low scores require medical attention.
artificial insemination (AI)	Placement of active semen into the vagina or cervix for the purpose of impregnation. The semen can be from a husband, partner, or donor.
cesarean section *se-ZAR-ē-an*	Incision of the abdominal wall and uterus for delivery of a fetus
culdocentesis *kul-dō-sen-TĒ-sis*	Puncture of the vaginal wall to sample fluid from the rectouterine space for diagnosis

TERMINOLOGY

Continued

Supplementary Terms

endometrial ablation *ab-LĀ-shun*	Selective destruction of the endometrium for therapeutic purpose; done to relieve excessive menstrual bleeding (menorrhagia)
extracorporeal membrane oxygenation **(ECMO)**	A technique for pulmonary bypass in which deoxygenated blood is removed, passed through a circuit that oxygenates the blood, and then returned. Used for selected newborn and pediatric patients in respiratory failure with an otherwise good prognosis.
in vitro fertilization (IVF)	Clinical procedure for achieving fertilization when it cannot be accomplished naturally. An oocyte (immature ovum) is removed, fertilized in the laboratory, and placed as a zygote into the uterus or fallopian tube (ZIFT, zygote intrafallopian transfer). Alternatively, an ovum can be removed and placed along with sperm cells into the fallopian tube (GIFT, gamete intrafallopian transfer).
obstetrics *ob-STET-riks*	The branch of medicine that treats women during pregnancy, childbirth, and the puerperium. Usually combined with the practice of gynecology.
pediatrics *pē-dē-AT-riks*	The branch of medicine that treats children and diseases of children (root: *ped/o* means "child")
pelvimetry *pel-VIM-e-trē*	Measurement of the pelvis by manual examination or radiographic study to determine whether delivery of a fetus through the vagina will be possible
Pitocin *pi-TŌ-sin*	Trade name for oxytocin; used to induce and hasten labor
presentation	Term describing the part of the fetus that can be felt by vaginal or rectal examination. Normally the head presents first (vertex presentation), but sometimes the buttocks (breech presentation), face, or other part presents first.
Rho-GAM *RŌ-gam*	Trade name for a preparation of antibody to the Rh(D) antigen; used to prevent hemolytic disease of the newborn in cases of Rh incompatibility

Go to the pronunciation glossary in Chapter 15 on the CD-ROM to hear these words pronounced.

TERMINOLOGY Abbreviations

Pregnancy and Birth

AB	Abortion	**GIFT**	Gamete intrafallopian transfer
AFP	Alpha-fetoprotein	**hCG**	Human chorionic gonadotropin
AGA	Appropriate for gestational age	**HDN**	Hemolytic disease of the newborn
AI	Artificial insemination	**IVF**	In vitro fertilization
ART	Assisted reproductive technology	**LMP**	Last menstrual period
C section	Cesarean section	**NB**	Newborn
CPD	Cephalopelvic disproportion	**NICU**	Neonatal intensive care unit
CVS	Chorionic villus sampling	**OB**	Obstetrics
D&E	Dilatation and evacuation	**PDA**	Patent ductus arteriosus
ECMO	Extracorporeal membrane oxygenation	**PIH**	Pregnancy-induced hypertension
EDC	Estimated date of confinement	**PKU**	Phenylketonuria
FHR	Fetal heart rate	**SVD**	Spontaneous vaginal delivery
FHT	Fetal heart tone	**UC**	Uterine contractions
FTND	Full-term normal delivery	**UTP**	Uterine term pregnancy
FTP	Full-term pregnancy	**VBAC**	Vaginal birth after cesarean section
GA	Gestational age	**ZIFT**	Zygote intrafallopian transfer

15

CHAPTER REVIEW

LABELING EXERCISE
Female Reproductive System

Write the name of each numbered part on the corresponding line of the answer sheet.

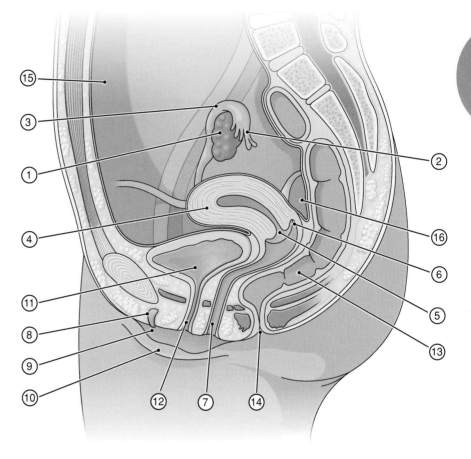

15

Anus   1. _____

Cervix   2. _____

Clitoris   3. _____

Cul-de-sac   4. _____

Fimbriae   5. _____

Labium majus   6. _____

Labium minus   7. _____

Ovary   8. _____

Oviduct (fallopian tube) 9. _____

(continued on next page)

15

Peritoneal cavity	10. _____
Posterior fornix	11. _____
Rectum	12. _____
Urethra	13. _____
Urinary bladder	14. _____
Uterus	15. _____
Vagina	16. _____

Ovulation and Fertilization

Write the name of each numbered part on the corresponding line of the answer sheet.

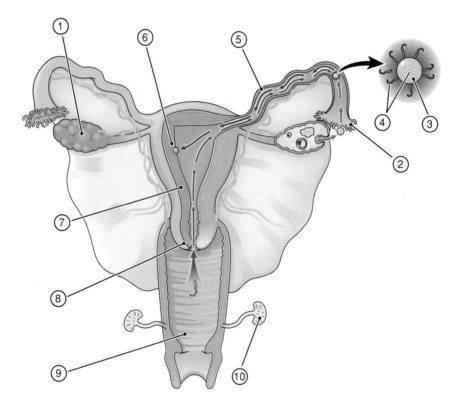

Cervix	1. _____
Corpus (body) of uterus	2. _____
Fimbriae	3. _____
Greater vestibular (Bartholin) gland	4. _____

Implanted embryo   5. _____

Ovary   6. _____

Oviduct (fallopian tube)   7. _____

Ovum   8. _____

Sperm cells (spermatozoa)   9. _____

Vagina   10. _____

15

TERMINOLOGY

Match the following terms and write the appropriate letter to the left of each number:

_____	1. vulva	a. fertilized egg
_____	2. gestation	b. female erectile tissue
_____	3. oxytocin	c. external female genitalia
_____	4. zygote	d. period of development in the uterus
_____	5. clitoris	e. hormone that stimulates labor

_____	6. menarche	a. producing female characteristics
_____	7. metrorrhagia	b. wasting of uterine tissue
_____	8. metratrophia	c. excess uterine bleeding
_____	9. gynecogenic	d. suppression of menstruation
_____	10. menostasis	e. first menstrual period

_____	11. eutocia	a. present at birth
_____	12. congenital	b. absence of a normal body opening
_____	13. atresia	c. normal labor
_____	14. rubella	d. genetic change
_____	15. mutation	e. German measles

Supplementary Terms

_____	16. hymen	a. uterine discharge after childbirth
_____	17. areola	b. period after childbirth
_____	18. meconium	c. first feces of the newborn
_____	19. lochia	d. a pigmented ring
_____	20. puerperium	e. membrane that covers the vaginal opening

_____	**21.** dyspareunia
_____	**22.** speculum
_____	**23.** leukorrhea
_____	**24.** umbilicus
_____	**25.** fontanel

a. whitish vaginal discharge

b. instrument used to enlarge an opening for examination

c. pain during intercourse

d. soft spot between cranial bones

e. navel

15

Fill in the blanks:

26. The female gonad is the _____.

27. The graafian follicle encloses a developing _____.

28. The tissue that nourishes and maintains the developing fetus is the _____.

29. The secretion of milk from the mammary glands is called _____.

30. Loss of an embryo or fetus before 20 weeks or 500 g is termed a(n) _____.

31. Parametritis (*par-a-mē-TRĪ-tis*) means inflammation of the tissue near the _____.

32. Polymastia (*pol-ē-MAS-tē-a*) means the presence of more than one pair of _____.

True–False. Examine the following statements. If the statement is true, write T in the first blank. If the statement is false, write F in the first blank and correct the statement by replacing the <u>underlined</u> word in the second blank.

33. Parturition is <u>childbirth</u>. _____ _____

34. The fallopian tube is the <u>oviduct</u>. _____ _____

35. The lining of the uterus is the <u>myometrium</u>. _____ _____

36. After ovulation, the ovarian follicle becomes a <u>fimbriae</u>. _____ _____

37. Fertilization of an ovum occurs in the <u>uterus</u>. _____ _____

38. Agalactia is the lack of <u>milk</u> production. _____ _____

39. For the first two months, the developing offspring is called a <u>fetus</u>. _____ _____

Eliminations. In each of the sets below, underline the word that does not fit in with the rest and explain the reason for your choice:

40. umbilical cord – labia majora – amniotic fluid – chorion – placenta

_____

41. colostrum – progesterone – LH – estrogen – FSH

_____

42. hemophilia – albinism – measles – PKU – cystic fibrosis

_____

43. amniocentesis – chorionic villus sampling – karyotype – ultrasonography – candidiasis

_____

44. placental abruption – spina bifida – pregnancy induced hypertension – placenta previa – eclampsia

_____

Define the following terms:

45. metromalacia (*mē-trō-ma-LĀ-shē-a*) _____

46. retrouterine (*re-trō-Ū-ter-in*) _____

47. hysteropathy (*his-te-ROP-a-thē*) _____

48. colpostenosis (*kol-pō-ste-NŌ-sis*) _____

49. pyosalpinx (*pī-ō-SAL-pinx*) _____

50. anovulatory (*an-OV-ū-la-tō-rē*) _____

51. submammary (*sub-MAM-a-rē*) _____

52. postnatal (*pōst-NĀ-tal*) _____

53. extraembryonic (*eks-tra-em-brē-ON-ik*) _____

54. nulligravida (*nul-i-GRAV-i-da*) _____

55. tripara (*TRIP-a-ra*) _____

56. teratogenic (*TER-at-ō-jen-ik*) _____

Write words for the following:

57. narrowing of the uterus (metr/o) _____

58. surgical removal of the uterus (hyster/o) and oviducts _____

59. suture of the vulva (episi/o-) _____

60. radiographic study of the breast (mamm/o) _____

61. hernia of an oviduct _____

62. inflammation of the cervix _____

63. rupture of the amniotic sac _____

64. study of the embryo _____

65. measurement of a fetus _____

66. abnormal or difficult labor _____

Synonyms. Write one word that means the same as the following:

67. neonate _____

68. para 1 _____

69. gravida 0 _____

Opposites. Write a word that means the opposite of the following:

70. antepartum _____

71. postnatal _____

72. dystocia _____

73. anovulatory _____

Adjectives. Write the adjective form of the following:

74. cervix _____

75. uterus _____

76. perineum _____

77. vagina _____

78. embryo _____

79. amnion _____

15

Plurals. Write the plural form of the following:

80. ovum   _____

81. cervix   _____

82. fimbria   _____

83. labium   _____

Write the meaning of the following abbreviations:

84. TSS _____

85. IUD _____

86. DUB _____

87. LMP _____

88. GIFT _____

89. GA _____

90. FHR _____

91. VBAC _____

Word analysis. Define the following words and give the meaning of the word parts in each. Use a dictionary if necessary.

92. gynecomastia (*jin-e-kō-MAS-tē-a*) _____

     a. gynec/o _____

     b. mast/o _____

     c. -ia _____

93. oxytocia _____

     a. oxy sharp, acute _____

     b. toc _____

     c. -ia _____

94. oligohydramnios _____

     a. oligo- _____

     b. hydr/o _____

     c. amnio(s) _____

Go to the word exercises in Chapter 15 on the CD-ROM for additional review exercises.

CASE STUDY 15–1: Total Abdominal Hysterectomy with Bilateral Salpingo-Oophorectomy

M.T., a 60-year-old gravida 2, para 2, had spent 3 months under the care of her gynecologist for treatment of postmenopausal bleeding and cervical dysplasia. She had had several vaginal examinations with Pap smears, a uterine ultrasound, colposcopy with endocervical biopsies, and a D&C with cone biopsy. She wanted to take hormone therapy, but her doctor thought she was at too much risk with the abnormal cells on her cervix and the excessive bleeding.

She had a TAH & BSO under general anesthesia with no complications and an uneventful recovery. Her uterus had been prolapsed on abdominal examination, but there was no sign of malignancy or PID. The pathology report revealed several uterine leiomyomas and stenosis of the right oviduct. She was discharged on the second postoperative day with few activity restrictions.

CASE STUDY 15–2: In Vitro Fertilization

C.A. had worked as a technologist in the IVF lab at University Medical Center for 4 years. Her department was the Advanced Reproductive Technology Program. Although her work was primarily in the laboratory, she followed each patient through all five phases of the IVF and embryo-transfer treatment cycle: follicular development, aspiration of the preovulatory follicles, sperm preparation, IVF, and embryo transfer. Her department does both GIFT and ZIFT.

While the female patient is in surgery having an ultrasound-guided transvaginal oocyte retrieval, C.A. examines the recently donated sperm for motility and quantity. She prepares to inoculate the sample into the cytoplasm of the ova as soon as she receives the cells from the OR. After inoculation, she places the sterile Petri dish with the fertilized oocytes into an incubator until they are ready to be introduced into the female patient.

CASE STUDY 15–3: Cesarean Section Birth

A.Y., a gravida 2, para 1 at 39 weeks' gestation, had been in active labor for several hours, fully effaced and dilated, yet unable to progress. She had had an uneventful pregnancy with good health, moderate weight gain, good fetal heart sounds, and no signs or symptoms of pregnancy-induced hypertension. X-ray pelvimetry revealed CPD with the fetus in the right occiput posterior position. Changes in fetal heart rate indicated fetal distress. A.Y. was transported to the OR for emergency C-section under spinal anesthesia.

After being placed in the supine position, A.Y. had a urethral catheter inserted and her abdomen was prepped with antimicrobial solution. After draping, a transverse suprapubic incision was made. Dissection was continued through the muscle layers to the uterus, with care not to

nick the bladder. The uterus was incised through the lower segment, 2 cm from the bladder. The fetal head was gently elevated through the incision while the assistant put gentle pressure on the fundus. The baby's mouth and nose were suctioned with a bulb syringe, and the umbilical cord was clamped and cut. The baby was handed off to an attending pediatrician and OB nurse and placed in a radiant neonate warmer bed. The Apgar score was 9/9. The placenta was gently delivered from the uterus, and the scrub nurse checked for three vessels and filled two sterile test tubes with cord blood for lab analysis. A.Y. was given an injection of Pitocin to stimulate uterine contraction. The uterus and abdomen were closed, and A.Y. was transported to the PACU (postanesthesia care unit).

CASE STUDY QUESTIONS

Multiple choice. Select the best answer and write the letter of your choice to the left of each number:

_____ 1. M.T. is a gravida 2, para 2. This means:
- **a.** she has four children from two pregnancies
- **b.** she has had two pregnancies and two births
- **c.** she has had four pregnancies and two births
- **d.** she has had two pregnancies and two sets of twins
- **e.** she has one set of twins

15

_____ 2. An endocervical biopsy is:
    a. a tissue sample from the cul-de-sac
    b. a cone-shaped tissue sample from the uterine fundus
    c. a tissue sample from within the neck
    d. a tissue sample from the lining of the cervix
    e. a scraping of tissue cells from the vaginal wall

_____ 3. A curettage is a(n):
    a. suturing
    b. scraping
    c. cutting
    d. examination
    e. incision

_____ 4. A colposcopy is an endoscopic examination of the:
    a. vagina
    b. fundus
    c. intraperitoneal pelvic floor
    d. pouch of Douglas
    e. uterus and fallopian tubes

_____ 5. Another name for a leiomyoma is a(n):
    a. ectopic pregnancy
    b. uterine fibroid
    c. myoma
    d. a and b
    e. b and c

_____ 6. Pregnancy-induced hypertension is also called:
    a. tubal pregnancy
    b. congenital mutation
    c. ectopic pregnancy
    d. preeclampsia
    e. placenta previa

_____ 7. The occiput of the fetus is the:
    a. forehead
    b. foot
    c. back of the head
    d. chin
    e. shoulder

_____ 8. Pitocin is the trade name for:
    a. progesterone
    b. estrogen
    c. chorionic gonadotropin
    d. FSH
    e. oxytocin

Write a term from the case studies with each of the following meanings:

9. displaced downward _____

10. cell produced by fertilization _____

11. measurement of the pelvis _____

12. upper rounded portion of the uterus _____

13. method for rating a newborn's physical condition _____

14. afterbirth _____

Define each of the following abbreviations:

15. D&C _____

16. BSO _____

17. PID _____

18. HRT _____

19. IVF _____

20. CPD _____

21. OB _____

22. GYN _____

23. GU _____

Female Reproductive System; Pregnancy and Birth

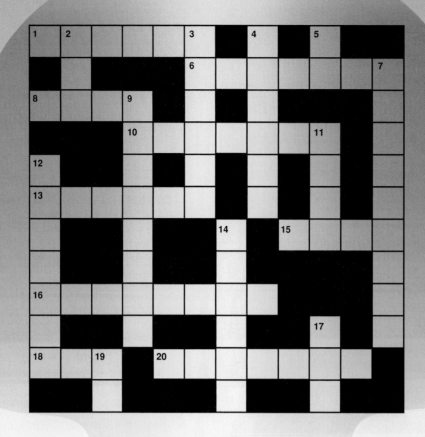

ACROSS

1. Neck of the uterus: root
6. Fallopian tube
8. Vagina: root
10. Outside the normal position
13. Tube between the uterus and the external genitalia
15. Developing infant in the uterus from the third month of gestation: combining form
16. Premature separation of the placenta: _____ placentae
18. In, within: prefix
20. The outermost layer of the embryo; forms the inner portion of the placenta

DOWN

2. Outside, away from: prefix
3. Against: prefix
4. Removal of tissue for laboratory study
5. The reproductive and urinary systems together: abbreviation
7. Substance or agent that causes birth abnormalities
9. The region between the thighs, including the genitalia
11. Hernia, localized dilation; suffix
12. To release an ovum from the ovary
14. Erectile tissue in the female: root
17. Labor: root
19. Down, without, removal: prefix

THE ENDOCRINE SYSTEM

16

OBJECTIVES

After study of this chapter you should be able to:

1. Define hormones.
2. Compare steroid and amino acid hormones.
3. Label a diagram of the endocrine system.
4. Name the hormones produced by the endocrine glands, and briefly describe the function of each.
5. Identify and use roots pertaining to the endocrine system.

6. Describe the main disorders of the endocrine system.
7. Interpret abbreviations used in endocrinology.
8. Analyze several case studies concerning disorders of the endocrine system.

PRETEST

1. The secretions of the endocrine glands are called _____.

2. The small gland in the brain that controls other glands is the _____.

3. The glands that are located above the kidneys are the _____.

4. Diabetes mellitus involves the hormone insulin, which is made by the _____.

5. A goiter involves the _____ gland.

*T*he endocrine system consists of a widely distributed group of glands that secrete regulatory substances called **hormones.** Because hormones are released directly into the blood, the **endocrine** glands are known as the *ductless glands,* as compared to glands that secrete through ducts, such as sweat glands and digestive glands. Despite the fact that hormones circulating in the blood reach all parts of the body, only certain tissues respond to a specific hormone. The tissue that is influenced by a specific hormone is called the **target tissue.** The cells in a target tissue have specific **receptors** on their membranes or within the cell to which the hormone attaches, enabling it to act.

Hormones

Hormones are produced in extremely small amounts and are highly potent. By means of their actions on various target tissues, they affect growth, metabolism, reproductive activity, and behavior. (Box 16-1 describes some old ideas about the effects of substances circulating in the blood.)

Chemically, hormones fall into two categories:

> ➤ **steroid hormones,** which are made from lipids. Steroids are produced by the sex glands (gonads) and the outer region (cortex) of the adrenal glands.
> ➤ hormones made of amino acids, which include proteins and proteinlike compounds. All of the endocrine glands aside from the gonads and adrenal cortex produce amino acid hormones.

The production of hormones is controlled mainly by negative feedback—that is, the hormone itself, or some product of hormone activity, acts as a control over further manufacture of the hormone—a self-regulating system. Hormone production also may be controlled by the nervous system or by other hormones.

The Endocrine Glands

Refer to Figure 16-1 to locate the endocrine glands described below. Box 16-2 lists the endocrine glands, along with the hormones they secrete and their functions.

Box 16•1 Focus on Words   *Are You in a Good Humor?*

*I*n ancient times, people accepted the theory that a person's state of health depended on the balance of four body fluids. These fluids, called "humors," were yellow bile, black bile, phlegm, and blood. A predominance of any one of these humors would determine a person's mood or temperament. Yellow bile caused anger; black bile caused depression; phlegm (mucus) made a person sluggish; blood resulted in cheerfulness and optimism.

Although we no longer believe in humoralism, we still have adjectives in our vocabulary that reflect these early beliefs. Choleric describes a person under the influence of yellow bile; melancholic describes the effects of black bile (melano- means black or dark); a phlegmatic person is slow to respond; a sanguine individual "goes with the flow." (*Sanguine* is from the Greek word for blood.)

The humors persist today in the adjective *humoral,* which describes substances carried in the blood or other body fluids. The term applies to hormones and other circulating materials that influence body responses. Humoral immunity is immunity based on antibodies carried in the bloodstream.

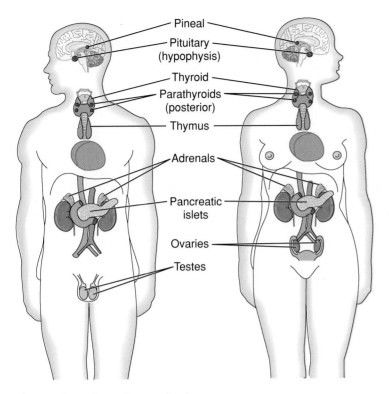

Figure 16-1 The endocrine glands.

Box 16•2 **For Your Reference**	*The Endocrine Glands and Their Hormones*

Gland	Hormone	Principal Functions
anterior pituitary	GH (growth hormone), also called somatotropin (*sō-ma-tō-TRŌ-pin*)	promotes growth of all body tissues
	TSH (thyroid-stimulating hormone)	stimulates thyroid gland to produce thyroid hormones
	ACTH (adrenocorticotropic hormone) (*a-drē-nō-kor-ti-kō-TRŌ-pik*)	stimulates adrenal cortex to produce cortical hormones; aids in protecting body in stress situations (injury, pain)
	FSH (follicle-stimulating hormone)	stimulates growth and hormone activity of ovarian follicles; stimulates growth of testes; promotes development of sperm cells
	LH (luteinizing hormone) (*LŪ-tē-in-ī-zing*)	causes development of corpus luteum at site of ruptured ovarian follicle in female; stimulates secretion of testosterone in male
	PRL (prolactin) (*prō-LAK-tin*)	stimulates milk secretion by mammary glands
posterior pituitary	ADH (antidiuretic hormone; vasopressin) (*an-tē-dī-ū-RET-ik; vā-sō-PRES-in*)	promotes reabsorption of water in kidney tubules; stimulates smooth muscle tissue of blood vessels to constrict
	oxytocin (*ok-sē-TŌ-sin*)	causes contraction of uterus; causes ejection of milk from mammary glands

Box 16•2 **For Your Reference** *Continued*

16

thyroid	thyroxine or tetraiodothyronine (T$_4$) and triiodothyronine (T$_3$) (thī-ROK-sēn; trī-ī-ō-dō-THĪ-rō-nēn)	increase metabolic rate and production of body heat, influencing both physical and mental activities; required for normal growth
	calcitonin (kal-si-TŌ-nin)	decreases calcium level in blood
parathyroids	parathyroid hormone (par-a-THĪ-royd)	regulates exchange of calcium between blood and bones; increases blood calcium level
adrenal cortex	cortisol (hydrocortisone) (KOR-ti-sol)	aids in metabolism of carbohydrates, proteins, and fats; active during stress
	aldosterone (al-DOS-ter-ōn)	aids in regulating electrolytes and water balance
	sex hormones	may influence secondary sexual characteristics
adrenal medulla	epinephrine (adrenaline) and norepinephrine (noradrenaline) (ep-i-NEF-rin; a-DREN-a-lin)	active in response to stress; increases respiration, blood pressure, and heart rate
pancreatic islets	insulin (IN-sū-lin)	aids transport of glucose into cells; required for cellular metabolism of foods, especially glucose; decreases blood sugar levels
	glucagon (GLŪ-ka-gon)	stimulates liver to release glucose, thereby increasing blood sugar levels
pineal	melatonin (mel-a-TŌN-in)	regulates mood, sexual development, and daily cycles in response to light in the environment
thymus	thymosin (THĪ-mō-sin)	important in development of T cells needed for immunity and in early development of lymphoid tissue
testes	testosterone (tes-TOS-te-rōn)	stimulates growth and development of sexual organs plus development of secondary sexual characteristics; stimulates maturation of sperm cells
ovaries	estrogens (ES-trō-jenz)	stimulate growth of primary sexual organs and development of secondary sexual characteristics
	progesterone (prō-JES-ter-ōn)	prepares uterine lining for implantation of fertilized ovum; aids in maintaining pregnancy; stimulates development of secretory parts of mammary glands

Pituitary

The **pituitary gland** (**hypophysis**) is a small gland beneath the brain. It is divided into an anterior lobe (adenohypophysis) and a posterior lobe (neurohypophysis). Both lobes are connected to and controlled by the **hypothalamus,** a part of the brain.

The anterior pituitary produces six hormones. One of these is growth hormone (somatotropin), which stimulates bone growth and acts on other tissues as well (see Box 16-3). The remainder of the pituitary hormones regulate other glands, including the thyroid, adrenals, gonads, and mammary glands (see Box 16-2). The ending *-tropin*, as in *gonadotropin,* indicates a hormone that acts on another gland. The adjective ending is *-tropic,* as in *adrenocorticotropic.*

Box 16•3 Clinical Perspectives — *Growth Hormone: Its Clinical Use Is Growing*

Growth hormone (GH) is produced by the anterior pituitary. It is released mainly at the beginning of deep sleep, so the old belief that you grow while you sleep has some basis in fact. Although GH affects primarily the development of bones and muscles during early growth, it has a general stimulating effect on most other tissues throughout life. Its alternative name, somatotropin, comes from *soma* meaning "body" and *tropin* meaning "acting on." GH is released during times of stress to boost liver output of energy-rich fatty acids when blood-glucose levels drop. A lack of GH in childhood results in dwarfism, and the hormone was initially prescribed only for children with a GH deficiency. Now it has also been approved for children who are in the lowest percentile of height for their age. If a child is still growing, as shown by x-rays of the hand and wrist, GH will lead to some ultimate increase in height. Because GH increases lean muscle mass, it is also touted as a body-building and anti-aging medication. However, it may have some side effects, and its long-term effects are not known. GH for clinical use was initially obtained from cadaver pituitaries, but it is now made by genetic engineering.

The posterior pituitary releases two hormones that are actually produced in the hypothalamus. These hormones are stored in the posterior pituitary until they are needed:

- Antidiuretic hormone (ADH) acts on the kidneys to conserve water and also promotes constriction of blood vessels. Both of these actions serve to increase blood pressure.
- Oxytocin stimulates uterine contractions and promotes milk "letdown" in the breasts during lactation.

Thyroid and Parathyroids

The **thyroid gland** consists of two lobes on either side of the larynx and upper trachea. The lobes are connected by a narrow band (isthmus) (Fig. 16-2). The thyroid secretes a mixture of hormones, mainly thyroxine (T_4) and triiodothyronine (T_3). Because thyroid hormones contain iodine, laboratories can measure their levels and study thyroid gland activity by following the uptake of iodine. Most thyroid hormone in the blood is bound to protein, primarily thyroxine-binding globulin (TBG).

On the posterior surface of the thyroid are four to six tiny **parathyroid glands** that affect calcium metabolism (Fig. 16-3). Parathyroid hormone increases the blood level of calcium. It works with the thyroid hormone thyrocalcitonin, which lowers blood calcium, to regulate calcium balance.

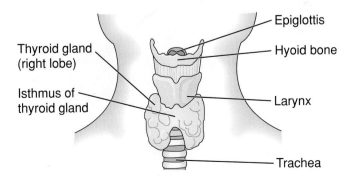

Figure 16-2 Thyroid gland. This anterior view shows the gland in relation to the larynx and trachea.

16

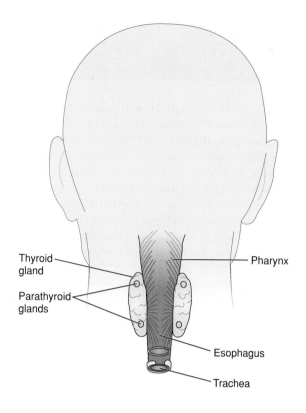

Figure 16-3 Parathyroid glands. A posterior view of the thyroid gland shows the parathyroid glands embedded in its surface.

Adrenals

The **adrenal glands,** located atop the kidneys, are divided into two distinct regions: an outer cortex and an inner medulla (Fig. 16-4). The hormones produced by this gland are involved in the body's response to stress. The cortex produces steroid hormones:

➤ Cortisol (hydrocortisone) mobilizes reserves of fats and carbohydrates to increase the levels of these nutrients in the blood. It also reduces inflammation and is used clinically for this purpose.
➤ Aldosterone causes the kidneys to conserve sodium and water while eliminating potassium.

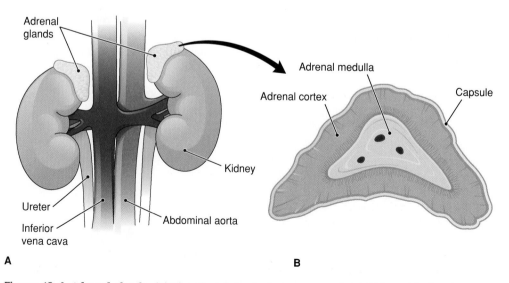

A   B

Figure 16-4 Adrenal glands. (*A*) The adrenal glands shown on top of each kidney. (*B*) The adrenal gland is divided into a medulla and cortex, each secreting different hormones.

16

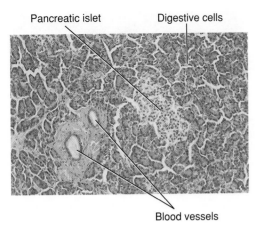

Pancreatic islet   Digestive cells

Blood vessels

Figure 16-5 Pancreatic cells, microscopic view. Light-staining islet cells are seen among the cell clusters that produce digestive juices.

> Sex hormones, mainly testosterone, are also produced in small amounts, but their importance is not well understood. Some athletes, illegally and dangerously, take testosterone-like steroids to increase muscle size, strength, and endurance (see Box 20-1).

The medulla of the adrenal gland produces two similar hormones that are released in response to stress. Epinephrine (adrenaline) and norepinephrine (noradrenaline) work with the nervous system to help the body meet challenges.

Pancreas

The endocrine portions of the pancreas are the **pancreatic islets**, small clusters of cells within the pancreatic tissue. The term *islet*, meaning "small island," is used because these cells look like little islands in the midst of the many pancreatic cells that secrete digestive juices (Fig. 16-5). The islet cells produce two hormones, insulin and glucagon, that regulate sugar metabolism. Insulin increases cellular use of glucose, thus decreasing sugar levels in the blood. Glucagon has the opposite effect, increasing blood sugar levels.

Other Endocrine Tissues

There are three additional types of endocrine glands:

> The **pineal** is a small gland in the brain (see Fig. 16-1). It regulates mood, daily rhythms, and sexual development in response to environmental light. Its hormone is melatonin, which some people take to help regulate sleep-wake cycles when they travel between time zones.
> The thymus, described in Chapter 9, is considered an endocrine gland because it secretes a hormone, thymosin, that stimulates the immune system's T lymphocytes.
> The gonads, the testes and ovaries described in Chapters 14 and 15, are also included because they secrete hormones in addition to producing the sex cells.

Other organs, including the stomach, kidney, heart, and small intestine, also produce hormones. However, they have other major functions and are discussed with the systems to which they belong.

Finally, **prostaglandins** are a group of hormones produced by many cells. They have a variety of effects, including stimulation of uterine contractions, promotion of inflammation, and vasomotor activities. They are called prostaglandins because they were first discovered in the prostate gland.

TERMINOLOGY Key Terms

NORMAL STRUCTURE AND FUNCTION

adrenal gland *a-DRĒ-nal*	A gland on the superior surface of the kidney. The outer region (cortex) secretes steroid hormones; the inner region (medulla) secretes epinephrine (adrenaline) and norepinephrine (noradrenaline) (root: *adren/o*)
endocrine *EN-dō-krin*	Pertaining to a ductless gland that secretes directly into the blood
hormone *HOR-mōn*	A secretion of an endocrine gland. A substance that travels in the blood and has a regulatory effect on tissues, organs, or glands.
hypophysis *hī-POF-i-sis*	The pituitary gland (root: *hypophys*); named from *hypo*, meaning "below," and *physis*, meaning "growing," because the gland grows below the hypothalamus
hypothalamus *hī-pō-THAL-a-mus*	A portion of the brain that controls the pituitary gland and is active in maintaining homeostasis
pancreatic islets *Ī-lets*	Clusters of endocrine cells in the pancreas that secrete hormones to regulate sugar metabolism; also called islets of Langerhans or islet cells (root *insul/o* means "island")
parathyroid glands *par-a-THĪ-royd*	Small endocrine glands on the posterior thyroid that act to increase blood calcium levels; there are usually four to six parathyroid glands (root: *parathyr/o, parathyroid/o*); the name literally means "near the thyroid"
pineal gland *PIN-ē-al*	A small gland in the brain (see Fig. 16-1). Appears to regulate mood, daily rhythms, and sexual development in response to environmental light. Secretes the hormone melatonin.
pituitary gland *pi-TŪ-i-tar-ē*	A small endocrine gland at the base of the brain. The anterior lobe secretes growth hormone and hormones that stimulate other glands; the posterior lobe releases ADH and oxytocin manufactured in the hypothalamus.
prostaglandins *pros-ta-GLAN-dinz*	A group of hormones produced throughout the body that have a variety of effects, including stimulation of uterine contractions and regulation of blood pressure, blood clotting, and inflammation
receptor	A site on the cell membrane or within the cell to which a substance, such as a hormone, attaches
steroid hormone *STER-oyd*	A hormone made from lipids and including the sex hormones and the hormones of the adrenal cortex
target tissue	The specific tissue on which a hormone acts; may also be called the target organ
thyroid gland *THĪ-royd*	An endocrine gland on either side of the larynx and upper trachea. It secretes hormones that affect metabolism and growth and a hormone (calcitonin) that regulates calcium balance (root: *thyr/o, thyroid/o*).

Go to the pronunciation glossary in Chapter 16 of the CD-ROM to hear these words pronounced.

Roots Pertaining to the Endocrine System

ROOT	MEANING	EXAMPLE	DEFINITION OF EXAMPLE
Table 16·1	**Roots Pertaining to the Endocrine System**		
endocrin/o	endocrine glands or system	endocrinology *en-dō-krin-OL-ō-jē*	study of the endocrine glands
pituitar	pituitary gland, hypophysis	pituitarism *pi-TŪ-i-ta-rizm*	condition caused by any disorder of pituitary function
hypophys	pituitary gland, hypophysis	hypophysectomy *hī-pōf-i-SEK-tō-mē*	excision of the pituitary gland
thyr/o, thyroid/o	thyroid gland	thyrolytic *thī-rō-LIT-ik*	destroying the thyroid gland
parathyr/o, parathyroid/o	parathyroid gland	hyperparathyroidism *hī-per-par-a-THĪ-royd-izm*	overactivity of a parathyroid gland
adren/o, adrenal/o	adrenal gland, epinephrine	adrenergic *ad-ren-ER-jik*	activated (erg-) by or related to epinephrine (adrenaline)
adrenocortic/o	adrenal cortex	adrenocorticotropic *a-drē-nō-kor-ti-kō-TRŌ-pik*	acting on the adrenal cortex
insul/o	pancreatic islets	insular *IN-sū-lar*	pertaining to islet cells

16

Exercise 16-1

Define the following words:

1. endocrinopathy (*en-dō-kri-NOP-a-thē*) _____

2. hypophysial (*hī-pō-FIZ-ē-al*) _____

3. thyrotropic (*thī-rō-TROP-ik*) _____

4. hypoadrenalism (*hī-pō-a-DRĒ-nal-izm*) _____

5. insulitis (*in-sū-LĪ-tis*) _____

*Words for conditions resulting from endocrine dysfunctions are formed by adding the suffix **-ism** to the name of the gland or its root and adding the prefix **hyper-** or **hypo-** for overactivity or underactivity of the gland. Use the full name of the gland to form words with the following definitions:*

6. condition of underactivity of the thyroid gland _____

7. condition of underactivity of the parathyroid gland _____

8. condition of overactivity of the adrenal gland _____

Use the word root for the gland to form words with the following definitions:

9. condition of overactivity of the adrenal cortex _____

10. condition of underactivity of the pituitary gland (use pituitar) _____

Word building. Write a word for the following definitions:

11. physician who specializes in study of the endocrine system

   _____

12. incision into the thyroid gland

   _____

13. any disease of the adrenal gland

   _____

14. inflammation of the adrenal gland

   _____

15. tumor of the pancreatic islets

   _____

16

Clinical Aspects of the Endocrine System

Endocrine diseases usually result from the overproduction (hypersecretion) or under-production (hyposecretion) of hormones. They also may result from secretion at the wrong time or from failure of the target tissue to respond. The causes of abnormal secretion may originate in the gland itself or may result from failure of the hypothalamus or the pituitary to release the proper amount of hormone stimulators. Some of the common endocrine disorders are described below. Conditions resulting from hypersecretion or hyposecretion of hormones are summarized in Box 16-4.

Pituitary

A pituitary **adenoma** (glandular tumor) usually increases secretion of growth hormone or adrenocorticotropic hormone (ACTH). Less commonly, a tumor affects the secretion of prolactin. An excess of growth hormone in children causes **gigantism.** In adults it causes **acromegaly,** characterized by enlargement of the hands, feet, jaw, and facial features. Treatment is by surgery to remove the tumor (adenomectomy) or by drugs to reduce the level of growth hormone in the blood. Excess ACTH overstimulates the adrenal cortex, resulting in **Cushing disease.** Increased prolactin causes milk secretion, or galactorrhea, in both males and females. Radiographic studies in cases of pituitary adenoma usually show enlargement of the skull's bony socket (sella turcica) that contains the pituitary.

Box 16•4 For Your Reference   *Disorders Associated with Endocrine Dysfunction**

Hormone	Hypersecretion	Hyposecretion
growth hormone	gigantism (children), acromegaly (adults)	dwarfism (children)
antidiuretic hormone	syndrome of inappropriate ADH (SIADH)	diabetes insipidus
aldosterone	aldosteronism	Addison disease
cortisol	Cushing syndrome	Addison disease
thyroid hormone	Graves disease, thyrotoxicosis	congenital hypothyroidism (children), myxedema (adults)
insulin	hypoglycemia	diabetes mellitus
parathyroid hormone	bone degeneration	tetany (muscle spasms)

*Refer to key terms for pronunciations and descriptions.

Pituitary hypofunction, as caused by tumor or interruption of the gland's supply, may involve a single hormone but usually affects all functions and is referred to as **panhypopituitarism.** The widespread effects of this condition include dwarfism (from lack of growth hormone), lack of sexual development and sexual function, fatigue, and weakness.

A specific lack of ADH from the posterior pituitary results in **diabetes insipidus,** in which the kidneys have a decreased ability to conserve water. Symptoms are polyuria (elimination of large amounts of urine) and polydipsia (excessive thirst). Diabetes insipidus should not be confused with diabetes mellitus, a disorder of glucose metabolism described below. The two diseases share the symptoms of polyuria and polydipsia but have entirely different causes. Diabetes mellitus is the more common disorder, and when the term *diabetes* is used alone, it generally refers to diabetes mellitus. The word *diabetes* is from the Greek meaning "siphon," referring to the large urinary output in both forms of diabetes.

Thyroid

Because the thyroid hormone affects the growth and function of many tissues, a deficiency of this hormone in infancy causes physical and mental retardation as well as other symptoms that together constitute **congenital hypothyroidism,** formerly called cretinism. The United States and other developed countries now require testing of newborns for hypothyroidism. If not diagnosed at birth and treated, hypothyroidism will lead to mental retardation within 6 months.

In adults, thyroid deficiency causes **myxedema,** in which there is weight gain; lethargy; rough, dry skin; hair loss; and facial swelling. There may be reproductive problems and muscular weakness, pain, and stiffness. A common cause of hypothyroidism in adults is autoimmune destruction of the thyroid. Hypothyroidism in both children and adults is easily treated with thyroid hormone.

The most common form of hyperthyroidism is **Graves disease,** also called diffuse toxic goiter. This is an autoimmune disorder in which antibodies stimulate an increased production of thyroid hormone. There is weight loss, irritability, hand tremor, and rapid heart rate (tachycardia). A most distinctive sign is a bulging of the eyeballs, termed **exophthalmos,** caused by swelling of the tissues behind the eyes (Fig. 16-6). Treatment for Graves disease may include antithyroid drugs, surgical removal of all or part of the thyroid, or radiation delivered in the form of radioactive iodine.

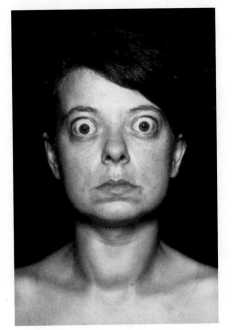

Figure 16-6 Graves disease. A young woman with hyperthyroidism showing a mass in the neck and exophthalmos.

A common sign in thyroid disease is an enlarged thyroid, or **goiter.** However, a goiter is not necessarily accompanied by thyroid malfunction. A simple or nontoxic goiter is caused by a deficiency of iodine in the diet. Such cases are rare in industrialized countries because of the addition of iodine to salt and other commercial foods.

Thyroid function is commonly tested by measuring the gland's radioactive iodine uptake (RAIU). Laboratories use radioimmunoassays to measure blood levels of pituitary thyroid-stimulating hormone (TSH), which varies with changing levels of thyroid hormones. Total and free thyroxine (T_4) and triiodothyronine (T_3) are also measured, as are the levels of TBG, a blood protein that bonds to thyroid hormones. Thyroid scans following administration of radioactive iodine are also used to study the activity of this gland.

Parathyroids

Overactivity of the parathyroid glands, usually from a tumor, causes a high level of calcium in the blood. Because this calcium is obtained from the bones, there is also degeneration of the skeleton and bone pain. A common side effect is the development of kidney stones from the high levels of circulating calcium.

Damage to the parathyroids or their surgical removal, as during thyroid surgery, results in a decrease in blood calcium levels. This causes numbness and tingling in the arms and legs and around the mouth (perioral), as well as **tetany** (muscle spasms). Treatment consists of supplying calcium.

Adrenals

Hypofunction of the adrenal cortex, or **Addison disease,** is usually caused by autoimmune destruction of the gland. It may also result from a deficiency of ACTH from the pituitary. The lack of aldosterone results in water loss, low blood pressure, and electrolyte imbalance. There is also weakness and nausea and an increase of brown pigmentation. This last symptom is caused by release of a hormone from the pituitary that stimulates the skin's pigment cells (melanocytes). Once diagnosed, Addison disease is treated with replacement cortical hormones.

An excess of adrenal cortical hormones results in **Cushing syndrome.** Patients with this syndrome have a moon-shaped face, obesity localized in the torso, weakness, excess hair growth (hirsutism), and fluid retention (Fig. 16-7). The most common cause of Cushing syndrome is the therapeutic administration of steroid hormones. An adrenal tumor is another possible cause. If the disorder is caused by a pituitary tumor that increases production of ACTH, it is referred to as **Cushing disease.**

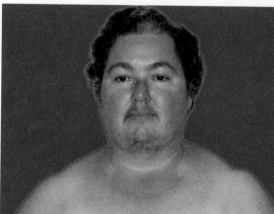

Figure 16-7 Cushing syndrome. The woman has a moon face, buffalo hump, increased facial hair, and thinning of the scalp hair.

The Pancreas and Diabetes

The most common endocrine disorder, and a serious public health problem, is **diabetes mellitus (DM),** a failure of the body cells to use glucose effectively. The excess glucose accumulates in the blood, causing **hyperglycemia.** Increased urination (polyuria) marks the effort to eliminate the excess glucose in the urine, a condition termed **glycosuria.** The result is dehydration and excessive thirst (polydipsia). There is also weakness, weight loss, and extreme hunger (polyphagia). Unable to use carbohydrates, the body burns more fat. This leads to accumulation of ketone bodies in the blood and a shift toward acidosis, a condition termed **ketoacidosis.** If untreated, diabetes will lead to starvation of the central nervous system and coma. Diabetic patients are prone to cardiovascular, neurologic, and visual problems, infections, and renal failure.

Types of Diabetes Mellitus

There are two main types of diabetes mellitus:

➤ Type 1 diabetes mellitus (T1DM) is caused by autoimmune destruction of pancreatic islet cells and failure of the pancreas to produce insulin. It has an abrupt onset and usually appears in children and teenagers. Because insulin levels are very low or absent, patients need careful monitoring and regular administration of this hormone. The former names for type 1 DM, juvenile-onset and insulin-dependent diabetes mellitus (IDDM) are not accurate, because this form of the disease may develop past early youth and also because many people with type 2 diabetes require insulin.

➤ Type 2 diabetes mellitus (T2DM) accounts for about 90 percent of diabetes cases. Heredity plays a much greater role in this form of diabetes than in type 1. Type 2 diabetes is initiated by cellular resistance to insulin. Feedback stimulation of the pancreatic islets leads to overproduction of insulin followed by a failure of the overworked cells to produce enough insulin to meet needs. Most cases of type 2 diabetes are linked to obesity, especially upper-body obesity. Although seen mostly in older people, the incidence of type 2 diabetes is increasing among younger generations, presumably because of increased obesity, poor diet, and sedentary habits. For this reason and also because of possible insulin need, the former names, adult-onset DM and non-insulin-dependent DM (NIDDM), have been dropped.

Metabolic syndrome (also called syndrome X or insulin resistance syndrome) is related to T2DM and describes a state of hyperglycemia caused by insulin resistance in association with some metabolic disorders, including high levels of plasma triglycerides (fats), low levels of high-density lipoproteins (HDLs), hypertension, and coronary heart disease.

Gestational diabetes mellitus (GDM) refers to glucose intolerance during pregnancy. This imbalance usually appears in women with a family history of diabetes and in those who are obese. Women, especially those with predisposing factors, must be monitored during pregnancy for signs of DM because this condition can cause complications for both the mother and the fetus. Gestational diabetes usually disappears after childbirth, but it may be a sign that diabetes will develop later in life. As with other forms of diabetes, a proper diet is a first step to management, with insulin treatment if needed.

Diabetes mellitus may also follow other endocrine disorders or treatment with corticosteroids and may be caused by a genetic disorder of the pancreatic islets.

Diagnosis

Diabetes is diagnosed by measuring glucose levels in blood plasma with or without fasting. The standard for diagnosis of diabetes in a random test is >200 mg/dL and for a fasting plasma glucose (FPG) >126 mg/dL. Measuring glucose levels in the blood after oral administration of glucose is an oral glucose tolerance test (OGTT). Categories of impaired fasting blood glucose (IFG) and impaired glucose tolerance (IGT) are stages between a normal response to glucose and diabetes.

Treatment

People with T1DM must monitor blood sugar levels four to eight times a day. Traditionally, this is done with blood obtained by a finger stick, but new methods of monitoring glucose through the skin are available. Systems for continuous monitoring are also available, and these can alert patients to high and low blood glucose levels. Insulin may be given in divided doses by injection or by means of an insulin pump that delivers the hormone around the clock (continuous subcutaneous insulin infusion; CSII). Newer computerized pumps monitor glucose levels and adjust insulin dosage automatically. Diet must be carefully regulated to keep glucose levels steady.

While managing diabetes, patients monitor their own glucose levels on a daily basis. Every few months, physicians obtain more precise indications of long-term glucose control with a **glycated hemoglobin (HbA1c) test.** This test is based on glucose uptake by red blood cells and reflects the average blood glucose levels for 2 to 3 months before the test.

Exercise and weight loss for those who are overweight are the first approaches to treating type 2 diabetes, and these measures often lead to management of the disorder. Drugs for increasing insulin production or improving cellular responses to insulin may also be prescribed, with insulin treatment given if necessary.

Insulin is now made by genetic engineering. There are various forms with different action times that can be alternated to achieve glucose regulation. Excess insulin may result from a pancreatic tumor, but more often it occurs after administration of too much hormone to a diabetic patient. The resultant **hypoglycemia** leads to **insulin shock,** which is treated by the administration of glucose.

Methods of administering insulin in pills or capsules, inhaler spray, or skin patches are still experimental. Researchers are also studying the possibility of transplanting healthy pancreas or islet cells to compensate for failed cells. Another area of research is the use of immunosuppression to halt type 1 DM.

Also used to diagnose endocrine disorders are imaging techniques, other measurements of hormones or their metabolites in plasma and urine, and studies involving hormone stimulation or suppression.

TERMINOLOGY   Key Terms

DISORDERS

acromegaly *ak-rō-MEG-a-lē*	Overgrowth of bone and soft tissue, especially in the hands, feet, and face, caused by an excess of growth hormone in an adult. The name comes from *acro* meaning "extremity" and *megal/o* meaning "enlargement."
Addison disease	A disease resulting from deficiency of adrenocortical hormones. It is marked by darkening of the skin, weakness, and alterations in salt and water balance.
adenoma *ad-e-NŌ-ma*	A neoplasm of a gland
congenital hypothyroidism	A condition caused by congenital lack of thyroid secretion and marked by arrested physical and mental development; formerly called cretinism (*KRĒ-tin-izm*)
Cushing disease	Overactivity of the adrenal cortex resulting from excess production of ACTH by the pituitary

TERMINOLOGY
Continued

Key Terms

Cushing syndrome	A condition resulting from an excess of hormones from the adrenal cortex. It is associated with obesity, weakness, hyperglycemia, hypertension, and hirsutism (excess hair growth).
diabetes insipidus *dī-a-BĒ-tēz in-SIP-i-dus*	A disorder caused by insufficient release of ADH from the posterior pituitary. It results in excessive thirst and production of large amounts of very dilute urine. The word insipidus means "tasteless," referring to the dilution of the urine.
diabetes mellitus *MEL-i-tus*	A disorder of glucose metabolism caused by deficiency of insulin production or failure of the tissues to respond to insulin. Type 1 results from autoimmune destruction of pancreatic islet cells; it generally appears in children and requires insulin administration. Type 2 generally occurs in obese adults; it is treated with diet, exercise, drugs to improve insulin production or activity, and sometimes insulin. The word *mellitus* comes from the Latin root for honey, referring to the sugar content of the urine.
exophthalmos *ek-sof-THAL-mos*	Protrusion of the eyeballs, as seen in Graves disease
gigantism *JĪ-gan-tizm*	Overgrowth caused by an excess of growth hormone from the pituitary during childhood; also called giantism
glycated hemoglobin (HbA1c) test *GLĪ-kā-ted*	A test that measures the binding of glucose to hemoglobin during the lifespan of a red blood cell. It reflects the average blood glucose level over 2 to 3 months and is useful in evaluating long-term therapy for diabetes mellitus. Also called A1c test.
glycosuria *glī-kō-SŪ-rē-a*	Excess sugar in the urine
goiter *GOY-ter*	Enlargement of the thyroid gland. May be toxic or nontoxic. Simple (nontoxic) goiter is caused by iodine deficiency.
Graves disease	An autoimmune disease resulting in hyperthyroidism. A prominent symptom is exophthalmos (protrusion of the eyeballs). Also called diffuse toxic goiter.
hyperglycemia *hī-per-glī-SĒ-mē-a*	Excess glucose in the blood
hypoglycemia *hī-pō-glī-SĒ-mē-a*	Abnormally low level of glucose in the blood
insulin shock	A condition resulting from an overdose of insulin, causing hypoglycemia
ketoacidosis *kē-tō-as-i-DŌ-sis*	Acidosis (increased acidity of body fluids) caused by an excess of ketone bodies, as in diabetes mellitus; diabetic acidosis
metabolic syndrome	A state of hyperglycemia caused by cellular resistance to insulin, as seen in type 2 diabetes, in association with other metabolic disorders; syndrome X or insulin resistance syndrome

16

TERMINOLOGY Key Terms

Continued

myxedema *miks-e-DĒ-ma*	A condition caused by hypothyroidism in an adult. There is dry, waxy swelling most notable in the face.
panhypopituitarism *pan-hī-pō-pi-TŪ-i-ta-rism*	Underactivity of the entire pituitary gland
tetany *TET-a-nē*	Irritability and spasms of muscles; may be caused by low blood calcium and other factors

Go to the pronunciation glossary in Chapter 16 on the CD-ROM to hear these words pronounced.

TERMINOLOGY Supplementary Terms

NORMAL STRUCTURE AND FUNCTION

sella turcica *SEL-a TUR-si-ka*	A saddle-shaped depression in the sphenoid bone that contains the pituitary gland (literally means "Turkish saddle")
sphenoid bone *SFĒ-noyd*	A bone at the base of the skull that houses the pituitary gland

SYMPTOMS AND CONDITIONS

adrenogenital syndrome *ad-rē-nō-JEN-i-tal*	Condition caused by overproduction of androgens from the adrenal cortex, resulting in masculinization; may be congenital or acquired, usually as a result of an adrenal tumor
Conn syndrome	Hyperaldosteronism caused by an adrenal tumor
craniopharyngioma *krā-nē-ō-far-in-jē-Ō-ma*	A tumor of the pituitary gland
Hashimoto disease *ha-shē-MŌ-tō*	A chronic thyroiditis of autoimmune origin
impaired glucose tolerance (IGT)	High blood glucose levels after glucose intake that may signal borderline diabetes mellitus

TERMINOLOGY Supplementary Terms

Continued

ketosis *kē-TŌ-sis*	Accumulation of ketone bodies, such as acetone, in the body. Usually results from deficiency or faulty metabolism of carbohydrates, as in cases of diabetes mellitus and starvation.
multiple endocrine neoplasia (MEN)	A hereditary disorder that causes tumors in several endocrine glands; classified according to the combination of glands involved
pheochromocytoma *fē-ō-krō-mō-sī-TŌ-ma*	A usually benign tumor of the adrenal medulla or other structures containing chromaffin cells (cells that stain with chromium salts); *phe/o* means "brown" or "dusky." The adrenal tumor causes increased production of epinephrine and norepinephrine.
pituitary apoplexy *AP-ō-plek-sē*	Sudden massive hemorrhage and degeneration of the pituitary gland associated with a pituitary tumor. Common symptoms include severe headache, visual problems, and loss of consciousness.
seasonal affective disorder (SAD)	A mood disorder with lethargy, depression, excessive need for sleep, and overeating that generally occurs in winter. Thought to be related to melatonin levels as influenced by environmental light. See Box 16-5
Simmonds disease	Hypofunction of the anterior pituitary (panhypopituitarism), usually because of an infarction; pituitary cachexia (*ka-KEK-sē-a*)
thyroid storm	A sudden onset of the symptoms of thyrotoxicosis occurring in patients with hyperthyroidism who are untreated or poorly treated. May be brought on by illness or trauma. Also called thyroid crisis.
thyrotoxicosis *thī-rō-tok-si-KŌ-sis*	Condition resulting from overactivity of the thyroid gland. Symptoms include anxiety, irritability, weight loss, and sweating. The main example of thyrotoxicosis is Graves disease.
von Recklinghausen disease	Degeneration of bone caused by excess production of parathyroid hormone. Also called Recklinghausen disease of bone.

DIAGNOSIS AND TREATMENT

fasting plasma glucose (FPG)	Measurement of glucose in the blood after a fast of at least 8 hours. A reading ≥126 mg/dL indicates diabetes. Also called fasting blood glucose (FBG) or fasting blood sugar (FBS).
free thyroxine index (FTI, T_7)	Calculation based on the amount of T_4 present and T_3 uptake, used to diagnose thyroid dysfunction
oral glucose tolerance test (OGTT)	Measurement of glucose levels in blood plasma after administration of a challenge dose of glucose to a fasting patient. Used to measure patient's ability to metabolize glucose. A value ≥200 mg/dL in the 2-hour sample indicates diabetes.
radioactive iodine uptake test (RAIU)	A test that measures thyroid uptake of radioactive iodine as an evaluation of thyroid function

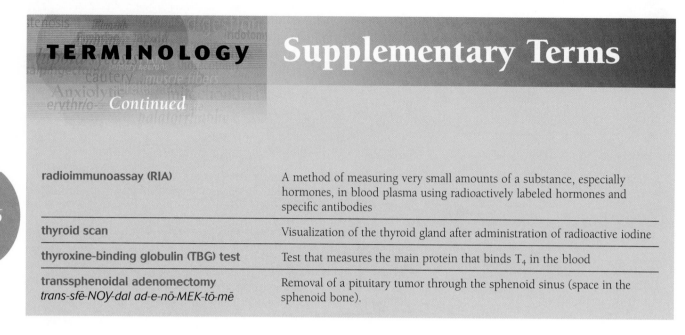

TERMINOLOGY Supplementary Terms

Continued

radioimmunoassay (RIA)	A method of measuring very small amounts of a substance, especially hormones, in blood plasma using radioactively labeled hormones and specific antibodies
thyroid scan	Visualization of the thyroid gland after administration of radioactive iodine
thyroxine-binding globulin (TBG) test	Test that measures the main protein that binds T_4 in the blood
transsphenoidal adenomectomy *trans-sfē-NOY-dal ad-e-nō-MEK-tō-mē*	Removal of a pituitary tumor through the sphenoid sinus (space in the sphenoid bone).

Go to the pronunciation glossary in Chapter 16 of the CD-ROM to hear these words pronounced.

Box 16•5 Clinical Perspectives — *Seasonal Affective Disorder: Some Light on the Subject*

We all sense that long dark days make us blue and sap our motivation. Are these learned responses, or is there a physical basis for them? Studies have shown that the amount of light in the environment does have a physical effect on behavior. Evidence that light alters mood comes from people who are intensely affected by the dark days of winter—people who suffer from **seasonal affective disorder,** aptly abbreviated SAD. When days shorten, these people feel sleepy, depressed, and anxious. They tend to overeat, especially carbohydrates.

As light strikes the retina of the eye, it starts nerve impulses that decrease the amount of melatonin produced by the pineal gland in the brain. Because melatonin depresses mood, the final effect of light is to elevate mood. Daily exposure to bright lights has been found to improve the mood of most people with SAD. Exposure for 15 minutes after rising in the morning may be enough, but some people require longer sessions both morning and evening. Other aids include aerobic exercise, stress-management techniques, and antidepressant medications.

TERMINOLOGY Abbreviations

A1c	Glycated hemoglobin (test)
ACTH	Adrenocorticotropic hormone
ADH	Antidiuretic hormone
BS	Blood sugar
CSII	Continuous subcutaneous insulin infusion
DM	Diabetes mellitus
FBG	Fasting blood glucose
FBS	Fasting blood sugar
FPG	Fasting plasma glucose
FTI	Free thyroxine index
GDM	Gestational diabetes mellitus
GH	Growth hormone
HbA1c	Hemoglobin A1c; glycated hemoglobin
^{131}I	Iodine-131 (radioactive iodine)
IFG	Impaired fasting blood glucose

IGT	Impaired glucose tolerance
MEN	Multiple endocrine neoplasia
NPH	Neutral protamine Hagedorn (insulin)
OGTT	Oral glucose tolerance test
RAIU	Radioactive iodine uptake
RIA	Radioimmunoassay
SIADH	Syndrome of inappropriate antidiuretic hormone (secretion)
T1DM	Type 1 diabetes mellitus
T2DM	Type 2 diabetes mellitus
T_3	Triiodothyronine
T_4	Thyroxine; tetraiodothyronine
T_7	Free thyroxine index
TBG	Thyroxine-binding globulin
TSH	Thyroid-stimulating hormone

16

Chapter Review

Labeling Exercise 16-1
Glands of the Endocrine System

Write the name of each numbered part on the corresponding line of the answer sheet.

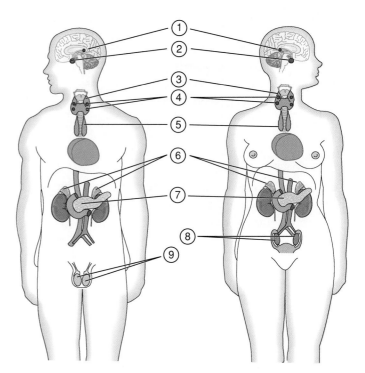

Adrenals	1.	_____
Ovaries	2.	_____
Pancreatic islets	3.	_____
Parathyroids	4.	_____
Pineal	5.	_____
Pituitary (hypophysis)	6.	_____
Testes	7.	_____
Thymus	8.	_____
Thyroid	9.	_____

TERMINOLOGY

Match the following terms and write the appropriate letter to the left of each number:

_____ 1. hypothalamus   **a.** gland important in immunity

_____ 2. posterior pituitary   **b.** pancreatic endocrine cells

_____ 3. pineal   **c.** part of the brain that controls the pituitary

_____ 4. islets   **d.** gland that is regulated by light

_____ 5. thymus   **e.** gland that releases ADH

_____ 6. growth hormone   **a.** pancreatic hormone that regulates sugar metabolism

_____ 7. epinephrine   **b.** hormone produced by the adrenal medulla

_____ 8. hydrocortisone   **c.** hormone that produces uterine contractions

_____ 9. glucagon   **d.** somatotropin

_____ 10. oxytocin   **e.** hormone produced by the adrenal cortex

_____ 11. RAIU   **a.** substance used to monitor blood glucose levels

_____ 12. T$_4$ **b.** test of thyroid function

_____ 13. ACTH   **c.** method for delivering insulin

_____ 14. CSII   **d.** thyroxine

_____ 15. HbA1c   **e.** hormone that stimulates the adrenal cortex

_____ 16. Graves disease   **a.** disorder that results from excess growth hormone

_____ 17. myxedema   **b.** disorder caused by underactivity of the adrenal cortex

_____ 18. Cushing syndrome   **c.** condition caused by hyperthyroidism

_____ 19. acromegaly   **d.** disorder caused by overactivity of the adrenal cortex

_____ 20. Addison disease   **e.** disorder caused by lack of thyroid hormone

Supplementary Terms

_____ 21. sphenoid   **a.** common effect of uncontrolled diabetes mellitus

_____ 22. Hashimoto disease   **b.** tumor of the pituitary gland

_____ 23. pheochromocytoma   **c.** chronic thyroiditis

_____ 24. ketosis   **d.** bone that encloses the pituitary

_____ 25. craniopharyngioma   **e.** tumor of the adrenal medulla

Fill in the blanks:

26. The gland under the brain that controls other glands is the _____.

27. The gland in the neck that affects metabolic rate is the _____.

28. The endocrine glands located above the kidneys are the _____.

29. The most common endocrine disorder is _____.

30. Excess sugar in the blood is called _____.

True-False. Examine the following statements. If the statement is true, write T in the first blank. If the statement is false, write F in the first blank and correct the statement by replacing the underlined word in the second blank.

31. The hypophysis is the <u>pituitary</u> gland.

_____ _____

32. The outer region of an organ is the <u>medulla</u>.

_____ _____

33. The thyroid and parathyroids regulate the element <u>sodium</u>.

_____ _____

34. Goiter is an enlargement of the <u>pineal</u> gland.

_____ _____

35. Thyroid hormones contain the element <u>iodine</u>.

_____ _____

36. The adrenal cortex produces <u>steroid</u> hormones.

_____ _____

37. <u>Type 1</u> diabetes mellitus always requires insulin.

_____ _____

Eliminations. In each of the sets below, underline the word that does not fit in with the rest and explain the reason for your choice:

38. GH — TSH — FSH — ADH — ACTH

_____

39. Cushing syndrome — gigantism — dwarfism — acromegaly — thyrotoxicosis

_____

40. TBG — GDM — FPG — IGT — IFG

_____

41. ovary — larynx — adrenals — parathyroids — pituitary

_____

Define the following words:

42. hypophysial (*hī-pō-FIZ-ē-al*) _____

43. hypopituitarism (*hī-pō-pi-TŪ-i-ta-rizm*) _____

44. adrenopathy (*a-drē-NOP-a-thē*) _____

45. thyroidectomy (*thī-roy-DEK-tō-mē*) _____

46. endocrinologist (*en-dō-kri-NOL-ō-jist*) _____

47. adrenomegaly (*a-drē-nō-MEG-a-lē*) _____

Word building. Write words for the following definitions:

48. inflammation of the hypophysis

_____

49. tumor of the pancreatic islets

_____

50. pertaining to the adrenal cortex

_____

Use the full name of the gland as the root to write words for the following definitions:

51. inflammation of the thyroid gland

_____

52. removal of one half (hemi-) of the thyroid gland

_____

53. surgical removal of parathyroid gland

_____

54. overactivity of the adrenal gland

_____

Use the root *thyr/o* to write words for the following definitions:

55. acting on the thyroid gland _____

56. destructive of (-lytic) thyroid tissue _____

57. any disease of the thyroid gland _____

Word analysis. Define each of the following words, and give the meaning of the word parts in each. Use a dictionary if necessary.

58. euthyroidism _____

    a. eu- _____

    b. thyroid _____

    c. -ism _____

59. panhypopituitarism _____

    a. pan- _____

    b. hypo- _____

    c. pituitar _____

    d. -ism _____

60. thyrotoxicosis _____

    a. thyr/o _____

    b. toxic/o _____

    c. -sis _____

Go to the word exercises in Chapter 16 of the CD-ROM for additional review exercises.

CASE STUDIES

CASE STUDY 16–1: Acute Pancreatitis

Two weeks after his emergency cardiac bypass surgery, R.B. was admitted to the hospital with acute pancreatitis, probably triggered by the trauma of the heart surgery. As a nurse, R.B. knew that the mild form of the disease was self-limiting, whereas severe pancreatitis has a mortality rate near 50 percent. Having survived heart surgery, he was now terrified of having multisystem organ failure develop. He had once cared for a patient who died of necrotizing hemorrhagic pancreatitis.

On admission, R.B. had severe stabbing midepigastric pain that radiated to his back, nausea, vomiting, abdominal distention and rigidity, and jaundice. He also had a low-grade fever, hypotension, tachycardia, and decreased breath sounds over all lung fields. His cardiac enzymes were normal, but he showed an increase in serum leukocytes, amylase, and lipase. CT scan of the abdomen showed pancreatic inflammation with edema. His chest radiograph showed bilateral pleural effusion and atelectasis.

R.B.'s treatments included NPO, an NG tube, medications to decrease his pain and gastric secretions, and supplemental oxygen. He was monitored for all physiologic parameters, with close attention paid to his fluid and electrolyte balance and intravascular volume. He recovered and was discharged after 6 days.

CASE STUDY 16–2: Hyperparathyroidism

B.E., a 58-year-old woman with a history of hypertension, had a partial nephrectomy 4 years ago for renal calculi. During a routine physical examination, her total serum calcium level was 10.8 mg/dL. Her parathyroid hormone level was WNL; she was in no apparent distress, and the remainder of her physical examination and laboratory data were noncontributory.

B.E. underwent exploratory surgery for an enlarged right superior parathyroid gland. The remaining three glands appeared normal. The enlarged gland was excised, and a biopsy was performed on the remaining glands. The pathology report showed an adenoma of the abnormal gland. On her first postoperative day, she reported perioral numbness and tingling. She had no other symptoms, but her serum calcium was subnormal. She was given one ampule of calcium gluconate. Within 2 days, her calcium level had improved and she was discharged.

CASE STUDY 16–3: Diabetes Treatment With an Insulin Pump

M.G., a 32-year-old marketing executive, was diagnosed with type 1 diabetes at the age of 3 years. She vividly remembers her mother taking her to the doctor because she had an illness that caused her to feel extremely tired and very thirsty and hungry. She also had a cut on her knee that would not heal and had begun to wet her bed. Her mother had had gestational diabetes during her pregnancy with M.G., and at birth M.G. was described as having "macrosomia" because she weighed 10 lb.

M.G. has managed her disease with meticulous attention to her diet, exercise, preventive health care, regular blood-glucose monitoring, and twice-daily injections of regular and NPH insulin, which she rotates among her upper arms, thighs, and abdomen. She continues in a smoking-cessation program supported by weekly acupuncture treatments. She maintains good control of her disease in spite of the inconvenience and time it consumes each day. She will be married next summer and would like to start a family. M.G.'s doctor suggested she try an insulin pump to give her more freedom and enhance her quality of life. After intensive training, she has received her pump. It is about the size of a beeper with a thin catheter that she introduces through a needle into her abdominal subcutaneous tissue. She can administer her insulin in a continuous subcutaneous insulin infusion (CSII) and in calculated meal bolus doses. She still has to test her blood for hyperglycemia and hypoglycemia and her urine for ketones when her blood sugar is too high. She hopes one day to have an islet transplantation.

CASE STUDY QUESTIONS

Multiple choice. Select the best answer and write the letter of your choice to the left of each number:

_____ 1. Necrotizing hemorrhagic pancreatitis can be described as:
   a. enlargement of the pancreas with anemia
   b. inflammation of the pancreas with tissue death and bleeding
   c. inflammation of the pancreas with overgrowth of tissue
   d. marsupialization of a pancreatic pseudocyst
   e. none of the above

_____ 2. R.B.'s midepigastric pain was located:
   a. inferior to the sternum
   b. periumbilical
   c. cephalad to the clavicle
   d. lateral to the anterior costal margins
   e. anterolateral

_____ 3. Intravascular volume and hemodynamic stability refer to:
   a. measured amount of urine in the drainage bag
   b. speed with which pancreatic fluid moves
   c. movement of cells through a flow cytometer
   d. body fluids and blood pressure
   e. blood count and clotting factors

_____ 4. Renal calculi are:
   a. kidney stones
   b. gallstones
   c. stomach ulcers
   d. bile obstructions
   e. muscle spasms

_____ 5. B.E.'s serum calcium was 10.8 mg/dL, which is:
   a. 5.4 micrograms of calcium in her serous fluid
   b. 10.8 grams of electrolytes in parathyroid hormone
   c. 10.8 milligrams calcium in 100 mL of blood
   d. 21.6 liters of calcium in 100 grams of serum
   e. 10.8 micrograms of calcium in 100 mL of serous parathyroid fluid

_____ 6. B.E. had perioral numbness and tingling. Perioral is:
   a. peripheral to any orifice
   b. lateral to the eye
   c. within the buccal mucosa
   d. around the mouth
   e. circumferential to the perineum

_____ 7. Gestational diabetes occurs:
   a. in a pregnant woman
   b. to any large fetus
   c. during menopause
   d. at the time of puberty
   e. in a large baby with high blood sugar

16

_____ 8. The term *macrosomia* describes:
   a. excessive weight gain during pregnancy
   b. a large body
   c. an excessive amount of sleep
   d. inability to sleep during pregnancy
   e. too much sugar in the amniotic fluid

_____ 9. M.G. injected the insulin into the subcutaneous tissue, which is:
   a. only present in the abdomen, thighs, and upper arms
   b. a topical application
   c. below the skin
   d. in a large artery
   e. above the pubic bone

_____ 10. An islet transplantation refers to:
   a. transfer of parathyroid cells to the liver
   b. excision of bovine pancreatic cells
   c. surgical insertion of an insulin pump into the abdomen
   d. a total pancreas and kidney transplantation
   e. transfer of insulin-secreting cells into a pancreas

Write terms from the case studies with the following meanings:

11. yellowish color of the skin _____

12. enzyme that digests fats _____

13. surgical excision of a kidney _____

14. tumor of a gland _____

15. single-use glass injectable medication container _____

16. high serum glucose _____

Abbreviations. Define the following abbreviations:

17. NPO _____

18. NG _____

19. BUN _____

20. WNL _____

21. NPH _____

22. CSII _____

Endocrine System

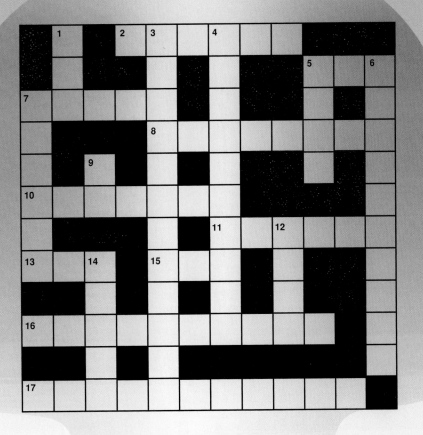

ACROSS

2. An islet is a small _____.
5. Measurement used to diagnose diabetes: abbreviation
7. Temperature: root
8. Sudden degeneration of the pituitary is pituitary _____.
10. Diabetes affects the metabolism of _____.
11. A form of hyperthyroidism is named for him.
13. Pituitary hormone that acts on the thyroid: abbreviation
15. Test for measuring hormones in the blood: abbreviation
16. Alternative name for the pituitary
17. Any disease of the adrenal gland

DOWN

1. Pituitary hormone that controls water loss: abbreviation
3. Alternative name for growth hormone
4. Disorder caused by excess growth hormone in adults
5. A form of thyroid hormones in the blood
6. Excess sugar in the urine
7. The cells or tissues a hormone acts on
9. True, normal: prefix
12. Against: prefix
14. Over, abnormally high: prefix

CHAPTER SEVENTEEN

THE NERVOUS SYSTEM AND BEHAVIORAL DISORDERS

CHAPTER CONTENTS

OBJECTIVES

After study of this chapter you should be able to:

1. Label diagrams showing components of the nervous system.
2. Briefly describe the functions of the regions of the brain.
3. Describe how the central nervous system is protected.
4. Compare the sympathetic and parasympathetic systems.
5. Identify and use word parts pertaining to the nervous system.
6. Describe the major disorders of the nervous system.
7. Describe the major behavioral disorders.
8. List some common symptoms of neurologic disorders.
9. Define abbreviations used in neurology.
10. Interpret case studies involving the nervous system.

PRETEST

1. The basic cell of the nervous system is a(n) _____.

2. The largest part of the brain is the _____.

3. The midbrain, pons, and medulla make up the _____.

4. Involuntary responses are controlled by the _____.

5. A simple response that requires few cells is a(n) _____.

6. A disorder, often of unknown cause, characterized by seizures is called _____.

7. An instrument used to study the electrical activity of the brain is the _____.

8. An extreme, persistent fear is a(n) _____.

*T*he nervous system and the endocrine system coordinate and control the body. Together they regulate our responses to the environment and maintain homeostasis. Whereas the endocrine system functions by means of circulating hormones, the nervous system functions by means of electric impulses and locally released chemicals called **neurotransmitters**.

Organization of the Nervous System

For study purposes, the nervous system may be divided into two parts:

> the **central nervous system (CNS)**, consisting of the brain and spinal cord (Fig 17-1)
> the **peripheral nervous system (PNS)**, consisting of all nervous tissue outside the brain and spinal cord

Functionally, the nervous system can be divided into:

> the **somatic nervous system**, which controls skeletal muscles
> the **visceral** or **autonomic nervous system (ANS)**, which controls smooth muscle, cardiac muscle, and glands. The ANS regulates responses to stress and helps to maintain homeostasis.

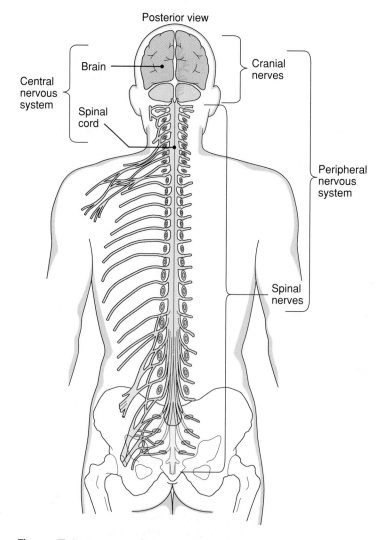

Figure 17-1 Anatomic divisions of the nervous system.

Two types of cells are found in the nervous system. **Neurons**, or nerve cells, make up the conducting tissue of the nervous system. **Neuroglia** are the cells that support and protect nervous tissue.

The Neuron

The neuron is the basic functional unit of the nervous system (Fig. 17-2). Each neuron has two types of fibers extending from the cell body:

> ➤ The **dendrite** carries impulses toward the cell body.
> ➤ The **axon** carries impulses away from the cell body.

Some axons are covered with **myelin**, a whitish, fatty material that insulates and protects the axon and speeds electric conduction. Axons so covered are described as myelinated, and they make up the **white matter** of the nervous system. Unmyelinated tissue makes up the **gray matter** of the nervous system.

Each neuron is part of a pathway that carries information through the nervous system. A neuron that transmits impulses toward the CNS is a **sensory**, or **afferent**, neuron; a neuron that transmits impulses away from the CNS is a **motor**, or **efferent**, neuron. There are also connecting cells within the CNS called **interneurons**.

A **synapse** is the point of contact between two nerve cells. At the synapse, energy is passed from one cell to another, usually by means of a neurotransmitter, and sometimes by direct transfer of electric current.

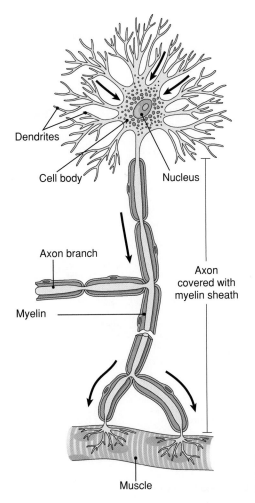

Dendrites

Cell body

Nucleus

Axon branch

Axon covered with myelin sheath

Myelin

Muscle

Figure 17-2 A motor neuron. The break in the axon denotes length. The *arrows* show the direction of the nerve impulse.

17

Nerves

Individual neuron fibers are held together in bundles like wires in a cable. If this bundle is part of the PNS, it is called a **nerve**. A collection of cell bodies along the pathway of a nerve is a **ganglion**. A few nerves (sensory nerves) contain only sensory neurons, and a few (motor nerves) contain only motor neurons, but most contain both types of fibers and are described as mixed nerves.

The Brain

The **brain** is nervous tissue contained within the cranium. It consists of the cerebrum, diencephalon, brainstem, and cerebellum. The **cerebrum** is the largest part of the brain (Fig. 17-3); it is composed largely of white matter with a thin outer layer of gray matter, the **cerebral cortex**. It is within the cortex that the higher brain functions of memory, reasoning, and abstract thought occur. The cerebrum's distinct surface is formed by grooves, or **sulci** (singular: sulcus), and raised areas, or **gyri** (singular: gyrus) that provide additional surface area (Fig. 17-4). The cerebrum is divided into two hemispheres by a deep groove, the longitudinal fissure. Each hemisphere is further divided into lobes with specialized functions (see Fig. 17-4). The lobes are named for the skull bones under which they lie.

The remaining parts of the brain are:

> the **diencephalon** contains the thalamus, the hypothalamus, and the pituitary gland (see Fig. 17-3). The **thalamus** receives sensory information and directs it to the proper portion of the cortex. The **hypothalamus** controls the pituitary and forms a link between the endocrine and nervous systems.
> The **brainstem** (see Fig.. 17-3) consists of:
>> the **midbrain**, which contains reflex centers for improved vision and hearing
>> the **pons**, which forms a bulge on the anterior surface of the brainstem. It contains fibers that connect the brain's different regions.

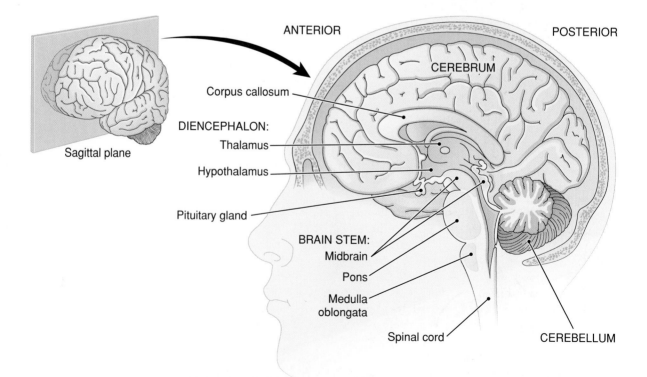

Figure 17-3 Brain, sagittal section. The main divisions are shown.

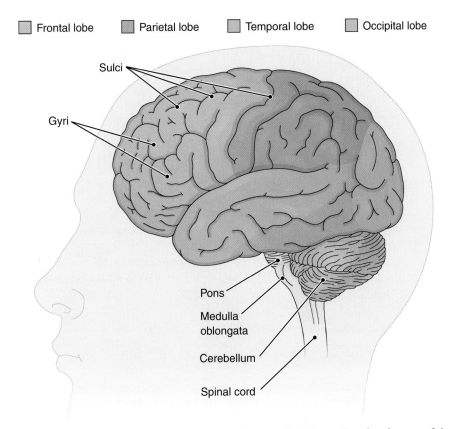

□ Frontal lobe   □ Parietal lobe   □ Temporal lobe   □ Occipital lobe

Sulci

Gyri

Pons

Medulla
oblongata

Cerebellum

Spinal cord

Figure 17-4 External surface of the brain, lateral view. The lobes and surface features of the cerebrum are shown as well as other divisions of the brain and the spinal cord.

> the **medulla oblongata**, which connects the brain with the spinal cord. All impulses passing to and from the brain travel through this region. The medulla also has vital centers for control of heart rate, respiration, and blood pressure.
> The **cerebellum** is under the cerebrum and dorsal to the pons and medulla (see Fig. 17-3). Like the cerebrum, it is divided into two hemispheres. It helps to control voluntary muscle movements and to maintain posture, coordination, and balance.

Protecting the Brain

Within the brain are four **ventricles** (cavities) in which **cerebrospinal fluid (CSF)** is produced. This fluid circulates around the brain and spinal cord, acting as a protective cushion for these tissues.

Covering the brain and the spinal cord are three protective layers, together called the **meninges** (Fig. 17-5). All are named with the Latin word *mater*, meaning "mother," to indicate their protective function.

> The **dura mater** is the outermost and toughest of the three. *Dura* means "hard."
> The **arachnoid mater** is the thin, weblike middle layer. It is named for the Latin word for spider, because it resembles a spider web.
> The **pia mater** is the thin, vascular inner layer, attached directly to the tissue of the brain and spinal cord. *Pia* means "tender."

Twelve pairs of **cranial nerves** connect with the brain (Fig. 17-6). These nerves are identified by Roman numerals and also by name. Box 17-1 is a summary chart of the cranial nerves.

17

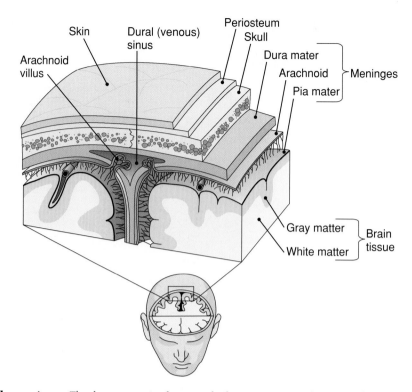

Figure 17-5 The meninges. The three protective layers and adjacent tissue are shown in a frontal section of the head.

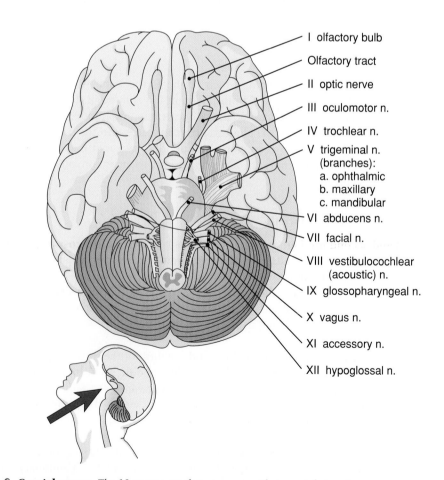

Figure 17-6 Cranial nerves. The 12 nerves are shown on one side in an inferior view.

Box 17·1	For Your Reference	The Cranial Nerves

Number	Name	Function
I	olfactory *ol-FAK-tō-rē*	carries impulses for the sense of smell
II	optic *OP-tik*	carries impulses for the sense of vision
III	oculomotor *ok-ū-lō-MŌ-tor*	controls movement of eye muscles
IV	trochlear *TROK-lē-ar*	controls a muscle of the eyeball
V	trigeminal *trī-JEM-i-nal*	carries sensory impulses from the face; controls chewing muscles
VI	abducens *ab-DŪ-sens*	controls a muscle of the eyeball
VII	facial *FĀ-shal*	controls muscles of facial expression, salivary glands, and tear glands; conducts some impulses for taste
VIII	vestibulocochlear *ves-tib-ū-lō-KOK-lē-ar*	conducts impulses for hearing and equilibrium; also called auditory or acoustic nerve
IX	glossopharyngeal *glos-ō-fa-RIN-jē-al*	conducts sensory impulses from tongue and pharynx; stimulates parotid salivary gland and partly controls swallowing
X	vagus *VĀ-gus*	supplies most organs of thorax and abdomen; controls digestive secretions
XI	spinal accessory *ak-SES-ō-rē*	controls muscles of the neck
XII	hypoglossal *hī-pō-GLOS-al*	controls muscles of the tongue

The Spinal Cord

The spinal cord begins at the medulla oblongata and tapers to an end between the first and second lumbar vertebrae (Fig 17-7). It has enlargements in the cervical and lumbar regions, where nerves for the arms and legs attach to the cord. Seen in cross section (Fig 17-8), the spinal cord has a central area of gray matter surrounded by white matter. The gray matter projects toward the posterior and the anterior as the dorsal and ventral horns. The white matter contains the ascending and descending **tracts** (fiber bundles) that carry impulses to and from the brain. A central canal contains CSF.

The Spinal Nerves

Thirty-one pairs of **spinal nerves** connect with the spinal cord (see Fig 17-7). These nerves are grouped in the segments of the cord as follows:

- ➤ Cervical: 8
- ➤ Thoracic: 12
- ➤ Lumbar: 5
- ➤ Sacral: 5
- ➤ Coccygeal: 1

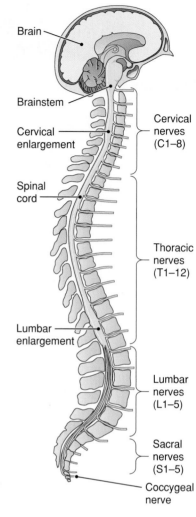

Figure 17-7 Spinal cord, lateral view. The divisions of the spinal nerves are shown.

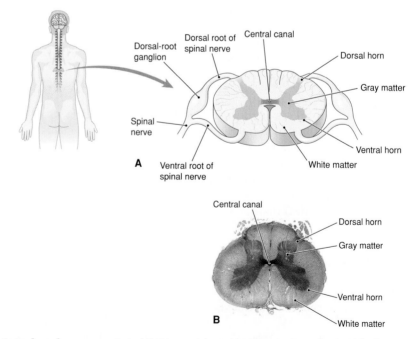

A

Figure 17-8 Spinal cord, cross section. (*A*) Diagram shows the organization of gray and white matter and the roots of the spinal nerves. (*B*) Microscopic view of the spinal cord in cross section (magnification, ×5).

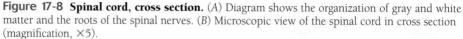

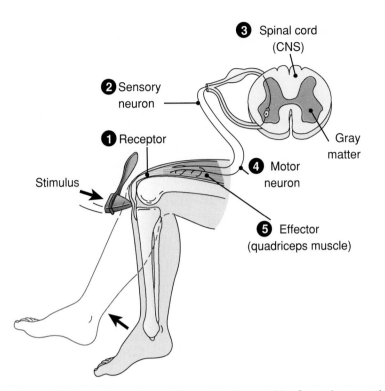

Figure 17-9 A reflex pathway. The patellar (knee-jerk) reflex is shown, with numbers indicating the sequence of impulses.

Each nerve joins the cord by two **roots** (see Fig. 17-8). The dorsal, or posterior, root carries sensory impulses into the cord; the ventral, or anterior, root carries motor impulses away from the cord and out toward a muscle or gland. An enlargement on the dorsal root, the dorsal-root ganglion, has the cell bodies of sensory neurons carrying impulses toward the CNS (see Fig. 17-8).

Reflexes

A simple response that requires few neurons is a **reflex** (Fig. 17-9). In a spinal reflex, impulses travel through the spinal cord only and do not reach the brain. An example of this type of response is the knee-jerk reflex used in physical examinations. Most neurologic responses, however, involve complex interactions among multiple neurons in the CNS.

The Autonomic Nervous System

The autonomic nervous system (ANS) is the division of the nervous system that controls the involuntary actions of muscles and glands (Fig. 17-10). The ANS itself has two divisions:

> The **sympathetic nervous system** motivates our response to stress, the so-called fight-or-flight response. It increases heart rate and respiration rate, stimulates the adrenal gland, and delivers more blood to skeletal muscles.
> The **parasympathetic system** returns the body to a steady state and stimulates maintenance activities, such as digestion of food. Most organs are controlled by both systems and, in general, the two systems have opposite effects on a given organ.

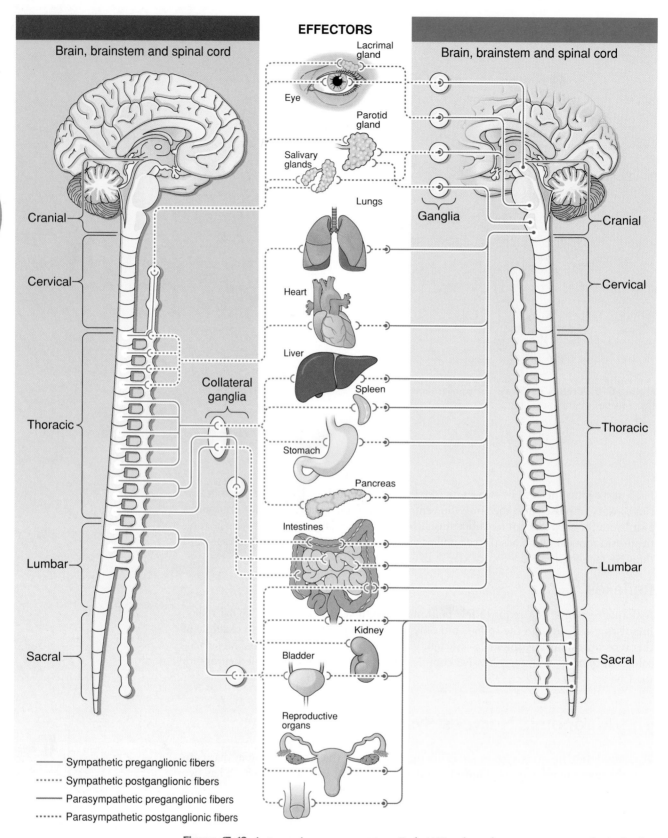

EFFECTORS

Brain, brainstem and spinal cord

Brain, brainstem and spinal cord

Lacrimal gland

Eye

Parotid gland

Salivary glands

Ganglia

Cranial

Cranial

Lungs

Cervical

Cervical

Heart

Liver

Collateral ganglia

Spleen

Thoracic

Thoracic

Stomach

Pancreas

Lumbar

Intestines

Lumbar

Sacral

Kidney

Bladder

Sacral

Reproductive organs

———— Sympathetic preganglionic fibers

·········· Sympathetic postganglionic fibers

———— Parasympathetic preganglionic fibers

·········· Parasympathetic postganglionic fibers

Figure 17-10 Autonomic nervous system. Each ANS pathway has two neurons, as shown by the solid and dashed lines. The diagram shows only one side of the body for each division (sympathetic and parasympathetic).

TERMINOLOGY Key Terms

NORMAL STRUCTURE AND FUNCTION

afferent *AF-er-ent*	Carrying toward a given point, such as the sensory neurons and nerves that carry impulses toward the CNS (root *fer* means "to carry")
arachnoid mater *a-RAK-noyd*	The middle layer of the meninges (from the Greek word for spider, because this tissue resembles a spider web)
autonomic nervous system (ANS) *aw-tō-NOM-ik*	The division of the nervous system that regulates involuntary activities, controlling smooth muscles, cardiac muscle, and glands; the visceral nervous system
axon *AK-son*	The fiber of a neuron that conducts impulses away from the cell body
brain	The nervous tissue contained within the cranium; consists of the cerebrum, diencephalon, brainstem, and cerebellum (root: *encephal/o*)
brainstem	The part of the brain that consists of the midbrain, pons, and medulla oblongata
central nervous system (CNS)	The brain and spinal cord
cerebellum *ser-e-BEL-um*	The posterior portion of the brain dorsal to the pons and medulla; helps to coordinate movement and to maintain balance and posture (*cerebellum* means "little brain") (root: *cerebell/o*)
cerebral cortex *SER-e-bral*	The cerebrum's thin surface layer of gray matter (the cortex is the outer region of an organ) (root: *cortic/o*)
cerebrum *SER-e-brum*	The large upper portion of the brain; it is divided into two hemispheres by the longitudinal fissure (root: *cerebr/o*)
cerebrospinal fluid (CSF) *ser-e-brō-SPĪ-nal*	The watery fluid that circulates in and around the brain and spinal cord as a protection
cranial nerves	The twelve pairs of nerves that are connected to the brain
dendrite *DEN-drīt*	A fiber of a neuron that conducts impulses toward the cell body
diencephalon *dī-en-SEF-a-lon*	The part of the brain that contains the thalamus, hypothalamus, and pituitary gland; located between the cerebrum and the brainstem
dura mater *DŪ-ra MĀ-ter*	The strong, fibrous outermost layer of the meninges
efferent *EF-er-ent*	Carrying away from a given point, such as the motor neurons and nerves that carry impulses away from the CNS (root *fer* means "to carry")
ganglion *GANG-glē-on*	A collection of nerve cell bodies outside the CNS (plural: ganglia; root: *gangli/o, ganglion/o*)
gray matter	Unmyelinated tissue of the nervous system
gyrus *JĪ-rus*	A raised convolution of the surface of the cerebrum (see Fig. 17-4) (plural: gyri)

17

17

hypothalamus *hī-pō-THAL-a-mus*	The part of the brain that controls the pituitary gland and maintains homeostasis
interneuron *in-ter-NŪR-on*	Any neuron located between a sensory and a motor neuron in a neural pathway, such as the neurons that transmit impulses within the CNS
medulla oblongata *me-DUL-la ob-long-GA-ta*	The portion of the brain that connects with the spinal cord. It has vital centers for control of respiration, heart rate, and blood pressure (root: *medull/o*). Often called simply medulla.
meninges *men-IN-jēz*	The three membranes that cover the brain and spinal cord (see Fig. 17-5) (singular: meninx; root: *mening/o, meninge/o*)
midbrain	The part of the brainstem between the diencephalon and the pons; contains centers for coordination of reflexes for vision and hearing
motor	Producing movement; describes neurons that carry impulses away from the CNS
myelin *MĪ-e-lin*	A whitish, fatty substance that surrounds certain axons of the nervous system
neuroglia *nū-ROG-lē-a*	The support cells of the nervous system; also called glial cells (from *glia* meaning "glue"; root: *gli/o*)
neuron *NŪ-ron*	The basic unit of the nervous system; a nerve cell
neurotransmitter	A chemical that transmits energy across a synapse. Examples are epinephrine, acetylcholine (*a-sē-til-KŌ-lēn*), serotonin (*ser-ō-TŌ-nin*), and dopamine (*DŌ-pa-mēn*).
nerve	A bundle of nerve cell fibers outside the CNS (root: *neur/o*)
parasympathetic nervous system	The part of the automatic nervous system that reverses the response to stress and restores homeostasis. It slows heart rate and respiration rate and stimulates activity of the digestive, urinary, and reproductive systems.
peripheral nervous system (PNS) *per-IF-er-al*	The portion of the nervous system outside the CNS
pia mater *PĒ-a MĀ-ter*	The innermost layer of the meninges
pons *ponz*	A rounded area on the ventral surface of the brainstem; contains fibers that connect regions of the brain (adjective: pontine [*PON-tēn*])
reflex *RĒ-fleks*	A simple, rapid, and automatic response to a stimulus
root	A branch of a spinal nerve that connects with the spinal cord; the dorsal (posterior) root joins the dorsal gray horn of the spinal cord; the ventral (anterior) root joins the ventral gray horn of the spinal cord (root: *radicul/o*)

TERMINOLOGY

Continued

Key Terms

sensory *SEN-so-rē*	Describing neurons that carry impulses toward the CNS
somatic nervous system	The division of the nervous system that controls skeletal (voluntary) muscles
spinal cord	The nervous tissue contained within the spinal column; extends from the medulla oblongata to the second lumbar vertebra (root: *myel/o*)
spinal nerves	The 31 pairs of nerves that connect with the spinal cord
sulcus *SUL-kus*	A shallow furrow or groove, as on the surface of the cerebrum (see Fig. 17-4) (plural: sulci)
sympathetic nervous system	The part of the autonomic nervous system that mobilizes a response to stress; increases heart rate and respiration rate and delivers more blood to skeletal muscles
synapse *SIN-aps*	The junction between two neurons
thalamus *THAL-a-mus*	The part of the brain that receives all sensory impulses, except those for the sense of smell, and directs them to the proper portion of the cerebral cortex (root: *thalam/o*)
tract *trakt*	A bundle of nerve cell fibers within the CNS
ventricle *VEN-trik-l*	A small cavity, such as one of the cavities in the brain in which CSF is produced (root: *ventricul/o*)
visceral nervous system	The autonomic nervous system
white matter	Myelinated tissue of the nervous system

Go to the pronunciation glossary in Chapter 17 on the CD-ROM to hear these words pronounced.

Word Parts Pertaining to the Nervous System

Table 17·1	Roots for the Nervous System and the Spinal Cord		
ROOT	**MEANING**	**EXAMPLE**	**DEFINITION OF EXAMPLE**
neur/o, neur/i	nervous system, nervous tissue, nerve	neurotrophin *nū-rō-TRŌ-fin*	factor that promotes nerve growth (*troph/o* = nourish)
gli/o	neuroglia	glioma *glī-Ō-ma*	a neuroglial tumor
gangli/o, ganglion/o	ganglion	ganglionectomy *gang-glē-o-NEK-tō-mē*	surgical removal of a ganglion
mening/o, meninge/o	meninges	meningococci *me-ning-gō-KOK-sī*	cocci (bacteria) that infect the meninges
myel/o	spinal cord (also bone marrow)	myelodysplasia *mī-e-lō-dis-PLĀ-sē-a*	abnormal development of the spinal cord
radicul/o	spinal nerve root	radiculitis *ra-dik-ū-LĪ-tis*	inflammation of a spinal nerve root

Exercise 17-1

Define the following adjectives:

1. neural (*NŪ-ral*) _____ pertaining to a nerve or the nervous system ____

2. glial (*GLĪ-al*) _____

3. ganglionic (*gang-glē-ON-ik*) _____

4. meningeal (*me-NIN-jē-al*) _____

5. radicular (*ra-DIK-ū-lar*) _____

Fill in the blanks:

6. Hematomyelia (*hē-ma-tō-mī-Ē-lē-a*) is hemorrhage into the _____

7. A neurotropic (*nū-rō-TROP-ik*) dye has an affinity for the _____

8. A meningocele (*me-NING-gō-sēl*) is hernia of the _____

9. polyradiculitis (*pol-ē-ra-dik-ū-LĪ-tis*) is inflammation of many _____

Define the following terms:

10. neurolysis (*nū-ROL-i-sis*) _____

11. myelography (*mī-e-LOG-ra-fē*) _____

12. meningioma (*me-nin-jē-Ō-ma*) (combining vowel is i) _____

13. radiculopathy (*ra-dik-ū-LOP-a-thē*) _____

Write words for the following definitions:

14. tumor of a ganglion _____

15. inflammation of the spinal cord _____

16. pain in a nerve _____

17. x-ray image of the spinal cord _____

18. any disease of the nervous system _____

Table 17·2	Roots for the Brain		
ROOT	**MEANING**	**EXAMPLE**	**DEFINITION OF EXAMPLE**
encephal/o	brain	anencephaly *an-en-SEF-a-lē*	absence of a brain
cerebr/o	cerebrum (loosely, brain)	cerebrovascular *ser-ē-brō-VAS-kū-lar*	pertaining to the blood vessels in the brain
cortic/o	cerebral cortex, outer portion	corticospinal *kor-ti-kō-SPĪ-nal*	pertaining to the cerebral cortex and spinal cord
cerebell/o	cerebellum	supracerebellar *sū-pra-ser-e-BEL-ar*	above the cerebellum
thalam/o	thalamus	thalamotomy *thal-a-MOT-ō-mē*	incision of the thalamus
ventricul/o	cavity, ventricle	intraventricular *in-tra-ven-TRIK-ū-lar*	within a ventricle
medull/o	medulla oblongata (also spinal cord)	medullary *MED-ū-lar-ē*	pertaining to the medulla
psych/o	mind	psychoactive *sī-kō-AK-tiv*	acting on the mind
narc/o	stupor, unconsciousness	narcosis *nar-KŌ-sis*	state of stupor induced by drugs
somn/o, somn/i	sleep	somnolence *SOM-nō-lens*	sleepiness

Exercise 17-2

Fill in the blanks:

1. An electroencephalogram (*ē-lek-trō-en-SEF-a-lō-gram*) (EEG) is a record of the electric activity of the

_____

2. The term decerebrate (*dē-SER-e-brāt*) refers to loss of function in the _____.

3. The hypothalamus (*hī-pō-THAL-a-mus*) is below the _____.

4. The term psychogenic (*sī-kō-JEN-ik*) means originating in the _____.

5. A narcotic (*nar-KOT-ik*) is a drug that causes _____.

6. Somnambulism (*som-NAM-bū-lizm*) means walking during _____.

Write an adjective for the following definitions. Note the endings.

7. pertaining to (-al) the cerebrum _____

8. pertaining to (-al) the cerebral cortex _____

9. pertaining to (-ic) the thalamus _____

10. pertaining to (-ar) the cerebellum _____

11. pertaining to (-ar) a ventricle _____

Define the following words:

12. encephalopathy (*en-sef-a-LOP-a-thē*) _____

13. extramedullary (*eks-tra-MED-ū-lar-ē*) _____

14. ventriculotomy (*ven-trik-ū-LOT-ō-mē*) _____

15. cerebrospinal (*ser-e-brō-SPĪ-nal*) _____

16. psychology (*sī-KOL-ō-jē*) _____

17. insomnia (*in-SOM-nē-a*) _____

Write words for the following definitions:

18. inflammation of the brain _____

19. within the cerebellum _____

20. pertaining to the cerebral cortex and the thalamus _____

21. radiograph of a ventricle _____

22. outside (extra-) the cerebrum _____

Table 17·3	Suffixes for the Nervous System		
SUFFIX	**MEANING**	**EXAMPLE**	**DEFINITION OF EXAMPLE**
-phasia	speech	heterophasia *het-er-ō-FĀ-zē-a*	uttering words that are different from those intended
-lalia	speech, babble	coprolalia *kop-rō-LĀ-lē-a*	compulsive use of obscene words (*copro-* means "feces")
-lexia	reading	dyslexia *dis-LEK-sē-a*	difficulty in reading
-plegia	paralysis	tetraplegia *tet-ra-PLĒ-jē-a*	paralysis of all four limbs
-paresis*	partial paralysis	hemiparesis *hem-i-pa-RĒ-sis*	partial paralysis of one side of the body
-lepsy	seizure	narcolepsy *NAR-kō-lep-sē*	condition marked by sudden episodes of sleep
-phobia*	persistent, irrational fear	agoraphobia *ag-o-ra-FŌ-bē-a*	fear of being in a public place (from Greek *agora*, meaning "marketplace")
-mania*	excited state, obsession	megalomania *meg-a-lō-MĀ-nē-a*	exaggerated self-importance; "delusions of grandeur"

*May be used alone as a word.

Exercise 17-3

Fill in the blanks:

1. Echolalia (*ek-ō-LĀ-lē-a*) refers to repetitive _____.

2. Epilepsy (*EP-i-lep-sē*) is a disease characterized by _____.

3. In myoparesis (*mī-ō-pa-RĒ-sis*), a muscle shows _____.

4. A person with alexia (*a-LEK-sē-a*) lacks the ability to _____.

5. Another term for quadriplegia is _____.

Define the following words:

6. aphasia (*a-FĀ-zē-a*) _____

7. bradylexia (*brad-ē-LEK-sē-a*) _____

8. pyromania (*pī-rō-MĀ-nē-a*) _____

9. gynephobia (*jin-e-FŌ-bē-a*) _____

Write words for the following definitions:

10. slowness in speech (-lalia) _____

11. paralysis of one side (hemi-) of the body _____

12. paralysis of the heart _____

13. fear of night and darkness _____

14. fear of (or abnormal sensitivity to) light _____

17

Clinical Aspects of the Nervous System

Vascular Disorders

The term **cerebrovascular accident (CVA)**, or **stroke**, applies to any occurrence that deprives brain tissue of oxygen. These events include blockage in a vessel that supplies the brain, a ruptured blood vessel, or some other damage that leads to hemorrhage within the brain. Stroke is the third leading cause of death in developed countries, after cancer and heart attack (myocardial infarction), and is a leading cause of **paralysis** and other neurologic disabilities. Risk factors for a stroke include hypertension, atherosclerosis, heart disease, diabetes mellitus, and cigarette smoking. Heredity is also a factor.

Thrombosis

Thrombosis is the formation of a blood clot in a vessel. Often, in cases of CVA, thrombosis occurs in the carotid artery, the large vessel in the neck that supplies the brain. Sudden blockage by an obstruction traveling from another part of the body is described as an **embolism**. In cases of stroke, the embolus usually originates in the heart.

These obstructions can be diagnosed by **cerebral angiography** with radiopaque dye, computed tomographic (CT) scans, and other radiographic techniques. In cases of thrombosis, surgeons can remove the blocked section of a vessel and insert a graft. If the carotid artery leading to the brain is involved, a **carotid endarterectomy** may be performed to open the vessel. Thrombolytic drugs for dissolving ("busting") such clots are also available.

17

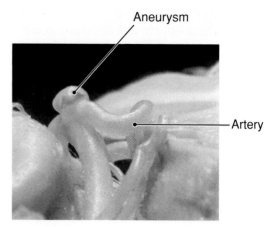

Figure 17-11 Aneurysm. A thin-walled aneurysm protrudes from an artery.

Aneurysm

An **aneurysm** (Fig. 17-11) is a localized dilation of a vessel that may rupture and cause hemorrhage. An aneurysm may be congenital or may arise from other causes, especially atherosclerosis, which weakens the vessel wall. Hypertension then contributes to its rupture.

The effects of cerebral hemorrhage vary from massive loss of function to mild impairment of sensory or motor activity, depending on the degree of damage. **Aphasia**, loss or impairment of speech communication, is a common aftereffect. **Hemiplegia** (paralysis of one side of the body) on the side opposite the damage is also seen. It has been found that in cases of hemorrhage, as in other forms of brain injury, that immediate retraining therapy may help to restore lost function.

Trauma

A **cerebral contusion** is a bruise to the surface of the brain, usually caused by a blow to the head. Blood escapes from local vessels, but the injury is not deep.

A more serious injury may cause bleeding into or around the meninges, resulting in a hematoma, a localized collection of clotted blood. Damage to an artery from a skull fracture, usually on the side of the head, may be the cause of an **epidural hematoma** (Fig. 17-12), which appears between the dura mater and the skull bone. The rapidly accumulating blood puts pressure on local vessels and interrupts blood flow to the brain. There may be headache, loss of consciousness, or **hemiparesis** (partial paralysis) on the side opposite the blow. Diagnosis is made by CT scan or magnetic resonance imaging (MRI). If pressure is not relieved within one or two days, death results.

A **subdural hematoma** (see Fig. 17-12) often results from a blow to the front or back of the head, as when the moving head hits a stationary object. The force of the blow

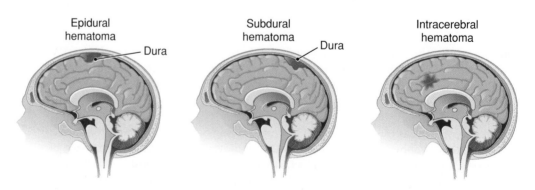

Figure 17-12 Cranial hematomas. Location of epidural, subdural, and intracerebral hematomas are shown.

separates the dura from the arachnoid below. Blood from a damaged vessel, usually a vein, slowly enters this space. The gradual accumulation of blood puts pressure on the brain, causing headache, weakness, and **dementia**. If there is continued bleeding, death results. Figure 17-12 also shows a site of bleeding into the brain tissue itself, forming an intracerebral hematoma.

A cerebral **concussion** results from a blow to the head or from a fall and is usually followed by temporary loss of consciousness and a short period of amnesia. Aftereffects of a concussion may include headache, dizziness, vomiting, fatigue, and even paralysis, among other symptoms. Damage that occurs on the side of the brain opposite a blow as the brain is thrown against the skull is described as a **contrecoup** (*kon-tre-KŪ*) **injury** (from French, meaning "counterblow").

Other injuries may damage the brain directly. Injury to the base of the brain may involve vital centers in the medulla and interfere with respiration and cardiac function.

Confusion and Coma

Confusion is a state of reduced comprehension, coherence, and reasoning ability resulting in inappropriate responses to environmental stimuli. Confusion may worsen to include loss of memory, loss of language ability, reduced alertness, and emotional changes. This condition may accompany a head injury, drug toxicity, extensive surgery, organ failure, infection, or degenerative disease.

Coma is a state of unconsciousness from which one cannot be aroused. Causes of coma include brain injury, epilepsy, toxins, metabolic imbalance (such as the ketoacidosis or sugar imbalances associated with diabetes mellitus), and respiratory, hepatic, or renal failure.

Health-care professionals use various responses to evaluate coma, for example, reflex behavior and responses to touch, pressure, and mild pain, as from a light pin prick. Laboratory tests, EEG, and sometimes CT and MRI scans help to identify the causes of coma.

Infection

Inflammation of the meninges, or **meningitis**, is usually caused by bacteria that enter through the ear, nose, or throat or are carried by the blood. One of these organisms, the meningococcus (*Neisseria meningitidis*), is responsible for meningitis epidemics among individuals living in close quarters. Other bacteria implicated in cases of meningitis include *Haemophilus influenzae, Streptococcus pneumoniae,* and *Escherichia coli*. A stiff neck is a common symptom. The presence of pus or lymphocytes in spinal fluid is also characteristic.

Physicians can withdraw fluid for diagnosis by a **lumbar puncture** (Fig. 17-13), using a needle to remove CSF from the meninges in the lumbar region of the spine. This

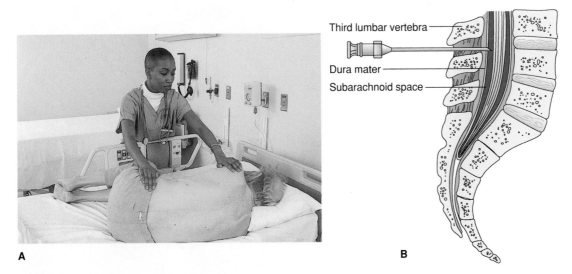

Third lumbar vertebra

Dura mater

Subarachnoid space

A   **B**

Figure 17-13 Lumbar puncture. (*A*) Position of the patient for a lumbar puncture. (*B*) CSF is withdrawn from the subarachnoid space between the third and fourth or fourth and fifth lumbar vertebrae.

fluid can be examined for white blood cells and bacteria in the case of meningitis, for red blood cells in the case of brain injury, or for tumor cells. The fluid also can be analyzed chemically. Normally, spinal fluid is clear, with glucose and chlorides but no protein and very few cells.

Other conditions that can cause meningitis and **encephalitis** (inflammation of the brain) include viral infections, tuberculosis, and syphilis. Viruses that can involve the central nervous system include the polio and rabies viruses; herpesvirus; human immunodeficiency virus (HIV; the cause of AIDS); tick- and mosquito-borne viruses, such as West Nile Virus; and, rarely, common infections such as measles and chickenpox. Aseptic meningitis is a benign, nonbacterial form of the disease caused by a virus.

Varicella-zoster virus, which causes chickenpox, is also responsible for **shingles**, a nerve infection. If someone had chickenpox as a child, the latent virus can become reactivated later in life and spread along peripheral nerves, causing an itching, blistering rash. The name *shingles* comes from the Latin word for belt, as the shingles rash is often near or around the waist. Childhood vaccinations for chickenpox will prevent shingles in the future.

Neoplasms

Almost all tumors that originate in the nervous system are tumors of nonconducting support cells, the neuroglia. These growths are termed **gliomas** and may be named for the specific type of cell involved, such as **astrocytoma**, oligodendroglioma, or **neurilemoma** (schwannoma). Because they tend not to metastasize, these tumors may be described as benign. However, they do harm by compressing brain tissue (Fig. 17-14). The symptoms they cause depend on their size and location. There may be **seizures**, headache, vomiting, muscle weakness, or interference with a special sense, such as vision or hearing. If present, edema and **hydrocephalus**, accumulation of excess CSF in the ventricles, add to the effects of the tumor (Fig 17-15).

A **meningioma** is a tumor of the meninges. Because a meningioma does not spread and is localized at the surface, a surgeon can usually remove it completely.

Tumors of neural tissue generally occur in childhood, and may even originate before birth, when nervous tissue is actively multiplying. Also, cancer may metastasize to the brain from elsewhere in the body. For unknown reasons, certain forms of cancer, especially melanoma, breast cancer, and lung cancer, tend to spread to the brain.

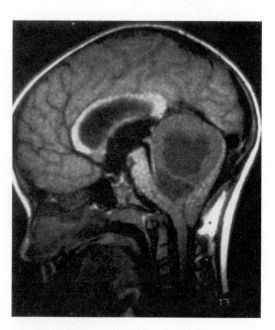

Figure 17-14 Brain tumor. MRI shows a large tumor that arises from the cerebellum and pushes the brainstem forward.

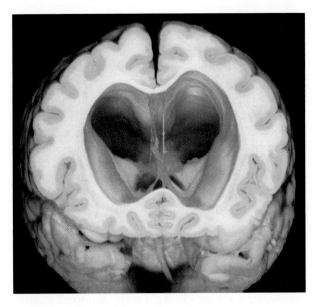

Figure 17-15 Hydrocephalus. Coronal section of the brain showing marked enlargement of the ventricles caused by a tumor that obstructed the flow of CSF.

Degenerative Diseases

Multiple sclerosis (MS) commonly attacks people in their 20s or 30s and progresses at intervals and at varying rates. It involves patchy loss of myelin with hardening (sclerosis) of tissue in the CNS. The symptoms include vision problems, tingling or numbness in the arms and legs, urinary incontinence, **tremor** (shaking), and stiff gait. MS is thought to be an autoimmune disorder, but the exact cause is not known.

Parkinsonism occurs when, for unknown reasons, certain neurons in the midbrain fail to secrete the neurotransmitter dopamine. This leads to tremors, muscle rigidity, flexion at the joints, akinesia (loss of movement), and emotional problems. Parkinsonism is treated with daily administration of the drug **L-dopa** (levodopa), a form of dopamine that can be carried by the blood into the brain.

Alzheimer disease (AD) results from unexplained degeneration of neurons and atrophy of the cerebral cortex (Fig. 17-16). These changes cause progressive loss of

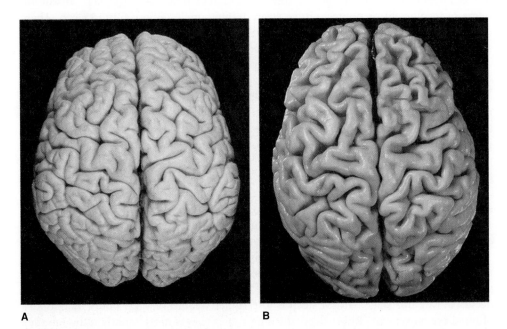

A   B

Figure 17-16 Effects of Alzheimer disease. (*A*) Normal brain. (*B*) Brain of a patient with Alzheimer disease, showing atrophy of the cortex with narrow gyri and enlarged sulci.

recent memory, confusion, and mood changes. Dangers associated with AD are injury, infection, malnutrition, and aspiration of food or fluids into the lungs. Originally called presenile dementia and used only to describe cases in patients about 50 years of age, the term is now applied to these same changes when they occur in elderly patients.

AD is diagnosed by CT or MRI scans and confirmed at autopsy. Histologic (tissue) studies show deposits of a substance called **amyloid** in the tissues. The disease may be hereditary. AD commonly develops in people with Down syndrome after age 40, indicating that AD is associated with abnormality on chromosome 21, the same chromosome that is involved in Down syndrome.

Multi-infarct dementia (MID) resembles AD in that it is a progressive cognitive impairment associated with loss of memory, loss of judgment, aphasia, altered motor and sensory function, repetitive behavior, and loss of social skills. The disorder is caused by multiple small strokes that interrupt blood flow to brain tissue and deprive areas of oxygen.

Epilepsy

A prime characteristic of **epilepsy** is recurrent seizures brought on by abnormal electric activity of the brain. These attacks may vary from brief and mild episodes known as absence (petit mal) seizures to major tonic–clonic (grand mal) seizures with loss of consciousness, **convulsion** (intervals of violent involuntary muscle contractions), and sensory disturbances. In other cases (psychomotor seizures), there is a 1- to 2-minute period of disorientation. Epilepsy may be the result of a tumor, injury, or neurologic disease, but in most cases the cause in unknown.

Electroencephalography (EEG) reveals abnormalities in brain activity and can be used in the diagnosis and treatment of epilepsy. The disorder is treated with antiepileptic and anticonvulsive drugs to control seizures, and sometimes surgery is of help. If seizures cannot be controlled, the individual with epilepsy may have to avoid certain activities that can lead to harm.

Sleep Disturbances

The general term *dyssomnia* includes a variety of possible disorders that result in excessive sleepiness or difficulty in beginning or maintaining sleep. Simple causes for such disorders include schedule changes or travel to different time zones (jet lag). **Insomnia** refers to insufficient or nonrestorative sleep despite ample opportunity to sleep. There may be physical causes for insomnia, but often it is related to emotional upset caused by stressful events. **Narcolepsy** is characterized by brief, uncontrollable attacks of sleep during the day. The disorder is treated with stimulants, regulation of sleep habits, and short daytime naps.

Sleep apnea refers to failure to breathe for brief periods during sleep. It usually results from upper airway obstruction, often associated with obesity, alcohol consumption, or weakened throat muscles, and is usually accompanied by loud snoring with brief periods of silence. Dental appliances that move the tongue and jaw forward may help to prevent sleep apnea. Other options are surgery to correct an obstruction or positive air pressure delivered through a mask.

Sleep disorders are diagnosed by physical examination, a sleep history, and a log of sleep habits, including details of the sleep environment and note of any substances consumed that may interfere with sleep. Study in a sleep laboratory with a variety of electric and other studies, composing a **polysomnography**, may also be needed.

Sleep studies identify two components of normal sleep, each showing a specific EEG pattern. Non-rapid eye movement (NREM) sleep has four stages, which take a person progressively into the deepest level of sleep. If sleepwalking (somnambulism) occurs, it occurs during this stage. NREM sleep is interrupted about every 1.5 hours by episodes of rapid eye movement (REM) sleep, during which the eyes move rapidly, although they are closed. Dreaming occurs during REM sleep and muscles lose tone, while heart rate, blood pressure, and brain activity increase.

Box 17·2 Health Professions *Careers in Occupational Therapy*

Occupational therapy (OT) helps people with physical or mental disability achieve independence at home and at work by teaching them "skills for living." Many people can benefit, including those:

➤ Recovering from traumas such as fractures, amputations, burns, spinal cord injury, stroke, and heart attack.
➤ With chronic conditions such as arthritis, multiple sclerosis, Alzheimer disease, and schizophrenia.
➤ With developmental disabilities such as Down syndrome, cerebral palsy, spina bifida, muscular dystrophy, and autism.

OTs work as part of multidisciplinary teams, which include physicians, nurses, physical therapists, speech pathologists, and social workers. They assess their clients' capabilities and develop individualized treatment programs that help them recover from injury or compensate for permanent disability. Treatment may include teaching activities ranging from work tasks to dressing, cooking, and eating, and using adaptive equipment such as wheelchairs and computers. OT assistants implement treatment plans and report results to a therapist. To perform these duties, OTs and assistants need a thorough understanding of anatomy and physiology. Most OTs in the United States have bachelor's or master's degrees and must pass a national licensing exam. Assistants typically train in a 2-year program and also take a licensing exam.

OTs and their assistants work in hospitals, clinics, and nursing care facilities, and also visit homes and schools. As the population continues to age and the need for rehabilitative therapy increases, job prospects remain good. The American Occupational Therapy Association has more information on OT careers.

Others

Many hereditary diseases affect the nervous system. Some of these are described in Chapter 15. Hormonal imbalances that involve the nervous system are described in Chapter 16. Finally, drugs, alcohol, toxins, and nutritional deficiencies may act on the nervous system in a variety of ways.

Box 17-2 has information on occupational therapists, who are often involved in treating people with neurologic disturbances.

Behavioral Disorders

This section is an introduction to some of the behavioral disorders that involve the nervous system. Criteria for clinical diagnosis of these and other behavioral and mental disorders are set forth in the *Diagnostic and Statistical Manual of Mental Disorders* (DSM) of the American Psychiatric Association.

Anxiety Disorders

Anxiety is a feeling of fear, worry, uneasiness, or dread. It may be associated with physical problems or drugs and is often prompted by feelings of helplessness or loss of self-esteem. Generalized anxiety disorder (GAD) is characterized by chronic excessive and uncontrollable worry about various life circumstances, often with no basis. It may be accompanied by muscle tensing, restlessness, dyspnea, palpitations, insomnia, irritability, or fatigue.

Panic disorder is a form of anxiety disorder marked by episodes of intense fear. A person with panic disorder may isolate himself or herself or avoid social situations for fear of having a panic attack or in response to attacks.

A **phobia** is an extreme, persistent fear of a specific object or situation (Box 17-3). It may center on social situations; particular objects, such as animals or blood; or activities, such as flying or driving through tunnels.

Box 17•3 Focus on Words *Phobias and Manias*

Some of the terms for phobias and manias are just as strange and interesting as the behaviors themselves.

Agoraphobia is fear of being in a public place. The agora in ancient Greece was the marketplace. Xenophobia is an irrational fear of strangers, taken from the Greek root *xen/o*, which means strange or foreign. Acrophobia, a fear of heights, is taken from the root *acro-*, meaning terminal, highest, or topmost. In most medical terms, this root is used to mean extremity, as in *acrocyanosis*. Hydrophobia is a fear of or aversion to water (*hydr/o*). The term was used as an alternative name for rabies, because people infected with this paralytic disease had difficulty swallowing water and other liquids.

Trichotillomania is the odd practice of compulsively pulling out one's hair in response to stress. The word comes from the root for hair (*trich/o*) plus a Greek word that means "to pull." Kleptomania, also spelled cleptomania, is from the Greek word for thief, and describes an irresistible urge to steal in the absence of need.

Obsessive–compulsive disorder (OCD) is a condition marked by disturbing thoughts or images that are persistent and intrusive. To relieve anxiety about these thoughts or images, the person with OCD engages in repetitive behavior that interferes with normal daily activities, although he or she knows that such behavior is unreasonable. These patterns include repeated washing; performing rituals; arranging, touching, or counting objects; and repeating words or phrases. OCD is associated with perfectionism and rigidity in behavior. Some specialists believe that OCD is related to low levels of the neurotransmitter serotonin in the brain. Treatment is with behavioral therapy and antidepressant drugs that increase the brain's serotonin levels (Box 17-4).

When a highly stressful, catastrophic event results in persistent emotional difficulties, the condition is described as **posttraumatic stress disorder (PTSD)**. People who are abused, whose lives are threatened, who witness a crime, who experience a natural disaster, and especially those who are combat veterans are subject to PTSD. Responses

Box 17•4 Clinical Perspectives *Psychoactive Drugs: Adjusting Neurotransmitters to Alter Mood*

Fluoxetine (Prozac) and related compounds are among the newest chemicals used to alter mood. Many psychoactive drugs used today operate by affecting levels and activities of neurotransmitters such as serotonin, norepinephrine, and dopamine in the brain.

Prozac increases serotonin's activity by blocking its reuptake–that is, it blocks transporters that carry serotonin back into the secreting cell at the synapse. Like other selective serotonin reuptake inhibitors (SSRIs), Prozac prolongs the neurotransmitter's activity at the synapse, producing a mood-elevating effect. Prozac is used to treat depression, anxiety, and symptoms of obsessive–compulsive disorder.

Other psychoactive drugs are less selective than Prozac. Venlafaxine (Effexor) blocks reuptake of serotonin and norepinephrine and is used to treat depression and generalized anxiety disorder. Bupropion (Zyban) inhibits reuptake of norepinephrine and dopamine and is prescribed for depression and smoking cessation. Another class of antidepressants, the monoamine oxidase inhibitors (MAOIs), prevent an enzyme from breaking down serotonin in the synapse. Like SSRIs, MAOIs increase the amount of serotonin available in the synapse. Examples are phenelzine (Nardil) and tranylcypromine (Parnate).

Some herbal remedies are also used to treat depression. St. John's wort contains the active ingredient hypericin, which appears to both nonselectively inhibit serotonin reuptake and block norepinephrine and dopamine reuptake. As with any drug, care must be taken when using St. John's Wort, especially if it is combined with other antidepressant medications, and health-care providers should always be informed of any drugs, including herbal preparations, that a person is taking.

include anger, fear, sleep disturbances, and physical symptoms, including changes in brain chemistry and hormone imbalances. PTSD is often associated with other emotional problems such as depression, withdrawal, substance abuse, and impaired social and family relationships. Patients need early treatment with emotional support, protection, psychotherapy, and drugs to treat depression and anxiety.

Mood Disorders

Depression is a mental state characterized by profound feelings of sadness, emptiness, hopelessness, inability to concentrate, and lack of interest or pleasure in activities. Depression is often accompanied by insomnia, loss of appetite, and suicidal tendencies. Depression frequently coexists with other physical or emotional conditions.

Dysthymia is a chronic mood disorder that lasts for several months to years and is often triggered by a serious event. Depression is a common symptom, as well as eating disorders, sleep disturbances, fatigue, lack of concentration, indecision, and feelings of hopelessness.

In **bipolar disorder** (formerly called manic depressive illness), normal moods alternate with episodes of depression and **mania**, a state of elation, which may include agitation, hyperexcitability, or hyperactivity. Treatment for bipolar disorder may differ from therapy for depression alone and includes mood-stabilizing drugs and professional mental health therapy.

Most of the drugs used to treat mood disorders affect the level of neurotransmitters in the brain, such as the selective serotonin reuptake inhibitors (SSRIs), which prolong the action of serotonin.

Psychosis

Psychosis is a mental state in which there is gross misperception of reality. This loss of touch with reality may be evidenced by **delusions** (false beliefs), including **paranoia**, delusions of persecution or threat, or **hallucinations**, imagined sensory experiences. Although the patient's condition makes it impossible for him or her to cope with the ordinary demands of life, there is lack of awareness that this behavior is inappropriate.

Schizophrenia is a form of chronic psychosis that may include bizarre behavior, paranoia, anxiety, delusions, withdrawal, and suicidal tendencies. The diagnosis of schizophrenia encompasses a broad category of disorders with many subtypes. The causes of schizophrenia are unknown, but there is evidence of hereditary factors and imbalance in brain chemistry.

Attention-Deficit/Hyperactivity Disorder

Attention-deficit/hyperactivity disorder (ADHD) is difficult to diagnose because many of its symptoms overlap or coexist with other behavioral disorders. Although inattention and hyperactivity usually appear together in these cases, one component may predominate. ADHD commonly begins in childhood and is characterized by attention problems, easy boredom, impatience, and impulsive behavior. Associated hyperactivity may be manifested by fidgeting, squirming, rapid motion, or excessive talking. In adults, the signs of ADHD may be confused with other disorders, such as mood disturbances, substance abuse, and endocrine problems.

ADHD has been correlated with alterations in brain structure and metabolism. Treatment is with psychotherapy or behavioral therapy and certain drugs. A stimulant, methylphenidate (Ritalin) has traditionally been prescribed for children with ADHD, but more recently the antidepressant atomoxetine (Strattera) has given positive results.

Pervasive Developmental Disorder

The term *pervasive developmental disorder* (PDD) applies to impairments that appear early in life and affect social interactions and communication skills. Some forms are commonly associated with a degree of mental retardation; however, people with PDD may be of normal or above average intelligence, and even brilliant. Each child with PDD is unique and has his or her own specific needs. All of these conditions fall into a continuum that includes, among others, autism and Asperger syndrome.

Autism is a complex disorder of unknown cause that usually appears between the ages of 2 and 6 years as a child does not reach appropriate developmental signposts. It is marked by self-absorption and lack of response to social contact and affection. An autistic child may have low intelligence and poor language skills. They often appear to be disconnected and out of place. They may overrespond to stimuli and may show self-destructive behavior. There may also be stereotyped (repetitive) behavior, preoccupations, mood swings, and resistance to change. Autism may be accompanied by neurologic problems and problems with sleeping and eating. Those with autism may need the help of mental health specialists, social workers, and occupational, physical, and speech therapists.

People with **Asperger syndrome** are often highly intelligent and verbal, but have trouble with social interactions and understanding others' behavior. Thus, as children, they are often isolated and bullied. Repetitive behaviors may develop. These children also may develop a strong interest in specific topics. They need help in learning to interpret social cues, but often can apply their talents in satisfying occupations.

Drugs Used in Treatment

A psychotropic or psychoactive drug is one that acts on the mental state. This category of drugs includes antianxiety drugs or anxiolytics, mood stabilizers, antidepressants, and antipsychotics, also called neuroleptics. Many of these drugs work by increasing the brain's levels of neurotransmitters. Note that psychoactive drugs do not work in the same way for everyone. It is often necessary to try different therapies until the right drug is found. Also, it may take several weeks for a drug to become effective. For more information, see descriptions and examples of specific types of psychoactive drugs in the supplementary terms.

TERMINOLOGY   Key Terms

NEUROLOGIC DISORDERS

Alzheimer disease (AD) *ALTS-hī-mer*	A form of dementia caused by atrophy of the cerebral cortex; presenile dementia (see Fig. 17-16)
amyloid *AM-i-loyd*	A starchlike substance of unknown composition that accumulates in the brain in Alzheimer and other diseases
aneurysm *AN-ū-rizm*	A localized abnormal dilation of a blood vessel that results from weakness of the vessel wall (see Fig. 17-11); an aneurysm may eventually burst
aphasia *a-FĀ-zē-a*	Specifically, loss or defect in speech communication (from Greek *phasis*, meaning "speech"). In practice, the term is applied more broadly to a range of language disorders, both spoken and written. May affect ability to understand speech (receptive aphasia) or the ability to produce speech (expressive aphasia). Both forms are combined in global aphasia.
astrocytoma *as-trō-sī-TŌ-ma*	A neuroglial tumor composed of astrocytes

TERMINOLOGY

Key Terms

Continued

17

cerebral contusion *kon-TŪ-zhun*	A bruise to the surface of the brain following a blow to the head
cerebrovascular accident (CVA)	Sudden damage to the brain resulting from reduction of cerebral blood flow; possible causes are atherosclerosis, thrombosis, or a ruptured aneurysm; commonly called stroke
coma *KŌ-ma*	State of deep unconsciousness from which one cannot be roused
concussion *kon-KUSH-un*	Injury resulting from a violent blow or shock; a concussion of the brain usually results in loss of consciousness
confusion *kon-FŪ-zhun*	A state of reduced comprehension, coherence, and reasoning ability resulting in inappropriate responses to environmental stimuli.
contrecoup injury *kon-tre-KŪ*	Damage to the brain on the side opposite the point of a blow as a result of the brain's hitting the skull (from French, meaning "counterblow")
convulsion *kon-VUL-shun*	A series of violent, involuntary muscle contractions. A tonic convulsion involves prolonged contraction of the muscles; in a clonic convulsion there is alternation of contraction and relaxation. Both forms appear in grand mal epilepsy.
dementia *dē-MEN-shē-a*	A gradual and usually irreversible loss of intellectual function
embolism *EM-bō-lizm*	Obstruction of a blood vessel by a blood clot or other material carried in the circulation
encephalitis *en-sef-a-LĪ-tis*	Inflammation of the brain
epidural hematoma	Accumulation of blood in the epidural space (between the dura mater and the skull; see Fig. 17-12)
epilepsy *EP-i-lep-sē*	A chronic disease involving periodic sudden bursts of electric activity from the brain, resulting in seizures
glioma *glī-Ō-ma*	A tumor of neuroglia cells
hemiparesis *hem-i-pa-RĒ-sis*	Partial paralysis or weakness of one side of the body
hemiplegia *hemi-i-PLĒ-jē-a*	Paralysis of one side of the body
hydrocephalus *hī-drō-SEF-a-lus*	Increased accumulation of CSF in or around the brain as a result of obstruction to flow. May be caused by tumor, inflammation, hemorrhage, or congenital abnormality (see Fig. 17-15)
insomnia *in-SOM-nē-a*	Insufficient or nonrestorative sleep despite ample opportunity to sleep

TERMINOLOGY
Continued

Key Terms

meningioma *men-nin-jē-Ō-ma*	Tumor of the meninges
meningitis *men-in-JĪ-tis*	Inflammation of the meninges
multi-infarct dementia (MID)	Dementia caused by chronic cerebral ischemia (lack of blood supply to the tissues) as a result of multiple small strokes. There is progressive loss of cognitive function, memory, and judgment as well as altered motor and sensory function.
multiple sclerosis (MS)	A chronic, progressive disease involving loss of myelin in the CNS
narcolepsy *NAR-kō-lep-sē*	Brief, uncontrollable episodes of sleep during the day
neurilemoma *nŭ-ri-lem-Ō-ma*	A tumor of the sheath (neurilemma) of a peripheral nerve; schwannoma
paralysis *pa-RAL-i-sis*	Temporary or permanent loss of function. Flaccid paralysis involves loss of muscle tone and reflexes and degeneration of muscles. Spastic paralysis involves excess muscle tone and reflexes but no degeneration.
parkinsonism	A disorder originating in the basal ganglia and characterized by slow movements, tremor, rigidity, and masklike face. Also called Parkinson disease.
seizure *SĒ-zhur*	A sudden attack, as seen in epilepsy. The most common forms of seizure are tonic–clonic, or grand mal (*gran mal*) (from French, meaning "great illness"); absence seizure, or petit mal (*pet-Ē mal*), meaning "small illness"; and psychomotor seizure.
shingles	An acute viral infection that follows nerve pathways causing small lesions on the skin. Caused by reactivation of the virus that also causes chickenpox (varicella–zoster virus). Also called herpes zoster (*HER-pēz ZOS-ter*).
sleep apnea *ap-NĒ-a*	Brief periods of breathing cessation during sleep
stroke	Sudden interference with blood flow in one or more cerebral vessels leading to oxygen deprivation and necrosis of brain tissue; caused by a blood clot in a vessel (ischemic stroke) or rupture of a vessel (hemorrhagic stroke). Cerebrovascular accident (CVA)
subdural hematoma	Accumulation of blood beneath the dura mater (see Fig. 17-12)
thrombosis *throm-BŌ-sis*	Development of a blood clot within a vessel
tremor *TREM-or*	A shaking or involuntary movement

TERMINOLOGY
Key Terms
Continued

DIAGNOSIS AND TREATMENT

carotid endarterectomy *end-ar-ter-EK-tō-mē*	Surgical removal of the lining of the carotid artery, the large artery in the neck that supplies blood to the brain
cerebral angiography	Radiographic study of the blood vessels of the brain after injection of a contrast medium
electroencephalography (EEG) *ē-lek-trō-en-sef-a-LOG-ra-fē*	Amplification, recording, and interpretation of the electric activity of the brain
L-dopa *DŌ-pa*	A drug used in the treatment of parkinsonism; levodopa
lumbar puncture	Puncture of the subarachnoid space in the lumbar region of the spinal cord to remove spinal fluid for diagnosis or to inject anesthesia (see Fig. 17-13); spinal tap
polysomnography *pol-ē-som-NOG-ra-fē*	Simultaneous monitoring of a variety of physiologic functions during sleep to diagnose sleep disorders

BEHAVIORAL DISORDERS

anxiety *ang-ZĪ-e-tē*	A feeling of fear, worry, uneasiness, or dread
Asperger syndrome *AHS-per-ger*	A behavioral condition on a continuum with autism that may include difficulty with social interactions and understanding, strong specific interests, and repetitive behaviors
attention-deficit/hyperactivity disorder (ADHD)	A condition that begins in childhood and is characterized by attention problems, easy boredom, impulsive behavior, and hyperactivity
autism *AW-tizm*	A disorder of unknown cause consisting of self-absorption, lack of response to social contact and affection, preoccupations, stereotyped behavior, and resistance to change (from *auto-*, "self" and *-ism*, "condition of")
bipolar disorder *bī-PŌ-lar*	A form of depression with episodes of mania (a state of elation); manic depressive illness
delusion *dē-LŪ-zhun*	A false belief inconsistent with knowledge and experience
depression *dē-PRESH-un*	A mental state characterized by profound feelings of sadness, emptiness, hopelessness, and lack of interest or pleasure in activities
dysthymia *dis-THĪ-mē-a*	A mild form of depression that usually develops in response to a serious life event (from *dys-* and Greek *thymos*, meaning "mind, emotion")
hallucination *ha-lū-si-NĀ-shun*	A false perception unrelated to reality or external stimuli

TERMINOLOGY   Key Terms
Continued

mania *MĀ-nē-a*	A state of elation, which may include agitation, hyperexcitability, or hyperactivity (adjective: manic)
obsessive-compulsive disorder (OCD)	A condition associated with recurrent and intrusive thoughts, images, and repetitive behaviors performed to relieve anxiety
panic disorder	A form of anxiety disorder marked by episodes of intense fear
paranoia *par-a-NOY-a*	A mental state characterized by jealousy, delusions of persecution, or perceptions of threat or harm
phobia *FŌ-bē-a*	An extreme, persistent fear of a specific object or situation
posttraumatic stress disorder (PTSD)	Persistent emotional disturbances that follow exposure to life-threatening, catastrophic events, such as trauma, abuse, natural disasters, and warfare
psychosis *sī-KŌ-sis*	A mental disorder extreme enough to cause gross misperception of reality with delusions and hallucinations
schizophrenia *skiz-ō-FRĒ-nē-a*	A poorly understood group of severe mental disorders with features of psychosis, delusions, hallucinations, and withdrawn or bizarre behavior (*schizo* means "split" and *phren* means "mind")

Go to the pronunciation glossary in Chapter 17 on the CD-ROM to hear these words pronounced.

TERMINOLOGY   Supplementary Terms

NORMAL STRUCTURE AND FUNCTION

acetylcholine *as-ē-til-KŌ-lēn*	A neurotransmitter; activity involving acetylcholine is described as cholinergic
basal ganglia	Four masses of gray matter in the cerebrum and upper brainstem that are involved in movement and coordination
blood–brain barrier	A special membrane between circulating blood and the brain that prevents certain damaging substances from reaching brain tissue

Supplementary Terms

Broca area *BRŌ-ka*	An area in the left frontal lobe of the cerebrum that controls speech production
circle of Willis	An interconnection (anastomosis) of several arteries supplying the brain, located at the base of the cerebrum
contralateral *kon-tra-LAT-er-al*	Affecting the opposite side of the body
corpus callosum *KOR-pus ka-LŌ-sum*	A large band of connecting fibers between the cerebral hemispheres
dermatome *DER-ma-tōm*	The area of the skin supplied by a spinal nerve; term also refers to an instrument used to cut skin for grafting (see Chapter 21)
epinephrine *ep-i-NEF-rin*	A neurotransmitter; also called adrenaline; activity involving epinephrine is described as adrenergic
ipsilateral *ip-si-LAT-er-al*	On the same side; unilateral
leptomeninges *lep-to-men-IN-jēz*	The pia mater and arachnoid together
nucleus *NŪ-klē-us*	A collection of nerve cells within the central nervous system
plexus *PLEKS-us*	A network, as of nerves or blood vessels
pyramidal tracts *pi-RAM-i-dal*	A group of motor tracts involved in fine coordination. Most of the fibers in these tracts cross in the medulla to the opposite side of the spinal cord and affect the opposite side of the body. Fibers not included in the pyramidal tracts are described as extrapyramidal.
reticular activating system (RAS) *re-TIK-ū-lar*	A widespread system in the brain that maintains wakefulness
Schwann cells *shvon*	Cells that produce the myelin sheath around peripheral axons
Wernicke area *VER-ni-kē*	An area in the temporal lobe concerned with speech comprehension

SYMPTOMS AND CONDITIONS

amyotrophic lateral sclerosis (ALS) *a-mī-ō-TROF-ik*	A disorder marked by muscular weakness, spasticity, and exaggerated reflexes caused by degeneration of motor neurons; Lou Gehrig disease
amnesia *am-NĒ-zē-a*	Loss of memory

17

TERMINOLOGY *Continued*

Supplementary Terms

apraxia *a-PRAK-sē-a*	Inability to move with purpose or to use objects properly
ataxia *a-TAK-sē-a*	Lack of muscle coordination; dyssynergia
athetosis *ath-e-TŌ-sis*	Involuntary, slow, twisting movements in the arms, especially the hands and fingers
Bell palsy *PAWL-zē*	Paralysis of the facial nerve
berry aneurysm *AN-ū-rizm*	A small saclike aneurysm of a cerebral artery
catatonia *kat-a-TŌ-nē-a*	A phase of schizophrenia in which the patient is unresponsive; there is a tendency to remain in a fixed position without moving or talking
cerebral palsy *SER-e-bral PAWL-zē*	A nonprogressive neuromuscular disorder usually caused by damage to the CNS near the time of birth. May include spasticity, involuntary movements, or ataxia.
chorea *KOR-ē-a*	A nervous condition marked by involuntary twitching of the limbs or facial muscles
claustrophobia *claws-trō-FŌ-bē-a*	Fear of being shut in or enclosed (from Latin *claudere*, "to shut")
compulsion *kom-PUL-shun*	A repetitive, stereotyped act performed to relieve tension
Creutzfeldt–Jakob disease (CJD) *KROITS-felt YA-kob*	A slow-growing degenerative brain disease caused by a prion (*PRĪ-on*), an infectious protein agent. Related to bovine spongiform encephalopathy (BSE, "mad cow disease") in cattle.
delirium *de-LIR-ē-um*	A sudden and temporary state of confusion marked by excitement, physical restlessness, and incoherence
dysarthria *dis-AR-thrē-a*	Defect in speech articulation caused by lack of control over the required muscles
dysmetria *dis-MĒ-trē-a*	Disturbance in the path or placement of a limb during active movement. In hypometria, the limb falls short; in hypermetria, the limb extends beyond the target.
euphoria *ū-FOR-ē-a*	An exaggerated feeling of well-being; elation
glioblastoma *glī-ō-blas-TŌ-ma*	A malignant astrocytoma
Guillain–Barré syndrome *gē-YAN-bar-RĀ*	An acute polyneuritis with progressive muscular weakness that usually occurs after a viral infection; in most cases recovery is complete, but *may* take several months to years

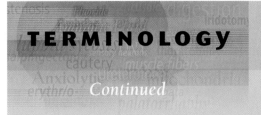

TERMINOLOGY
Continued

Supplementary Terms

hematomyelia *hē-ma-tō-mī-Ē-lē-a*	Hemorrhage of blood into the spinal cord, as from an injury
hemiballism *hem-ē-BAL-izm*	Jerking, twitching movements of one side of the body
Huntington disease	A hereditary disease of the CNS that usually appears between ages 30 and 50. The patient shows progressive dementia and chorea, and death occurs within 10 to 15 years.
hypochondriasis *hī-pō-kon-DRĪ-a-sis*	Abnormal anxiety about one's health
ictus *IK-tus*	A blow or sudden attack, such as an epileptic seizure
lethargy *LETH-ar-jē*	A state of sluggishness or stupor
migraine *MĪ-grān*	Chronic intense, throbbing headache that may result from vascular changes in cerebral arteries. Possible causes include genetic factors, stress, trauma, and hormonal fluctuations. Headache might be signaled by visual disturbances, nausea, photophobia, and tingling sensations.
neurofibromatosis *nū-rō-fi-brō-ma-TŌ-sis*	A condition involving multiple tumors of peripheral nerves
neurosis *nū-RŌ-sis*	An emotional disorder caused by unresolved conflicts, with anxiety as a main characteristic
paraplegia *par-a-PLĒ-jē-a*	Paralysis of the legs and lower part of the body
parasomnia *par-a-SOM-nē-a*	Condition of having undesirable phenomena, such as nightmares, occur during sleep or become worse during sleep
quadriplegia *kwod-ri-PLĒ-jē-a*	Paralysis of all four limbs; tetraplegia
Reye syndrome *rī*	A rare acute encephalopathy occurring in children after viral infections. The liver, kidney, and heart may be involved. Linked to administration of aspirin during a viral illness.
sciatica *sī-AT-i-ka*	Neuritis characterized by severe pain along the sciatic nerve and its branches
somatoform disorders *sō-MA-tō-form*	Conditions associated with symptoms of physical disease, such as pain, hypertension, or chronic fatigue, with no physical basis
somnambulism *som-NAM-bū-lizm*	Walking or performing other motor functions while asleep and out of bed; sleepwalking
stupor *STŪ-por*	A state of unconsciousness or lethargy with loss of responsiveness

17

TERMINOLOGY

Supplementary Terms

Continued

syringomyelia *sir-in-gō-mī-Ē-lē-a*	A progressive disease marked by formation of fluid-filled cavities in the spinal cord
tic	Involuntary, spasmodic, recurrent, and purposeless motor movements or vocalizations
tic douloureux *tik dū-lū-RŪ*	Episodes of extreme pain in the area supplied by the trigeminal nerve; also called trigeminal neuralgia
tabes dorsalis *TĀ-bēz dor-SAL-is*	Destruction of the dorsal (posterior) portion of the spinal cord with loss of sensation and awareness of body position, as seen in advanced cases of syphilis
Tourette syndrome *tū-RET*	A tic disorder with intermittent motor and vocal manifestations that begins in childhood. There also may be obsessive and compulsive behavior, hyperactivity, and distractibility.
transient ischemic attack (TIA) *is-KĒ-mik*	A sudden, brief, and temporary cerebral dysfunction usually caused by interruption of blood flow to the brain
Wallerian degeneration *wahl-LĒ-rē-an*	Degeneration of a nerve distal to an injury
whiplash	Cervical injury caused by rapid acceleration and deceleration resulting in damage to muscles, ligaments, disks, and nerves

Additional terms related to neurologic symptoms can be found in Chapters 18 (on the senses) and 20 (on the muscular system).

DIAGNOSIS AND TREATMENT

Babinski reflex	A spreading of the outer toes and extension of the big toe over the others when the sole of the foot is stroked. This response is normal in infants but indicates a lesion of specific motor tracts in adults.
evoked potentials	Record of the electric activity of the brain after sensory stimulation. Included are visual evoked potentials (VEPs), brainstem auditory evoked potentials (BAEPs), and somatosensory evoked potentials (SSEPs), obtained by stimulating the hand or leg. These tests are used to evaluate CNS function.
Glasgow coma scale	A system for assessing level of consciousness by assigning a score to each of three responses: eye opening, motor responses, and verbal responses
Positron emission tomography (PET)	Use of radioactive glucose or other metabolically active substance to produce images of biochemical activity in tissues. Used for study of the living brain, both healthy and diseased, and also in cardiology. Figure 17-17 compares CT, MRI, and PET scans.
Romberg sign	Inability to maintain balance when the eyes are shut and the feet are close together

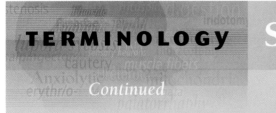

TERMINOLOGY
Continued

Supplementary Terms

sympathectomy *sim-pa-THEK-tō-mē*	Interruption of sympathetic nerve transmission either surgically or chemically
trephination *tref-i-NĀ-shun*	Cutting a piece of bone out of the skull; the instrument used is a trepan (*tre-PAN*) or trephine (*tre-FĪN*)

PSYCHOACTIVE DRUGS

antianxiety agents *an-tē-ang-ZĪ-e-tē*	Relieve anxiety by means of a calming, sedative effect on the CNS; e.g. chlordiazepoxide (Librium), diazepam (Valium), alprazolam (Xanax); anxiolytic
antidepressants (other than those listed in separate categories below)	Block the reuptake of neurotransmitters such as serotonin, norepinephrine, dopamine, alone or in combination; e.g. bupropion (Wellbutrin, Zyban), mirtazapine (Remeron), nefazodone (Serzone), venlafaxine (Effexor XR), atomoxetine (Strattera)
monoamine oxidase inhibitors (MAOI) *mō-nō-A-mēn OK-si-dās*	Block an enzyme that breaks down norepinephrine and serotonin, thus prolonging their action; e.g. phenelzine (Nardil), tranylcypromine (Parnate), isocarboxazid (Marplan)
neuroleptics *nū-rō-LEP-tiks*	Drugs used to treat psychosis, including schizophrenia; e.g. clozapine (Clozaril), haloperidol (Haldol), risperidone (Risperdal), olanzapine (Zyprexa); antipsychotic. Action mechanism unknown, but may interfere with neurotransmitter action.
selective serotonin reuptake inhibitors (SSRIs) *ser-ō-TŌ-nin*	Block the reuptake of serotonin in the brain, thus increasing levels; e.g. fluoxetine (Prozac), citalopram (Celexa), paroxetine (Paxil), sertraline (Zoloft)
stimulants *STIM-ū-lants*	Promote activity and a sense of well-being; e.g. methylphenidate (Ritalin), dextroamphetamine (Dexedrine), amphetamine + dextroamphetamine (Adderall)
tricyclic antidepressants (TCA) *trī-SĪ-klik*	Block the reuptake of norepinephrine, serotonin, or both; e.g. amitriptyline (Elavil), clomipramine (Anafril), imipramine (Tofranil), doxepin (Sinequan), trimipramine (Surmontil)

Go to the pronunciation glossary in Chapter 17 of the CD-ROM to hear these words pronounced.

17

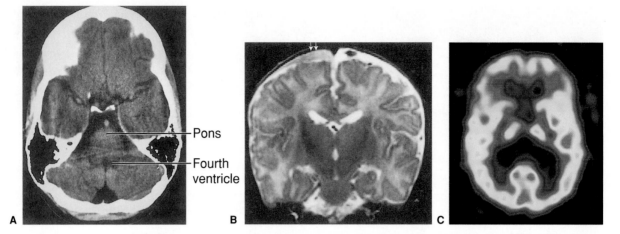

Figure 17-17 Brain images. (*A*) CT scan of a normal adult brain. (*B*) MRI of the brain showing a subdural hematoma (arrows). (*C*) PET scan showing regions of different metabolic activity.

TERMINOLOGY Abbreviations

ACh	Acetylcholine	**LOC**	Level of consciousness
AD	Alzheimer disease	**LP**	Lumbar puncture
ADHD	Attention-deficit/hyperactivity disorder	**MAOI**	Monoamine oxidase inhibitor
ALS	Amyotrophic lateral sclerosis	**MID**	Multi-infarct dementia
ANS	Autonomic nervous system	**MS**	Multiple sclerosis
BAEP	Brainstem auditory evoked potentials	**NICU**	Neurological intensive care unit
CBF	Cerebral blood flow	**NPH**	Normal pressure hydrocephalus
CJD	Creutzfeldt–Jakob disease	**NREM**	Non–rapid eye movement (sleep)
CNS	Central nervous system	**OCD**	Obsessive–compulsive disorder
CP	Cerebral palsy	**PDD**	Pervasive developmental disorder
CSF	Cerebrospinal fluid	**PET**	Positron emission tomography
CVA	Cerebrovascular accident	**PNS**	Peripheral nervous system
CVD	Cerebrovascular disease	**PTSD**	Posttraumatic stress disorder
DSM	*Diagnostic and Statistical Manual of Mental Disorders*	**RAS**	Reticular activating system
DTR	Deep tendon reflexes	**REM**	Rapid eye movement (sleep)
EEG	Electroencephalogram; electroencephalograph(y)	**SSEP**	Somatosensory evoked potentials
		SSRI	Selective serotonin reuptake inhibitor
		TCA	Tricyclic antidepressant
GAD	Generalized anxiety disorder	**TIA**	Transient ischemic attack
ICP	Intracranial pressure	**UMN**	Upper motor neuron
LMN	Lower motor neuron	**VEP**	Visual evoked potentials

CHAPTER REVIEW

LABELING EXERCISE
Anatomic Divisions of the Nervous System

Write the name of each numbered part on the corresponding line of the answer sheet.

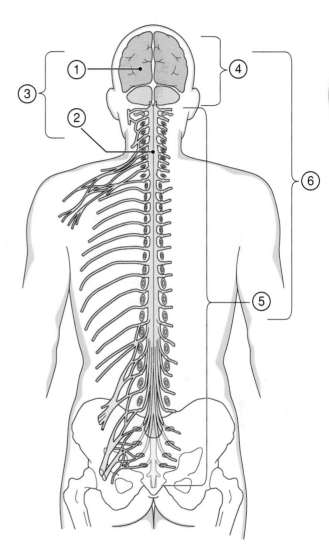

17

Brain	1. _____
Central nervous system	2. _____
Cranial nerves	3. _____
Peripheral nervous system	4. _____
Spinal cord	5. _____
Spinal nerves	6. _____

Motor Neuron

Write the name of each numbered part on the corresponding line of the answer sheet.

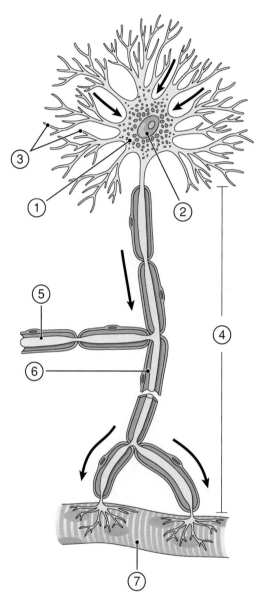

Axon branch	1. _____
Axon covered with myelin sheath	2. _____
Cell body	3. _____
Dendrites	4. _____
Muscle	5. _____
Myelin	6. _____
Nucleus	7. _____

17

External Surface of the Brain

Write the name of each numbered part on the corresponding line of the answer sheet.

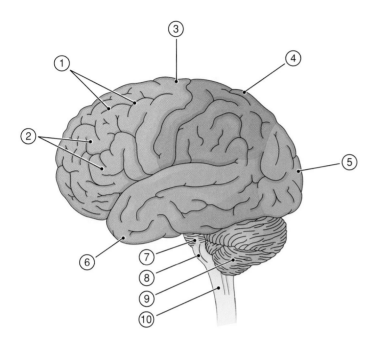

Cerebellum   1. _____

Frontal lobe   2. _____

Gyri   3. _____

Medulla oblongata   4. _____

Occipital lobe   5. _____

Parietal lobe   6. _____

Pons   7. _____

Spinal cord   8. _____

Sulci   9. _____

Temporal lobe   10. _____

17

Spinal Cord, Lateral View

Write the name of each numbered part on the corresponding line of the answer sheet.

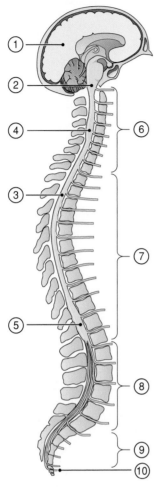

Brain   1. _____

Brainstem   2. _____

Cervical enlargement 3. _____

Cervical nerves   4. _____

Coccygeal nerve   5. _____

Lumbar enlargement   6. _____

Lumbar nerves   7. _____

Sacral nerves   8. _____

Spinal cord   9. _____

Thoracic nerves   10. _____

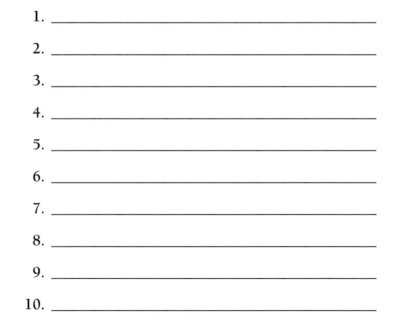

Spinal Cord, Cross Section

Write the name of each numbered part on the corresponding line of the answer sheet.

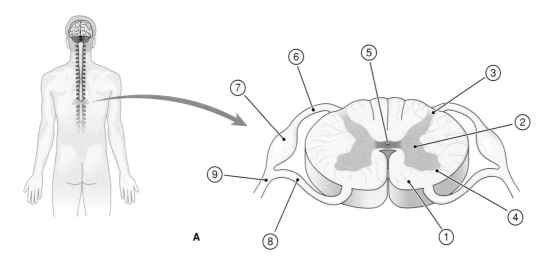

A

Central canal

Dorsal horn

Dorsal root ganglion

Dorsal root of spinal nerve

Gray matter

Spinal nerve

Ventral horn

Ventral root of spinal nerve

White matter

1. _____

2. _____

3. _____

4. _____

5. _____

6. _____

7. _____

8. _____

9. _____

Reflex Pathway

Write the name of each numbered part on the corresponding line of the answer sheet.

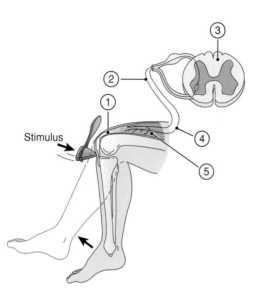

Stimulus

Effector	1. _____
Motor neuron	2. _____
Receptor	3. _____
Sensory neuron	4. _____
Spinal cord (CNS)	5. _____

TERMINOLOGY

Match the following terms and write the appropriate letter to the left of each number:

_____	1. neuroglia	**a.**	region that connects the brain and spinal cord
_____	2. ganglion	**b.**	largest part of the brain
_____	3. pons	**c.**	support cells of the nervous system
_____	4. medulla oblongata	**d.**	rounded area on the ventral surface of the brain
_____	5. cerebrum	**e.**	collection of neuron cell bodies
_____	6. hypersomnia	**a.**	inducing stupor
_____	7. concussion	**b.**	excessive fear of pain
_____	8. narcotic	**c.**	excessive sleepiness
_____	9. paranoia	**d.**	mental disorder associated with delusions of persecution
_____	10. odynophobia	**e.**	injury caused by a violent blow

_____	11. monoplegia	**a.** partial paralysis of a muscle
_____	12. aphasia	**b.** paralysis of the bladder
_____	13. meningomyelocele	**c.** loss of speech communication
_____	14. myoparesis	**d.** paralysis of one limb
_____	15. cystoplegia	**e.** hernia of the meninges and spinal cord

Supplementary Terms

_____	16. plexus	**a.** network
_____	17. Broca area	**b.** area of skin supplied by a spinal nerve
_____	18. dermatome	**c.** a neurotransmitter
_____	19. acetylcholine	**d.** a portion of the brain that controls speech
_____	20. claustrophobia	**e.** fear of being enclosed

_____	21. lethargy	**a.** sudden blow or attack
_____	22. ataxia	**b.** state of sluggishness
_____	23. ictus	**c.** loss of memory
_____	24. euphoria	**d.** lack of muscle coordination
_____	25. amnesia	**e.** sense of elation

_____	26. MID	**a.** type of psychoactive drug
_____	27. SSRI	**b.** stage of sleep
_____	28. DSM	**c.** dementia caused by many small strokes
_____	29. REM	**d.** reference for diagnosis of mental disorders
_____	30. EEG	**e.** study of brain waves

17

Fill in the blanks:

31. The scientific name for a nerve cell is _____.

32. The junction between two nerve cells is a(n) _____.

33. A simple, rapid, automatic response to a stimulus is a(n) _____.

34. The membranes that cover the brain and spinal cord are the _____.

35. The sympathetic and parasympathetic systems make up the _____.

36. A chemical that acts at a synapse is a(n) _____.

37. The posterior portion of the brain that coordinates muscle movement is the _____.

True–False. Examine the following statements. If the statement is true, write T in the first blank. If the statement is false, write F in the first blank and correct the statement by replacing the <u>underlined</u> word in the second blank.

38. The cervical nerves are in the region of the <u>neck</u>.　　　_____　_____

39. CSF forms in the <u>ventricles</u> of the brain.　　　_____　_____

40. Myelinated neurons make up the <u>gray</u> matter of the CNS.　　　_____　_____

41. The fiber that caries impulses away from the neuron cell body is the <u>dendrite</u>. _____ _____

42. <u>Sensory</u> fibers conduct impulses toward the CNS. _____ _____

43. There are <u>twelve</u> pairs of cranial nerves. _____ _____

44. The outermost layer of the meninges is the <u>pia</u> mater. _____ _____

Eliminations. In each of the sets below, underline the word that does not fit in with the rest and explain the reason for your choice:

45. CVA — lumbar puncture — embolism — thrombus — aneurysm

_____

46. glioma — astrocytoma — meningioma — hematoma — neurilemmoma

_____

47. gyri — sulci — mania — ventricles — lobes

_____

48. PTSD — CNS — ADHD — OCD — GAD

_____

Define the following words:

49. anencephaly (*an-en-SEF-a-lē*) _____

50. corticothalamic (*kor-ti-kō-tha-LAM-ik*) _____

51. polyneuritis (*pol-ē-nū-RĪ-tis*) _____

52. psychotherapy (*sī-kō-THER-a-pē*) _____

53. encephalomalacia (*en-sef-a-lō-ma-LĀ-shē-a*) _____

54. hemiparesis (*hem-i-pa-RĒ-sis*) _____

55. panplegia (*pan-PLĒ-jē-a*) _____

56. radicular (*ra-DIK-ū-lar*) _____

57. dyssomnia (*dis-SOM-nē-a*) _____

Word building. Write words for the following definitions:

58. any disease of the nervous system _____

59. study of the nervous system _____

60. inflammation of the spinal cord and meninges _____

61. excision of a ganglion _____

62. creation of an opening into a brain ventricle _____

63. within the cerebellum _____

64. paralysis of one side of the body _____

65. difficulty in reading _____

66. fear of water _____

Opposites. Write a word that means the opposite of the following words:

67. intramedullary _____

68. ipsilateral _____

69. preganglionic _____

70. bradylalia _____

71. motor _____

72. ventral _____

73. afferent _____

Adjectives. Write the adjective form of the following words:

74. ganglion _____

75. cortex _____

76. dura _____

77. meninges _____

78. psychosis _____

Plurals. Write the plural form of the following words:

79. ganglion _____

80. ventricle _____

81. meninx _____

82. gyrus _____

Word analysis. Define each of the following words, and give the meaning of the word parts in each. Use a dictionary if necessary.

83. myelodysplasia (*mī-e-lō-dis-PLĀ-sē-a*) _____

    a. myel/o _____

    b. dys- _____

    c. -plas _____

    d. -ia _____

84. polyneuroradiculitis (*pol-ē-nū-rō-ra-dik-ū-LĪ-tis*) _____

    a. poly- _____

    b. neur/o _____

    c. radicul/o _____

    d. -itis _____

85. dyssynergia (*dis-sin-ER-jē-a*) _____

    a. dys- _____

    b. syn- _____

    c. erg _____

    d. -ia _____

Go to the word exercises in Chapter 17 of the CD-ROM for additional review exercises.

CASE STUDY 17-1: Pediatric Brain Tumor

B.C., a 6-year-old first-grade student, was referred to a pediatric neurologist by his primary pediatrician for a neuro consult. He had presented with an acute onset of headaches, vomiting on waking in the morning, and progressive ataxia. The neurologist conducted a thorough neuro exam and ordered a CT scan, MRI, and lumbar puncture (LP) to look for possible tumor cells. When the LP revealed suspicious cells and the scans showed a tissue density, he was referred to a neurosurgeon for treatment of a suspected infratentorial astrocytoma (neuroglial tumor) of the posterior fossa.

B.C. had a craniotomy with tumor resection 5 days later. The cerebellar tumor was found to be noninfiltrating and was enclosed within a cyst, which was totally removed. B.C. spent 2 days in the neurological intensive care unit (NICU) because he was on seizure precautions and monitoring for increased intracranial pressure (ICP). A regimen of focal radiation followed after recovery from surgery. His spine was also treated because of the potential spread of tumor cells in the CSF. B.C. did not have chemotherapy because of the danger that hydrocephalus might develop, which generally requires a ventriculoperitoneal (VP) shunt.

B.C. was discharged 6 days after his surgery with a mild hemiparesis, which was expected to resolve within the next few weeks. He was scheduled for 6 weeks of outpatient rehabilitation, and his prognosis was good.

CASE STUDY 17-2: Cerebrovascular Accident (CVA)

A.R., a 62-year-old man, was admitted to the ER with right hemiplegia and aphasia. He had a history of hypertension and recent transient ischemic attacks (TIAs), yet was in good health when he experienced a sudden onset of right-sided weakness. He arrived in the ER via ambulance within 15 minutes of onset and was received by a member of the hospital's stroke team. He had a rapid general assessment and neuro exam, including a Glasgow Coma Scale (GCS) rating, to determine his candidacy for fibrinolytic (clot-dissolving) therapy.

He was sent for a noncontrast CT scan to look for evidence of hemorrhagic or ischemic stroke, post-cardiac arrest ischemia, hypertensive encephalopathy, craniocerebral or cervical trauma, meningitis, encephalitis, brain abscess, tumor, and subdural or epidural hematoma. The CT scan, read by the radiologist, did not show intracerebral or subarachnoid hemorrhage. A.R. was diagnosed with probable acute ischemic stroke within 1 hour of the onset of symptoms and cleared as a candidate for immediate fibrinolytic treatment.

He was admitted to the NICU for 48-hour observation to monitor his neuro status and vital signs. He was discharged after 3 days with a prognosis of full recovery.

CASE STUDY 17-3: Neuroleptic Malignant Syndrome

J.N., a 21-year-old woman with chronic paranoid schizophrenia, was admitted to the hospital with a diagnosis of pneumonia. She was brought to the ER by her mother, who said J.N. had been very lethargic, had a temperature of 104°F, and had had muscular rigidity for 3 days. She took Haldol (haloperidol) and Cogentin (benztropine mesylate). Her mother stated that J.N.'s psychiatrist had changed her neuroleptic medication the week before. Her secondary diagnosis was stated as neuroleptic malignant syndrome, a rare and life-threatening disorder associated with the use of antipsychotic medications. This drug-induced condition is usually characterized by alterations in mental status, temperature regulation, and autonomic and extrapyramidal functions.

J.N. was monitored for potential hypotension, tachycardia, diaphoresis, dyspnea, dysphagia, and changes in her level of consciousness (LOC). Her medications were discontinued, she was hydrated with IV fluids, and her body temperature was monitored for fluctuations. She was treated with bromocriptine, a dopamine antagonist, and dantrolene, a muscle relaxant and antispasmodic.

After 5 days, J.N. was transferred to a mental health facility and restarted on low-dose neuroleptics. She was monitored to prevent a recurrence. Both J.N. and her family were educated about neuroleptic malignant syndrome in preparation for her discharge back home in 2 weeks.

CASE STUDIES

CASE STUDY QUESTIONS

Multiple choice. Select the best answer and write the letter of your choice to the left of each number:

_____ 1. A neurologist is a physician who:
   a. performs brain surgery
   b. practices psychiatry
   c. practices psychology
   d. treats with natural and herbal medicine
   e. treats disorders of the nervous system

_____ 2. A diagnostic procedure in which fluid is withdrawn from the spinal subarachnoid space is a(n):
   a. thoracentesis
   b. lumbar puncture
   c. ventriculogram
   d. intracranial window
   e. trephine

_____ 3. B.C.'s tumor was in the cerebellum, which controls voluntary movement, balance, and coordination. His motor dysfunction is called:
   a. ataxia
   b. neurolepsis
   c. dysphagia
   d. dyspnea
   e. seizure

_____ 4. A VP shunt is a surgical treatment for hydrocephalus. Excess CSF is shunted (drained) from the _____ by way of tubing tunneled to the _____ cavity.
   a. vortex, ventricular
   b. ventricles, peritoneal
   c. peritoneum, ventricular
   d. ventricles, thoracic
   e. midbrain, stomach

_____ 5. Ischemic stroke is generally caused by:
   a. hemorrhage
   b. hematoma
   c. thrombosis
   d. hemiparesis
   e. hemangioma

_____ 6. Thrombolytic therapy is directed toward:
   a. stabilizing blood cells
   b. destroying RBCs
   c. triggering blood clotting
   d. decreasing CSF
   e. dissolving a blood clot

_____ 7. A general term for any disorder or alteration of brain tissue is:
   a. cerebrocyst
   b. encephalopathy
   c. neurocytoma

17

d. dysencephaloma

e. psychosomatic

_____ 8. J.N. had disease manifestations related to involuntary functions and to movement controlled by motor fibers outside the pyramidal tracts. These functions are:

17

a. antispasmodic and voluntary

b. autonomic and neuroleptic

c. autonomic and voluntary

d. extrapyramidal and pyramidal

e. autonomic and extrapyramidal

Write a term from the case studies with each of the following meanings:

9. tumor of astrocytes _____

10. surgical opening into the skull _____

11. sudden attack typical of epilepsy _____

12. partial paralysis on one side _____

13. inability to speak or understand speech _____

14. inflammation of the meninges _____

15. collection of blood below the dura mater _____

16. perceived feeling of threat or harm _____

17. drug that relieves muscle spasms _____

18. antipsychotic medications _____

19. a physician who treats psychiatric disorders _____

Define each of the following abbreviations:

20. CT _____

21. LP _____

22. NICU _____

23. ICP _____

24. CSF _____

25. CVA _____

26. TIA _____

27. LOC _____

Nervous System

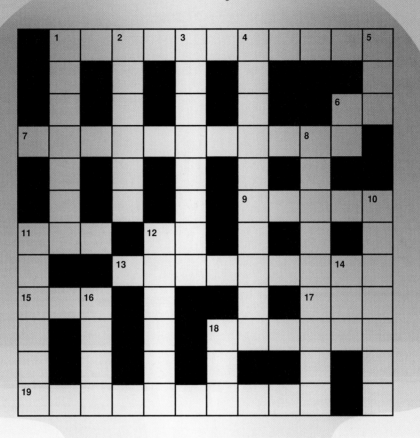

ACROSS

1. A division of the autonomic nervous system
6. Dementia caused by multiple small strokes (abbreviation): __ I __
7. Inflammation of a spinal nerve root
9. Drug used to treat Parkinson disease
11. Electric study of the brain (abbreviation)
12. Fluid around the brain and spinal cord (abbreviation): __ __ F
13. Instrument used for making computerized radiographic images
15. Order related to a patient's activity (abbreviation)
17. A sudden, brief interruption of blood flow to brain tissue (abbreviation)
18. Episodes associated with anxiety disorder
19. Mental state associated with sadness and loss of pleasure in life

DOWN

1. Junction between two neurons
2. Membranes around the brain and spinal cord: ____ root
3. Localized dilation of a blood vessel
4. Paralysis of one side of the body
5. Slow-growing viral disease of the brain (abbreviation)
6. Disease causing progressive loss of myelin in neurons (abbreviation)
8. Feeling associated with depression and other behavioral disorders
10. Loss or defect in speech communication
11. Methods for study of the nervous system: __ __ __ __ __ __ potentials
12. Type of brain injury caused by a blow: __ __ __ __ __ coup
14. Type of catheter (abbreviation): __ __ __ C
16. Method for studying the brain involving auditory stimulation (abbreviation)
18. All of the nervous system except the brain and spinal cord (abbreviation)

THE SENSES

18

OBJECTIVES

After study of this chapter you should be able to:

1. Explain the role of the sensory system.
2. Label diagrams of the ear and the eye, and briefly describe the function of each part.
3. Describe the pathway of nerve impulses from the ear to the brain.
4. Roots Pertaining to the Ear and Hearing
5. Describe the roles of the retina and the optic nerve in vision.

6. Identify and use word parts pertaining to the senses.
7. Describe the main disorders pertaining to the ear and the eye.
8. Interpret abbreviations used in the study of the ear and the eye.
9. Analyze several case studies pertaining to vision or hearing.

PRETEST

1. The scientific name for the sense of smell is _____.

2. The two senses located in the ear are _____ and _____.

3. Otitis is _____.

4. The receptor layer of the eye is the _____.

5. The scientific name for the white of the eye is _____.

6. Clouding of the lens is termed _____.

*T*he sensory system is our network for detecting stimuli from the internal and external environments. It is needed to maintain homeostasis, provide us with pleasure, and protect us from harm. Pain, for example, is an important warning sign of tissue damage. The signals generated in the various **receptors** of the sensory system must be transmitted to the central nervous system for interpretation.

The Senses

The senses are divided according to whether they are widely distributed or localized in special sense organs. The receptors for the general senses are found throughout the body. Many are located in the skin (Fig. 18-1). These senses include:

➤ Pain. These receptors are found in the skin and also in muscles, joints, and internal organs.
➤ Touch, the **tactile** sense, located in the skin. Sensitivity to touch depends on the concentration of these receptors in different areas, high on the fingers, lips and tongue, for example, but low at the back of the neck or back of the hand.
➤ Pressure, or deep touch, located beneath the skin and in deeper tissues.
➤ Temperature. Receptors for heat and cold are located in the skin and also in the hypothalamus, which regulates body temperature
➤ **Proprioception**, the awareness of body position. Receptors in muscles, tendons, and joints help to judge body position and coordinate muscle activity. They also help to maintain muscle tone.

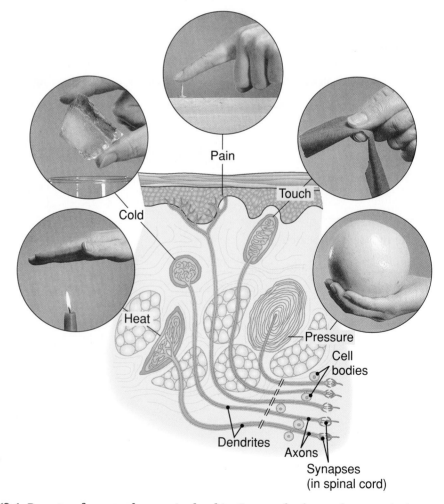

Figure 18-1 Receptors for general senses in the skin. Synapses for these pathways are in the spinal cord.

The special senses are localized within complex sense organs in the head. These include:

- ➤ **Gustation** (taste) is located in receptors in taste buds on the tongue. These receptors basically detect only sweet, sour, bitter, and salty, although researchers have recently identified receptors for alkali (bases), metallic taste, and the amino acid glutamate, as found in the flavor enhancer MSG. The senses of smell and taste are chemical senses, that is, they respond to chemicals in solution.
- ➤ **Olfaction** (smell) is located in receptors in the nose. Many more chemicals can be discriminated by smell than by taste. Both senses are important in stimulating appetite and warning of harmful substances.
- ➤ **Hearing** receptors are located in the ear. These receptors respond to movement created by sound waves as they travel through the ear.
- ➤ **Equilibrium** receptors are also located in the ear. These receptors are activated by changes in the position of cells as we move.
- ➤ **Vision** receptors are light-sensitive and located deep within the eye, protected by surrounding bone and other support structures. The coordinated actions of external and internal eye muscles help in the formation of a clear image.

The remainder of this chapter concentrates on hearing and vision, the senses that have received the most clinical attention.

18

TERMINOLOGY Key Terms

Senses

NORMAL STRUCTURE AND FUNCTION

equilibrium ē-kwi-LIB-rē-um	The sense of balance
gustation gus-TĀ-shun	The sense of taste
hearing HĒR-ing	The sense or perception of sound
olfaction ol-FAK-shun	The sense of smell
proprioception prō-prē-ō-SEP-shun	The awareness of posture, movement, and changes in equilibrium; receptors are located in muscles, tendons, and joints
receptor rē-SEP-tor	A sensory nerve ending or a specialized structure associated with a sensory nerve that responds to a stimulus
tactile TAK-til	Pertaining to the sense of touch
vision VIZH-un	The sense by which the shape, size, and color of objects are perceived by means of the light they give off

Go to the pronunciation glossary in Chapter 18 of the CD-ROM to hear these words pronounced.

Table 18·1	Suffixes Pertaining to the Senses		
SUFFIX	**MEANING**	**EXAMPLE**	**DEFINITION OF EXAMPLE**
-esthesia	sensation	cryesthesia *krī-es-THĒ-zē-a*	sensitivity to cold
-algesia	pain	hypalgesia* *hī-pal-JĒ-zē-a*	decreased sensitivity to pain
-osmia	sense of smell	pseudosmia *sū-DOS-mē-a*	false sense of smell
-geusia	sense of taste	parageusia *par-a-GŪ-zē-a*	abnormal (para-) sense of taste

*Prefix hyp/o.

Exercise 18-1

Define the following words:

1. dysesthesia *(dis-es-thē-zē-a)* _____

2. parosmia *(par-OZ-mē-a)* _____

3. ageusia *(a-Gū-zē-a)* _____

Synonyms. Write words that mean the same as the following:

4. lack (an-) of sensation _____

5. false sense of taste _____

6. sensitivity to temperature _____

7. excess sensitivity to pain _____

8. abnormal (dys-) sense of taste _____

9. muscular (my/o-) sensation _____

The Ear

The ear has the receptors for both hearing and equilibrium. For study purposes, it may be divided into three parts: the outer, middle, and inner ear (Fig. 18-2).

The outer ear consists of the projecting **pinna** (auricle) and the **external auditory canal** (meatus). This canal ends at the **tympanic membrane**, or eardrum, which transmits sound waves to the middle ear. Glands in the external canal produce a waxy material, **cerumen**, which protects the ear and helps to prevent infection.

Spanning the middle ear cavity are three **ossicles** (small bones), each named for its shape: the **malleus** (hammer), **incus** (anvil), and **stapes** (stirrup) (Fig. 18-3). Sound waves traveling over the ossicles are transmitted from the footplate of the stapes to the inner ear. The **eustachian tube** connects the middle ear with the nasopharynx and serves to equalize pressure between the outer ear and the middle ear.

The inner ear, because of its complex shape, is described as a **labyrinth**, which means "maze" (Fig. 18-4). It consists of an outer bony framework containing a similarly shaped membranous channel. The entire labyrinth is filled with fluid.

The **cochlea**, shaped like the shell of a snail, has the specialized **organ of Corti**, which is concerned with hearing. Cells in this receptor organ respond to sound waves traveling through the fluid-filled ducts of the cochlea. Sound waves enter the cochlea

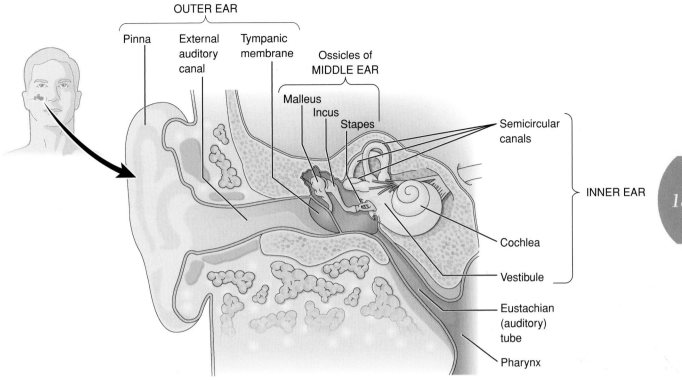

Figure 18-2 The ear. Structures in the outer, middle, and inner divisions are shown.

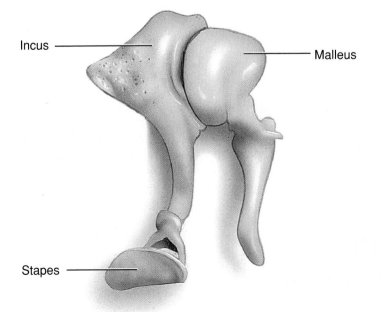

Figure 18-3 The ossicles of the middle ear. The malleus is in contact with the tympanic membrane. The base of the stapes is in contact with the oval window of the inner ear.

18

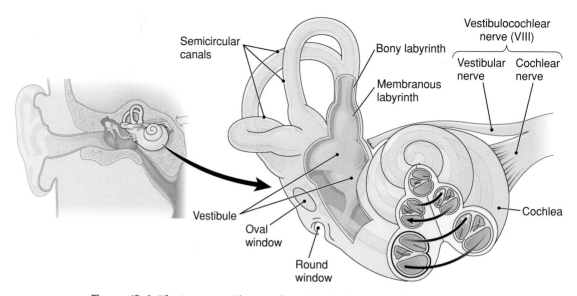

Figure 18-4 The inner ear. The outer bony labyrinth contains the membranous labyrinth. Receptors for equilibrium are in the vestibule and the semicircular canals. The cochlea contains the hearing receptor, the organ of Corti. Sound waves enter the cochlea through the oval window, travel through the cochlea, and exit through the round window. The inner ear transmits impulses to the brain in the vestibulocochlear nerve (VIIIth cranial nerve).

from the base of the stapes through an opening called the oval window and leave through another opening called the round window (see Fig. 18-4).

The sense of equilibrium is localized in the **vestibular apparatus**. This structure consists of the chamberlike **vestibule** and three projecting **semicircular canals**. Special cells within the vestibular apparatus respond to movement. (The senses of vision and proprioception are also important in maintaining balance.)

Nerve impulses are transmitted from the ear to the brain by way of the **vestibulocochlear nerve**, the eighth cranial nerve, also called the acoustic or auditory nerve. The cochlear branch of this nerve transmits impulses for hearing from the cochlea; the vestibular branch transmits impulses concerned with equilibrium from the vestibular apparatus (see Fig. 18-4).

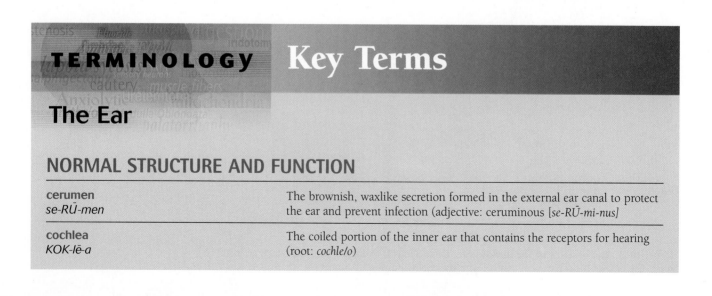

TERMINOLOGY Key Terms

The Ear

NORMAL STRUCTURE AND FUNCTION

cerumen *se-RŪ-men*	The brownish, waxlike secretion formed in the external ear canal to protect the ear and prevent infection (adjective: ceruminous [*se-RŪ-mi-nus*]
cochlea *KOK-lē-a*	The coiled portion of the inner ear that contains the receptors for hearing (root: *cochle/o*)

TERMINOLOGY Key Terms

The Ear
Continued

eustachian tube *ū-STĀ-shen*	The tube that connects the middle ear with the nasopharynx and serves to equalize pressure between the outer and middle ear (root: *salping/o*); auditory tube
external auditory canal	Tube that extends from the pinna of the ear to the tympanic membrane; external auditory meatus
incus *ING-kus*	The middle ossicle of the ear
labyrinth *LAB-i-rinth*	The inner ear, named for its complex structure, which resembles a maze
malleus *MAL-ē-us*	The ossicle of the middle ear that is in contact with the tympanic membrane and the incus
ossicles *OS-i-klz*	The small bones of the middle ear, the malleus, incus, and stapes
organ of Corti *KOR-tē*	The hearing receptor, which is located in the cochlea
pinna *PIN-a*	The projecting part of the outer ear; auricle (*AW-ri-kl*)
semicircular canals	The three curved channels of the inner ear that hold receptors for equilibrium
stapes *STĀ-pēz*	The ossicle that is in contact with the inner ear (root: *staped, stapedi/o*)
tympanic membrane *tim-PAN-ik*	The membrane between the external auditory canal and the middle ear (tympanic cavity); the eardrum. It serves to transmit sound waves to the ossicles of the middle ear (root: *myring/o, tympan/o*).
vestibular apparatus *ves-TIB-ū-lar*	The portion of the inner ear that is concerned with the sense of equilibrium; consists of the vestibule and the semicircular canals (root: *vestibul/o*)
vestibule *VES-ti-būl*	The chamber in the inner ear that holds some of the receptors for equilibrium
vestibulocochlear nerve *ves-tib-ū-lō-KOK-lē-ar*	The nerve that transmits impulses for hearing and equilibrium from the ear to the brain; eighth cranial nerve; auditory or acoustic nerve

Go to the pronunciation glossary in Chapter 18 of the CD-ROM to hear these words pronounced.

Table 18·2 Roots Pertaining to the Ear and Hearing

ROOT	MEANING	EXAMPLE	DEFINITION OF EXAMPLE
audi/o	hearing	audition *aw-DISH-un*	act of hearing
acous, acus, cus	sound, hearing	acoustic *a-KŪ-stik*	pertaining to sound or hearing
ot/o	ear	otogenic *ō-tō-JEN-ik*	originating in the ear
myring/o	tympanic membrane	myringotome *mi-RING-gō-tōm*	knife used for surgery on the eardrum
tympan/o	tympanic cavity (middle ear), tympanic membrane	tympanometry *tim-pa-NOM-e-trē*	measurement of transmission through the tympanic membrane and middle ear
salping/o	tube, eustachian tube	salpingoscope *sal-PING-go- skōp*	endoscope for examination of the eustachian tube
staped/o, stapedi/o	stapes	stapedoplasty *stā-pē-dō-PLAS-tē*	plastic repair of the stapes
labyrinth/o	labyrinth (inner ear)	labyrinthitis *lab-i-rin-THĪ-tis*	inflammation of the inner ear (labyrinth)
vestibul/o	vestibule, vestibular apparatus	vestibulotomy *ves-tib-ū-LOT-ō-mē*	incision of the vestibule of the inner ear
cochle/o	cochlea of inner ear	retrocochlear *ret-rō-KOK-lē-ar*	behind the cochlea

Exercise 18-2

Fill in the blanks:

1. Audiology (*aw- dē-OL-ō-jē*) is the study of _____.

2. Hyperacusis (*hī-per-a-Kū-sis*) is abnormally high sensitivity to _____.

3. Ototoxic (*ō-tō-TOKS-ik*) means poisonous or harmful to the _____.

Define the following adjectives:

4. auditory (*AW-di-tor-ē*) _____

5. otic (*Ō-tik*) _____

6. labyrinthine (*lab-i-RIN-thēn*) _____

7. vestibular (*ves-TIB-ū-lar*) _____

8. cochlear (*KOK-lē-ar*) _____

9. stapedial (*stā-PĒ-dē-al*) _____

Word building. Write words for the following definitions:

10. measurement of hearing (audi/o-) _____

11. pain in the ear _____

12. plastic repair of the middle ear _____

13. incision of the tympanic membrane _____

14. excision of the stapes _____

15. pertaining to the vestibular apparatus and cochlea _____

16. incision of the labyrinth _____

17. endoscopic examination of the eustachian tube _____

18. within the cochlea _____

18

Define the following terms:

19. audiometer (*aw-dē-OM-e-ter*) _____

20. vestibulopathy (*ves-tib-ū-LOP-a-thē*) _____

21. salpingopharyngeal (*sal-ping-gō-fa-RIN-jē-al*) _____

22. myringoscope (*mi-RING-gō-skōp*) _____

23. otitis (*ō-TĪ-tis*) _____

Clinical Aspects of Hearing

Hearing Loss

Hearing impairment may result from disease, injury, or developmental problems that affect the ear itself or any nervous pathways concerned with the sense of hearing.

Sensorineural hearing loss results from damage to the inner ear, the eighth cranial nerve, or central auditory pathways. Heredity, toxins, exposure to loud noises, and the aging process are possible causes for this type of hearing loss. It may range from inability to hear certain sound frequencies to a complete loss of hearing (deafness). People with extreme hearing loss that originates in the inner ear may benefit from a cochlear implant. This prosthesis stimulates the cochlear nerve directly, bypassing the receptor cells of the inner ear, and may allow the recipient to hear medium to loud sounds.

Conductive hearing loss results from blockage in sound transmission to the inner ear. Causes include obstruction, severe infection, or fixation of the middle ear ossicles. Often, physicians can successfully treat the conditions that cause conductive hearing loss.

Box 18-1 has information on careers in audiology, the study and treatment of hearing disorders.

Box 18•1 Health Professions *Audiologists*

Audiologists specialize in preventing, diagnosing, and treating hearing disorders that may be caused by injury, infection, birth defects, noise, or aging. They take a complete patient history to diagnose hearing disorders and use specialized equipment to measure hearing acuity. Audiologists design and implement individualized treatment plans, which may include fitting clients with assistive listening devices, such as hearing aids, or teaching alternative communication skills, such as lip reading. Audiologists also measure workplace and community noise levels and teach the public how to prevent hearing loss. Most audiologists in the United States have master's degrees or the equivalent from an accredited college or university and must pass a national licensing exam.

Audiologists work in a variety of settings, such as hospitals, nursing care facilities, schools, and clinics. Job prospects are good, as the need for audiologists' specialized skills will increase as populations age. The American Academy of Audiology has more information on this career.

Otitis

Otitis is any inflammation of the ear. **Otitis media** refers to an infection that leads to the accumulation of fluid in the middle ear cavity. One cause is malfunction or obstruction of the eustachian tube, as by allergy, enlarged adenoids, injury, or congenital abnormalities. Another cause is infection that spreads to the middle ear, most commonly from the upper respiratory tract. Continued infection may lead to accumulation of pus and perforation of the eardrum. Otitis media usually affects children under 5 years of age and may result in hearing loss. If not treated with antibiotics, the infection may spread to other regions of the ear and head. An incision, a **myringotomy**, and placement of a tube in the tympanic membrane helps to ventilate and drain the middle ear cavity in cases of otitis media.

Otitis externa is inflammation of the external auditory canal. Infections in this region may be caused by a fungus or bacterium and are most common among those living in hot climates and among swimmers, leading to the alternative name, "swimmer's ear."

Otosclerosis

In **otosclerosis**, the bony structure of the inner ear deteriorates and then reforms into spongy bone tissue that may eventually harden. Most commonly, the stapes becomes fixed against the inner ear and is unable to vibrate, resulting in conductive hearing loss. The cause of otosclerosis is unknown, but some cases are hereditary. Surgeons usually can remove the damaged bone. In a **stapedectomy**, the stapes is removed and a prosthetic bone is inserted.

Ménière Disease

Ménière disease is a disorder that affects the inner ear. It seems to involve production and circulation of the fluid that fills the inner ear, but the cause is unknown. The symptoms are **vertigo** (dizziness), hearing loss, pronounced **tinnitus** (ringing in the ears), and a feeling of pressure in the ear. The course of the disease is uneven, and symptoms may become less severe with time. Ménière disease is treated with drugs to control nausea and dizziness, such as those used to treat motion sickness. In severe cases, the inner ear or part of the eighth cranial nerve may be destroyed surgically.

Acoustic Neuroma

An **acoustic neuroma** (also called a schwannoma or neurilemoma) is a tumor that arises from the neurilemma (sheath) of the eighth cranial nerve. As the tumor enlarges, it presses on surrounding nerves and interferes with blood supply. This leads to tinnitus, dizziness, and progressive hearing loss. Other symptoms develop as the tumor presses on the brainstem and other cranial nerves. Usually it is necessary to remove the tumor surgically.

TERMINOLOGY Key Terms

The Ear

DISORDERS

acoustic neuroma *a-KŪ-stik nū-RŌ-ma*	A tumor of the eighth cranial nerve sheath; although benign, it can press on surrounding tissue and produce symptoms; also called a schwannoma or neurilemoma
conductive hearing loss	Hearing impairment that results from blockage of sound transmission to the inner ear
Ménière disease *men-NYĀR*	A disease associated with increased fluid pressure in the inner ear and characterized by hearing loss, vertigo, and tinnitus
otitis externa *ō-TĪ-tis ex-TER-na*	Inflammation of the external auditory canal; swimmer's ear
otitis media *ō-TĪ-tis MĒ-dē-a*	Inflammation of the middle ear with accumulation of serous (watery) or mucoid fluid
otosclerosis *ō-tō-skle-RŌ-sis*	Formation of abnormal and sometimes hardened bony tissue in the ear. It usually occurs around the oval window and the footplate (base) of the stapes, causing immobilization of the stapes and progressive loss of hearing.
sensorineural hearing loss *sen-sō-rē-NŪ-ral*	Hearing impairment that results from damage to the inner ear, eighth cranial nerve, or auditory pathways in the brain
tinnitus *tin-Ī-tus*	A sensation of noises, such as ringing or tinkling, in the ear
vertigo *VER-ti-gō*	An illusion of movement, as of the body moving in space or the environment moving about the body; usually caused by disturbances in the vestibular apparatus. Used loosely to mean dizziness or lightheadedness.

TREATMENT

myringotomy *mir-in-GOT-ō-mē*	Surgical incision of the tympanic membrane; performed to drain the middle ear cavity or to insert a tube into the tympanic membrane for drainage
stapedectomy *stā-pē-DEK-tō-mē*	Surgical removal of the stapes; it may be combined with insertion of a prosthesis to correct otosclerosis

Go to the pronunciation glossary in Chapter 18 of the CD-ROM to hear these words pronounced.

TERMINOLOGY Supplementary Terms

NORMAL STRUCTURE AND FUNCTION

aural *AW-ral*	Pertaining to or perceived by the ear
decibel (dB) *DES-i-bel*	A unit for measuring the relative intensity of sound
hertz (Hz)	A unit for measuring the frequency (pitch) of sound
mastoid process	A small projection of the temporal bone behind the external auditory canal; it consists of loosely arranged bony material and small, air-filled cavities
stapedius *stā-PĒ-dē-us*	A small muscle attached to the stapes. It contracts in the presence of a loud sound, producing the acoustic reflex.

SYMPTOMS AND CONDITIONS

cholesteatoma *kō-lē-stē-a-TŌ-ma*	A cystlike mass containing cholesterol that is most common in the middle ear and mastoid region; a possible complication of chronic middle ear infection
labyrinthitis *lab-i-rin-THĪ-tis*	Inflammation of the labyrinth of the ear (inner ear); otitis interna
mastoiditis *mas-toyd-Ī-tis*	Inflammation of the air cells of the mastoid process
presbycusis *prez-bē-KŪ-sis*	Loss of hearing caused by aging; also presbyacusis

DIAGNOSIS AND TREATMENT

audiometry *aw-de-OM-e-trē*	Measurement of hearing
electronystagmography (ENG) *ē-lek-trō-nis-tag-MOG-ra-fē*	A method for recording eye movements by means of electrical responses; such movements may reflect vestibular dysfunction
otorhinolaryngology (ORL) *ō-tō-rī-nō-lar-in-GOL-ō-jē*	The branch of medicine that deals with diseases of the ear(s), nose, and throat (ENT); also called otolaryngology (OL)
otoscope *Ō-tō-skōp*	Instrument for examining the ear (see Fig. 7-6)
Rinne test	Test that measures hearing by comparing results of bone conduction and air conduction (Fig. 18-5)
spondee *spon-dē*	A two-syllable word with equal stress on each syllable; used in hearing tests; examples are toothbrush, baseball, cowboy, pancake
Weber test	Test for hearing loss that uses a vibrating tuning fork placed at the center of the head (Fig. 18-6)

18

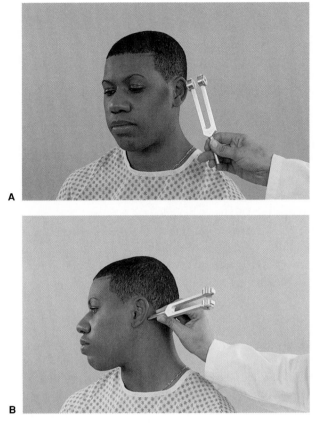

A

B

Figure 18-5 The Rinne test.
This test assesses both air and
bone conduction of sound.

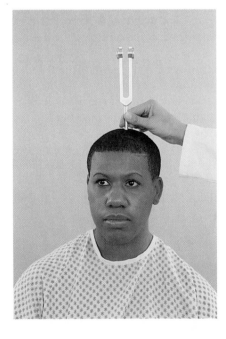

Figure 18-6 The Weber test. This test assesses
bone conduction of sound.

TERMINOLOGY Abbreviations

The Ear

ABR	Auditory brainstem response	HL	Hearing level
AC	Air conduction	Hz	Hertz
AD	Right ear (*Latin, auris dexter*)	OL	Otolaryngology
AS	Left ear (*Latin, auris sinistra*)	OM	Otitis media
BAEP	Brainstem auditory evoked potentials	ORL	Otorhinolaryngology
BC	Bone conduction	ST	Speech threshold
dB	Decibel	TM	Tympanic membrane
ENG	Electronystagmography	TTS	Temporary threshold shift
ENT	Ear(s), nose, and throat		

The Eye and Vision

The eye is protected by its position within a bony socket or **orbit**. It is also protected by the eyelids, or **palpebrae**, eyebrows, and eyelashes (Fig. 18-7). The **lacrimal (tear) glands** (Fig. 18-8) constantly bathe and cleanse the eyes with a lubricating fluid that drains into the nose. The protective **conjunctiva** is a thin membrane that lines the eyelids and covers the anterior portion of the eye. This membrane folds back to form a narrow space between the eyeball and the eyelids. Medications can be instilled into this conjunctival sac.

The wall of the **eye** is composed of three layers (Fig. 18-9). Named from outermost to innermost they are as follows:

1. The **sclera**, commonly called the *white of the eye*, is the tough surface protective layer. The sclera extends over the eye's anterior portion as the transparent **cornea**.
2. The **uvea** is the middle layer, which consists of:
   ➤ **the choroid**, a vascular and pigmented layer located in the posterior portion of the eyeball. The choroid provides nourishment for the retina.
   ➤ the **ciliary body**, which contains a muscle that controls the shape of the **lens** to allow for near and far vision, a process known as **accommodation** (Fig 18-10). The lens must become more rounded for viewing close objects.
   ➤ the **iris**, a muscular ring that controls the size of the **pupil**, thus regulating the amount of light that enters the eye (Fig. 18-11). The genetically controlled pigments of the iris determine eye color.
3. The **retina** is the innermost layer and the actual visual receptor. It consists of two types of specialized cells that respond to light:

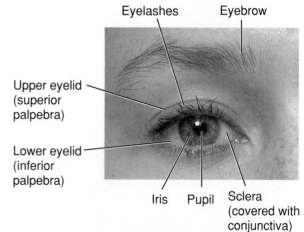

Figure 18-7 **Protective structures of the eye.**

18

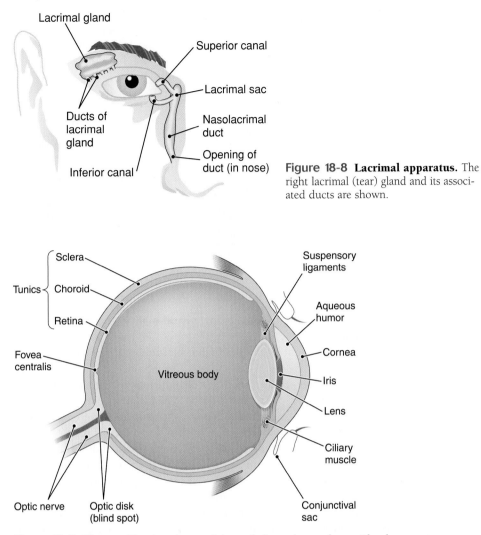

Lacrimal gland
Superior canal
Lacrimal sac
Ducts of lacrimal gland
Nasolacrimal duct
Inferior canal
Opening of duct (in nose)

Figure 18-8 Lacrimal apparatus. The right lacrimal (tear) gland and its associated ducts are shown.

Sclera
Choroid
Tunics
Retina
Suspensory ligaments
Aqueous humor
Fovea centralis
Vitreous body
Cornea
Iris
Lens
Ciliary muscle
Optic nerve
Optic disk (blind spot)
Conjunctival sac

Figure 18-9 The eye. The three layers of the eyeball are shown along with other structures involved in vision.

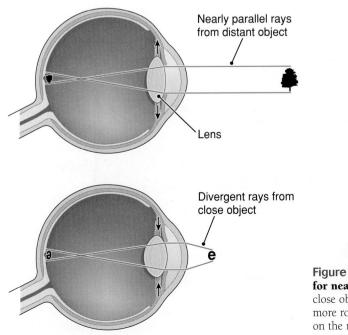

Nearly parallel rays from distant object

Lens

Divergent rays from close object

Figure 18-10 Accommodation for near vision. When viewing a close object, the lens must become more rounded to focus light rays on the retina.

18

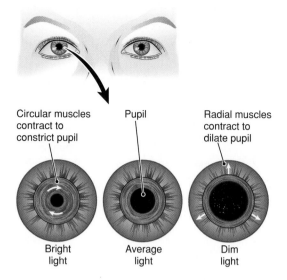

Figure 18-11 Function of the iris. In bright light, muscles in the iris constrict the pupil, limiting the light that enters the eye. In dim light, the iris dilates the pupil to allow more light to enter the eye.

Circular muscles contract to constrict pupil

Pupil

Radial muscles contract to dilate pupil

Bright light

Average light

Dim light

> ➤ **The rods** function in dim light, provide low **visual acuity** (sharpness), and do not respond to color.
> ➤ The **cones** are active in bright light, have high visual acuity, and respond to color.

Proper vision requires the **refraction** (bending) of light rays as they pass through parts of the eye to focus on a specific point on the retina. The impulses generated within the rods and cones are transmitted to the brain by way of the optic nerve (second cranial nerve). Where the optic nerve connects to the retina, there are no rods or cones. This point, at which there is no visual perception, is called the **optic disk**, or blind spot (Fig. 18-12). The **fovea** is a tiny depression in the retina near the optic nerve that has a high concentration of cone cells and is the point of greatest visual acuity. The fovea is surrounded by a yellowish spot called the **macula** (see Fig. 18-12).

The eyeball is filled with a jellylike **vitreous body** (see Fig. 18-9), which helps maintain the shape of the eye and also refracts light. The **aqueous humor** is the fluid that fills the eye anterior to the lens, maintaining the shape of the cornea and refracting light. This fluid is constantly produced and drained from the eye.

Six muscles attached to the outside of each eye coordinate eye movements to achieve **convergence**, that is, coordinated movement of the eyes so that they both are fixed on the same point.

Box 18-2 explores the Greek origins of some medical words, including some pertaining to the eye.

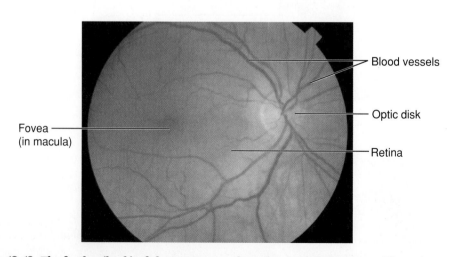

Fovea (in macula)

Blood vessels

Optic disk

Retina

Figure 18-12 The fundus (back) of the eye as seen through an ophthalmoscope. The optic disk (blind spot) is shown as well as the fovea, the point of sharpest vision, in the retina.

Box 18•2 Focus on Words — *The Greek Influence*

Some of our most beautiful (and difficult to spell and pronounce) words come from Greek. *Esthesi/o* means sensation. It appears in the word *anesthesia*, a state in which there is lack of sensation, particularly pain. It is found in the word *esthetics* (also spelled aesthetics), which pertains to beauty, artistry, and appearance. The prefix *presby*, in the terms *presbycusis* and *presbyopia*, means "old," and these conditions appear with aging. The root *cycl/o*, pertaining to the ringlike ciliary body of the eye, is from the Greek word for circle or wheel. The same root appears in the words *bicycle* and *tricycle*. Also pertaining to the eye, the term iris means "rainbow" in Greek, and the iris is the colored part of the eye.

The root *sthen/o* means "strength," and occurs in the words *asthenia*, meaning lack of strength or weakness, and *neurasthenia*, an old term for vague "nervous exhaustion,"

now applied to conditions involving chronic symptoms of generalized fatigue, anxiety, and pain. The root also appears in the word *calisthenics* in combination with the root *cali-*, meaning "beauty." So the rhythmic strengthening and conditioning exercises that are done in calisthenics literally give us beauty through strength.

The Greek root *steth/o* means "chest," although a stethoscope is used to listen to sounds in other parts of the body as well as the chest.

Asphyxia is derived from the Greek root *sphygm/o* meaning "pulse." The word is literally "stoppage of the pulse," which is exactly what happens when one suffocates. This same root is found in *sphygmomanometer*, the apparatus used to measure blood pressure. One look at the word and one attempt to pronounce it make clear why most people call the device a blood pressure cuff!

TERMINOLOGY Key Terms

The Eye

NORMAL STRUCTURE AND FUNCTION

accommodation *a-kom-ō-DĀ-shun*	Adjustment of the curvature of the lens to allow for vision at various distances
aqueous humor *AK-wē-us*	Fluid that fills the eye anterior to the lens
choroid *KOR-oyd*	The dark, vascular, middle layer of the eye (**roots:** *chori/o, choroid/o*); part of the uvea (see below)
ciliary body *SIL-ē-ar-ē*	The muscular portion of the uvea that surrounds the lens and adjusts its shape for near and far vision (root: *cycl/o*)
cone	A specialized cell in the retina that responds to light; cones have high visual acuity, function in bright light, and can discriminate colors
conjunctiva *kon-junk-TĪ-va*	The mucous membrane that lines the eyelids and covers the anterior portion of the eyeball
convergence *kon-VER-jens*	Coordinated movement of the eyes toward fixation on the same point
cornea *KOR-nē-a*	The clear, anterior portion of the sclera (root: *corne/o, kerat/o*)
eye	The organ of vision (root: *opt/o, ocul/o, ophthalm/o*)
fovea *FŌ-vē-a*	The tiny depression in the retina that is the point of sharpest vision; fovea centralis, central fovea

TERMINOLOGY Key Terms

The Eye *Continued*

iris *Ī-ris*	The muscular colored ring between the lens and the cornea; regulates the amount of light that enters the eye by altering the size of the pupil at its center (roots: *ir, irid/o, irit/o*; plural: irides [*IR-i-dēz*])
lacrimal glands *LAK-ri-mal*	Pertaining to tears (roots: *lacrim/o, dacry/o*)
lens *lenz*	The transparent, biconvex structure in the anterior portion of the eye that refracts light and functions in accommodation (roots: *lent/i, phak/o*)
macula *MAK-ū-la*	A small spot or colored area; used alone to mean the yellowish spot in the retina that contains the fovea
optic disk	The point where the optic nerve joins the retina; at this point there are no rods or cones; also called the blind spot or optic papilla
orbit *OR-bit*	The bony cavity that contains the eyeball
palpebra *PAL-pe-bra*	An eyelid; a protective fold (upper or lower) that closes over the anterior surface of the eye (root: *palpebr/o, blephar/o*; adjective" palpebral; plural: palpebrae [*pal-PĒ-brē*])
pupil *PŪ-pil*	The opening at the center of the iris (root: *pupill/o*)
refraction *rē-FRAK-shun*	The bending of light rays as they pass through the eye to focus on a specific point on the retina; also the determination and correction of ocular refractive errors
retina *RET-i-na*	The innermost, light-sensitive layer of the eye; contains the rods and cones, the specialized receptor cells for vision (root: *retin/o*)
rod	A specialized cell in the retina of the eye that responds to light; rods have low visual acuity, function in dim light, and do not discriminate color
sclera *SKLĒR-a*	The tough, white, fibrous outermost layer of the eye; the white of the eye (root: *scler/o*)
uvea *Ū-vē-a*	The middle, vascular layer of the eye (root: *uve/o*); consists of the choroid, ciliary body, and iris
visual acuity *a-KŪ-i-tē*	Sharpness of vision
vitreous body *VIT-rē-us*	The transparent jellylike mass that fills the main cavity of the eyeball; also called vitreous humor

Go to the pronunciation glossary in Chapter 18 of the CD-ROM to hear these words pronounced.

Word Parts Pertaining to the Eye and Vision

Table 18•3	Roots for External Eye Structures		
ROOT	**MEANING**	**EXAMPLE**	**DEFINITION OF EXAMPLE**
blephar/o	eyelid	symblepharon *sim-BLEF-a-ron*	adhesion of the eyelid to the eyeball (*sym-* = together)
palpebr/o	eyelid	palpebral *PAL-pe-bral*	pertaining to an eyelid
dacry/o	tear, lacrimal apparatus	dacryolith *DAK-rē-ō-lith*	stone in the lacrimal apparatus
dacryocyst/o	lacrimal sac	dacryocystocele *dak-rē-ō-SIS-tō-sēl*	hernia of the lacrimal sac
lacrim/o	tear, lacrimal apparatus	lacrimation *lak-ri-MĀ-shun*	secretion of tears

18

Exercise 18-3

Define the following words:

1. dacryocystectomy (*dak-rē-ō-sis-TEK-tō-mē*) _____

2. blepharoplegia (*BLEF-a-rō-plē-jē-a*) _____

3. interpalpebral (*in-ter-PAL-pe-bral*) _____

4. nasolacrimal (*nā-zō-LAK-ri-mal*) _____

Word building. Use the roots indicated to write words with the following meanings:

5. spasm of the eyelid (blephar/o) _____

6. discharge from the lacrimal apparatus (dacry/o) _____

7. inflammation of a lacrimal sac _____

Table 18•4	Roots for the Eye and Vision		
ROOT	**MEANING**	**EXAMPLE**	**DEFINITION OF EXAMPLE**
opt/o	eye, vision	optometer *op-TOM-e-ter*	instrument for measuring the refractive power of the eye
ocul/o	eye	sinistrocular *si-nis-TROK-ū-lar*	pertaining to the left eye
ophthalm/o	eye	exophthalmos *eks-of-THAL-mos*	protrusion of the eyeball
scler/o	sclera	episcleritis *ep-i-skle-RĪ-tis*	inflammation of the tissue on the surface of the sclera
corne/o	cornea	circumcorneal *sir-kum-KOR-nē-al*	around the cornea

Table 18•4	Continued		
kerat/o	cornea	keratoplasty *KER-a-tō-plas-tē*	plastic repair of the cornea; corneal transplant
lent/i	lens	lentiform *LEN-ti-form*	resembling a lens
phak/o, phac/o	lens	aphakia *a-FĀ-kē-a*	absence of a lens
uve/o	uvea	uveal *Ū-vē-al*	pertaining to the uvea
chori/o, choroid/o	choroid	subchoroidal *sub-kor-OYD-al*	below the choroid
cycl/o	ciliary body, ciliary muscle	cycloplegic *sī-klō-PLĒ-jik*	pertaining to or causing paralysis of the ciliary muscle
ir, irit/o, irid/o	iris	iridoschisis *ir-i-DOS-ki-sis*	splitting of the iris
pupill/o	pupil	iridopupillary *ir-i-dō-PŪ-pi-ler-ē*	pertaining to the iris and the pupil
retin/o	retina	retinoscopy *ret-in-OS-kō-pē*	examination of the retina

Exercise 18-4

Fill in the blanks:

1. The oculomotor (*ok-ū-lō-MŌ-tor*) nerve controls movements of the _____.

2. The term *phacolysis* (*fa-KOL-i-sis*) means destruction of the _____.

3. A keratometer (*ker-a-TOM-e-ter*) is an instrument for measuring the curves of the _____.

4. The science of orthoptics (*or-THOP-tiks*) deals with correcting defects in _____.

5. Lenticonus (*LEN-ti-kō-nus*) is conical protrusion of the _____.

Identify and define the roots pertaining to the eye in the following words:

	Root	**Meaning of Root**
6. microphthalmos (*mī-krof-THAL-mus*)	_____	_____
7. interpupillary (*in-ter-PŪ-pi-ler-ē*)	_____	_____
8. retrolental (*ret-rō-LEN-tal*)	_____	_____
9. uveitis (*ū-vē-Ī-tis*)	_____	_____
10. phacotoxic (*fak-ō-TOK-sik*)	_____	_____
11. iridodilator (*ir-id-ō-DĪ-lā-tor*)	_____	_____
12. optometrist (*op-TOM-e-trist*)	_____	_____

Write words for the following definitions:

13. surgical fixation of the retina _____

14. inflammation of the uvea and sclera _____

15. pertaining to the pupil _____

16. softening of the lens (use phac/o) _____

17. inflammation of the ciliary body _____

Use the root ophthalm/o to write words for the following definitions:

18. an instrument used to examine the eye _____

19. the medical specialty that deals with the eye and diseases of the eye _____

Use the root irid/o to write words for the following definitions:

20. surgical removal of (part of) the iris _____

21. paralysis of the iris _____

Define the following words:

22. optical (*OP-ti-kal*) _____

23. retinoschisis (*ret-i-NOS-ki-sis*) _____

24. sclerotome (*SKLĒR-ō-tōm*) _____

25. lenticular (*len-TIK-ū-lar*) _____

26. keratitis (*ker-a-TĪ-tis*) _____

27. cyclotomy (*sī-KLOT-ō-mē*) _____

28. iridocyclitis (*ir-i-dō-sī-KLĪ-tis*) _____

29. chorioretinal (*kor-ē-ō-RET-i-nal*) _____

30. dextrocular (*deks-TROK-ū-lar*) _____

Table 18·5	Suffixes for the Eye and Vision*		
SUFFIX	**MEANING**	**EXAMPLE**	**DEFINITION OF EXAMPLE**
-opsia	vision	heteropsia *het-er-OP-sē-a*	unequal vision in the two eyes
-opia	eye, vision	hemianopia *hem-ē-an-Ō-pē-a*	blindness in half the visual field

Compounds of -ops (eye) + -ia.

Exercise 18-5

Use the suffix -opsia to write words for the following definitions:

1. a visual defect in which objects seem larger (macr/o) than they are _____

2. lack of (a-) color (chromat/o) vision (complete color blindness) _____

Use the suffix -opia to write words for the following definitions:

3. double vision _____

4. changes in vision due to old age (use the prefix *presby-* meaning "old") _____

The suffix -opia is added to the root **metr/o** *(measure) to form words pertaining to the refractive power of the eye. Add a prefix to* **-metropia** *to form words for the following:*

5. a lack of perfect refractive power in the eye _____

6. unequal refractive powers in the two eyes _____

Clinical Aspects of Vision

Errors of Refraction

If the eyeball is too long, images will form in front of the retina. To focus clearly, one must bring an object closer to the eye. This condition of nearsightedness is technically called **myopia** (Fig. 18-13). The opposite condition is **hyperopia**, or farsightedness, in which the eyeball is too short and images form behind the retina. One must move an object away from the eye for the focus to be clear. The same effect is produced by **presbyopia**, which accompanies aging. The lens loses elasticity and can no longer accommodate for near vision, so a person becomes increasingly farsighted.

An **astigmatism** is an irregularity in the curve of the cornea or lens that distorts light entering the eye and blurs vision.

Glasses can compensate for most of these refractive impairments, as shown for nearsightedness and farsightedness in Figure 18-13. See also Box 18-3 for information on a surgical technique to correct refractive errors.

Infection

Several microorganisms can cause **conjunctivitis** (inflammation of the conjunctiva). This is a highly infectious disease commonly called "pinkeye."

The bacterium *Chlamydia trachomatis* causes **trachoma**, inflammation of the cornea and conjunctiva that results in scarring. This disease is rare in the United States but is a common cause of blindness in underdeveloped countries, although it is easily cured with sulfa drugs and antibiotics.

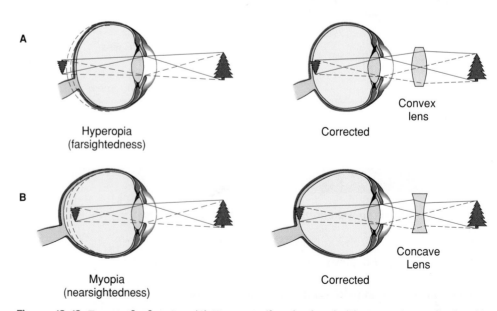

Figure 18-13 Errors of refraction. (*A*) Hyperopia (farsightedness). (*B*) Myopia (nearsightedness). A convex (outwardly curved) lens corrects for hyperopia; a concave (inwardly curved) lens corrects for myopia.

Box 18•3 Clinical Perspectives · *Eye Surgery: A Glimpse of the Cutting Edge*

Cataracts, glaucoma, and refractive errors are common eye disorders. In the past, cataract and glaucoma treatments concentrated on managing the diseases. Refractive errors were corrected using eyeglasses and, more recently, contact lenses. Today, laser and microsurgical techniques can remove cataracts, reduce glaucoma, and allow people with refractive errors to put their eyeglasses and contacts away. These cutting-edge procedures include:

➤ LASIK (laser in situ keratomileusis) to correct refractive errors. During this procedure, a surgeon uses a laser to reshape the cornea so that it refracts light directly onto the retina, rather than in front of or behind it. A microkeratome (surgical knife) is used to cut a flap in the outer layer of the cornea. A computer-controlled laser sculpts the middle layer of the cornea and then the flap is replaced. The procedure takes only a few minutes and patients recover their vision quickly and usually with little postoperative pain.

➤ Phacoemulsification to remove cataracts. During this procedure, a surgeon makes a very small incision (approximately 3 mm long) through the sclera near the outer edge of the cornea. An ultrasonic probe is inserted through this opening and into the center of the lens. The probe uses sound waves to emulsify the central core of the lens, which is then suctioned out. Then, an artificial lens is permanently implanted in the lens capsule (see Fig. 18-17). The procedure is typically painless, although the patient may feel some discomfort for 1 to 2 days afterward.

➤ Laser trabeculoplasty to treat glaucoma. This procedure uses a laser to help drain fluid from the eye and lower intraocular pressure. The laser is aimed at drainage canals located between the cornea and iris and makes several burns that are believed to open the canals and allow fluid to drain better. The procedure is typically painless and takes only a few minutes.

Gonorrhea is the usual cause of an acute conjunctivitis in newborns called **ophthalmia neonatorum**. An antibiotic ointment is routinely used to prevent such eye infections in newborns.

Disorders of the Retina

Retinal detachment, separation of the retina from the underlying layer of the eye (the choroid), may be caused by a tumor, hemorrhage, or injury to the eye (Fig. 18-14). This condition interferes with vision and is commonly repaired with laser surgery.

Degeneration of the macula, the point of sharpest vision, is a common cause of visual problems in the elderly. When associated with aging, this deterioration is described as **age-related macular degeneration (AMD)**. In one form of macular degeneration ("dry"), material accumulates on the retina. Vitamins C and E, beta carotene, and zinc

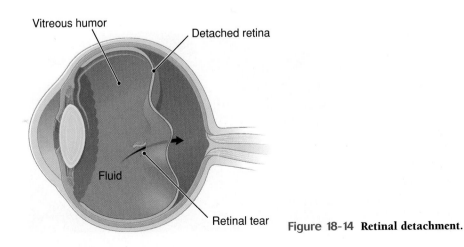

Figure 18-14 Retinal detachment.

18

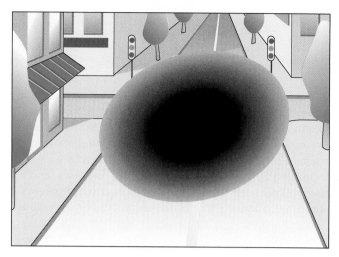

Figure 18-15 Visual loss associated with macular degeneration. The center of the visual field is affected, but peripheral vision is usually unaffected.

supplements may delay this process. In another form ("wet"), abnormal blood vessels grow under the retina, causing it to detach. Laser surgery may stop the growth of these vessels and delay vision loss. Macular degeneration typically affects central vision but not peripheral vision (Fig. 18-15). Other causes of macular degeneration are drug toxicity and hereditary diseases.

Circulatory problems associated with diabetes mellitus eventually cause changes in the retina referred to as **diabetic retinopathy**. In addition to vascular damage, there is a yellowish, waxy exudate high in lipoproteins. With time, new blood vessels form and penetrate the vitreous humor, causing hemorrhage, detachment of the retina, and blindness.

Cataract

A **cataract** is an opacity (cloudiness) of the lens (Fig 18-16). Causes of cataract include disease, injury, chemicals, and exposure to physical forces, especially the ultraviolet radiation in sunlight. The cataracts that frequently appear with age may result from exposure to environmental factors in combination with degeneration attributable to aging.

To prevent blindness, an ophthalmologist must remove the cloudy lens surgically. Commonly, the anterior capsule of the lens is removed along with the cataract, leaving the posterior capsule in place (Fig. 18-17). In **phacoemulsification**, the lens is fragmented with high-frequency ultrasound and extracted through a small incision (see Box 18-3). After cataract removal an artificial intraocular lens (IOL) usually is implanted to compensate for the missing lens. The original type of implant provides vision only within a fixed distance; newer implants are designed to allow for near and far accommodation. Alternatively, a person can wear a contact lens or special glasses.

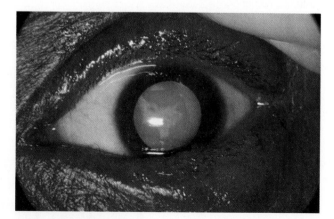

Figure 18-16 Cataract. The white appearance of the pupil in this eye is due to complete opacity of the lens.

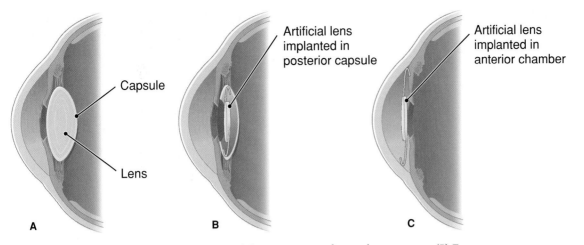

Figure 18-17 Cataract extraction surgeries. (*A*) Cross section of normal eye anatomy. (*B*) Extracapsular lens extraction involves removing the lens but leaving the posterior capsule intact to receive a synthetic intraocular lens. (*C*) Intracapsular lens extraction involves removing the lens and lens capsule and implanting a synthetic intraocular lens in the anterior chamber.

Glaucoma

Glaucoma is an abnormal increase in pressure within the eyeball. It occurs when more aqueous humor is produced than can be drained away from the eye. There is pressure on blood vessels in the eye and on the optic nerve, leading to blindness. There are many causes of glaucoma, and screening for this disorder should be a part of every routine eye examination. Fetal infection with German measles (rubella) early in pregnancy can cause glaucoma, as well as cataracts and hearing impairment. Glaucoma is usually treated with medication to reduce pressure in the eye and occasionally is treated with surgery (see Box 18-3).

TERMINOLOGY Key Terms

The Eye

DISORDERS

age-related macular degeneration (AMD)	Deterioration of the macula associated with aging; macular degeneration impairs central vision
astigmatism *a-STIG-ma-tizm*	An error of refraction caused by irregularity in the curvature of the cornea or lens
cataract *KAT-a-rakt*	Opacity of the lens of the eye
conjunctivitis *kon-junk-ti-VI-tis*	Inflammation of the conjunctiva; pinkeye
diabetic retinopathy *ret-i-NOP-a-thē*	Degenerative changes in the retina associated with diabetes mellitus

TERMINOLOGY Key Terms

The Eye   *Continued*

glaucoma *glaw-KŌ-ma*	A disease of the eye caused by increased intraocular pressure that damages the optic disk and causes loss of vision. Usually results from faulty fluid drainage from the anterior portion of the eye.
hyperopia *hī-per-Ō-pē-a*	An error of refraction in which light rays focus behind the retina and objects can be seen clearly only when far from the eye; farsightedness; also called hypermetropia
myopia *mī-Ō-pē-a*	An error of refraction in which light rays focus in front of the retina and objects can be seen clearly only when very close to the eye; nearsightedness
ophthalmia neonatorum *of-THAL-mē-a nē-ō-nā-TOR-um*	Severe conjunctivitis usually caused by infection with gonococcus during birth
phacoemulsification *fak-ō-ē-mul-si-fi-KĀ-shun*	Removal of a cataract by ultrasonic destruction and extraction of the lens
presbyopia *prez-bē-Ō-pē-a*	Changes in the eye that occur with age; the lens loses elasticity and the ability to accommodate for near vision
retinal detachment	Separation of the retina from the underlying layer of the eye
trachoma *tra-KŌ-ma*	An infection caused by *Chlamydia trachomatis* leading to inflammation and scarring of the cornea and conjunctiva; a common cause of blindness in underdeveloped countries

Go to the pronunciation glossary in Chapter 18 of the CD-ROM to hear these words pronounced.

TERMINOLOGY Supplementary Terms

The Eye

NORMAL STRUCTURE AND FUNCTION

canthus *KAN-thus*	The angle at either end of the slit between the eyelids
diopter *DĪ-op-ter*	A measurement unit for the refractive power of a lens
emmetropia *em-e-TRŌ-pē-a*	The normal condition of the eye in refraction, in which parallel light rays focus exactly on the retina

TERMINOLOGY

Supplementary Terms

The Eye

Continued

fundus *FUN-dus*	A bottom or base; the region farthest from the opening of a structure. The fundus of the eye is the back portion of the inside of the eyeball as seen with an ophthalmoscope.
meibomian gland *mī-BŌ-mē-an*	A sebaceous gland in the eyelid
tarsus *TAR-sus*	The framework of dense connective tissue that gives shape to the eyelid; tarsal plate
zonule *ZON-ūl*	A system of fibers that holds the lens in place; also called suspensory ligaments

SYMPTOMS AND CONDITIONS

amblyopia *am-blē-Ō-pē-a*	A condition that occurs when visual acuity is not the same in the two eyes in children (prefix *ambly* means "dim"). Disuse of the poorer eye will result in blindness if not corrected. Also called "lazy eye."
anisocoria *an-ī-sō-KŌ-rē-a*	Condition in which the two pupils (root: *cor/o*) are not of equal size
blepharoptosis *blef-a-rop-TŌ-sis*	Drooping of the eyelid
chalazion *ka-LĀ-zē-on*	A small mass on the eyelid resulting from inflammation and blockage of a meibomian gland
druzen *DRŪ-zen*	Small growths that appear as tiny yellowish spots beneath the retina of the eye; typically occur with age but also occur in certain abnormal conditions
hordeolum *hor-DĒ-ō-lum*	Inflammation of a sebaceous gland of the eyelid; a sty
keratoconus *ker-a-tō-KŌ-nus*	Conical protrusion of the corneal center
miosis *mī-Ō-sis*	Abnormal contraction of the pupils (from Greek, meaning "diminution")
mydriasis *mi-DRĪ-a-sis*	Pronounced or abnormal dilation of the pupil
nyctalopia *nik-ta-LŌ-pē-a*	Night blindness. Inability to see well in dim light or at night (root: *nyct/o*); often due to lack of vitamin A, which is used to make the pigment needed for vision in dim light
nystagmus *nis-TAG-mus*	Rapid, involuntary, rhythmic movements of the eyeball; may occur in neurologic diseases or disorders of the inner ear's vestibular apparatus
papilledema *pap-il-e-DĒ-ma*	Swelling of the optic disk (papilla); choked disk

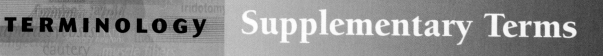

The Eye

Continued

phlyctenule *FLIK-ten-ūl*	A small blister or nodule on the cornea or conjunctiva
pseudophakia *sū-dō-FĀ-kē-a*	A condition in which a cataractous lens has been removed and replaced with a plastic lens implant
retinitis *ret-in-Ī-tis*	Inflammation of the retina; causes include systemic disease, infection, hemorrhage, exposure to light
retinitis pigmentosa *ret-in-Ī-tis pig-men-TŌ-sa*	A hereditary chronic degenerative disease of the retina that begins in early childhood. There is atrophy of the optic nerve and clumping of pigment in the retina.
retinoblastoma *ret-in-ō-blas-TŌ-ma*	A malignant glioma of the retina; usually appears in early childhood and is sometimes hereditary; fatal if untreated, but current cure rates are high
scotoma *skō-TŌ-ma*	An area of diminished vision within the visual field
strabismus *stra-BIZ-mus*	A deviation of the eye in which the visual lines of each eye are not directed to the same object at the same time. Also called heterotropia or squint. The various forms are referred to as *-tropias*, with the direction of turning indicated by a prefix, such as esotropia (inward), exotropia (outward), hypertropia (upward), and hypotropia (downward). The suffix *-phoria* is also used, as in esophoria.
synechia *sin-EK-ē-a*	Adhesion of parts, especially adhesion of the iris to the lens and cornea (plural: synechiae)
xanthoma *zan-THŌ-ma*	A soft, slightly raised, yellowish patch or nodule usually on the eyelids; occurs in the elderly; also called xanthelasma

DIAGNOSIS AND TREATMENT

canthotomy *kan-THOT-ō-mē*	Surgical division of a canthus
cystitome *SIS-ti-tōm*	Instrument for incising the lens capsule
electroretinography (ERG) *ē-lek-trō-ret-i-NOG-ra-fē*	Study of the electrical response of the retina to light stimulation
enucleation *ē-nū-klē-Ā-shun*	Surgical removal of the eyeball
gonioscopy *gō-nē-OS-kō-pē*	Examination of the angle between the cornea and the iris (anterior chamber angle) in which fluids drain out of the eye (root *goni/o* means "angle")
keratometer *ker-a-TOM-e-ter*	An instrument for measuring the curvature of the cornea

TERMINOLOGY Supplementary Terms

The Eye

Continued

mydriatic *mid-rē-AT-ik*	A drug that causes dilation of the pupil
phorometer *fo-ROM-e-ter*	An instrument for determining the degree and kind of strabismus
retinoscope *RET-in-ō-skōp*	An instrument used to determine refractive errors of the eye; also called a skiascope (*SKĪ-a-skōp*)
slit-lamp biomicroscope	An instrument for examining the eye under magnification
Snellen chart *SNEL-en*	A chart printed with letters of decreasing size used to test visual acuity when viewed from a set distance; results reported as a fraction giving a subject's vision compared with normal vision at a distance of 20 feet
tarsorrhaphy *tar-SOR-a-fē*	Suturing together of all or part of the upper and lower eyelids
tonometer *tō-NOM-e-ter*	An instrument used to measure fluid pressure in the eye

 Go to the pronunciation glossary in Chapter 18 of the CD-ROM to hear these words pronounced.

TERMINOLOGY Abbreviations

The Eye

A, Acc	Accommodation		**IOP**	Intraocular pressure
AMD	Age-related macular degeneration		**NRC**	Normal retinal correspondence
ARC	Abnormal retinal correspondence		**NV**	Near vision
As, AST	Astigmatism		**OD**	Right eye (Latin, *oculus dexter*)
cc	With correction		**ORL**	Otorhinolaryngology
Em	Emmetropia		**OS**	Left eye (Latin, *oculus sinister*)
EOM	Extraocular movement, muscles		**OU**	Both eyes (Latin, *oculi unitas*); also each
ERG	Electroretinography			eye (Latin, *oculus uterque*)
ET	Esotropia		**sc**	Without correction
FC	Finger counting		**VA**	Visual acuity
HM	Hand movements		**VF**	Visual field
IOL	Intraocular lens		**XT**	Exotropia

18

CHAPTER REVIEW

LABELING EXERCISE
The Ear

Write the name of each numbered part on the corresponding line of the answer sheet.

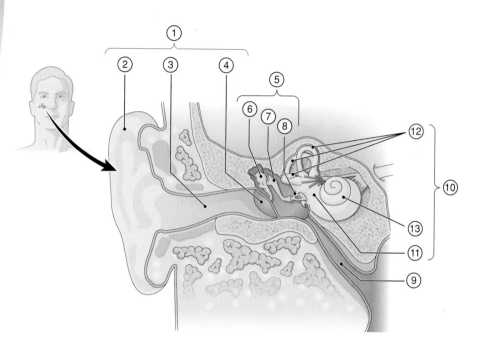

cochlea

eustachian (auditory) tube

external auditory canal

incus

inner ear

malleus

ossicles of middle ear

outer ear

pinna

semicircular canals

stapes

tympanic membrane

vestibule

1. _____

2. _____

3. _____

4. _____

5. _____

6. _____

7. _____

8. _____

9. _____

10. _____

11. _____

12. _____

13. _____

The Eye
Write the name of each numbered part on the corresponding line of the answer sheet.

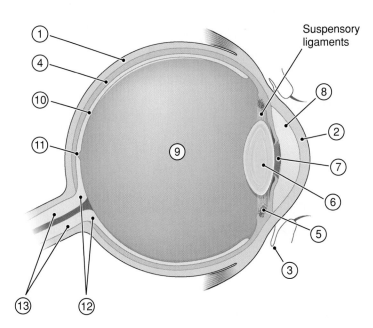

18

aqueous humor	1. _____
choroid	2. _____
ciliary muscle	3. _____
conjunctival sac	4. _____
cornea	5. _____
fovea	6. _____
iris	7. _____
lens	8. _____
optic disk (blind spot)	9. _____
optic nerve	10. _____
retina	11. _____
sclera	12. _____
vitreous body	13. _____

TERMINOLOGY

Match the following terms and write the appropriate letter to the left of each number:

_____	1. tactile	a.	increased sensation
_____	2. parosmia	b.	blindness in half the visual field
_____	3. hyperesthesia	c.	small bone
_____	4. ossicle	d.	pertaining to touch
_____	5. hemianopia	e.	abnormal smell perception

_____	6. lens	a.	point of sharpest vision
_____	7. fovea	b.	structure that changes shape for near and far vision
_____	8. rods and cones	c.	muscular ring that regulates light entering the eye
_____	9. vestibular apparatus	d.	location of equilibrium receptors
_____	10. iris	e.	vision receptors

_____	11. phacosclerosis	a.	corneal transplant
_____	12. ophthalmoplegia	b.	sensation of noises in the ear
_____	13. anacusis	c.	paralysis of an eye muscle
_____	14. tinnitus	d.	hardening of the lens
_____	15. keratoplasty	e.	total loss of hearing

Supplementary Terms

_____	16. tarsus	a.	instrument used to measure pressure in the eye
_____	17. mastoid process	b.	small muscle attached to an ear ossicle
_____	18. stapedius	c.	projection of the temporal bone
_____	19. tonometer	d.	unit for measuring the frequency of sound
_____	20. hertz	e.	framework of the eyelid

_____	21. emmetropia	a.	rapid, involuntary eye movements
_____	22. nystagmus	b.	normal refraction of the eye
_____	23. mydriasis	c.	deviation of the eye
_____	24. diopter	d.	abnormal dilation of the pupil
_____	25. strabismus	e.	unit for measuring the refractive power of the lens

_____	26. AMD	a.	irregularity in the curve of the eye
_____	27. AD	b.	right ear
_____	28. AST	c.	unit for measuring the intensity of sound
_____	29. dB	d.	eye disorder associated with aging
_____	30. OU	e.	both eyes

Fill in the blanks:

31. The outermost layer of the eye wall is the _____.

32. The term *ceruminous* applies to _____.

33. The sense of awareness of body position is _____.

34. The ossicle that is in contact with the inner ear is the _____.

35. The bending of light rays as they pass through the eye is _____.

36. The innermost layer of the eye that contains the receptors for vision is the _____.

37. The transparent extension of the sclera that covers the front of the eye is the _____.

38. The scientific name for the eardrum is _____.

18

Eliminations. In each of the sets below, underline the word that does not fit in with the rest and explain the reason for your choice:

39. pain – temperature – taste – touch – pressure

_____

40. vestibule – pinna – cochlea – oval window – semicircular canals

_____

41. incus – lacrimal gland – conjunctiva – eyelash – palpebra

_____

42. cataract – myopia – glaucoma – macular degeneration – presbycusis

_____

True–False. Examine the following statements. If the statement is true, write T in the first blank. If the statement is false, write F in the first blank and correct the statement by replacing the <u>underlined</u> word in the second blank.

43. In bright light the pupils <u>dilate</u>. _____ _____

44. Olfaction is the sense of <u>smell</u>. _____ _____

45. The malleus is located in the <u>middle ear</u>. _____ _____

46. Hypergeusia is an abnormal increase in the sense of <u>touch</u>. _____ _____

47. The eustachian tube is also called the <u>auditory tube</u>. _____ _____

48. The organ of Corti is located in the <u>cochlea</u>. _____ _____

49. A myringotomy is incision of the <u>vitreous body</u>. _____ _____

50. The lacrimal gland produces <u>aqueous humor</u>. _____ _____

Define the following words:

51. audiologist _____

52. aphakia _____

53. subscleral _____

54. ophthalmometer _____

55. keratoiritis _____

56. iridotomy _____

57. perilental _____

58. chorioretinal _____

59. dacryorrhea _____

60. myringotomy _____

Word building. Write words for the following definitions:

61. pertaining to the vestibular apparatus and cochlea _____

62. surgical removal of the stapes _____

63. plastic repair of the ear _____

64. absence of pain _____

65. drooping of the eyelid _____

66. any disease of the retina _____

67. measurement of the pupil _____

68. hardening of the tympanic membrane _____

69. pertaining to tears _____

70. endoscopic examination of the auditory tube _____

71. excision of (part of) the ciliary body _____

Adjectives. Write the adjective form of the following words:

72. cochlea _____

73. palpebra _____

74. vestibule _____

75. uvea _____

76. cornea _____

77. sclera _____

78. pupil _____

Opposites. Write words that mean the opposite of the following:

79. mydriasis _____

80. esotropia _____

81. sc _____

82. hyperopia _____

83. hypoesthesia _____

84. OS _____

Word analysis. Define the following words and give the meaning of the word parts in each. Use a dictionary if necessary.

85. anisometropia (*an-ī-sō-me-TRŌ-pē-a*) _____

   a. an- _____

   b. iso- _____

   c. metr/o _____

   d. -opia _____

86. asthenopia (*as-the-NŌ-pē-a*) _____

    a. a- _____

    b. sthen/o- _____

    c. -opia _____

87. otorhinolaryngology (*ō-tō-rī-nō-lar-in-GOL-ō-jē*) _____

    a. oto- _____

    b. rhin/o _____

    c. laryng/o _____

    d. -logy _____

18

Go to the word exercises in Chapter 18 of the CD-ROM for additional review exercises.

CASE STUDY 18-1: Medical Records

An electrical fire in the physicians' dictation room left a charred mass of burned and water-damaged medical records. Discharge charts had been stacked awaiting physician sign-off before they could be returned to Medical Records for storage. Several medical transcriptionists spent 3 days sorting through the remains to reassemble the charts, all of which were from the patients of the large otorhinolaryngology practice. In addition to patient identification information, the transcriptionists matched word cues to create piles of similar documents. Patients treated for middle and inner ear problems were identified with words such as stapedectomy, tympanoplasty, myringotomy, cochlear, cholesteatoma, otosclerosis, labyrinth, otitis media, and acoustic neuroma. Patients treated for external ear conditions were grouped using terms such as otoplasty, pinna, postauricular, and otitis externa. Mastoid, laryngeal, and nasal surgery patients were grouped separately. Restoring the charts was an impossible task, and the records were determined to be either incomplete or a total loss. The only document to survive the fire was an audiology report.

CASE STUDY 18-2: Audiology Report

S.R., a 55-year-old man, reported decreased hearing sensitivity in his left ear for the past 3 years. In addition to hearing loss, he was experiencing tinnitus and aural fullness. Pure-tone test results revealed normal hearing sensitivity for the right ear and a moderate sensorineural hearing loss in the left ear. Speech thresholds were appropriate for the degree of hearing loss noted. Word recognition was excellent for the right ear and poor for the left ear when the signal was present at a suprathreshold level. Tympanograms were characterized by normal shape, amplitude, and peak pressure points bilaterally. The contralateral acoustic reflex was normal for the right ear but absent for the left ear at the frequencies tested (500 to 4000 Hz). The ipsilateral acoustic reflex was present with the probe in the right ear and absent with the probe in the left ear. Brainstem auditory evoked potentials (BAEPs) were within normal range for the right ear. No repeatable response was observed from the left ear. A subsequent MRI showed a 1-cm acoustic neuroma.

CASE STUDY 18-3: Phacoemulsification with Intraocular Lens Implant

W.S., a 68-year-old woman, was scheduled for surgery for a cataract and relief from "floaters," which she had noticed in her visual field since her surgery for a retinal detachment the previous year. She reported to the ambulatory surgery center an hour before her scheduled procedure. Before transfer to the operating room, she spoke with her ophthalmologist and reviewed the surgical plan. Her right eye was identified as the operative eye and it was marked with a "yes" and the surgeon's initials on the lid. She was given anesthetic drops in the right eye and an intravenous bolus of 2.0 mg of midazolam (Versed).

In the OR, W.S. and her operative eye were again identified by the surgeon, anesthetist, and nurses. After anesthesia and akinesia were achieved, the eye area was prepped and draped in sterile sheets. An operating microscope with video system was positioned over her eye. A 5-0 silk suture was placed through the superior rectus muscle to retract the eye. A lid speculum was placed to open the eye. A minimal conjunctival peritotomy was performed, and hemostasis was achieved with wet-field cautery. The anterior chamber was entered at the 10:30 o'clock position. A capsulotomy was performed after Healon was placed in the anterior chamber. Phacoemulsification was carried out without difficulty. The remaining cortex was removed by irrigation and aspiration.

An intraocular lens (IOL) was placed into the posterior chamber. Miochol was injected to achieve papillary miosis, and the wound was closed with one 10-0 suture. Subconjunctival Celestone and Garamycin were injected. The lid speculum and retraction suture were removed. After application of Eserine and Bacitracin ointments, the eye was patched and a shield was applied. W.S. left the OR in good condition and was discharged to home 4 hours later.

CASE STUDY QUESTIONS

Multiple choice. Select the best answer and write the letter of your choice to the left of each number:

_____ 1. The medical specialty of otorhinolaryngology is most often referred to as:
  a. ENT, or ear, nose, and throat
  b. optometry
  c. PERLA
  d. oral surgery
  e. EENT/dental

_____ 2. The surgery to remove one of the microscopic bones of the middle ear is a(n):
  a. stapedectomy
  b. mastoidectomy
  c. myringotomy
  d. tympanoplasty
  e. otoplasty

_____ 3. The procedure in question 2 may require construction of a new eardrum, a procedure called a(n):
  a. otoplasty
  b. myringotomy
  c. stapes transfer
  d. tympanoplasty
  e. otoscope

_____ 4. Mastoid surgery incisions are made postauricularly, which is:
  a. anterior to the ear drum
  b. over the left ear
  c. behind the ear
  d. inferior to the tympanic membrane
  e. between the ears

_____ 5. The study of hearing is termed:
  a. acousticology
  b. radio frequency
  c. light spectrum
  d. otology
  e. audiology

_____ 6. Sensorineural hearing loss may result from:
  a. damage to the second cranial nerve
  b. otitis media
  c. otosclerosis
  d. damage to the eighth cranial nerve
  e. stapedectomy

_____ 7. Ultrasound destruction and aspiration of the lens is called:
  a. catarectomy
  b. phacoemulsification
  c. stapedectomy
  d. radial keratotomy
  e. refraction

18

_____ 8. The term akinesia means:
   a. movement
   b. lack of sensation
   c. washing
   d. lack of movement
   e. incision

_____ 9. The term that means "on the same side" is:
   a. contralateral
   b. bilateral
   c. distal
   d. ventral
   e. ipsilateral

_____ 10. Another name for an acoustic neuroma is:
   a. macular degeneration
   b. neurilemoma
   c. otosclerosis
   d. labyrinthitis
   e. glaucoma

Write terms from the case studies with the following meanings:

11. record obtained by tympanometry _____

12. pertaining to or perceived by the ear _____

13. inflammation of the middle ear _____

14. inflammation of the external ear _____

15. physician who specializes in conditions of the eye _____

16. within the eye _____

17. abnormal contraction of the pupil _____

18. generic drug name for Versed _____

Abbreviations. Define the following abbreviations:

19. Hz _____

20. BAEP _____

21. OD _____

22. IOL _____

The Senses

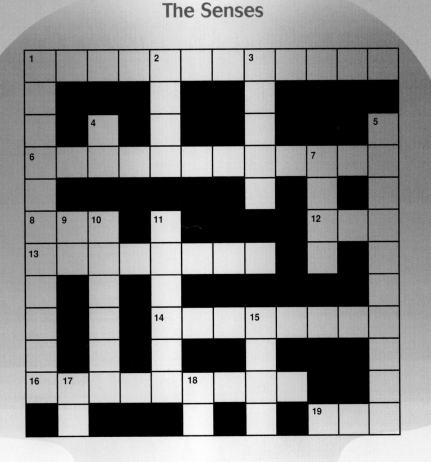

18

ACROSS

1. Membranes that line the eyelids and cover the fronts of the eyes
6. Sharpness of vision
8. A light-sensitive cell of the retina
12. Lens implant: abbreviation
13. Eye disorder caused by increased pressure
14. Pertaining to tears
16. Inward deviation of the eye
19. Three: prefix

DOWN

1. Coordinated movement of the eyes toward fixation on the same point
2. The middle layer of the eye
3. The tactile sense
4. Left ear: abbreviation
5. Paralysis of the ciliary body: _ _ _ _ _ _ _ _ _ _ <u>a</u>
7. Iris: root
9. Medical specialty treating the ear and throat: abbreviation
10. Tear, lacrimal apparatus: combining form
11. Pertaining to the eye
15. Nose: root
17. Without correction: abbreviation
18. Right eye: abbreviation

CHAPTER NINETEEN

THE SKELETON

CHAPTER CONTENTS

OBJECTIVES

After study of this chapter you should be able to:

1. Compare the axial skeleton and the appendicular skeleton.
2. Briefly describe the formation of bone tissue.
3. Describe the structure of a long bone.
4. Compare a suture, a symphysis, and a synovial joint.
5. Identify and use roots pertaining to the skeleton.

6. Describe the main disorders that affect the skeleton and joints.
7. Describe the common methods used to diagnose and treat disorders of the skeleton.
8. Interpret abbreviations used in relation to the skeleton.
9. Label diagrams of the skeleton.

PRETEST

1. The root *oste/o* means _____.

2. The root *myel/o* refers to the spinal cord. Used in reference to bones it means _____.

3. A bone of the spinal column is a(n) _____.

4. The large, flared superior bone of the pelvis is the _____.

5. The bones of the wrist are the _____.

6. The bone of the thigh is the _____.

7. A general term for inflammation of a joint is _____

8. Chondrosarcoma is a tumor that originates in _____.

*T*he **skeleton** forms the framework of the body, protects vital organs, and works with the muscular system to produce movement at the joints. The human adult skeleton is composed of 206 **bones**, which are organized for study into two divisions.

Divisions of the Skeleton

The axial skeleton forms the central core or "axis" of the body's bony framework (Fig. 19-1). It consists of:

> ➤ the skull, made up of the eight cranial bones and the 14 bones of the face (Fig. 19-2). The skull bones are joined by nonmovable joints (sutures), except for the joint between the lower jaw (mandible) and the temporal bone of the cranium, the temporomandibular joint (TMJ).
> ➤ the spinal column (Fig. 19-3) consisting of 26 vertebrae. Between the vertebrae are disks of cartilage that add strength and flexibility to the spine. The five groups of vertebrae, listed from superior to inferior with the number of bones in each group are:

> *1.* cervical (7), designated C1 to C7. The first and second cervical vertebrae also have specific names, the **atlas** and the **axis**, respectively (see Fig 19-3).
> *2.* thoracic (12), designated T1 to T12

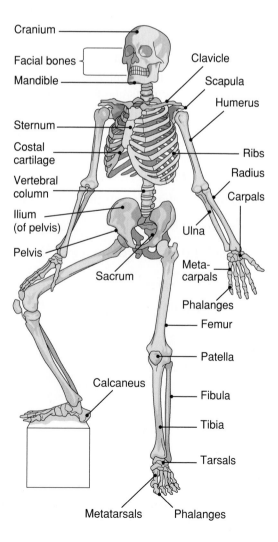

Figure 19-1 The skeleton. The axial skeleton is shown in yellow; the appendicular, in blue.

Bones of the skull:

- ▨ Frontal
- ☐ Parietal
- ☐ Sphenoid
- ☐ Temporal
- ▨ Nasal
- ▨ Maxilla
- ▨ Occipital
- ☐ Zygomatic
- ☐ Mandible

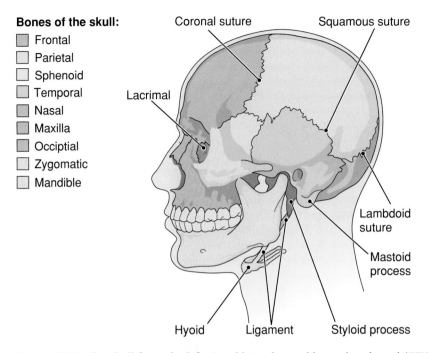

Figure 19-2 The skull from the left. An additional cranial bone, the ethmoid (*ETH-moyd*), is visible mainly from the interior of the skull. The hyoid is considered part of the axial skeleton but is not attached to any other bones. The tongue and other muscles are attached to the hyoid.

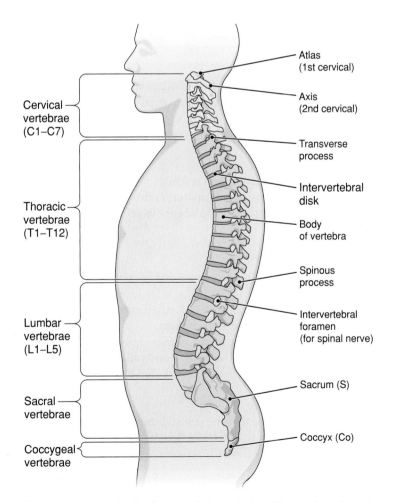

Figure 19-3 Vertebral column, left lateral view. The number of vertebrae in each group and the abbreviations for each are shown. The sacrum and coccyx are formed from fused bones.

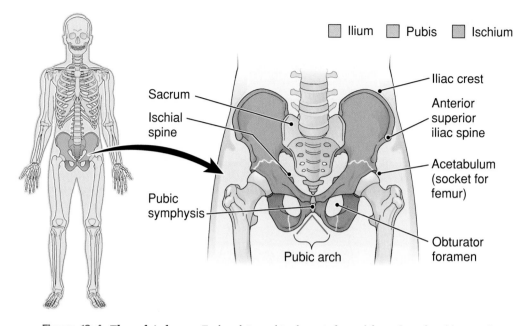

Figure 19-4 The pelvic bones. Each pelvic, or hip, bone is formed from three fused bones, the ilium, ischium, and pubis. Together with the sacrum and coccyx, they form the bony pelvis. The acetabulum is the socket for the femur.

3. lumbar (5), designated L1 to L5
4. the sacrum (S), composed of five fused bones
5. the coccyx (Co), composed of four to five fused bones

➤ the **thorax**, consisting of 12 pairs of ribs joined by cartilage to the sternum (breast bone). The rib cage encloses and protects the thoracic organs.

The appendicular skeleton is attached or "appended" to the axial skeleton (see Fig 19-1). The upper division includes:

➤ the bones of the shoulder girdle, the clavicle and scapula
➤ the bones of the upper extremities (arms), the humerus, radius, ulna, carpals (wrist bones), metacarpals (bones of the palm), and phalanges (finger bones)

The lower division includes:

➤ the **pelvic bones**, two large bones that join the sacrum and coccyx to form the bony pelvis. Each pelvic or hip bone (os coxae) is formed by three fused bones, the large, flared **ilium**, the ischium, and the pubis (Fig. 19-4). The deep socket in the hip bone that holds the head of the femur is the **acetabulum**.
➤ the bones of the lower extremities (legs), the femur, patella (kneecap), tibia, fibula, tarsals (ankle bones), metatarsals (bones of the instep), and phalanges (toe bones). The large tarsal bone that forms the heel is the calcaneus (*kal-KĀ-nē-us*), shown in Figure 19-1.

All of these bone groups, and also the hyoid under the jaw and the ear ossicles, are listed with phonetic pronunciations and described in Reference Box 19-1.

Box 19•1	For Your Reference	*Bones of the Skeleton*

Region	Bones	Description
Axial Skeleton *(AK-sē-al)*		

SKULL

Region	Bones	Description
Cranium *(KRĀ-nē-um)*	Cranial bones (8)	Chamber enclosing the brain; houses the ear and forms part of the eye socket
Facial portion *(FĀ-shal)*	Facial bones (14)	Form the face and chambers for sensory organs
Hyoid *(HĪ-oyd)*		U-shaped bone under mandible (lower jaw); used for muscle attachments
Ossicles *(OS-i-klz)*	Ear bones (3)	Transmit sound waves in inner ear

TRUNK

Region	Bones	Description
Vertebral column *(VER-te-bral)*	Vertebrae (26) *(VER-te-brē)*	Encloses the spinal cord
Thorax *(THŌ-raks)*	Sternum *(STER-num)*	Anterior bone of the thorax
	Ribs (12 pair)	Enclose the organs of the thorax
Appendicular Skeleton *(ap-en-DIK-ū-lar)*		

UPPER DIVISION

Region	Bones	Description
Shoulder girdle	Clavicle *(KLAV-i-kel)*	Anterior; between sternum and scapula
	Scapula *(SKAP-ū-la)*	Posterior, anchors muscles that move arm
Upper extremity	Humerus *(HŪ-mer-us)*	Proximal arm bone
	Ulna *(UL-na)*	Medial bone of forearm
	Radius *(RĀ-dē-us)*	Lateral bone of forearm
	Carpals (8) *(KAR-palz)*	Wrist bones
	Metacarpals (5) *(met-a-KAR-palz)*	Bones of palm
	Phalanges (14) *(fa-LAN-jēz)*	Bones of fingers

19

Box 19•1 **For Your Reference** *Continued*

LOWER DIVISION

Pelvic bones *(PEL-vic)*	Os coxae (2) *(os KOK-sē)*	Join sacrum and coccyx of vertebral column to form the bony pelvis.
Lower extremity	Femur *(FĒ-mur)*	Thigh bone
	Patella *(pa-TEL-a)*	Kneecap
	Tibia *(TIB-ē-a)*	Medial bone of leg
	Fibula *(FIB-ū-la)*	Lateral bone of leg
	Tarsal bones (7) *(TAR-sal)*	Ankle bones. The large heel bone is the calcaneus *(kal-KĀ-nē-us)*.
	Metatarsals (5) *(met-a-TAR-salz)*	Bones of instep
	Phalanges (14) *(fa-LAN-jēz)*	Bones of toes

Bone Formation

Bone is formed by the gradual addition of calcium and phosphorus salts to **cartilage**, a type of dense connective tissue. This process of **ossification** begins before birth and continues to adulthood. Although bone appears to be inert, it is actually living tissue that is constantly being replaced and remodeled throughout life. Three types of cells are involved in these changes:

> ➤ **osteoblasts**, the cells that produce bone
> ➤ **osteocytes**, mature bone cells that help to maintain bone tissue
> ➤ **osteoclasts**, involved in the breakdown of bone tissue to release needed minerals or to allow for reshaping and repair.

The process of destroying bone so that its components can be taken into the circulation is called **resorption**. This activity occurs continuously and is normally in balance with bone formation. In disease states, resorption may occur more rapidly or more slowly than bone production.

Structure of a Long Bone

A typical long bone (Fig. 19-5) has a shaft or **diaphysis** composed of compact bone tissue. Within the shaft is a medullary cavity containing the yellow form of **bone marrow**, which is high in fat. The irregular **epiphysis** at either end is made of a less dense, spongy bone tissue (Fig. 19-6). The spaces in spongy bone contain the blood-forming red bone marrow. A layer of cartilage covers the epiphysis to protect the bone surface at a joint. The thin layer of fibrous tissue, or **periosteum**, that covers the bone's outer surface nourishes and protects the bone and also generates new bone cells for growth and repair.

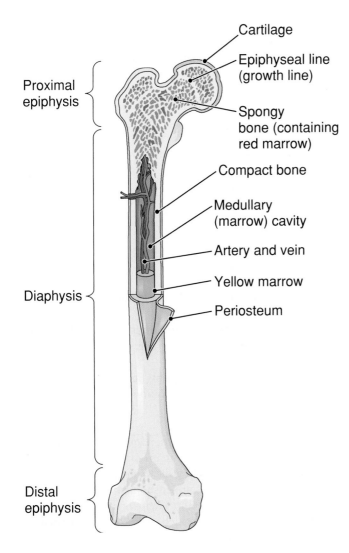

Cartilage

Epiphyseal line (growth line)

Proximal epiphysis

Spongy bone (containing red marrow)

Compact bone

Medullary (marrow) cavity

Artery and vein

Diaphysis

Yellow marrow

Periosteum

Distal epiphysis

Figure 19-5 Structure of a long bone

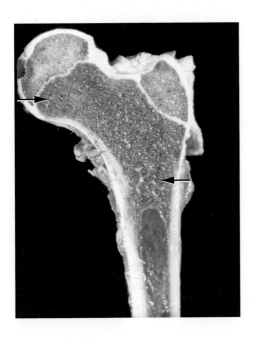

Figure 19-6 Bone tissue, longitudinal section. Spongy bone makes up most of the epiphysis (end) of this long bone, shown by the arrows. A thin layer of compact bone is seen at the surface.

Between the diaphysis and the epiphysis at each end, in a region called the **metaphysis**, is the growth region or **epiphyseal plate**. Long bones continue to grow in length at these regions throughout childhood and into early adulthood. When the bone stops elongating, this area becomes fully calcified but remains visible as the epiphyseal line (see Fig. 19-5).

Long bones are found in the arms, legs, hands, and feet. Other bones are described as:

> ➤ flat (i.e., cranial bones, ribs, scapulae)
> ➤ short (i.e., wrist and ankle bones)
> ➤ irregular (i.e., facial bones, vertebrae)

Joints

The **joints**, or **articulations**, are classified according to the degree of movement they allow:

> ➤ A **suture** is an immovable joint held together by fibrous connective tissue, as is found between the bones of the skull (see Fig. 19-2).
> ➤ A **symphysis** is a slightly movable joint connected by fibrous cartilage. Examples are the joints between the bodies of the vertebrae (see Fig. 19-3) and the joint between the pubic bones (see Fig. 19-4).
> ➤ A **synovial joint**, or **diarthrosis**, is a freely movable joint. Such joints allow for a wide range of movements, as described in Chapter 20. **Tendons** attach muscles to bones to produce movement at the joints.

Freely movable joints are subject to wear and tear, and they therefore have some protective features (Fig. 19-7). The cavity of a diarthrotic joint contains **synovial fluid**, which cushions and lubricates the joint. This fluid is produced by the synovial membrane that lines the joint cavity. The ends of the articulating bones are cushioned and protected by cartilage. A fibrous capsule, continuous with the periosteum, encloses the joint. Synovial joints are stabilized and strengthened by **ligaments**, which connect the articulating bones. A **bursa** is a small sac of synovial fluid that cushions the area around a joint. Bursae are found at stress points between tendons, ligaments, and bones (see Fig. 19-7).

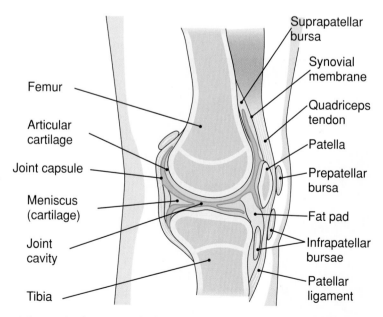

Figure 19-7 The knee joint, sagittal section. The knee joint is an example of a freely movable, synovial, joint, also called a diarthrosis. Synovial fluid fills the joint cavity. Other protective structures, such as cartilage, joint capsule, ligaments, and bursae are also shown.

TERMINOLOGY Key Terms

NORMAL STRUCTURE AND FUNCTION

acetabulum *as-e-TAB-ū-lum*	The bony socket in the hip bone that holds the head of the femur (from the Latin word for vinegar because it resembles the base of a vinegar cruet).
articulation *ar-tik-ū-LĀ-shun*	A joint (adjective: articular)
atlas *AT-las*	The first cervical vertebra (see Fig. 19-3) (root: *atlant/o*)
axis *AK-sis*	The second cervical vertebra (see Fig. 19-3)
bone	A calcified form of dense connective tissue; osseous tissue; also an individual unit of the skeleton made of such tissue (root: *oste/o*)
bone marrow	The soft material that fills the cavities of bones. Yellow marrow fills the central cavity of the long bones; blood cells are formed in red bone marrow, which is located in spongy bone tissue (root: *myel/o*).
bursa *BUR-sa*	A fluid-filled sac that reduces friction near a joint (root: *burs/o*)
cartilage *KAR-ti-lij*	A type of dense connective tissue that is found in the skeleton, larynx, trachea, and bronchi. It is the precursor to most bone tissue (root: *chondr/o*).
diarthrosis *di-ar-THRŌ-sis*	A freely movable joint; also called a synovial joint (adjective: diarthrotic)
diaphysis *dī-AF-i-sis*	The shaft of a long bone
epiphyseal plate *ep-i-FIZ-ē-al*	The growth region of a long bone; located in the metaphysis, between the diaphysis and epiphysis. When bone growth ceases, this area appears as the epiphyseal line.
epiphysis *e-PIF-i-sis*	The irregularly shaped end of a long bone
ilium *IL-ē-um*	The large, flared, superior portion of the pelvic bone (adjective: iliac; root: *ili/o*)
joint	The junction between two bones; articulation (root: *arthr/o*)
ligament *LIG-a-ment*	A strong band of connective tissue that joins one bone to another
metaphysis *me-TAF-i-sis*	The region of a long bone between the diaphysis (shaft) and epiphysis (end); during development, the growing region of a long bone
ossification *os-i-fi-KĀ-shun*	The formation of bone tissue (from Latin os, meaning "bone")
osteoblast *OS-tē-ō-blast*	A cell that produces bone tissue

TERMINOLOGY *Continued*

Key Terms

osteoclast *OS-tē-ō-clast*	A cell that destroys bone tissue
osteocyte *OS-tē-ō-sīt*	A mature bone cell that nourishes and maintains bone tissue
pelvis	The large ring of bone at the inferior trunk. Formed of the two hip bones (os coxae) joined to the sacrum and coccyx (plural: pelves). Each os coxae is formed of three bones, the superior, flared ilium (*IL-ē-um*), ischium (*IS-kē-um*), and pubis (*PŪ-bis*).
periosteum *per-ē-OS-tē-um*	The fibrous membrane that covers the surface of a bone
resorption *rē-SORP-shun*	Removal of bone by breakdown and absorption into the circulation
skeleton *SKEL-e-ton*	The bony framework of the body, consisting of 206 bones. The axial portion (80 bones) is composed of the skull, spinal column, ribs, and sternum. The appendicular skeleton (126 bones) contains the bones of the arms and legs, shoulder girdle, and pelvis.
suture *SŪ-chur*	An immovable joint, such as the joints between the bones of the skull
symphysis *SIM-fi-sis*	A slightly movable joint
synovial fluid *sin-O-vē-al*	The fluid contained in a freely movable (diarthrotic) joint; synovia (root: *synov/i*)
synovial joint	A freely movable joint; has a joint cavity containing synovial fluid; a diarthrosis
tendon *TEN-don*	A fibrous band of connective tissue that attaches a muscle to a bone
thorax *THŌ-raks*	The upper part of the trunk between the neck and the abdomen; formed by the 12 pairs of ribs and sternum

 Go to the pronunciation glossary in Chapter 19 of the CD-ROM to hear these words pronounced.

Roots Pertaining to the Skeleton, Bones, and Joints

Table 19•1	Roots for Bones and Joints		
ROOT	**MEANING**	**EXAMPLE**	**DEFINITION OF EXAMPLE**
oste/o	bone	osteoid *OS-tē-oyd*	resembling bone or bone tissue
myel/o	bone marrow; also, spinal cord	myelogenous *mī-e-LOJ-e-nus*	originating in bone marrow
chondr/o	cartilage	chondromalacia *kon-drō-ma-LĀ-shē-a*	softening of cartilage
arthr/o	joint	arthrosis *ar-THRŌ-sis*	joint; condition affecting a joint
synov/i	synovial fluid, joint, or membrane	asynovia *a-sin-Ō-vē-a*	lack of synovial fluid
burs/o	bursa	peribursal *per-i-BER-sal*	around a bursa

19

Exercise 19-1

Fill in the blanks:

1. The term *osteogenesis* (*os-tē-ō-JEN-i-sis*) means formation of _____.

2. A myeloblast is an immature cell found in _____.

3. Arthrodesis (*ar-THROD-e-sis*) is fusion of a(n) _____.

4. A chondrocyte (*KON-drō-sīt*) is a cell found in _____.

5. A bursolith (*BUR-sō-lith*) is a stone in a(n) _____.

Define the following words:

6. osteolysis (*os-tē-OL-i-sis*) _____

7. myelopoiesis (*mī-e-lō-poy-Ē-sis*) _____

8. chondroma (*kon-DRŌ-ma*) _____

9. arthrocentesis (*ar-thrō-sen-TĒ-sis*) _____

10. bursitis (*bur-SĪ-tis*) _____

11. myeloid (*MĪ-e-loyd*) _____

Word building. Write words for the following definitions:

12. inflammation of bone and bone marrow _____

13. deficiency (-penia) of bone tissue _____

14. plastic repair of a joint _____

15. tumor of bone marrow _____

16. incision of a bursa _____

17. inflammation of a synovial membrane _____

18. instrument for examining the interior of a joint _____

19. pertaining to or resembling cartilage _____

20. any disease of a joint _____

The word ostosis means "bone growth." Use this as a suffix for the following two words:

21. excess growth of bone _____

22. abnormal growth of bone _____

Table 19·2	Roots for the Skeleton		
ROOT	**MEANING**	**EXAMPLE**	**DEFINITION OF EXAMPLE**
crani/o	skull, cranium	craniometry *krā-ne-OM-e-trē*	measurement of the cranium
spondyl/o	vertebra	spondylolysis *spon-di-LOL-i-sis*	destruction and separation of a vertebra
vertebr/o	vertebra, spinal column	prevertebral *prē-VER-te-bral*	before or in front of the spinal column
rachi/o	spine	rachischisis *rā-KIS-ki-sis*	fissure (-schisis) of the spine; spina bifida
cost/o	rib	costochondral *kos-tō-KON-dral*	pertaining to a rib and its cartilage
sacr/o	sacrum	perisacral *per-i-SĀ-kral*	around the sacrum
coccy, coccyg/o	coccyx	coccygeal* *kok-SIJ-ē-al*	pertaining to the coccyx
pelvi/o	pelvis	pelviscope *PEL-vi-skōp*	endoscope for examining the pelvis
ili/o	ilium	iliopelvic *il-ē-ō-PEL-vik*	pertaining to the ilium and pelvis

*Note spelling.

Exercise 19-2

Adjectives. Write adjectives for the following definitions:

1. pertaining to (-al) the skull _____

2. pertaining to (-al) a rib _____

3. pertaining to (-ic) the pelvis _____

4. pertaining to (-ac) the ilium _____

5. pertaining to (-al) the spinal column _____

6. pertaining to (-al) the sacrum _____

Define the following terms:

7. craniotomy (*krā-nē-OT-ō-mē*) _____

8. paravertebral (*pa-ra-VER-te-bral*) _____

9. spondylodynia (*spon-di-lō-DIN-ē-a*) _____

10. suprapelvic (*sū-pra-PEL-vik*) _____

Word building. Write words for the following definitions:

11. fissure of the skull _____

12. inflammation of the vertebrae (use spondyl/o) _____

13. surgical excision of a rib _____

14. surgical puncture of the spine; spinal tap _____

15. pertaining to the sacrum and ilium _____

16. pertaining to the cranium and sacrum _____

17. measurement of the pelvis _____

18. before or in front of the sacrum _____

19. excision of the coccyx _____

20. pertaining to the ilium and coccyx _____

21. below the ribs _____

Clinical Aspects of the Skeleton

Disorders of the skeleton often involve surrounding tissues—ligaments, tendons, and muscles—and may be studied together as diseases of the musculoskeletal system. (The muscular system is described in Chapter 20.) The medical specialty that concentrates on diseases of the skeletal and muscular systems is **orthopedics**. Physical therapists and occupational therapists must also understand these systems. (Some colorful terms used to describe musculoskeletal abnormalities are given in Box 19-2).

Box 19·2 Focus on Words   *Names That Are Like Pictures*

Some conditions are named by terms that are very descriptive. In orthopedics, several names for types of bursitis are based on the repetitive stress that leads to the irritation. For example, "tailor's bottom" involves the ischial ("sit") bones of the pelvis, as might be irritated by sitting tailor-fashion to sew. "Housemaid's knee" comes from the days of scrubbing floors on hands and knees, and "tennis elbow" is named for the sport that is its most common cause. "Student's elbow" results from leaning to pore over books while studying, although today a student is more likely to have neck and wrist problems from sitting at a computer.

The term *knock-knee* describes genu valgum, in which the knees are abnormally close and the space between the ankles is wide. The opposite is genu varum, in which the knees are far apart and the bottom of the legs are close together, giving rise to the term *bowleg*. A dowager's hump appears dorsally between the shoulders as a result of osteoporosis and is most commonly seen in elderly women.

Injury to the roots of nerves that supply the arm may cause the arm to abduct slightly and rotate medially with the wrist flexed and the fingers pointing backward, a condition colorfully named "waiter's tip position." "Popeye's shoulder" is sign of a separation or tear at the head of the biceps tendon. The affected arm, when abducted with the elbow flexed, reveals a bulge on the upper arm—just like Popeye's!

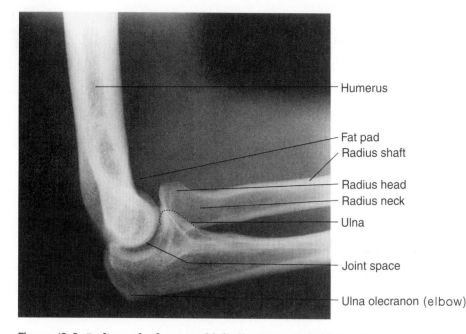

Figure 19-8 Radiograph of a normal left elbow joint, lateral view. The olecranon (ō-LEK-ra-non) is the proximal enlargement of the ulna that forms the prominent bone of the elbow.

Most abnormalities of the bones and joints appear on simple radiographs (see Fig. 19-8 for a radiograph of a normal joint). Radioactive bone scans, computed tomography (CT), and magnetic resonance imaging (MRI) scans are used as well. Also indicative of disorders are changes in blood levels of calcium and **alkaline phosphatase**, an enzyme needed for calcification of bone.

Infection

Osteomyelitis is an inflammation of bone caused by pus-forming bacteria that enter through a wound or are carried by the blood. Often the blood-rich ends of the long bones are invaded, and the infection then spreads to other regions, such as the bone marrow and even the joints. The use of antibiotics has greatly reduced the threat of osteomyelitis.

Tuberculosis may spread to bone, especially the long bones of the arms and legs and the bones of the wrist and ankle. Tuberculosis of the spine is **Pott disease**. Infected vertebrae are weakened and may collapse, causing pain, deformity, and pressure on the spinal cord. Antibiotics can control tuberculosis as long as the strains are not resistant to these drugs and the host is not weakened by other diseases.

Fractures

A **fracture** is a break in a bone, usually caused by trauma. The effects of a fracture depend on the location and severity of the break; the amount of associated injury; possible complications, such as infections; and success of healing, which may take months. In a closed or simple fracture, the skin is not broken. If the fracture is accompanied by a wound in the skin, it is described as an open fracture. Various types of fractures are listed in Reference Box 19-3 and illustrated in Figure 19-9.

Reduction of a fracture refers to realignment of the broken bone. If no surgery is required, the reduction is described as closed; an open reduction is one that requires surgery to place the bone in proper position. Rods, plates, or screws might be needed to ensure proper healing. A splint or cast is often needed during the healing phase to immobilize the bone. **Traction** refers to using pulleys and weights to maintain alignment of a fractured bone during healing. A traction device may be attached to the skin or attached to the bone itself by means of a pin or wire.

Box 19•3 For Your Reference | *Types of Fractures*

Fracture	Description
closed	a simple fracture with no open wound
Colles *KOL-ēz*	fracture of the distal end of the radius with backward displacement of the hand
comminuted *COM-i-nū-ted*	fracture in which the bone is splintered or crushed
compression	fracture caused by force from both ends, as to a vertebra
greenstick	one side of the bone is broken and the other side is bent
impacted	one fragment is driven into the other
oblique	break occurs at an angle across the bone; usually one fragment slips by the other
open	fracture is associated with an open wound, or broken bone protrudes through the skin
Pott	fracture of the distal end of the fibula with injury to the tibial joint
spiral	fracture is in a spiral or S shape; usually caused by twisting injuries
transverse	a break at right angles to the long axis of a bone

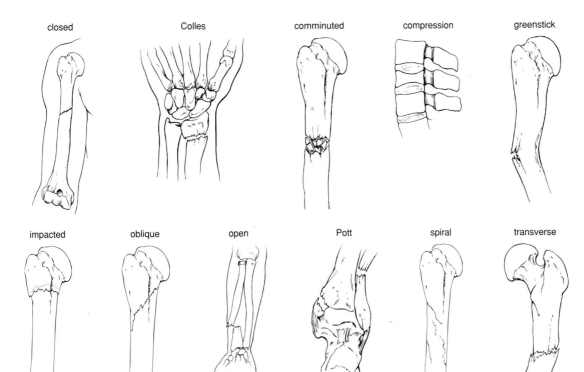

closed   Colles   comminuted   compression   greenstick

impacted   oblique   open   Pott   spiral   transverse

Figure 19-9 Types of fractures.

19

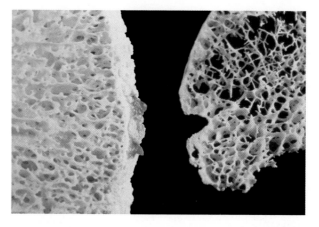

Figure 19-10 Osteoporosis.
Femoral head showing osteoporosis (*right*) compared with a normal control (*left*).

Metabolic Bone Diseases

Osteoporosis is a loss of bone mass that results in weakening of the bones (Fig. 19-10). A decrease in estrogens after menopause makes women over age 50 most susceptible to the effects of this disorder. Efforts to prevent osteoporosis include a healthful diet, adequate intake of calcium and vitamin D, and engaging in regular weight-bearing exercises, such as walking, running, aerobics, and weight training. These exercises stimulate bone growth and also contribute to the muscle strength and balance needed to prevent falls. Perimenopausal hormone replacement therapy (HRT) prevents bone loss, but because of safety concerns, this treatment is currently being reevaluated. Some drugs are available for reducing bone resorption and increasing bone density. These include the **bisphosphonates** and **selective estrogen receptor modulators (SERMs)** described in Chapter 15.

Osteoporosis is diagnosed and monitored using a DEXA (dual-energy x-ray absorptiometry) scan, an imaging technique that measures bone mineral density (BMD). The diagnostic term **osteopenia** refers to a lower-than-average bone density, which is not considered to be abnormal. Osteopenia may progress to osteoporosis, but does not necessarily need treatment.

Other conditions that can lead to bone loss include nutritional deficiencies; disuse, as in paralysis or immobilization in a cast; and excess steroids from the adrenal cortex. Overactivity of the parathyroid glands also leads to osteoporosis because parathyroid hormone releases calcium from bones to raise blood calcium levels. Certain drugs, smoking, lack of exercise, and high intake of alcohol, caffeine, and proteins may also contribute to the development of osteoporosis.

In **osteomalacia** there is a softening of bone tissue because of diminished calcium salt formation. Possible causes include deficiency of vitamin D, needed to absorb calcium and phosphorus from the intestine; renal disorders; liver disease; and certain intestinal disorders. When osteomalacia occurs in children, the disease is called **rickets** (Fig. 19-11). Rickets is usually caused by a vitamin D deficiency.

Paget disease (osteitis deformans) is a disorder of aging in which bones become overgrown and thicker, but deformed. The disease results in bowing of the long bones and distortion of the flat bones, such as those of the skull. Paget disease usually involves the bones of the axial skeleton, causing pain, fractures, and hearing loss. With time, there may be neurologic signs, heart failure, and predisposition to bone cancer.

Neoplasms

Osteogenic sarcoma (osteosarcoma) most commonly occurs in the growing region of a bone, especially around the knee. This is a highly malignant tumor that often requires amputation. It most commonly metastasizes to the lungs.

Chondrosarcoma usually appears in midlife. As the name implies, this tumor arises in cartilage. It may require amputation and most frequently metastasizes to the lungs.

In cases of malignant bone tumors, early surgical removal is important for prevention of metastasis. Signs of bone tumors are pain, easy fracture, and increases in serum

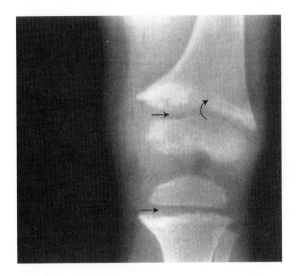

Figure 19-11 Rickets. Radiograph of the left knee joint showing widening of the growth regions of the bones *(arrows)*.

calcium and alkaline phosphatase levels. Aside from primary tumors, neoplasms at other sites often metastasize to bone, most commonly to the spine.

Joint Disorders

Some sources of joint problems include congenital malformations, infectious disease of the joint or adjacent bones, injury leading to degeneration, and necrosis resulting from loss of blood supply. **Arthritis** is a term broadly used to mean any inflammation of a joint. Based on cause, several types are recognized.

Arthritis

The most common form of arthritis is **osteoarthritis (OA)** or **degenerative joint disease (DJD)** (Fig. 19-12). This involves a gradual degeneration of articular (joint) cartilage as a result of wear and tear. Predisposing factors for OA are age, heredity, injury, congenital skeletal abnormalities, and endocrine disorders. It usually appears at midlife and beyond and involves the weight-bearing joints, such as the knees, hips, and finger joints. Radiographs show a narrowing of the joint cavity and bone thickening. Cartilage may crack and break loose, causing inflammation in the joint and exposing the underlying bone.

Osteoarthritis is treated with analgesics to relieve pain, **antiinflammatory agents**, such as corticosteroids, **nonsteroidal antiinflammatory drugs (NSAIDs)**, and physical therapy. Steroids can be injected directly into an arthritic joint, but because they may ultimately cause cartilage damage, only a few injections can be given within a year at

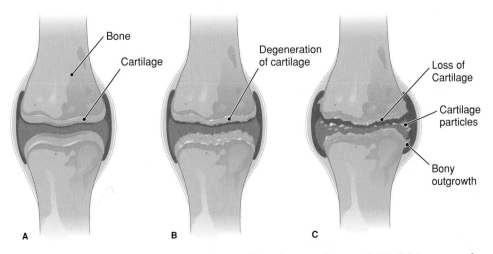

Figure 19-12 Osteoarthritis. (*A*) Normal joint. (*B*) Early stage of osteoarthritis. (*C*) Late stage of disease.

19

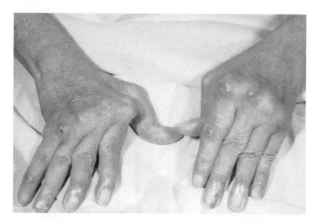

Figure 19-13 Advanced rheumatoid arthritis. The hands show swelling of the joints and deviation of the fingers.

intervals of several months. Treatment may include drainage of excess fluid from the joint in an **arthrocentesis**. Application of ice, elevation, and acupuncture may also help to relieve pain in cases of joint inflammation.

Rheumatoid arthritis (RA) is a systemic inflammatory joint disease that commonly appears in young adult women. Its exact causes are unknown, but it may involve immunologic reactions. A group of antibodies called **rheumatoid factor** often appears in the blood, but is not always specific for rheumatoid arthritis, as it may occur in other systemic diseases as well. There is an overgrowth of the synovial membrane that lines the joint cavity. As this membrane covers and destroys the joint cartilage, synovial fluid accumulates, causing joint swelling (Fig. 19-13). There is degeneration of the underlying bones, eventually causing fusion, or **ankylosis**. Treatment includes rest, physical therapy, analgesics, and antiinflammatory drugs.

Gout is caused by an increased level of uric acid in the blood, salts of which are deposited in the joints. It mostly occurs in middle-aged men and almost always involves pain at the base of the great toe. Gout may result from a primary metabolic disturbance or may be a secondary effect of another disease, as of the kidneys. It is treated with drugs to suppress formation of uric acid or to increase elimination of uric acid (uricosuric agent).

Joint Repair

In **arthroscopy**, orthopedic surgeons use a type of endoscope called an arthroscope to examine the interior of a joint and perform surgical repairs if needed (Fig. 19-14). With an arthroscope, it is possible to smooth articular surfaces and to remove loose tissue that is causing pain and irritation.

If more conservative treatments don't bring relief, orthopedists may recommend an **arthroplasty**. This term generally means any reconstruction of a joint, but usually applies to a total or partial joint replacement. Hips, knees, shoulders, and other joints can be replaced with prostheses to eliminate pain and restore mobility, as explained in Box 19-4.

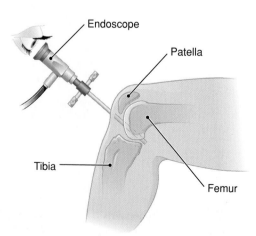

Figure 19-14 Arthroscopic examination of the knee. An endoscope (arthroscope) is inserted between projections at the end of the femur to view the posterior of the knee.

Box 19·4 Clinical Perspectives   *Arthroplasty: Bionic Parts for a Better Life*

Since the first total hip replacement in the early 1960s, millions of joint replacements, called arthroplasties, have been performed successfully. Most are done to decrease joint pain in older people with arthritis and other chronic degenerative bone diseases after other treatments such as weight loss, physical therapy, and medication have been tried. Hips and knees are most commonly restored, with 300,000 hip arthroplasties and an equal number of knee replacements performed each year in the United States. Orthopedic surgeons can also replace shoulder, elbow, wrist, hand, ankle, and foot joints.

Artificial, or *prosthetic,* joints are engineered to be strong, nontoxic, corrosion-resistant, and firmly bondable to the patient. Computer-controlled machines now produce individualized joints in less time and at less cost than in the past. Ball-and-socket joint prostheses, like those used in total hip replacement, consist of a cup, ball, and stem. The cup replaces the hip socket (acetabulum)

and is bonded to the pelvis using screws or glue. The cup is usually plastic but may also be made of longer-lasting ceramic or metal. The ball, made of metal or ceramic, replaces the femoral head and is attached to the stem, which is implanted into the femoral shaft. Stems are made of various metal alloys such as cobalt and titanium and are often glued into place. Stems designed to promote bone growth into them are commonly used in younger, more active patients because it is believed that they will remain firmly attached for a longer time.

Until recently, arthroplasty was rarely performed on young people because prosthetics had a lifespan of only about 10 years. Today's materials and surgical techniques could increase this lifespan to 20 years or more, and young people who undergo arthroplasty will require fewer replacements later on. This improvement is important because the incidence of sports-related joint injuries in young adults is increasing.

19

A final alternative to relieve pain and provide stability at a joint is fusion, or **arthrodesis**, which results in total loss of joint mobility. Surgeons use pins or bone grafts to stabilize the joint and allow bone surfaces to adhere.

Disorders of the Spine

Ankylosing spondylitis is a disease of the spine that appears mainly in males. Joint cartilage is destroyed; eventually the disks between the vertebrae calcify and there is ankylosis (fusion) of the bones (Fig. 19-15). Changes begin low in the spine and progress upward, limiting mobility.

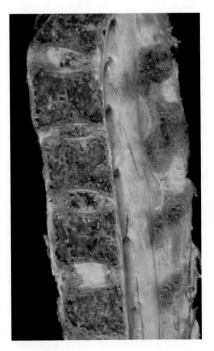

Figure 19-15 Ankylosing spondylitis. Bone bridges fuse one vertebra to the next across the intervertebral disks and fuse the posterior portions of the vertebrae. Osteoporosis results from disuse.

19

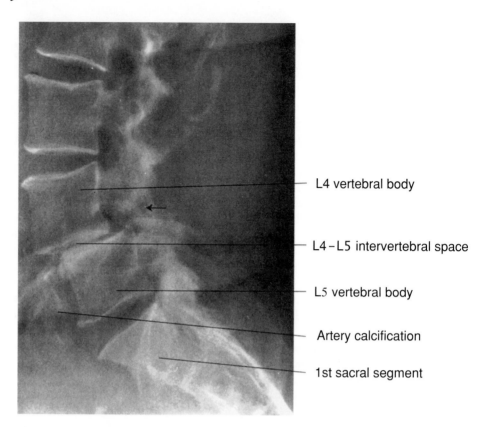

L4 vertebral body

L4 – L5 intervertebral space

L5 vertebral body

Artery calcification

1st sacral segment

Figure 19-16 Spondylolisthesis. The L4 vertebral body has slid forward over L5 and there is marked narrowing of the L4–5 intervertebral disk space.

Spondylolisthesis is a forward sliding of a vertebra over the vertebra below (-listhesis means "slipping") (Fig. 19-16). The condition follows **spondylolysis**, degeneration of the joint structures that normally stabilize the vertebrae. Spondylolisthesis is most common in the weight-bearing lumbar region of the spine, where it causes low back pain and sometimes leg pain resulting from irritation of spinal nerve roots.

Herniated Disk

In cases of a **herniated disk** (Fig. 19-17), the central mass (nucleus pulposus) of an intervertebral disk protrudes through the disk's weakened outer ring (annulus fibrosus) into the spinal canal. This commonly occurs in the lumbosacral or cervical regions of the spine as a result of injury or heavy lifting. The herniated or "slipped" disk puts pressure on the spinal cord or spinal nerves, often causing **sciatica**, which is pain along the sciatic nerve. There may be spasms of the back muscles, leading to disability.

A herniated disk is diagnosed by myelography, CT scan, MRI, and neuromuscular tests. Treatment is bed rest; drugs to reduce pain, muscle spasms, and inflammation; followed by an exercise program to strengthen muscles. In severe cases, it may be necessary to remove the disk surgically in a **diskectomy**, sometimes followed by vertebral fusion with a bone graft to stabilize the spine. Using techniques of microsurgery, surgery done under magnification through a small incision, it is now possible to remove an exact amount of extruded disk tissue instead of the entire disk.

Curvatures of the Spine

The spine has four normal curves—two directed toward the anterior in the cervical and lumbar regions, and two directed toward the posterior in the thoracic and sacral regions (see Fig. 19-3). Any exaggeration or deviation of these curves is described as **curvature**

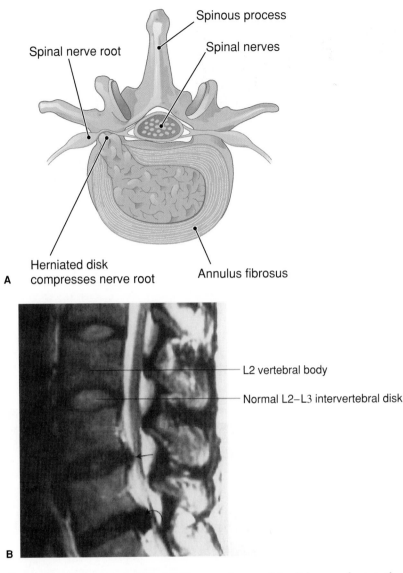

A

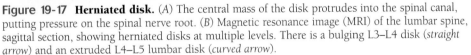

B

Figure 19-17 Herniated disk. (*A*) The central mass of the disk protrudes into the spinal canal, putting pressure on the spinal nerve root. (*B*) Magnetic resonance image (MRI) of the lumbar spine, sagittal section, showing herniated disks at multiple levels. There is a bulging L3–L4 disk (*straight arrow*) and an extruded L4–L5 lumbar disk (*curved arrow*).

of the spine. Three common types of spinal curvatures are shown in Figure 19-18 and described as follows:

> **Kyphosis** is an exaggerated curve in the thoracic region, popularly known as "hunchback."
> **Lordosis** is an exaggerated curve in the lumber region, popularly known as "swayback."
> **Scoliosis** is a sideways curvature of the spine in any region.

Spinal curvatures may be congenital or may result from muscle weakness or paralysis, poor posture, joint problems, disk degeneration, extreme obesity, or disease, such as tuberculosis of the spine, rickets, or osteoporosis. Extreme cases may cause pain, breathing problems, or degenerative changes.

Bracing the spine during childhood may help to correct a curvature. If surgery is needed, vertebrae are fused and bone grafts and implants are used to stabilize the spine. It is now sometimes possible for surgeons to make these corrections endoscopically.

19

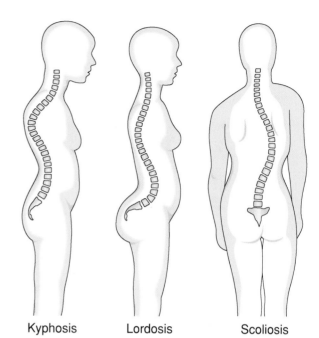

Figure 19-18 Curvatures of the spine. Kyphosis is an exaggerated thoracic curve; lordosis is an exaggerated lumbar curve; scoliosis is a sideways curve in any region.

Kyphosis   Lordosis   Scoliosis

TERMINOLOGY | Key Terms

DISORDERS

ankylosing spondylitis *ang-ki-LŌ-sing spon-di-LĪ-tis*	A chronic, progressive inflammatory disease involving the joints of the spine and surrounding soft tissue, most common in young males; also called rheumatoid spondylitis
ankylosis *ang-ki-LŌ-sis*	Immobility and fixation of a joint
arthritis *ar-THRĪ-tis*	Inflammation of a joint
chondrosarcoma *kon-drō-sar-KŌ-ma*	A malignant tumor of cartilage
curvature of the spine	An exaggerated spinal curve, such as scoliosis, lordosis, or kyphosis (see Fig. 19-18)
degenerative joint disease (DJD)	Osteoarthritis (see below)
fracture	A break in a bone. In a closed or simple fracture, the broken bone does not penetrate the skin; in an open fracture, there is an accompanying wound in the skin.
gout *gowt*	A form of acute arthritis, usually beginning in the knee or foot, caused by deposit of uric acid salts in the joints
herniated disk	Protrusion of the center (nucleus pulposus) of an intervertebral disk into the spinal canal; ruptured or "slipped" disk

Key Terms

kyphosis *kī-FŌ-sis*	An exaggerated curve of the spine in the thoracic region; hunchback, humpback (see Fig. 19-18)
lordosis *lor-DŌ-sis*	An exaggerated curve of the spine in the lumbar region; swayback (see Fig. 19-18)
osteoarthritis (OA) *os-tē-ō-ar-THRĪ-tis*	Progressive deterioration of joint cartilage with growth of new bone and soft tissue in and around the joint; the most common form of arthritis; results from wear and tear, injury, or disease; also called degenerative joint disease (DJD)
osteogenic sarcoma *os-tē-ō-JEN-ik*	A malignant bone tumor; osteosarcoma
osteomalacia *os-tē-ō-ma-LĀ-shē-a*	A softening and weakening of the bones due to vitamin D deficiency or other disease
osteomyelitis *os-tē-ō-mī-e-LĪ-tis*	Inflammation of bone and bone marrow caused by infection, usually bacterial
osteopenia *os-tē-ō-PĒ-nē-a*	A lower-than-average bone density, which may foreshadow osteoporosis
osteoporosis *os-tē-ō-po-RŌ-sis*	A condition characterized by reduction in bone density, most common in white women past menopause; predisposing factors include poor diet, inactivity, and low estrogen levels
Paget disease *PAJ-et*	Skeletal disease of the elderly characterized by bone thickening and distortion with bowing of long bones; osteitis deformans
Pott disease	Inflammation of the vertebrae, usually caused by tuberculosis
rheumatoid arthritis *RŪ-ma-toyd*	A chronic autoimmune disease of unknown origin resulting in inflammation of peripheral joints and related structures; more common in women than in men
rheumatoid factor	A group of antibodies found in the blood in cases of rheumatoid arthritis and other systemic diseases
rickets *RIK-ets*	Faulty bone formation in children, usually caused by a deficiency of vitamin D
sciatica *sī-AT-i-ka*	Severe pain in the leg along the course of the sciatic nerve, usually related to spinal nerve-root irritation
scoliosis *skō-lē-Ō-sis*	A sideways curvature of the spine in any region (see Fig. 19-18)
spondylolisthesis *spon-di-lō-LIS-the-sis*	A forward displacement of one vertebra over another (*-listhesis* means "a slipping")
spondylolysis *spon-di-LOL-i-sis*	Degeneration of the articulating portions of a vertebra allowing for spinal distortion, specifically in the lumbar region

19

TERMINOLOGY Key Terms

Continued

TREATMENT

alkaline phosphatase *AL-ka-lin FOS-fa-tās*	An enzyme needed in the formation of bone; serum activity of this enzyme is useful in diagnosis
arthrocentesis *ar-thrō-sen-TĒ-sis*	Aspiration of fluid from a joint by needle puncture
arthrodesis *ar-THROD-e-sis*	Surgical immobilization (fusion) of a joint; artificial ankylosis
arthroplasty *AR-thrō-plas-tē*	Partial or total replacement of a joint with a prosthesis
arthroscopy *ar-THROS-kō-pē*	Use of an endoscope to examine the interior of a joint or to perform surgery on the joint (see Fig. 19-14); the instrument used is an arthroscope
diskectomy *dis-KEK-tō-mē*	Surgical removal of a herniated intervertebral disk; also spelled discectomy
orthopedics *or-thō-PĒ-diks*	The study and treatment of disorders of the skeleton, muscles, and associated structures; literally "straight" (ortho) "child" (ped); also spelled orthopaedics
reduction of a fracture	Return of a fractured bone to a normal position; may be closed (not requiring surgery) or open (requiring surgery)
traction *TRAK-shun*	The process of drawing or pulling, such as traction of the head in the treatment of injuries to the cervical vertebrae

DRUGS

antiinflammatory agent	Drug that reduces inflammation; includes steroids, such as cortisone, and nonsteroidal antiinflammatory drugs (NSAIDs)
bisphosphonate *bis-FOS-fō-nāt*	Agent used to prevent and treat osteoporosis; increases bone mass by decreasing bone turnover. Examples are alendronate (Fosamax) and risedronate (Actonel)
nonsteroidal antiinflammatory drug (NSAID)	Drug that reduces inflammation but is not a steroid; examples include aspirin and ibuprofen and other inhibitors of prostaglandins, naturally produced substances that promote inflammation
selective estrogen receptor modulator (SERM)	Drug that acts on estrogen receptors. Raloxifene (Avista) is used to prevent bone loss after menopause. Other SERMs are used to prevent and treat estrogen-sensitive breast cancer.

Go to the pronunciation glossary in Chapter 19 of the CD-ROM to hear these words pronounced.

TERMINOLOGY Supplementary Terms

NORMAL STRUCTURE AND FUNCTION*

annulus fibrosus *AN-ū-lus fī-BRŌ-sus*	The outer ringlike portion of an intervertebral disk
calvaria *kal-VAR-ē-a*	The domelike upper portion of the skull
coxa *KOK-sa*	Hip
cruciate ligaments *KRŪ-shē-āt*	Ligaments that cross in the knee joint to connect the tibia and fibula. They are the anterior cruciate ligament (ACL) and the posterior cruciate ligament (PCL). *Cruciate* means "shaped like a cross."
genu *JE-nu*	The knee
glenoid cavity *GLEN-oyd*	The bony socket in the scapula that articulates with the head of the humerus
hallux *HAL-uks*	The great toe
malleolus *ma-LĒ-ō-lus*	The projection of the tibia or fibula on either side of the ankle
meniscus *me-NIS-kus*	Crescent-shaped disk of cartilage found in certain joints, such as the knee joint. In the knee, the medial meniscus and the lateral meniscus separate the tibia and femur. (plural: menisci (*me-NIS-kī*); meniscus means "crescent")
olecranon *ō-LEK-ra-non*	The process of the ulna that forms the elbow
os	Bone (plural: ossa)
osseous *OS-ē-us*	Pertaining to bone
symphysis pubis *SIM-fi-sis*	The anterior joint of the pelvis, formed by the union of the two pubic bones (see Fig. 19-4); also called pubic symphysis

See Box 19-5 for a list of bone markings.

SYMPTOMS AND CONDITIONS

achondroplasia *a-kon-drō-PLĀ-zha*	Decreased growth of cartilage in the growth plate of long bones resulting in dwarfism; a genetic disorder
Baker cyst	Mass formed at the knee joint by distention of a bursa with excess synovial fluid resulting from chronic irritation
bunion *BUN-yun*	Inflammation and enlargement of the metatarsal joint of the great toe, usually with displacement of the great toe toward the other toes

TERMINOLOGY *Continued*

Supplementary Terms

bursitis *bur-SĪ-tis*	Inflammation of a bursa, a small fluid-filled sac near a joint; causes include injury, irritation, and joint disease; the shoulder, hip, elbow, and knee are common sites
carpal tunnel syndrome	Numbness and weakness of the hand caused by pressure on the median nerve as it passes through a tunnel formed by carpal bones
chondroma *kon-DRŌ-ma*	A benign tumor of cartilage
Ewing tumor	A bone tumor that usually appears in children 5 to 15 years of age. It begins in the shaft of a bone and spreads readily to other bones. It may respond to radiation therapy, but then returns. Also called Ewing sarcoma.
exostosis *eks-os-TŌ-sis*	A bony outgrowth from the surface of a bone
giant-cell tumor	A bone tumor that usually appears in children and young adults. The ends of the bones are destroyed, commonly at the knee, by a large mass that does not metastasize.
hammertoe *HAM-er-tō*	Change in position of the toe joints so that the toe takes on a clawlike appearance and the first joint protrudes upward, causing irritation and pain on walking.
hallux valgus	Painful condition involving lateral displacement of the great toe at the metatarsal joint. There is also enlargement of the metatarsal head and bunion formation.
Heberden nodes *HĒ-ber-den*	Small, hard nodules formed in the cartilage of the distal joints of the fingers in osteoarthritis
hemarthrosis *hē-mar-THRŌ-sis*	Bleeding into a joint cavity
Legg–Calvé–Perthes disease *leg-kahl-vā-PER-tez*	Degeneration (osteochondrosis) of the proximal growth center of the femur. The bone is eventually restored, but there may be deformity and weakness. Most common in young boys. Also called coxa plana.
multiple myeloma *mī-e-LŌ-ma*	A cancer of blood-forming cells in bone marrow (see Chapter 10)
neurogenic arthropathy *nū-rō-JEN-ik ar-THROP-a-thē*	Degenerative disease of joints caused by impaired nervous stimulation; most common cause is diabetes mellitus; Charcot arthropathy
Osgood-Schlatter disease *oz-good-SHLAHT-er*	Degeneration (osteochondrosis) of the proximal growth center of the tibia causing pain and tendinitis at the knee
osteochondroma *os-tē-ō-kon-DRŌ-ma*	A benign tumor consisting of cartilage and bone
osteochondrosis *os-tē-ō-kon-DRŌ-sis*	Disease of a bone's growth center in children; degeneration of the tissue is followed by recalcification
osteodystrophy *os-tē-ō-DIS-trō-fē*	Abnormal bone development

19

osteogenesis imperfecta (OI) *os-tē-ō-JEN-e-sis im-per-FEK-ta*	A hereditary disease resulting in the formation of brittle bones that fracture easily. There is faulty synthesis of collagen, the main structural protein in connective tissue.
osteoma	A benign bone tumor that usually remains small and localized
Reiter syndrome	Chronic polyarthritis that usually affects young men; occurs after a bacterial infection and is common in those infected with HIV; may also involve the eyes and genitourinary tract
spondylosis *spon-di-LŌ-sis*	Degeneration and ankylosis of the vertebrae resulting in pressure on the spinal cord and nerve roots; often applied to any degenerative lesion of the spine
sprain	Trauma to a joint involving the ligaments
subluxation *sub-luk-SĀ-shun*	A partial dislocation
talipes *TAL-i-pēz*	A deformity of the foot, especially one occurring congenitally; clubfoot
valgus *VAL-gus*	Bent outward
varus *VAR-us*	Bent inward
von Recklinghausen disease	Loss of bone tissue caused by increased parathyroid hormone; bones become decalcified and deformed, and fracture easily

DIAGNOSIS AND TREATMENT

allograft *AL-ō-graft*	Graft of tissue between individuals of the same species but different genetic makeup; homograft, allogenic graft (see autograft)
arthroclasia *ar-thrō-KLĀ-zha*	Surgical breaking of an ankylosed joint to provide movement
aspiration *as-pi-RĀ-shun*	Removal by suction, as removal of fluid from a body cavity; also inhalation, such as accidental inhalation of material into the respiratory tract
autograft *AW-tō-graft*	Graft of tissue taken from a site on or in the body of the person receiving the graft; autologous graft (see allograft)
calcitonin *kal-si-TŌ-nin*	A hormone from the thyroid gland that decreases resorption (loss) of bone tissue; used in the treatment of Paget disease and osteoporosis; also called thyrocalcitonin
chondroitin *kon-DRŌ-i-tin*	A complex polysaccharide found in connective tissue; used as a dietary supplement, usually with glucosamine, for treatment of joint pain
glucosamine	A dietary supplement used in the treatment of joint pain

19

TERMINOLOGY Supplementary Terms
Continued

goniometer *gō-nē-OM-e-ter*	A device used to measure joint angles and movements (root *goni/o* means "angle")
iontophoresis *ī-on-tō-for-Ē-sis*	Introduction into the tissue by means of electric current, using the ions of a given drug; used in the treatment of musculoskeletal disorders
laminectomy *lam-i-NEK-tō-mē*	Excision of the posterior arch (lamina) of a vertebra
meniscectomy *men-i-SEK-tō-mē*	Removal of the crescent-shaped cartilage (meniscus) of the knee joint
myelogram *MĪ-e-lō-gram*	Radiograph of the spinal canal after injection of a radiopaque dye; used to evaluate a herniated disk
osteoplasty *OS-tē-ō-plas-tē*	Scraping and removal of damaged bone from a joint
prosthesis *PROS-thē-sis*	An artificial organ or part, such as an artificial limb

Go to the pronunciation glossary in Chapter 19 of the CD-ROM
to hear these words pronounced.

Box 19•5 For Your Reference *Bone Markings*

Marking	Description
Condyle *KON-dīl*	smooth, rounded protuberance at a joint
crest	raised, narrow ridge (see iliac crest in Fig. 19-4)
epicondyle *ep-i-KON-dīl*	projection above a condyle
facet *FAS-et*	small, flattened surface
foramen *for-Ā-men*	rounded opening (see foramen for spinal nerve in Fig. 19-3)
fossa *FOS-a*	hollow cavity

Box 19•5	**For Your Reference**	*Continued*

meatus *mē-Ā-tus*	long channel within a bone
process	projection (see mastoid process and styloid process in Fig. 19-2)
sinus *SĪ-nus*	air-filled space or channel
spine	sharp projection (see ischial spine in Fig. 19-4)
trochanter *trō-KAN-ter*	large, blunt projection as at the top of the femur
tubercle *TŪ-ber-kl*	small, rounded projection
tuberosity *tū-ber-OS-i-tē*	large, rounded projection

19

TERMINOLOGY Abbreviations

ACL	Anterior cruciate ligament	**MTP**	Metatarsophalangeal (joint)
AE	Above the elbow	**NSAID(s)**	Nonsteroidal antiinflammatory drug(s)
AK	Above the knee	**OA**	Osteoarthritis
ASF	Anterior spinal fusion	**OI**	Osteogenesis imperfecta
BE	Below the elbow	**ORIF**	Open reduction internal fixation
BK	Below the knee	**ortho, ORTH**	Orthopedics
BMD	Bone mineral density	**PCL**	Posterior cruciate ligament
C	Cervical vertebra; numbered C1 to C7	**PIP**	Proximal interphalangeal (joint)
Co	Coccyx; coccygeal	**PSF**	Posterior spinal fusion
DEXA	Dual-energy x-ray absorptiometry (scan)	**RA**	Rheumatoid arthritis
DIP	Distal interphalangeal (joint)	**S**	Sacrum; sacral
DJD	Degenerative joint disease	**SERM**	Selective estrogen receptor modulator
Fx	Fracture	**T**	Thoracic vertebra; numbered T1 to T12
HNP	Herniated nucleus pulposus	**THA**	Total hip arthroplasty
IM	Intramedullary	**TKA**	Total knee arthroplasty
L	Lumbar vertebra; numbered L1 to L5	**TMJ**	Temporomandibular joint
MCP	Metacarpophalangeal (joint)	**Tx**	Traction

CHAPTER REVIEW

19

LABELING EXERCISE
The Skeleton

Write the name of each numbered part on the corresponding line of the answer sheet.

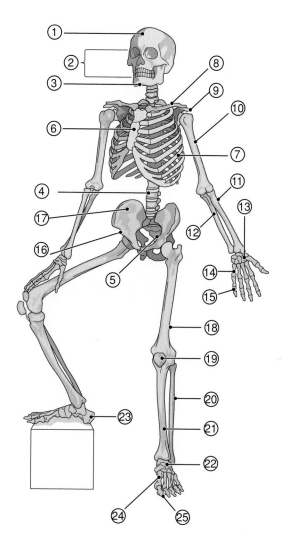

calcaneus	1. _____
carpals	2. _____
clavicle	3. _____
cranium	4. _____
facial bones	5. _____
femur	6. _____
fibula	7. _____

humerus

ilium

mandible

metacarpals

metatarsals

patella

pelvis

phalanges

phalanges

radius

ribs

sacrum

scapula

sternum

tarsals

tibia

ulna

vertebral column

8. _____

9. _____

10. _____

11. _____

12. _____

13. _____

14. _____

15. _____

16. _____

17. _____

18. _____

19. _____

20. _____

21. _____

22. _____

23. _____

24. _____

25. _____

19

Skull from the Left

Write the name of each numbered part on the corresponding line of the answer sheet.

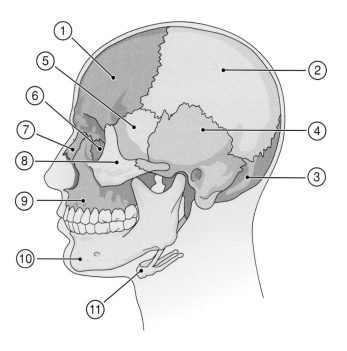

frontal

hyoid

lacrimal

mandible

maxilla

nasal

occipital

parietal

sphenoid

temporal

zygomatic

1. _____

2. _____

3. _____

4. _____

5. _____

6. _____

7. _____

8. _____

9. _____

10. _____

11. _____

Vertebral Column

Write the name of each numbered part on the corresponding line of the answer sheet.

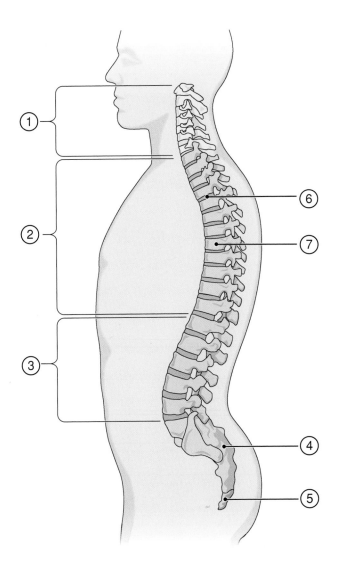

body of vertebra   1. _____

cervical vertebrae   2. _____

coccyx   3. _____

intervertebral disk   4. _____

lumbar vertebrae   5. _____

sacrum   6. _____

thoracic vertebrae   7. _____

The Pelvic Bones

Write the name of each numbered part on the corresponding line of the answer sheet.

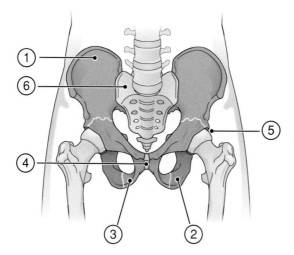

ilium

ischium

pubis

pubic symphysis

acetabulum

sacrum

1. _____

2. _____

3. _____

4. _____

5. _____

6. _____

Structure of a Long Bone

Write the name of each numbered part on the corresponding line of the answer sheet.

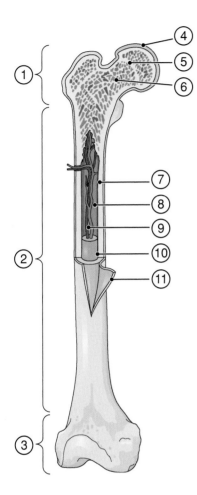

19

artery and vein   1. _____

cartilage   2. _____

compact bone   3. _____

diaphysis   4. _____

distal epiphysis   5. _____

epiphyseal line (growth line)   6. _____

medullary cavity   7. _____

periosteum   8. _____

proximal epiphysis   9. _____

spongy bone (containing red marrow)   10. _____

yellow marrow   11. _____

TERMINOLOGY

Multiple choice. Select the best answer and write the letter of your choice to the left of each number:

_____	1. periosteum	**a.** growth region of a long bone
_____	2. metaphysis	**b.** breakdown and removal of bone tissue
_____	3. symphysis	**c.** cell that breaks down bone
_____	4. osteoclast	**d.** membrane that covers a bone
_____	5. resorption	**e.** slightly movable joint
_____	6. scoliosis	**a.** immobility of a joint
_____	7. ankylosis	**b.** spinal tap
_____	8. osteoporosis	**c.** displacement of a vertebra
_____	9. spondylolisthesis	**d.** sideways curvature of the spine
_____	10. rachiocentesis	**e.** loss of bone mass

Supplementary Terms

_____	11. laminectomy	**a.** knee
_____	12. calvaria	**b.** part of the ulna that forms the elbow
_____	13. subluxation	**c.** excision of part of a vertebra
_____	14. genu	**d.** upper portion of the skull
_____	15. olecranon	**e.** partial dislocation
_____	16. exostosis	**a.** removal of knee cartilage
_____	17. hallux	**b.** device used to measure joint angles
_____	18. prosthesis	**c.** great toe
_____	19. goniometer	**d.** outgrowth of bone
_____	20. meniscectomy	**e.** artificial part

Fill in the blanks:

21. The study and treatment of disorders of the skeleton, muscles, and associated structures is _____.

22. The type of tissue that covers the ends of the bones at the joints is _____.

23. A band of connective tissue that connects a bone to another bone is a(n) _____.

24. The part of the vertebral column that articulates with the ilium is the _____.

25. A fluid-filled sac near a joint is a(n) _____.

26. The fluid that fills a freely movable joint is _____.

27. Hemarthrosis is bleeding into a(n) _____.

28. The term *costochondral* refers to a rib and its _____.

29. Spondylarthritis (*spon-dil-ar-THRĪ-tis*) is arthritis of the _____.

30. Rachischisis (*rā-KIS-ki-sis*) is fissure of the _____.

19

True–False. Examine each of the following statements. If the statement is true, write T in the first blank. If the statement is false, write F in the first blank and correct the statement by replacing the <u>underlined</u> word in the second blank.

31. The shaft of a long bone is the <u>epiphysis</u>. _____ _____

32. The carpal bones are found in the <u>wrist</u>. _____ _____

33. An immovable joint is a <u>suture</u>. _____ _____

34. The ulna is part of the <u>axial</u> skeleton. _____ _____

35. The <u>thoracic</u> vertebrae are located in the neck. _____ _____

36. The cells that produce bone tissue are <u>osteoblasts</u>. _____ _____

37. Blood cells are formed in <u>red</u> bone marrow. _____ _____

38. An exaggerated lumbar curve of the spine is <u>kyphosis</u>. _____ _____

39. The term *valgus* means bent <u>outward</u>. _____ _____

Eliminations. In each of the sets below, underline the word that does not fit in with the rest and explain the reason for your choice:

40. foramen – process – hyoid – crest – condyle

_____

41. coronal – occipital – parietal – frontal – sphenoid

_____

42. rachi/o – sacr/o – sponodyl/o – vertebr/o – cost/o

_____

43. Colles – sciatic – impacted – comminuted – greenstick

_____

44. L – C – T – Co – RA

_____

Define each of the following words:

45. myelogenous (*mī-e-LOJ-e-nus*) _____

46. osteitis (*os-tē-Ī-tis*) _____

47. arthrodesis (*ar-THROD-e-sis*) _____

48. synovectomy (*sin-ō-VEK-tō-mē*) _____

49. intraosseous (*in-tra-OS-ē-us*) _____

50. peribursal (*per-i-BER-sal*) _____

51. spondylodynia (*spon-di-lō-DIN-ē-a*) _____

52. polyarticular (*pol-ē-ar-TIK-ū-lar*) _____

53. subcostal (*sub-KOS-tal*) _____

54. coccygeal (*kok-SIJ-ē-al*) _____

Word building. Write words for the following definitions:

55. formation of cartilage _____

56. death (-necrosis) of bone tissue _____

57. incision into the cranium _____

58. tumor of bone and cartilage _____

59. narrowing of a joint _____

60. surgical excision of cartilage _____

61. stone in a bursa _____

62. breaking of a joint _____

63. instrument for incising a joint _____

64. measurement of the pelvis _____

65. endoscopic examination of a joint _____

66. pertaining to the sacrum and ilium _____

67. dissolving or destruction of bone _____

68. surgical excision of the coccyx _____

69. near the sacrum _____

Adjectives. Write the adjective form of the following words:

70. cranium _____

71. ilium _____

72. coccyx _____

73. pelvis _____

74. vertebra _____

Word analysis. Define the following words and give the meaning of the word parts in each. Use a dictionary if necessary.

75. chondroblastoma (*kon-drō-blas-TŌ-ma*) _____

    a. chondr/o _____

    b. blast _____

    c. -oma _____

76. spondylosyndesis (*spon-di-lō-SIN-de-sis*) _____

    a. spondyl/o _____

    b. syn- _____

    c. -desis _____

77. achondroplasia (*a-kon-drō-PLĀ-zha*) _____

    a. a- _____

    b. chondr/o _____

    c. -plasia _____

Go to the word exercises in Chapter 19 of the CD-ROM for additional review exercises.

CASE STUDY 19-1: Arthroplasty of the Right TMJ

S.A., a 38-year-old teacher, was admitted for surgery for degenerative joint disease (DJD) of her right temporo-mandibular joint (TMJ). She has experienced chronic pain in her right jaw, neck, and ear since her automobile accident the previous year. S.A.'s diagnosis was confirmed by CT scan and was followed up with conservative therapy, which included a bite plate, NSAIDs, and steroid injections. She had also tried hypnosis in an attempt to manage her pain but was not able to gain relief. Her doctor referred her to an oral surgeon who specializes in TMJ disorders. S.A. was scheduled for an arthroplasty of the right TMJ to remove diseased bone on the articular surface of the right mandibular condyle.

On the following day, she was transported to the OR for surgery. She was given general endotracheal anesthesia, and a vertical incision was made from the superior aspect of the right ear down to the base of the attachment of the right earlobe. After appropriate dissection and retraction, the posterior–superior aspect of the right zygomatic arch was bluntly dissected anteroposteriorly. With a nerve stimulator, the zygomatic branch of the facial nerve was identified

and retracted from the surgical field with a vessel loop. The periosteum was then incised along the superior aspect of the arch. An inferior dissection was then made along the capsular ligament and retracted posteriorly. With a Freer elevator, the meniscus was freed, and a horizontal incision was made to the condyle. With a Hall drill and saline coolant, a high condylectomy of approximately 3 mm of bone was removed while conserving function of the external pterygoid muscle. The stump of the condyle was filed smooth and irrigated copiously with NSS. The lateral capsule, periosteum, subcutaneous tissue, and skin were then closed with sutures. The facial nerve was tested before closing and confirmed to be intact. A pressure pack and Barton bandage were applied. The sponge, needle, and instrument counts were correct. Estimated blood loss (EBL) was approximately 50 mL.

S.A. was discharged on the second postoperative day with instructions for a soft diet; daily mouth-opening exercises; an antibiotic (Keflex 500 mg po q6h); Tylenol no. 3 po q4h prn for pain; and four weekly postoperative appointments.

CASE STUDY 19-2: Osteogenesis Imperfecta

M.H., a 3-year-old boy with osteogenesis imperfecta (OI) type III, was admitted to the pediatric orthopedic hospital for treatment of yet another fracture. Since birth he has had 15 arm and leg fractures as a result of his congenital disease. This latest fracture occurred when he twisted at the hip while standing in his wheeled walker. He has been in a research study and receives a bisphosphonate infusion every 2 months. He is short in stature with short limbs for his age, and has bowing of both legs.

M.H. was transferred to the OR and carefully lifted to the OR table by the staff. After he was anesthetized, he was positioned with gentle manipulation, and his left hip was

elevated on a small gel pillow. After skin preparation and sterile draping, a stainless steel rod was inserted into the medullary canal of his left femur to reduce and stabilize the femoral fracture. The muscle, fascia, subcutaneous tissue, and skin were sutured closed. Three nurses gently held M.H. in position on a pediatric spica box while the surgeon applied a hip spica (body cast) to stabilize the fixation, protect the leg, and maintain abduction. M.H. was transferred to the PACU for recovery. The surgeon dictated the procedure as an open reduction internal fixation (ORIF) of the left femur with intramedullary (IM) rodding and application of spica cast.

CASE STUDY 19-3: Idiopathic Adolescent Scoliosis

Four years ago, L.R., who is now 15, had a posterior spinal fusion (PSF) for correction of idiopathic adolescent scoliosis in a pediatric orthopedic hospital in another state. Her spinal curvature had been surgically corrected with the insertion of bilateral laminar and pedicle hooks and two 3/16-inch rods. A bone autograft was taken from her right posterior superior ilium and applied along the lateral processes of T4 to L2 to complete the fusion.

During a follow-up visit, she presented with a significant prominence of the right scapula and back pain in the mid and lower back. She denied numbness or tingling of the lower extremities, bowel or bladder problems, chest pain, and shortness of breath. A CT scan of the upper thoracic spine showed a prominent rotatory scoliosis deformity of the right posterior thorax with acute angulation of the ribs. Her deformity is a common consequence of overcorrection of prior spinal fusion surgery, called crank shaft phenomenon.

L.R. was referred to the chief spinal surgeon of a local pediatric orthopedic hospital for removal of the spinal instrumentation, posterior spinal osteotomies from T4 to L2, insertion of replacement hooks and rods, bilateral rib resections, autograft bone from the resected ribs, partial scapulectomy and possible bone allograft, and bilateral chest-tube placement. The surgical plan was explained to her and her mother and consent was obtained and signed. The surgical procedure as well as the potential benefits versus risks were discussed. L.R. and her mother stated that they fully understood and provided consent to proceed with the plan for surgery.

CASE STUDY QUESTIONS

Multiple choice. Select the best answer and write the letter of your choice to the left of each number:

_____ 1. A condylectomy is:
   a. removal of a joint capsule
   b. plastic repair of a vertebra
   c. removal of a rounded bone protuberance
   d. enlargement of a cavity
   e. removal of a tumor

_____ 2. The articulating surface of a bone is located:
   a. under the epiphysis
   b. in a joint
   c. around the bone marrow
   d. at a muscle attachment
   e. at a tendon attachment

_____ 3. The dissection directed anteroposteriorly was done:
   a. posterior–superior
   b. circumferential
   c. front to back
   d. top to bottom
   e. perpendicular to the mandible

_____ 4. Another term for bow-legged is:
   a. internal rotation
   b. knock-kneed
   c. adduction
   d. varus
   e. valgus

_____ 5. An IM rod is placed:
   a. inferior to the femoral condyle
   b. into the acetabulum
   c. within the medullary canal
   d. on top of the periosteum
   e. lateral to the epiphyseal growth plates

_____ 6. The anatomic area described as thoracic or as the thorax is the:
   a. chest
   b. lower pelvis
   c. between sternum and umbilicus

    d. shoulders

    e. posterior abdomen

_____ 7. L.R.'s spinal fusion will immobilize the spinal levels of T4 to L2. These segments describe the _____ and _____ vertebrae.

    a. cervical, lumbar

    b. sacral, cranial

    c. lamina, disks

    d. thoracic, lumbar

    e. lumbar, thoracic

_____ 8. The grafted bone for L.R.'s fusion came from her own right ilium. The proper name for this is a(n):

    a. allograft

    b. autograft

    c. heterograft

    d. iliograft

    e. homograft

Write terms from the case studies with the following meanings:

9. pertaining to the cheekbone _____

10. the membrane around the bone _____

11. a crescent-shaped cartilage in a joint _____

12. on both sides _____

13. plastic repair of a joint _____

14. term for a disease of unknown origin _____

15. removal of the shoulder blade _____

16. a break in a bone _____

17. surgical openings into bones _____

Abbreviations. Define the following abbreviations:

18. DJD _____

19. MRI _____

20. NSAIDs _____

21. CT _____

22. NSS _____

23. TMJ _____

24. OI _____

25. ORIF _____

26. PSF _____

27. EBL _____

19

The Skeleton

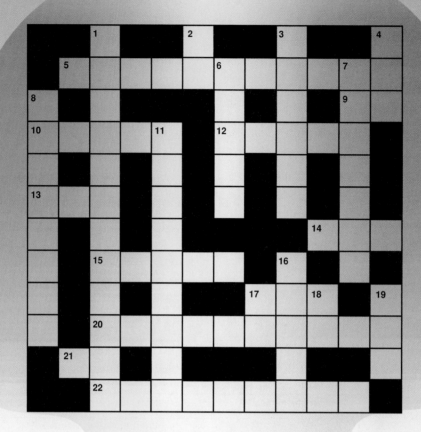

ACROSS

5. Study and treatment of the skeleton, muscles, and associated structures
9. Abbreviation used in taking medical histories
10. Deficiency of: suffix
12. Instrument for measuring joint angles: _____ meter
13. New: prefix
14. Cold: root
15. First cervical vertebra
17. Twice per day: abbreviation
20. Breakdown and removal of bone
21. Type of arthritis: abbreviation
22. Slipping of a vertebra: spondylo _____

DOWN

1. Pertaining to the cranium and sacrum
2. Last portion of the spinal column: abbreviation
3. Pain: suffix
4. Same, equal: prefix
6. A bone disease is named for him
7. Cartilage: combining form
8. Vertebra: combining form
11. Immobility of a joint
16. Stones: suffix
17. Blood pressure: abbreviation
18. Two, twice: prefix
19. Meaning of the prefix tel/o

CHAPTER TWENTY

THE MUSCULAR SYSTEM

CHAPTER CONTENTS

OBJECTIVES

After study of this chapter you should be able to:

1. Compare the location and function of smooth, cardiac, and skeletal muscle.
2. Describe the typical structure of a skeletal muscle.
3. Briefly describe the mechanism of muscle contraction.
4. Explain how muscles work together to produce movement.
5. Describe the main types of movements produced by muscles.
6. List some of the criteria for naming muscles.
7. Identify and use the roots pertaining to the muscular system.
8. Describe the main disorders that affect muscles.
9. Label diagrams of the superficial anterior and posterior muscles.
10. Interpret abbreviations pertaining to muscles.
11. Analyze several case studies involving muscles.

PRETEST

1. The neuromuscular junction is between a muscle and a(n) _____.

2. In muscle anatomy, the opposite of the origin is the _____.

3. The quadriceps femoris muscle forms the anterior part of the _____.

4. The opposite of pronation is _____.

5. The band of connective tissue that attaches a muscle to a bone is a(n) _____.

6. Polymyositis is inflammation of many _____.

The main characteristic of **muscle** tissue is its ability to contract. When stimulated, muscles shorten to produce movement of the skeleton, vessels, or internal organs. Muscles also may remain partially contracted to maintain posture. In addition, the heat generated by muscle contraction is the main source of body heat.

Types of Muscle

There are three types of muscle tissue in the body (Fig. 20-1):

> **Smooth (visceral) muscle** makes up the walls of the hollow organs, such as the stomach, intestines, and uterus, and the walls of ducts, such as the blood vessels and bronchioles. Smooth muscle operates involuntarily and is responsible for peristalsis, the wavelike movements that propel materials through the systems.
> **Cardiac muscle** makes up the myocardium of the heart wall. It functions involuntarily and is responsible for the heart's pumping action.
> **Skeletal muscle** is attached to bones and is responsible for voluntary movement. It also maintains posture and generates a large proportion of body heat. All of these voluntary muscles together make up the muscular system.

Skeletal Muscle

The discussion that follows describes the characteristics of skeletal muscle, which has been the most extensively studied of the three muscle types.

Muscle Structure

Muscles are composed of individual cells, often referred to as fibers because they are so long and threadlike. These cells are held together in **fascicles** (bundles) by connective tissue (Fig. 20-2). Covering each muscle is a sheath of connective tissue or **fascia**. These supporting tissues merge to form the **tendons** that attach the muscle to bones.

Muscle Action

Skeletal muscles are stimulated to contract by motor neurons of the nervous system (Fig. 20-3). At the **neuromuscular junction (NMJ)**, the synapse (junction) where a branch of a neuron meets a muscle cell, the neurotransmitter **acetylcholine (ACh)** is released from small vesicles (sacs) in an axon branch. ACh interacts with the muscle cell membrane to prompt cellular contraction. Two special protein filaments in muscle cells, **actin** and **myosin**, interact to produce the contraction. ATP (the cell's energy compound)

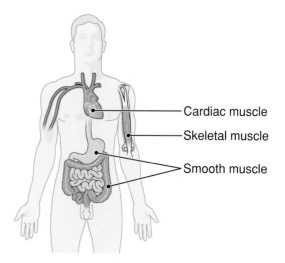

Figure 20-1 Muscle types. Smooth muscle makes up the wall of ducts and hollow organs, such as the stomach and intestine; cardiac muscle makes up the wall of the heart; skeletal muscle is attached to bones.

20

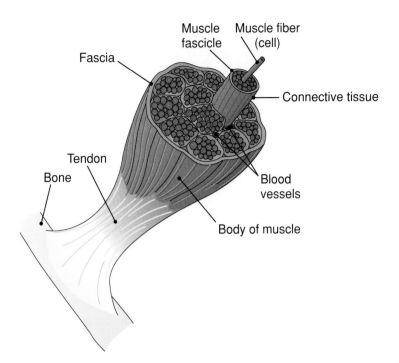

Figure 20-2 Structure of a skeletal muscle. Connective tissue coverings are shown as is the tendon that attaches the muscle to a bone.

and calcium are needed for this response. Box 20-1 discusses the use of steroids to increase muscle development and strength.

Most skeletal muscles contract rapidly to produce movement and then relax rapidly unless stimulation continues. Sometimes muscles are kept in a steady partially contracted state, to maintain posture, for example. This state of firmness is called **tonus**, or muscle tone.

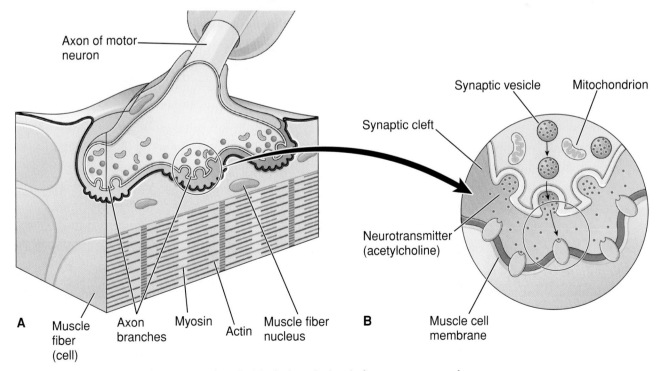

Figure 20-3 Neuromuscular junction (NMJ). (*A*) The branched end of a motor neuron makes contact with the membrane of a muscle fiber (cell). (*B*) Enlarged view of the NMJ showing release of neurotransmitter (acetylcholine) from a neuron and its attachment to a muscle-cell membrane. Mitochondria generate ATP, the cells' energy compound.

20

Anabolic Steroids: Winning at All Costs?

Anabolic steroids mimic the effects of the male sex hormone testosterone by promoting metabolism and stimulating growth. These drugs are legally prescribed to promote muscle regeneration and prevent atrophy from disuse after surgery. However, athletes also purchase them illegally, using them to increase muscle size and strength and improve endurance.

When steroids are used illegally to enhance athletic performance, the doses needed are large enough to cause serious side effects. They increase blood cholesterol levels, which may lead to atherosclerosis, heart disease, kidney failure, and stroke. Steroids damage the liver, making it more susceptible to disease and cancer, and they suppress the immune system, increasing the risk of infection and cancer. In men, steroids cause impotence, testicular atrophy, low sperm count, infertility, and the development of female sex characteristics such as breasts (gynecomastia). In women, steroids disrupt ovulation and menstruation and produce male sex characteristics such as breast atrophy, enlargement of the clitoris, increased body hair, and deepening of the voice. In both sexes, steroids increase the risk for baldness and, especially in men, they cause mood swings, depression, and violence.

Muscles work in pairs to produce movement at the joints. As one muscle, the **prime mover**, contracts, an opposing muscle, the **antagonist**, must relax. For example, when the biceps brachii on the anterior surface of the upper arm contracts to flex the arm, the triceps brachii on the posterior surface must relax (Fig. 20-4). When the arm is extended, these actions are reversed. In a given movement, the point where the muscle is attached to a stable part of the skeleton is the **origin**; the point where a muscle is attached to a moving part of the skeleton is the **insertion**.

Box 20-2 describes various types of movements at the joints; these are illustrated in Fig. 20-5.

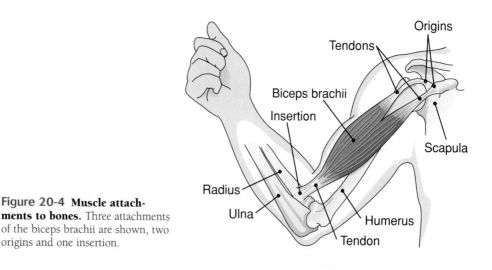

Figure 20-4 Muscle attachments to bones. Three attachments of the biceps brachii are shown, two origins and one insertion.

Types of Movement

Movement	Definition	Example
flexion *FLEK-shun*	closing the angle at a joint	bending at the knee or elbow
extension *eks-TEN-shun*	opening the angle at a joint	straightening at the knee or elbow

Box 20•2 **For Your Reference** *Continued*

20

abduction *ab-DUK-shun*	movement away from the midline of the body	outward movement of the arms at the shoulders
adduction *a-DUK-shun*	movement toward the midline of the body	return of lifted arms to the body
rotation *rō-TĀ-shun*	turning of a body part on its own axis	turning of the forearm from the elbow
circumduction *ser-kum-DUK-shun*	circular movement from a central point	describing a circle with an outstretched arm
pronation *prō-NĀ-shun*	turning downward	turning the palm of the hand downward
supination *sū-pin-Ā-shun*	turning upward	turning the palm of the hand upward
eversion *ē-VER-zhun*	turning outward	turning the sole of the foot outward
inversion *in-VER-zhun*	turning inward	turning the sole of the foot inward
dorsiflexion *dor-si-FLEK-shun*	bending backward	moving the foot so that the toes point upward, away from the sole of the foot
plantar flexion	bending the sole of the foot	pointing the toes downward

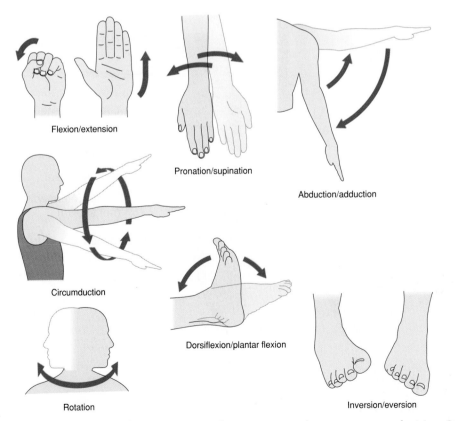

Flexion/extension

Pronation/supination

Abduction/adduction

Circumduction

Dorsiflexion/plantar flexion

Rotation

Inversion/eversion

Figure 20-5 Types of movement. Muscle contraction produces movement at the joints. Some muscles are named for the type of movement they produce, such as flexor, extensor, and adductor.

Naming of Muscles

A muscle can be named by its location (near a bone, for example), by the direction of its fibers, or by its size, shape, or number of attachment points (heads), as indicated by the suffix -ceps. It may also be named for its action, adding the suffix -or to the root for the action. For example, a muscle that produces flexion at a joint is a flexor. Examine the muscle diagrams in Figures 20-6 and 20-7. See how many of these criteria you can find in the muscle names. Note that sometimes more than one criterion is used in the name.

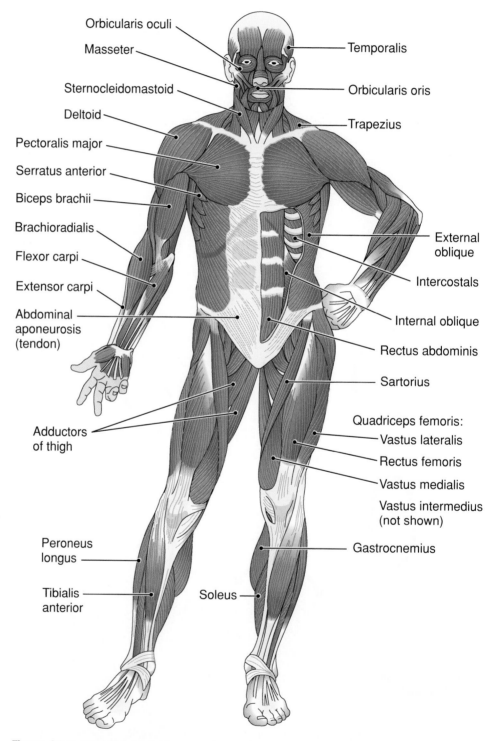

Figure 20-6 Superficial muscles, anterior view.

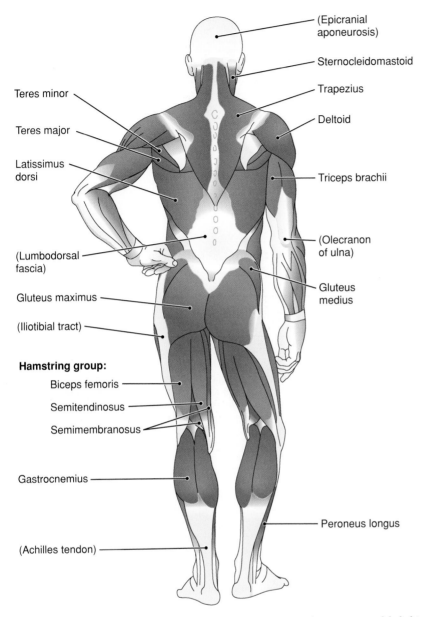

Figure 20-7 Superficial muscles, posterior view. Associated structures are labeled in parentheses.

20

TERMINOLOGY Key Terms

NORMAL STRUCTURE AND FUNCTION

acetylcholine (ACh) *as-e-til-KŌ-lēn*	A neurotransmitter that stimulates contraction of skeletal muscles
actin *AK-tin*	One of the two contractile proteins in muscle cells; the other is myosin

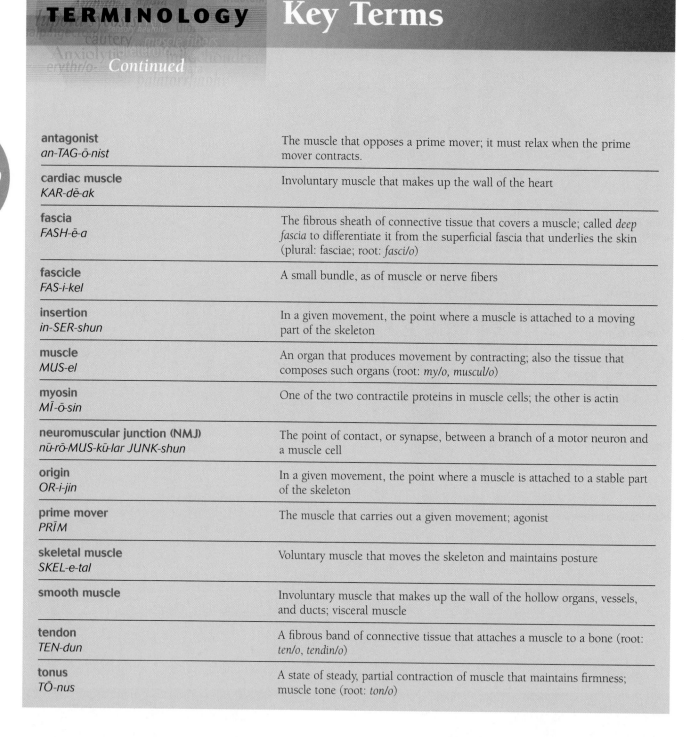

Key Terms

Continued

antagonist *an-TAG-ō-nist*	The muscle that opposes a prime mover; it must relax when the prime mover contracts.
cardiac muscle *KAR-dē-ak*	Involuntary muscle that makes up the wall of the heart
fascia *FASH-ē-a*	The fibrous sheath of connective tissue that covers a muscle; called *deep fascia* to differentiate it from the superficial fascia that underlies the skin (plural: fasciae; root: *fasci/o*)
fascicle *FAS-i-kel*	A small bundle, as of muscle or nerve fibers
insertion *in-SER-shun*	In a given movement, the point where a muscle is attached to a moving part of the skeleton
muscle *MUS-el*	An organ that produces movement by contracting; also the tissue that composes such organs (root: *my/o, muscul/o*)
myosin *MĪ-ō-sin*	One of the two contractile proteins in muscle cells; the other is actin
neuromuscular junction (NMJ) *nū-rō-MUS-kū-lar JUNK-shun*	The point of contact, or synapse, between a branch of a motor neuron and a muscle cell
origin *OR-i-jin*	In a given movement, the point where a muscle is attached to a stable part of the skeleton
prime mover *PRĪM*	The muscle that carries out a given movement; agonist
skeletal muscle *SKEL-e-tal*	Voluntary muscle that moves the skeleton and maintains posture
smooth muscle	Involuntary muscle that makes up the wall of the hollow organs, vessels, and ducts; visceral muscle
tendon *TEN-dun*	A fibrous band of connective tissue that attaches a muscle to a bone (root: *ten/o, tendin/o*)
tonus *TŌ-nus*	A state of steady, partial contraction of muscle that maintains firmness; muscle tone (root: *ton/o*)

Go to the pronunciation glossary in Chapter 20 on the CD-ROM to hear these words pronounced.

Roots Pertaining to Muscles

Table 20·1	Roots Pertaining to Muscles		
ROOT	**MEANING**	**EXAMPLE**	**DEFINITION OF EXAMPLE**
my/o	muscle	myositis* *mī-ō-SĪ-tis*	inflammation of muscle
muscul/o	muscle	musculotropic *mus-kyū-lō-TROP-ik*	acting on or attracted to muscle tissue
in/o	fiber	inosclerosis *in-ō-skle-RŌ-sis*	hardening of tissue from an increase of fibers
fasci/o	fascia	fasciodesis *fash-ē-OD-e-sis*	binding (suture) of a fascia to a tendon or other fascia
ten/o, tendin/o	tendon	tenostosis *ten-os-TŌ-sis*	ossification of a tendon
ton/o	tone	cardiotonic *kar-dē-ō-TON-ik*	having a strengthening action on the heart
erg/o	work	ergonomics	study of the efficient use of energy during work
kin/o-, kine, kinesi/o, kinet/o	movement	kinesis *ki-NĒ-sis*	movement (adjective: kinetic)

*Note addition of s to this root before the suffix -itis.

Exercise 20-1

Define the following adjectives:

1. muscular _____

2. fascial _____

3. tendinous _____

4. kinetic _____

5. tonic _____

Fill in the blanks:

6. Myoglobin (*mī-Ō-GLŌ-bin*) is a type of protein (globin) found in _____.

7. An ergograph (*ER-gō-graf*) is an instrument for measuring muscle _____.

8. Dystonia (*dis-TŌ-nē-a*) is abnormal muscle _____.

9. Kinesia (*kī-NĒ-sē-a*) is a term for sickness caused by _____.

10. Fasciitis (*fash-ē-Ī-tis*) is inflammation of _____.

11. Inotropic (*in-ō-TROP-ik*) means acting on _____.

12. Myofibrils (*mī-ō-FĪ-brils*) are small fibers found in _____.

13. The muscularis layer in the wall of a hollow organ or duct is composed of _____.

Exercise 20-1

Define the following terms:

14. atony (AT-ō-nē) _____

15. tenodesis (ten-OD-e-sis) _____

16. dyskinesia (dis-kī-NĒ-zē-a) _____

17. myalgia (mī-AL-jē-a) _____

18. musculotendinous (mus-kū-lō-TEN-di-nus) _____

19. tendinitis (ten-di-NĪ-tis), also tendonitis (ten-don-Ī-tis) _____

20. hypermyotonia (hī-per-mī-ō-TŌ-nē-a) _____

21. kinesitherapy (ki-nē-si-THER-a-pē) _____

22. fasciorrhaphy (fash-ē-OR-a-fē) _____

23. ergogenic (er-gō-JEN-ik) _____

24. myofascial (mī-ō-FASH-ē-al) _____

25. tenomyoplasty (ten-ō-MĪ-ō-plas-tē) _____

Write words for the following definitions:

26. inflammation of many (poly-) muscles _____

27. any disease of muscle _____

28. excision of fascia _____

29. study of movement (use kinesi/o) _____

30. incision of a tendon (use ten/o) _____

31. inflammation of a muscle and its tendon (use ten/o) _____

Clinical Aspects of the Muscular System

Muscle function may be affected by disorders elsewhere, particularly in the nervous system and connective tissue. The conditions described below affect the muscular system directly or involve the muscles and have not been described in other chapters. Any disorder of muscles is described as a myopathy.

Techniques for diagnosing muscle disorders include electrical studies of muscle in action, **electromyography (EMG)**, and serum assay of enzymes released in increased amounts from damaged muscles, mainly **creatine kinase (CK)**.

Muscular Dystrophy

Muscular dystrophy refers to a group of hereditary diseases involving progressive, noninflammatory degeneration of muscles. There is weakness and wasting of muscle tissue with its gradual replacement by connective tissue and fat. There also may be cardiomyopathy (disease of cardiac muscle) and mental impairment.

The most common form is Duchenne muscular dystrophy, a sex-linked disease passed from mother to son. This appears at 3 to 4 years of age, and patients are incapacitated by age 10 to 15. Death is commonly caused by respiratory failure or infection.

Multiple System Disorders Involving Muscles

Polymyositis

Polymyositis is inflammation of skeletal muscle leading to weakness, frequently associated with dysphagia (difficulty in swallowing) or cardiac problems. The cause is unknown and may be related to viral infection or autoimmunity. Often the disorder is associated with some other systemic disease such as rheumatoid arthritis or lupus erythematosus.

When the skin is involved, the condition is termed **dermatomyositis**. In this case, there is erythema (redness of the skin), dermatitis (inflammation of the skin), and a typical lilac-colored rash, predominantly on the face. In addition to enzyme studies and EMG, muscle biopsy is used in diagnosis.

Fibromyalgia Syndrome

Fibromyalgia syndrome (FMS) is a difficult-to-diagnose condition involving the muscles. It is associated with widespread muscle aches, tenderness, and stiffness, along with fatigue and sleep disorders in the absence of neurologic abnormalities or any other known cause. The disorder may coexist with other chronic diseases, may follow a viral infection, and may involve immune system dysfunction. A current theory is that FMS results from hormonal or neurotransmitter imbalances that increase sensitivity to pain. Treatments for FMS include a carefully planned exercise program and medication with pain relievers, muscle relaxants, or antidepressants.

Chronic Fatigue Syndrome

Chronic fatigue syndrome (CFS) involves persistent fatigue of no known cause that may be associated with impaired memory, sore throat, painful lymph nodes, muscle and joint pain, headaches, sleep problems, and immune disorders. The condition often occurs after a viral infection. Epstein-Barr virus (the agent that causes mononucleosis), herpesvirus, and other viruses have been suggested as possible causes of CFS. No traditional or alternative therapies have been consistently successful in treating CFS.

Myasthenia Gravis

Myasthenia gravis is an acquired autoimmune disease in which antibodies interfere with muscle stimulation at the neuromuscular junction. There is a progressive loss of muscle power, especially in the external eye muscles and other muscles of the face.

Amyotrophic Lateral Sclerosis

Also named Lou Gehrig disease after a famous baseball player who died of the disorder, **amyotrophic lateral sclerosis (ALS)** is a progressive degeneration of motor neurons that leads to muscle atrophy (amyotrophy). Early signs are weakness, cramping, and muscle twitching. The facial or respiratory muscles may be affected early depending on the site of degeneration. Mental function, sensory perception, and bowel and bladder function usually remain intact. The disease progresses and eventually leads to death from respiratory muscle paralysis in 3 to 5 years.

Stress Injuries

Not as grave as the above diseases perhaps, but much more common, are musculoskeletal disorders caused by physical stress. These include accidental injuries and work- or sports-related damage caused by overexertion or repetitive motion, so called **repetitive strain injury (RSI)**. Damages to soft tissues include muscle **strain**, inflammation or tearing of ligaments and tendons, and bursitis. **Tenosynovitis**, commonly called **tendinitis**, is inflammation of a tendon, tendon sheath, and the synovial membrane at a joint. The signs of these injuries are pain, fatigue, weakness, stiffness, numbness, and reduced range of motion (ROM). (The origins of some colorful terms for such conditions are given in Box 20-3.)

Box 20·3 Focus on Words — *Some Colorful Musculoskeletal Terms*

Some common terms for musculoskeletal disorders have interesting origins. A charley horse describes muscular strain and soreness, especially in the legs. The term comes from common use of the name Charley for old lame horses that were kept around for family use when they could no longer be used for hard work. Wryneck, technically torticollis, uses the word *wry* meaning twisted or turned, as in the word awry (*a-RĪ*), meaning amiss or out of position.

A bunion, technically called hallux valgus, is an enlargement of the first joint of the great toe with bursitis at the joint. It probably comes from the word bony, changed to bunny, and used to mean a bump on the head and then a swelling on a joint. A clavus is commonly called a corn because it is a hardened or horny thickening of the skin in an area of friction or pressure.

Stress injuries may involve any muscles or joints, but some common upper extremity conditions are:

➤ Rotator cuff (RTC) injury—The rotator cuff, which strengthens the shoulder joint, is formed by four muscles, the supraspinatus, infraspinatus, teres minor, and subscapularis, the "SITS" muscles (Fig. 20-8). Inflammation or tearing of the rotator cuff can occur in people who repeatedly perform overhead activities, such as swimming, painting, or pitching.

➤ Epicondylitis—The medial and lateral epicondyles (projections) of the distal humerus are attachment points for muscles that flex and extend the wrist and fingers. Inflammation of these tendons of origin causes pain at the elbow and forearm on lifting, carrying, squeezing, or typing. These stress injuries are often sports-related, leading to the terms "golfer's elbow" and "tennis elbow" for medial and lateral epicondylitis, respectively. A brace worn below the elbow to distribute stress on the joint may be helpful.

➤ Carpal tunnel syndrome (CTS)—CTS involves the tendons of the flexor muscles of the fingers and the nerves that supply the hand and fingers (Fig. 20-9). Hand numbness and weakness is caused by pressure on the median nerve as it passes through a tunnel formed by the carpal (wrist) bones. CTS commonly appears in people who use their hands and fingers strenuously, such as musicians and keyboarders.

➤ Trigger finger—This is a painful snapping, triggering, or locking of a finger as it is moved. It is caused by inflammation and swelling of the flexor tendon sheath at the metacarpophalangeal joint that prevents the tendon from sliding back and forth.

Some stress injuries that involve the lower extremities are:

➤ Hamstring strain—The hamstring is a large muscle group in the posterior thigh that extends from the hip to the knee and flexes the knee (see Fig. 20-7). A "pulled hamstring" is common in athletes who stop and start running suddenly. It is treated with stretching and strengthening activities.

➤ Shin splint—This is pain in the anterior portion of the leg, in the region of the tibia, from running on hard surfaces or overuse of the foot flexors, as in athletes and dancers. Help comes from good shoes with adequate support and avoidance of hard surfaces for exercise.

➤ Achilles tendinitis—The Achilles (*a-KIL-ēz*) tendon is a large tendon that attaches the calf muscles to the heel and is used to plantar flex the foot at the ankle (see Fig. 20-7). Damage to the Achilles tendon hampers or prevents walking and running.

Treatment

Orthopedists diagnose musculoskeletal disorders by MRI and other imaging techniques, range of motion (ROM) measurements, and strength testing. Treatment of stress injuries

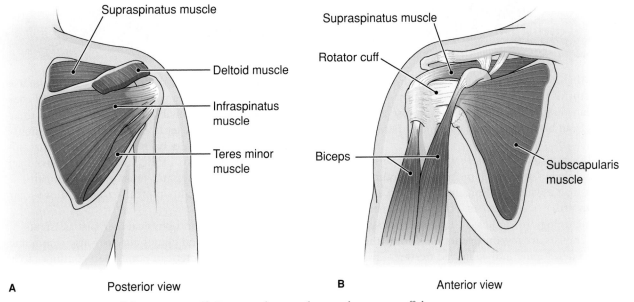

A   Posterior view   **B**   Anterior view

Figure 20-8 Anatomy of the rotator cuff. Four muscles contribute to the rotator cuff that strengthens the shoulder. (*A*) Posterior. (*B*) Anterior

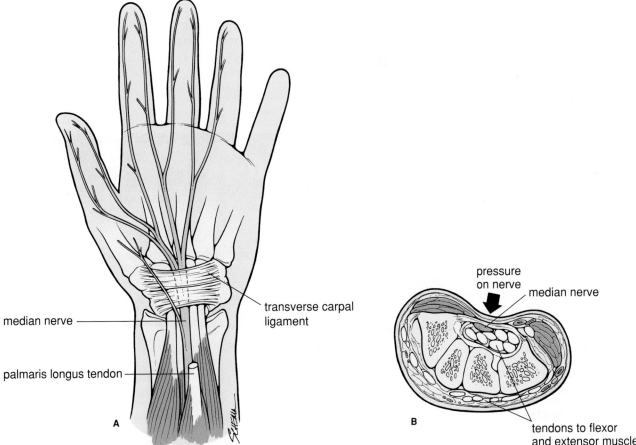

Figure 20-9 Carpal tunnel syndrome. (*A*) Pressure on the median nerve as it passes through the carpal (wrist) bones causes numbness and weakness in the areas of the hand supplied by the nerve. (*B*) Cross section of the wrist showing compression of the median nerve.

Box 20•4 Health Professions — *Careers in Physical Therapy*

Physical therapy restores mobility and relieves back pain, arthritis, and joint and muscle injuries. Individuals with heart disease and brain injury, or those who are recovering from burns or major surgery, may benefit as well.

Physical therapists work closely with physicians, nurses, occupational therapists, speech pathologists, and audiologists. Some treat a wide range of ailments, whereas others specialize in pediatrics, geriatrics, orthopedics, sports medicine, neurology, or cardiology. Regardless of specialty, physical therapists are responsible for examining their patients and developing individualized treatment programs. The examination includes a medical history and tests measuring strength, mobility, balance, coordination, and endurance. The treatment plan may include stretching and exercise to improve mobility; hot packs, cold compresses, and massage to reduce pain; as well as the use of crutches, prostheses, and wheelchairs. Physical therapy assistants are responsible for implementing a treatment plan, teaching patients exercises and equipment use, and reporting results back to the physical therapist. Most physical therapists in the United States have bachelor's or master's degrees and must pass a national licensing exam. Assistants typically train in a two-year program.

Physical therapists and physical therapist assistants practice in hospitals and clinics and may also visit homes and schools. As the American population continues to age and the need for rehabilitative therapy increases, job prospects are good. For more information about careers in physical therapy, contact the American Physical Therapy Association.

usually begins conservatively with rest, elevation, ice packs, bracing, and medications, such as analgesics, antiinflammatory agents, and muscle relaxants. (The acronym PRICE represents this simple approach—protection, rest, ice, compression, elevation.) Treatment may progress to steroid injections, ultrasound therapy for deep heat, strengthening exercises, or even surgery. Physical therapists often are involved in the various stages of treatment and rehabilitation (see Box 20-4).

TERMINOLOGY — Key Terms

DISORDERS

amyotrophic lateral sclerosis (ALS) *a-mī-ō-TROF-ik*	A disease caused by degeneration of motor neurons resulting in muscular weakness and atrophy; Lou Gehrig disease
chronic fatigue syndrome (CFS)	A disease of unknown cause that involves persistent fatigue, along with muscle and joint pain and other symptoms; may be virally induced
dermatomyositis *der-ma-tō-mī-ō-SĪ-tis*	A disease of unknown origin involving inflammation of muscles as well as dermatitis and skin rashes
fibromyalgia syndrome (FMS) *fi-brō-mī-AL-jē-a*	A disorder associated with widespread muscular aches and stiffness and having no known cause
muscular dystrophy *DIS-trō-fē*	A group of hereditary muscular disorders marked by progressive weakness and atrophy of muscles
myasthenia gravis (MG) *mī-as-THĒ-nē-a GRA-vis*	A disease characterized by progressive muscular weakness; an autoimmune disease affecting the neuromuscular junction

TERMINOLOGY Key Terms

Continued

polymyositis *pol-ē-mī-ō-SĪ-tis*	A disease of unknown cause involving muscle inflammation and weakness
repetitive strain injury	Tissue damage caused by repeated motion, usually overuse of the arm or hand in occupational activities such as writing, typing, painting, or using hand tools; also called repetitive motion injury, cumulative trauma injury, overuse syndrome.
strain *strān*	Trauma to a muscle because of overuse or excessive stretch; if severe, may involve tearing of muscle, bleeding, or separation of muscle from its tendon or separation of a tendon from bone
tendinitis *ten-di-NĪ-tis*	Inflammation of a tendon, usually caused by injury or overuse; the shoulder, elbow, and hip are common sites; also spelled tendonitis
tenosynovitis *ten-ō-sin-ō-VĪ-tis*	Inflammation of a tendon sheath

DIAGNOSIS

creatine kinase (CK) *KRĒ-a-tin KĪ-nās*	An enzyme found in muscle tissue; the serum level of CK increases in cases of muscle damage; creatine phosphokinase (CPK)
electromyography (EMG) *ē-lek-trō-mī-OG-ra-fē*	Study of the electrical activity of muscles during contraction

Go to the pronunciation glossary in Chapter 20 on the CD-ROM to hear these words pronounced.

TERMINOLOGY Supplementary Terms

NORMAL STRUCTURE AND FUNCTION

aponeurosis *ap-ō-nū-RŌ-sis*	A flat, white, sheetlike tendon that connects a muscle with the part that it moves (see abdominal aponeurosis, Fig. 20-6)
creatine *KRĒ-a-tin*	A substance in muscle cells that stores energy for contraction
glycogen *GLĪ-kō-jen*	A complex sugar that is stored for energy in muscles and in the liver

Supplementary Terms

isometric ī-sō-MET-rik	Pertaining to a muscle action in which the muscle tenses but does not shorten (literally: same measurement)
isotonic ī-sō-TON-ik	Pertaining to a muscle action in which the muscle shortens to accomplish movement (literally: same tone)
kinesthesia kin-es-THĒ-zē-a	Awareness of movement; perception of the weight, direction, and degree of movement (*-esthesia* means "sensation")
lactic acid LAK-tik	An acid that accumulates in muscle cells functioning without enough oxygen (anaerobically), as in times of great physical exertion. The lactic acid leads to muscle fatigue, after which it is gradually removed from the tissues.
motor unit	A single motor neuron and all of the muscle cells that its branches stimulate
myoglobin mī-ō-GLŌ-bin	A pigment similar to hemoglobin that stores oxygen in muscle cells
oxygen debt	The period during which muscles are functioning without enough oxygen. Lactic acid accumulates and leads to fatigue.

SYMPTOMS AND CONDITIONS

asterixis as-ter-IK-sis	Rapid, jerky movements, especially in the hands, caused by intermittent loss of muscle tone
asthenia as-THĒ-nē-a	Weakness (prefix a- meaning "without" with root *sthen/o* meaning "strength")
ataxia a-TAK-sē-a	Lack of muscle coordination (from root *tax/o* meaning "order, arrangement"; adjective: ataxic)
athetosis ath-e-TŌ-sis	A condition marked by slow, irregular, twisting movements, especially in the hands and fingers (adjective: athetotic)
atrophy AT-rō-fē	A wasting away; a decrease in the size of a tissue or organ, such as the wasting of muscle from disuse
avulsion a-VUL-shun	Forcible tearing away of a part
clonus KLŌ-nus	Alternating spasmodic contraction and relaxation in a muscle (adjective: clonic)
contracture kon-TRAK-chur	Permanent contraction of a muscle
fasciculation fa-sik-ū-LĀ-shun	Involuntary small contractions or twitching of muscle fiber groups (fasciculi)
fibromyositis fi-brō-mī-ō-SĪ-tis	A nonspecific term for pain, tenderness, and stiffness in muscles and joints
fibrositis fi-brō-SĪ-tis	Inflammation of fibrous connective tissue, especially the muscle fasciae; marked by pain and stiffness

TERMINOLOGY
Supplementary Terms

Continued

20

restless legs syndrome (RLS)	Uneasiness, twitching, or restlessness in the legs that occurs after going to bed and often leading to insomnia; may be caused by poor circulation or drug side effects
rhabdomyolysis *rab-dō-mī-OL-i-sis*	An acute disease involving diffuse destruction of skeletal muscle cells (root *rhabd/o* means "rod," referring to the long, rodlike muscle cells)
rhabdomyoma *rab-dō-mī-Ō-ma*	A benign tumor of skeletal muscle
rhabdomyosarcoma *rab-dō-mī-ō-sar-KŌ-ma*	A highly malignant tumor of skeletal muscle
rheumatism *RŪ-ma-tizm*	A general term for inflammation, soreness, and stiffness of muscles associated with pain in joints (adjective: rheumatic, rheumatoid)
spasm	A sudden, involuntary muscle contraction; may be clonic (contraction alternating with relaxation) or tonic (sustained); a strong and painful spasm may be called a cramp (adjectives, spastic, spasmodic)
spasticity *spas-TIS-i-tē*	Increased tone or contractions of muscles causing stiff and awkward movements
tetanus *TET-a-nus*	An acute infectious disease caused by the anaerobic bacillus *Clostridium tetani*. It is marked by persistent painful spasms of voluntary muscles; lockjaw.
tetany *TET-a-nē*	A condition marked by spasms, cramps, and muscle twitching caused by a metabolic imbalance, such as low blood calcium caused by underactivity of the parathyroid glands
torticollis *tor-ti-KOL-is*	Spasmodic contraction of the neck muscles causing stiffness and twisting of the neck; wryneck

DIAGNOSIS AND TREATMENT

Chvostek sign *VOS-tek*	Spasm of facial muscles after a tap over the facial nerve; evidence of tetany
occupational therapy	Health profession concerned with increasing function and preventing disability through work and play activities. The goal of occupational therapy is to increase the patient's independence and quality of daily life.
physical therapy	Health profession concerned with physical rehabilitation and prevention of disability. Exercise, massage, and other therapeutic methods are used to restore proper movement (see Box 20-4).
rheumatology *rū-ma-TOL-ō-jē*	The study and treatment of rheumatic diseases
Trousseau sign *tru-SŌ*	Spasmodic contractions caused by pressing the nerve supplying a muscle; seen in tetany

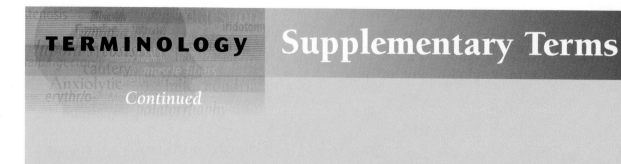

TERMINOLOGY Supplementary Terms

Continued

DRUGS

antiinflammatory agent	Drug that reduces inflammation; includes steroids, such as cortisone, and nonsteroidal antiinflammatory drugs
COX-2 inhibitor	Nonsteroidal antiinflammatory drug that does not cause the stomach problems associated with other NSAIDs. Inhibits the cyclooxygenase (COX)-2 enzyme without affecting the COX-1 enzyme, a lack of which can cause stomach ulcers. These drugs are under study, and some have been withdrawn from the market because of cardiac risk. Example is celecoxib (Celebrex).
muscle relaxant *rē-LAX-ant*	A drug that reduces muscle tension; different forms may be used to relax muscles during surgery, to control spasticity, or to relieve pain of musculoskeletal disorders
nonsteroidal antiinflammatory drug (NSAID)	Drug that reduces inflammation but is not a steroid; examples include aspirin, ibuprofen, naproxen, and other inhibitors of prostaglandins, naturally produced substances that promote inflammation

Go to the pronunciation glossary in Chapter 20 on the CD-ROM to hear these words pronounced.

TERMINOLOGY Abbreviations

ACh	Acetylcholine	**OT**	Occupational therapy/therapist
ALS	Amyotrophic lateral sclerosis	**PRICE**	Protection, rest, ice, compression, elevation
CFS	Chronic fatigue syndrome	**PT**	Physical therapy/therapist
C(P)K	Creatine (phospho)kinase	**RLS**	Restless legs syndrome
CTS	Carpal tunnel syndrome	**ROM**	Range of motion
EMG	Electromyography, electromyogram	**RSI**	Repetitive strain injury
FMS	Fibromyalgia syndrome	**RTC**	Rotator cuff
MG	Myasthenia gravis	**SITS**	Supraspinatus, infraspinatus, teres minor, subscapularis (muscles)
MMT	Manual muscle test(ing)		
NMJ	Neuromuscular junction		

CHAPTER REVIEW

LABELING EXERCISE
Superficial Muscles, Anterior View

Write the name of each numbered part on the corresponding line of the answer sheet.

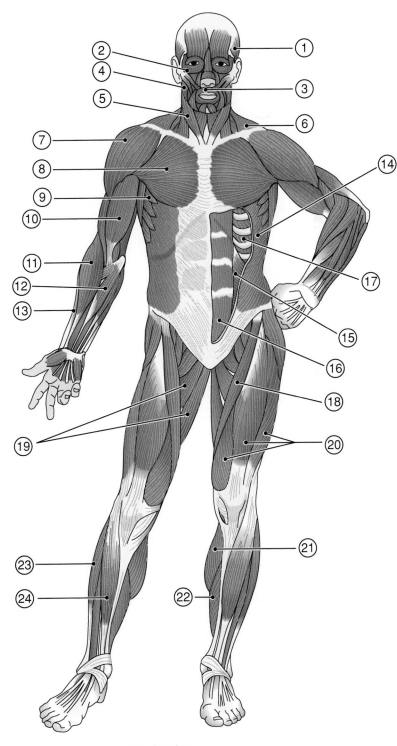

Anterior view

(continued on next page)

20

adductors of thigh

1. _____

biceps brachii

2. _____

brachioradialis

3. _____

deltoid

4. _____

extensor carpi

5. _____

external oblique

6. _____

flexor carpi

7. _____

gastrocnemius

8. _____

intercostals

9. _____

internal oblique

10. _____

masseter

11. _____

orbicularis oculi

12. _____

orbicularis oris

13. _____

pectoralis major

14. _____

peroneus longus

15. _____

quadriceps femoris

16. _____

rectus abdominis

17. _____

sartorius

18. _____

serratus anterior

19. _____

soleus

20. _____

sternocleidomastoid

21. _____

temporalis

22. _____

tibialis anterior

23. _____

trapezius

24. _____

Superficial Muscles, Posterior View

Write the name of each numbered part on the corresponding line of the answer sheet.

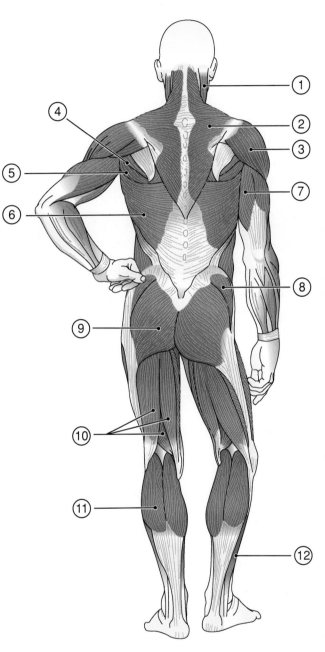

Posterior view

deltoid

gastrocnemius

gluteus maximus

gluteus medius

hamstring group

1. _____

2. _____

3. _____

4. _____

5. _____

(continued on next page)

20

latissimus dorsi	6. _____
peroneus longus	7. _____
sternocleidomastoid	8. _____
teres major	9. _____
teres minor	10. _____
trapezius	11. _____
triceps brachii	12. _____

TERMINOLOGY

Match the following terms and write the appropriate letter to the left of each number:

_____	1. pectoralis major	**a.** main muscle of the calf
_____	2. deltoid	**b.** triangular muscle that covers the shoulder
_____	3. latissimus dorsi	**c.** main muscle of the buttocks
_____	4. gastrocnemius	**d.** large muscle of the upper chest
_____	5. gluteus maximus	**e.** large muscle across the back below the trapezius

_____	6. dystrophy	**a.** instrument for measuring muscle work
_____	7. ergograph	**b.** slowness of movement
_____	8. inotropic	**c.** wasting of tissue
_____	9. bradykinesia	**d.** acting on muscle fibers
_____	10. dystonia	**e.** abnormal muscle tone

Supplementary Terms

_____	11. glycogen	**a.** substance that stores energy in muscle cells
_____	12. tetany	**b.** a type of muscle contraction
_____	13. isometric	**c.** muscular spasms and cramps
_____	14. creatine	**d.** complex sugar stored in muscles
_____	15. lactic acid	**e.** substance that accumulates in muscles working anaerobically

_____	16. aponeurosis	**a.** intermittent muscle contractions
_____	17. ataxia	**b.** lack of muscle coordination
_____	18. rhabdomyolysis	**c.** awareness of movement
_____	19. clonus	**d.** flat, white, sheetlike tendon
_____	20. kinesthesia	**e.** disease involving destruction of muscle cells

_____ 21. torticollis   **a.** forcible tearing away of a part

_____ 22. athetosis   **b.** acute infectious disease that affects muscles

_____ 23. spasm   **c.** wryneck

_____ 24. tetanus   **d.** sudden involuntary muscle contraction

_____ 25. avulsion   **e.** condition marked by slow, twisting movements

Fill in the blanks:

26. The neurotransmitter released at the neuromuscular junction is _____.

27. The sheath of connective tissue that covers a muscle is called _____.

28. The number of origins (heads) in the biceps brachii muscle is _____.

29. A muscle that produces flexion at a joint is called a(n) _____.

30. A band of connective tissue that attaches a muscle to a bone is a(n) _____.

31. The strong, cordlike tendon that attaches the calf muscle to the heel is the _____.

32. Movement away from the midline of the body is termed _____.

Eliminations. In each of the sets below, underline the word that does not fit in with the rest and explain the reason for your choice:

33. fascicle – fiber – tendon – osteoblast – fascia

_____

34. soleus – flexor carpi – biceps brachii – brachioradialis – extensor carpi

_____

35. vastus intermedius – intercostals – vastus lateralis – vastus medialis – rectus femoris

_____

36. circumduction – inversion – actin – dorsiflexion – rotation

_____

37. EMG – ALS – FMS – CFS – MG

_____

True-False. Examine the following statements. If the statement is true, write T in the first blank. If the statement is false, write F in the first blank and correct the statement by replacing the underlined word in the second blank.

38. The <u>origin</u> of a muscle is attached to a moving part.   _____   _____

39. The hamstring group is in the <u>anterior</u> thigh.   _____   _____

40. <u>Pronation</u> means turning downward.   _____   _____

41. Smooth muscle is also called <u>visceral muscle</u>.   _____   _____

42. The quadriceps muscle has <u>three</u> components.   _____   _____

43. The part of a neuron that contacts a muscle cell is the <u>axon</u>.   _____   _____

Define the following words:

44. myalgia (*mī-AL-jē-a*) _____

45. myofascial (*mī-ō-FASH-ē-al*) _____

46. tenoplasty (*ten-ō-PLAS-tē*) _____

47. inositis (*in-ō-SĪ-tis*) _____

48. hypotonia (*hī-pō-TŌ-nē-a*) _____

49. hyperkinesia (*hī-per-ki-NĒ-sē-a*) _____

Word building. Write words for the following definitions:

50. study of muscles (use my/o-)   _____

51. death of muscle tissue   _____

52. incision of fascia   _____

53. absence of muscle tone   _____

54. inflammation of fascia   _____

55. study of movement   _____

56. suture of a tendon (use ten/o-)   _____

57. pertaining to a tendon   _____

Opposites. Write a word that means the opposite of the following terms as they pertain to muscles:

58. prime mover   _____

59. origin   _____

60. abduction   _____

61. pronation   _____

62. extension   _____

Adjective. From the supplementary terms, write the adjective form of the following words:

63. ataxia   _____

64. athetosis   _____

65. spasm   _____

66. clonus   _____

Abbreviations. Write the meaning of each of the following:

67. EMG _____

68. ACh _____

69. OT _____

70. NMJ _____

71. CK _____

Word analysis. Define each of the following words, and give the meaning of the word parts in each. Use a dictionary if necessary.

72. dyssynergia (*dis-in-ER-jē-a*) _____

    a. dys- _____

    b. syn- _____

    c. erg/o _____

    d. -ia _____

20

73. amyotrophic (*a-mī-ō-TRŌ-fik*) _____

    a. a- _____

    b. my/o _____

    c. troph/o _____

    d. -ic _____

74. myasthenia (*mī-as-THĒ-nē-a*) _____

    a. my/o _____

    b. a- _____

    c. sthen/o _____

    d. -ia _____

20

Go to the word exercises in Chapter 20 of the CD-ROM for additional review exercises.

CASE STUDY 20-1: Rotator Cuff Tear

M.L., a 56-year-old business executive and former college football player, was referred to an orthopedic surgeon for recurrent shoulder pain. M.L. was unable to abduct his right arm without pain even after six months of physical therapy and NSAIDs. In addition, he had taken supplements of glucosamine, chondroitin, and S-adenosylmethionine for several months in an effort to protect the flexibility of his shoulder joint. M.L. recalled a shoulder dislocation resulting from a football injury 35 years earlier. An MRI scan confirmed a complete rotator cuff tear. The surgeon recommended the Bankart procedure for M.L.'s injury to restore his joint stability, alleviate his pain, and permit him to return to his former normal activities, including golf.

After anesthesia induction and positioning in a semi-sitting (beach chair) position, the surgeon made an antero-superior deltoid incision (the standard deltopectoral approach) and divided the coracoacromial ligament at the acromial attachment. The rotator cuff was identified after the deltoid was retracted and the clavipectoral fascia was incised. The subscapularis tendon was incised proximal to its insertion. After incision of the capsule, inspection showed a large pouch inferiorly in the capsule, consistent with laxity (instability). The torn edges of the capsule were anchored to the rim of the glenoid fossa with heavy non-absorbable sutures. A flap from the subscapularis tendon was transposed and sutured to the supraspinatus and infraspinatus muscles to bridge the gap. An intraoperative ROM examination showed that the external rotation could be performed past neutral and that the shoulder did not dislocate. The wound was closed, and a shoulder immobilizer sling was applied. M.L. was referred to PT to begin therapy in three weeks and was assured he would be able to play golf in six months.

CASE STUDY 20-2: Brachial Plexus Injury

T.D., a 16-year-old high school student, had a severe football accident three months before his admission. He sustained a right brachial plexus injury, resulting in a flail arm. He had no recovery and was on medication for neurologic pain. He reported that he had no feeling or motion in his right shoulder or arm. He had atrophy over the supraspinatus and infraspinatus muscles and also subluxation of his shoulder and deltoid atrophy. He had no active motion of the right upper extremity and no sensation. The rest of his orthopedic exam showed full ROM of his hips, knees, and ankles with intact sensation and palpable distal pulses as well as normal motor function. He was diagnosed with a possible middle trunk brachial plexus injury from C7. He was scheduled for an EMG, nerve-conduction studies, and somatosensory evoked potentials (SSEPs). His diaphragm was examined under fluoroscopy to R/O phrenic nerve injury.

With middle trunk brachial plexus injury, damage to the subscapular nerve will interrupt conduction to the subscapularis and teres major muscles. Damage to the long thoracic nerve prevents conduction to the serratus anterior muscles. Injury to the pectoral nerves affects the pectoralis major and minor muscles.

T.D. was scheduled for a brachial plexus exploration with possible nerve graft, nerve transfer, bilateral sural (calf) nerve harvest, or gracilis muscle graft from his right thigh.

CASE STUDY 20-3: "Wake Up" Test during Spinal Fusion Surgery

L.N.'s somatosensory evoked potentials (SSEPs) were monitored throughout her spinal fusion surgery to provide continuous information on the functional state of her sensory pathways from the median and posterior tibial nerves through the dorsal column to the primary somatosensory cortex. Before surgery, needle electrodes were inserted into L.N.'s right and left quadriceps muscles to determine nerve conduction through L2 to L4, into the anterior tibialis muscles to measure passage through L5, and into the gastrocnemius muscles to measure S1 to S2. Electrodes were placed in her rectus abdominis to monitor S1 to S2. All electrodes were taped in place, and the wires were plugged into a transformer box with feedback to a computer. A neuromonitoring technologist placed the electrodes and attended the computer monitor throughout the case. During the procedure, selected muscle groups were stimulated with 15 to 40 milliamps (mA) of current to test the nerves and muscles. Data fed back into the computer confirmed the neuromuscular integrity and status of the spinal fixation, the instrumentation, and implants.

After the pedicle screws, hooks, and wires were in place and the spinal rods were cinched down to straighten the spine, L.N. was permitted to emerge temporarily from anesthesia and muscle paralysis medication to a lightly sedated but pain-free state. She was given commands to move her feet, straighten her legs, and wiggle her toes to test all neuromuscular groups that could be affected by misplaced or compressed spinal fixation devices. Her feet were watched, and movement was announced to the team.

Dorsiflexion cleared the tibialis anterior muscles; plantar flexion cleared the gastrocnemius muscles. Knee flexion cleared the hamstring muscle group, and knee extension determined function of the quadriceps group. L.N. had a successful "wake-up" test. She was put back into deep anesthesia, and her incision was closed. A postoperative "wake-up" test was repeated after she was moved to her bed. The surgical instruments and tables were kept sterile until after all of the monitored muscle groups were tested and showed voluntary movement. The electrodes were removed, and she was taken to PACU for recovery.

CASE STUDY QUESTIONS

Multiple choice: Select the best answer and write the letter of your choice to the left of each number.

_____ 1. The insertion of the muscle is:
   a. the thick middle portion
   b. the point of attachment to the moving bone
   c. the point of attachment to the stable bone
   d. the fibrous sheath
   e. the connective tissue

_____ 2. M.L. was unable to abduct his affected arm. This motion is:
   a. toward the midline
   b. circumferential
   c. in the same direction as the muscle fibers
   d. away from the midline
   e. a position with the palm facing upward

_____ 3. An anterosuperior deltoid incision would be made:
   a. perpendicular to the muscle fibers
   b. below the fascia sheath
   c. behind the glenoid fossa
   d. in the best area
   e. at the top and to the front of the deltoid muscle

_____ 4. The subscapularis tendon arises from the subscapularis:
   a. fascia
   b. nerve
   c. bone
   d. extensor
   e. flexor

_____ 5. The intraoperative ROM examination was performed:
   a. in the OR corridor
   b. during surgery
   c. before surgery
   d. after surgery
   e. in the interventional radiology suite

20

_____ 6. M.L.'s arm and shoulder were immobilized after surgery to:
   a. encourage movement beyond the point of pain
   b. minimize rapid ROM
   c. maintain adduction and external rotation
   d. prevent movement
   e. stop bleeding

_____ 7. T.D. had atrophy of the supraspinatus and infraspinatus muscles. The term *atrophy* here refers to:
   a. hypercontraction
   b. intermittent contraction and relaxation
   c. muscle tissue wasting
   d. paralysis
   e. painful discoloration

_____ 8. Another term for subluxation is:
   a. dislocation
   b. hyperextension
   c. turning inside out
   d. overlapping
   e. stretched beyond original shape

_____ 9. A palpable distal pulse means that the pulse can be:
   a. heard at the foot
   b. felt at the top of the thigh
   c. felt at the foot
   d. obliterated with light
   e. undetectable

_____ 10. The pectoralis major and pectoralis minor muscles are located:
   a. below the knees
   b. behind the thighs
   c. in the lower back
   d. in the upper chest
   e. on the lateral side of the arms

_____ 11. The quadriceps muscle group is made up of:
   a. smooth and cardiac muscle fibers
   b. four muscles in the thigh
   c. three muscles in the leg and one in the anterior chest
   d. fascia and tendon sheaths
   e. tendons and fascia around the shoulder

_____ 12. The nerve supply for the rectus abdominis muscle runs through S1–S2. This anatomic region is:
   a. the first and second sural sheath
   b. subluxation and suppuration
   c. sacral disk space 1 and 2
   d. sacral disk space 3
   e. somatosensory electrodes 1 and 2

____ 13. The movement of elevating the toes toward the anterior ankle is:
   a. supination
   b. pronation
   c. dorsiflexion
   d. plantar flexion
   e. external rotation

____ 14. Knee extension results in:
   a. a bent knee
   b. a ballet position with the toes turned out
   c. bilateral abduction
   d. inversion
   e. a straight leg

Write terms from the case studies with the following meanings:

15. pertaining to the arm _____

16. pertaining to treatment of skeletal and muscular disorders _____

17. bending at a joint _____

18. to point the toes downward _____

Define the following abbreviations:

19. PT _____

20. ROM_____

21. R/O _____

22. EMG _____

23. SSEP_____

24. PACU _____

Muscular System

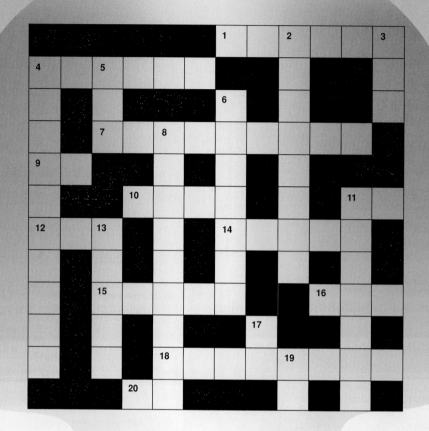

ACROSS

1. Around: prefix
4. Rod, such as a muscle cell: combining form
7. Muscle group at the back of the thigh
9. Not: prefix
10. Muscle tone: combining form
11. Down, without, removal: prefix
12. Disease caused by degeneration of motor neurons, with weakness, atrophy, and spasticity: abbreviation
14. Muscle that carries out a given movement, _ _ _ _ _ mover
15. Lack of muscle tone
16. Referring to a joint in the foot: abbreviation
18. Adjective for a type of muscle contraction
20. Fiber: root

DOWN

2. Muscle of the forearm, brachio _ _ _ _ _ _ _ _
3. Muscle: combining form
4. Like or resembling a systemic form of arthritis
5. Neurotransmitter active in the muscular system: abbreviation
6. Wasting of tissue
8. Substance that stores oxygen in muscles
11. Muscle that covers the shoulder
13. Sudden involuntary muscle contraction
17. Health profession concerned with physical rehabilitation and prevention of disability: abbreviation
19. Health profession concerned with working to increase function and independence in daily life: abbreviation

THE SKIN

21

OBJECTIVES

After study of this chapter you should be able to:

1. Compare the epidermis, dermis, and subcutaneous tissue.
2. Describe the roles of keratin and melanin in the skin.
3. Name and describe the glands in the skin.
4. Describe the structure of hair and of nails.

5. Identify and use roots pertaining to the skin.
6. Describe the main disorders that affect the skin.
7. Label a diagram of the skin.
8. Analyze several case studies involving the skin.

PRETEST

1. The uppermost portion of the skin is called the

   _____.

2. A hair grows within a sheath called the

   _____.

3. The skin glands that secrete an oily substance

   that lubricates the skin are the _____.

4. The rule of nines is a system used to evaluate

   _____.

5. A pigmented tumor of the skin is a(n)

   _____.

6. The root hidr/o pertains to _____.

7. Onychomycosis is a fungal infection of a(n)

   _____.

L ike the eyes, the **skin** is a readily visible reflection of one's health. Its color, texture, and resilience reveal much, as does the condition of the **hair** and **nails**. The skin and its associated structures make up the **integumentary system**. This body-covering system protects against infection, dehydration, ultraviolet radiation, and injury. Extensive damage to the skin, such as by burns, can result in a host of dangerous complications.

The skin helps to regulate temperature by evaporation of sweat and by changes in the diameter of surface blood vessels, which control how much heat is lost to the environment. The skin also contains receptors for the sensory perceptions of touch, temperature, pressure, and pain. Medication can be delivered through the skin from patches, as explained in Box 21-1.

The word **derma** (from Greek) means skin and is used as an ending in words pertaining to the skin, such as xeroderma (dryness of the skin) and scleroderma (hardening of the skin). The adjective **cutaneous** refers to the skin and is from the Latin word *cutis* for skin.

Anatomy of the Skin

The outermost portion of the skin is the **epidermis**, consisting of four to five layers (strata) of epithelial cells (Fig. 21-1). The deepest layer, the stratum basale, or basal layer, produces new cells. As these cells gradually rise toward the surface, they die and become filled with **keratin**, a protein that thickens and toughens the skin. The outermost layer of the epidermis, the stratum corneum or horny layer, is composed of flat, dead, protective cells that are constantly being shed and replaced. Some of the cells in the epidermis produce **melanin**, a pigment that gives the skin color and protects against sunlight.

The **dermis** is beneath the epidermis. It is composed of connective tissue, nerves, blood vessels, and lymphatics. This layer supplies nourishment and support for the skin. The **subcutaneous tissue** beneath the dermis is composed mainly of connective tissue and fat.

Box 21•1 Clinical Perspectives *Medication Patches: No Bitter Pill to Swallow*

F or most people, pills are a convenient way to take medication, but for some, they have drawbacks. Pills must be taken at regular intervals to ensure consistent dosing, and they must be digested and absorbed into the bloodstream before they can begin to work. For those who have difficulty swallowing or digesting pills, transdermal (TD) patches offer an effective alternative to oral medications.

TD patches deliver a consistent dose of medication that diffuses at a constant rate through the skin into the bloodstream. There is no daily schedule to follow, nothing to swallow, and no stomach upset. TD patches can also deliver medication to unconscious patients, who would otherwise require intravenous drug delivery. TD patches are used in hormone-replacement therapy, to treat heart disease, to manage pain, and to suppress motion sickness. Nicotine patches are also used as part of programs to quit smoking.

TD patches must be used carefully. Drug diffusion through the skin takes time, so it is important to know how long the patch must be in place before it is effective. It is also important to know when the medication's effects

disappear after the patch is removed. Because the body continues to absorb what has already diffused into the skin, removing the patch does not entirely remove the medicine. There is also a danger that patches may become unsafe when heated, as by exercise, high fever, or a hot environment, such as a hot tub, heating pad, or sauna. When heat dilates the capillaries in the skin, a dangerous increase in dosage may result as more medication enters the blood.

A recent advance in TD drug delivery is *iontophoresis*. Based on the principle that like charges repel each other, this method uses a mild electrical current to move ionic drugs through the skin. A small electrical device attached to the patch uses positive current to "push" positively charged drug molecules through the skin, and a negative current to push negatively charged ones. Even though very low levels of electricity are used, people with pacemakers should not use iontophoretic patches. Another disadvantage of these patches is that they can move only ionic drugs through the skin.

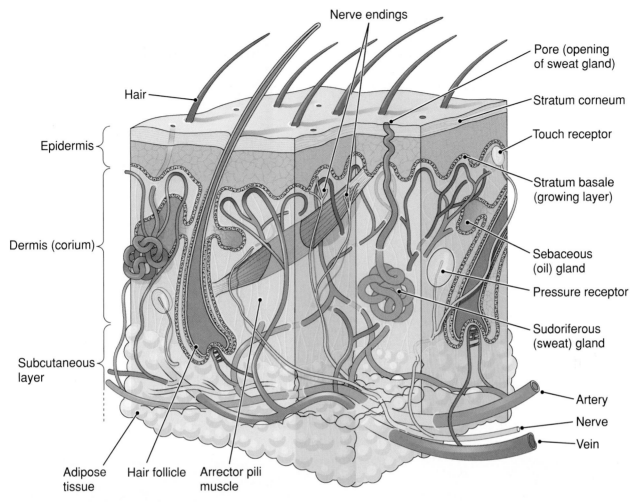

Figure 21-1 Cross-section of the skin. The skin layers and associated structures are shown.

Associated Skin Structures

Specialized structures within the skin are part of the integumentary system:

> ➤ The **sudoriferous (sweat) glands** act mainly in temperature regulation by releasing a watery fluid that evaporates to cool the body.
> ➤ The **sebaceous glands** release an oily fluid, **sebum**, that lubricates the hair and skin and prevents drying.
> ➤ Hair is widely distributed over the body. Each hair develops within a sheath or **hair follicle** and grows from its base within the skin's deep layers. A small muscle (arrector pili) attached to the follicle raises the hair to produce "goosebumps" when one is frightened or cold. In animals this is a warning sign and a means of insulating the body.
> ➤ Nails develop from a growing region at the proximal end (Fig. 21-2). The cuticle, technically named the eponychium (*ep-ō-NIK-ē-um),* is an extension of the epidermis onto the surface of the nail plate. A lighter region distal to the cuticle is called the lunula because it looks like a half moon. Here the underlying skin is thicker and blood doesn't show as much through the nail.

Hair and nails are composed of nonliving material consisting mainly of keratin. Both function in protection.

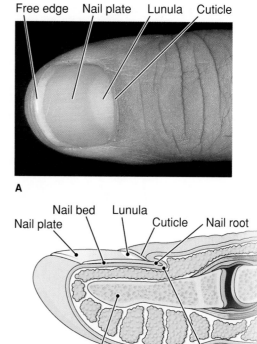

Figure 21-2 **Nail structure.** (*A*) Photograph of a nail, superior view. (*B*) Midsagittal section of a fingertip showing the growth region and tissue surrounding the nail plate.

TERMINOLOGY Key Terms

NORMAL STRUCTURE AND FUNCTION

cutaneous *kū-TĀ-nē-us*	Pertaining to the skin (from Latin *cutis*, meaning "skin")
derma	Skin (from Greek)
dermis *DER-mis*	The layer of the skin between the epidermis and the subcutaneous tissue; the true skin or corium
epidermis *ep-i-DER-mis*	The outermost layer of the skin (from *epi-*, meaning "upon or over" and *derm*, meaning "skin")
hair	A threadlike keratinized outgrowth from the skin (root: *trich/o*)
hair follicle *FOL-i-kel*	The sheath in which a hair develops
integumentary system *in-teg-ū-MEN-ta-rē*	The skin and its associated glands, hair, and nails
keratin *KER-a-tin*	A protein that thickens and toughens the skin and makes up hair and nails (root: *kerat/o*)
melanin *MEL-a-nin*	A dark pigment that gives color to the hair and skin and protects the skin against the sun's radiation (root *melan/o*)

TERMINOLOGY Key Terms

Continued

nail	A platelike keratinized outgrowth of the skin that covers the dorsal surface of the terminal phalanges (root: *onych/o*)
sebaceous gland *se-BĀ-shus*	A gland that produces sebum; usually associated with a hair follicle (root: *seb/o*)
sebum *SĒ-bum*	A fatty secretion of the sebaceous glands that lubricates the hair and skin (root: *seb/o*)
skin	The tissue that covers the body; the integument (root: *derm/o, dermat/o*)
subcutaneous tissue *sub-kū-TĀ-nē-us*	The layer of tissue beneath the skin; also called the hypodermis
sudoriferous gland *sū-dor-IF-er-us*	A sweat gland (root: *hidr/o*)

Go to the pronunciation glossary in Chapter 21 of the CD-ROM to hear these words pronounced.

Roots Pertaining to the Skin

Table 21·1 Roots Pertaining to the Skin

ROOT	MEANING	EXAMPLE	DEFINITION OF EXAMPLE
derm/o, dermat/o	skin	dermabrasion *derm-a-BRĀ-zhun*	surgical procedure used to resurface the skin and remove imperfections
kerat/o	keratin, horny layer of the skin	keratolysis *ker-a-TOL-i-sis*	loosening or separation of the horny layer of the skin
melan/o	dark, black, melanin	melanocyte *MEL-a-nō-sīt*	a cell that produces melanin
hidr/o	sweat, perspiration	anhidrosis *an-hī-DRŌ-sis*	absence of sweating
seb/o	sebum, sebaceous gland	seborrhea *seb-or-Ē-a*	excess flow of sebum
trich/o	hair	trichomycosis *trik-ō-mī-KŌ-sis*	fungal infection of the hair
onych/o	nail	onychia *ō-NIK-ē-a*	inflammation of the nail and nail bed (not an *-itis* ending)

Exercise 21-1

Identify and define the roots in the following words:

	Root	Meaning of Root
1. hypodermis (*hī-pō-DER-mis*)	_____	_____
2. hypermelanosis (*hī-per-mel-a-NŌ-sis*)	_____	_____
3. seborrheic (*seb-ō-RĒ-ik*)	_____	_____
4. keratosis (*ker-a-TŌ-sis*)	_____	_____
5. hypohidrosis (*hī-pō-hī-DRŌ-sis*)	_____	_____
6. eponychium (*ep-ō-NIK-ē-um*)	_____	_____
7. hypertrichosis (*hī-per-tri-KŌ-sis*)	_____	_____

Fill in the blanks:

8. Dermatopathology (*der-ma-tō-pa-THOL-ō-jē*) refers to any disease of the _____.

9. Dyskeratosis (*dis-ker-a-TŌ-sis*) is an abnormality in the skin's formation of _____.

10. A melanosome (*MEL-a-nō-sōm*) is a small cellular body in the cell that produces _____.

11. Hidradenitis (*hī-drad-e-NĪ-tis*) is inflammation of a gland that produces _____.

12. Onychomycosis (*on-i-kō-mī-KŌ-sis*) is a fungal infection of a(n) _____.

13. Trichoid (*TRIK-oyd*) means resembling a(n) _____.

14. A hypodermic (*hī-pō-DER-mik*) injection is given under the _____.

Word building. Write words for the following definitions:

15. instrument for cutting the skin _____

16. formation (-genesis) of keratin _____

17. a tumor containing melanin _____

18. loosening or separation of the skin _____

19. study of the hair _____

20. excess production of sweat _____

21. softening of a nail _____

22. study of the skin and skin diseases _____

Use -derma as a suffix meaning skin to write words with the following meanings:

23. hardening of the skin _____

24. presence of pus in the skin _____

Clinical Aspects of the Skin

Many diseases are manifested by changes in the quality of the skin or by specific lesions. Some types of skin lesions are described and illustrated in Box 21-2 and appear later in photographs of specific skin disorders. The study of the skin and skin diseases is **dermatology**, but careful observation of the skin, hair, and nails should be part of every physical examination. The skin should be examined for color, unusual pigmentation,

Box 21•2 For Your Reference — *Types of Skin Lesions*

Lesion	Description
bulla *BUL-a*	raised, fluid-filled lesion larger than a vesicle (plural: bullae)
fissure *FISH-ūr*	crack or break in the skin
macule *MAK-ū-l*	flat, colored spot
nodule *NOD-ūl*	solid, raised lesion larger than a papule; often indicative of systemic disease
papule *PAP-ūl*	small, circular, raised lesion at the surface of the skin
plaque *plak*	superficial, flat, or slightly raised differentiated patch more than 1 cm in diameter
pustule *PUS-tūl*	raised lesion containing pus; often in a hair follicle or sweat pore
ulcer *UL-ser*	lesion resulting from destruction of the skin and perhaps subcutaneous tissue
vesicle *VES-i-kal*	small, fluid-filled, raised lesion; a blister or bleb
wheal *wēl*	smooth, rounded, slightly raised area often associated with itching; seen in urticaria (hives), such as that resulting from allergy

Bulla Fissure

Macule Nodule

Papule Plaque

Pustule Ulcer

Vesicle Wheal

21

and lesions. It should be palpated to evaluate its texture, temperature, moisture, firmness, and any tenderness.

Wounds

Wounds are caused by trauma, as in cases of accidents or attacks, or by surgery and other therapeutic or diagnostic procedures. Wounds may affect not only the injured area but also other body systems. Infection and hemorrhage may complicate wounds, as do **dehiscence**, disruption of the wound layers, and **evisceration**, protrusion of internal organs through the lesion.

21

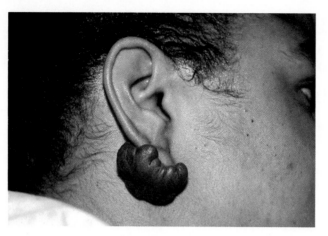

Figure 21-3 Keloid. Marked overgrowth of scar tissue following earlobe piercing.

As a wound heals, fluid and cells drain from the damaged tissue. This drainage, called **exudate**, may be clear, bloody (sanguinous), or pus-containing (purulent). Tubes may be used to remove exudate from the site of a wound.

Proper wound healing depends on cleanliness and care of the lesion and also on proper circulation, good general health, and good nutrition. The edges of a deep wound should be joined by sutures, either stitches, or for simple cuts in areas that can be kept dry and immobilized, with a tissue adhesive (glue). Healing is accompanied by scar formation or **cicatrization** (an alternative name for a scar is a cicatrix). Permanent scarring is lessened by appropriate wound care, but some people, especially those of African or Asian descent, may tend to form **keloids** because of excess collagen formation during healing (Fig. 21-3). Plastic surgery often can improve keloids and other unsightly scars.

Various types of dressings are used to protect wounded areas and promote healing. Vacuum-assisted closure (VAC) uses negative pressure to close the tissues and begin the healing process. Healing may be promoted by **débridement**, the removal of dead or damaged tissue from a wound (Box 21-3 mentions the origin of the word débridement and gives the meaning of other medical terms taken from French). Débridement may be accomplished by cutting or scrubbing away the dead tissue or by means of enzymes. A thick, dark crust or scab (eschar) may be removed in an **escharotomy**.

Deep wounds may require skin grafting for proper healing. Grafts may be a full-thickness skin graft (FTSG), which consists of the epidermis and dermis, or a split-

---

Box 21•3 Focus on Words   *The French Connection*

Many scientific and medical terms are adapted from foreign languages. Most of the roots come from Latin and Greek; others are derived from German or French. Sometimes a foreign word is used "as is." Débridement, removal of dead or damaged tissue from a wound, comes from the French, meaning removal of a restraint, such as the bridle of a harness. Also from French, a contrecoup injury occurs when the head is thrown forward and back, as in a car accident, and the brain is injured by hitting the skull on the side opposite the blow. Contrecoup in French means "counterblow." Tic douloureux, a disorder causing pain along the path of the trigeminal nerve in the face, translates literally as "painful spasm." A sound heard while listening to the body with a stethoscope is a bruit, a word in French that literally means "noise." Lavage, which refers to irrigation of a cavity, is a French word meaning "washing."

thickness skin graft (STSG), consisting of the epidermis only. Skin is cut for grafting with a **dermatome**.

Burns

Most burns are caused by hot objects, explosions, or scalding. They may also be caused by electricity, contact with harmful chemicals, or abrasion. Burns are assessed in terms of the depth of damage and the percentage of body-surface area (BSA) involved. Depth of tissue destruction is categorized as follows:

1. Superficial partial-thickness involves the epidermis and perhaps a portion of the dermis. The tissue is reddened and may blister, as in cases of sunburn.
2. Deep partial-thickness involves the epidermis and portions of the dermis. The tissue is blistered and broken and has a weeping surface. Causes include scalding and flash flame.
3. Full-thickness involves the full skin and sometimes subcutaneous tissue and underlying tissues as well. The tissue is broken and is dry and pale or charred. These injuries may result in loss of digits or limbs and require skin grafting.

The above classification replaces an older system of ranking burns as first-, second-, and third-degree according to the depth of tissue damage.

The amount of BSA involved in a burn may be estimated by using the **rule of nines**, in which areas of body surface are assigned percentages in multiples of nine (Fig. 21-4). The more accurate Lund and Browder method divides the body into small areas and estimates the proportion of BSA contributed by each.

Infection is a common complication of burns because a major defense against invasion of microorganisms is damaged. Respiratory complications and shock may also occur.

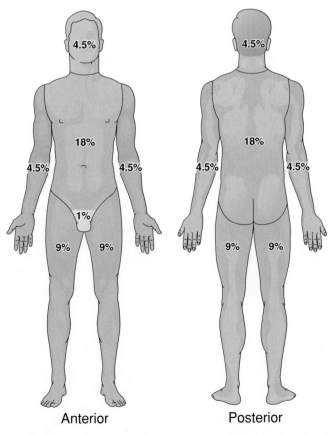

Anterior   Posterior

Figure 21-4 The rule of nines. Percentage of body-surface area (BSA) in the adult is estimated by sectioning the body surface into areas with numerical values related to nine. This method is used to evaluate the extent of skin burns.

Treatment of burns includes respiratory care, administration of fluids, wound care, and pain control. Monitoring for cardiovascular complications, infections, and signs of posttraumatic stress are also important.

Pressure Ulcers

Pressure ulcers are necrotic skin lesions that appear where the body rests on skin that covers bony projections, such as the sacrum, heel, elbow, ischial bone of the pelvis, or greater trochanter of the femur (see *ulcer*, Box 21-2). The pressure interrupts circulation, leading to thrombosis, ulceration, and death of tissue. Poor general health, malnutrition, age, obesity, and infection contribute to the development of pressure ulcers.

Pressure ulcer lesions first appear as redness of the skin. If ignored, they may penetrate the skin and underlying muscle, extending even to bone, and may require months to heal.

Pads or mattresses to relieve pressure, regular cleansing and drying of the skin, frequent change in position, and good nutrition help to prevent pressure ulcers. Other terms for pressure ulcers are *decubitus ulcer* and *bedsore*. Both of these terms refer to lying down in bed, although pressure ulcers may appear in anyone with limited movement, not only those who are confined to bed.

Dermatitis

Dermatitis is a general term for inflammation of the skin, which may be acute or chronic. Mild forms show **erythema** (redness) and edema, and sometimes **pruritus** (itching), but the condition may worsen to include deeper lesions and secondary bacterial infections. A chronic allergic form of this disorder that appears early in childhood is called **eczema** or **atopic dermatitis** (Fig. 21-5). Although its exact cause is unknown, atopic dermatitis is made worse by allergies, infection, temperature extremes, and skin irritants.

Other forms of dermatitis include contact dermatitis, caused by allergens or chemical irritants (see Fig. 21-5B); seborrheic dermatitis, which involves areas with large numbers of sebaceous glands such as the scalp and face; and stasis dermatitis, caused by poor circulation.

Psoriasis

Psoriasis is a chronic overgrowth (hyperplasia) of the epidermis, producing large, erythematous (red) plaques with silvery scales (Fig. 21-6; see also, *plaques*, Box 21-2). The cause is unknown, but there is sometimes a hereditary pattern, and autoimmunity may be involved.

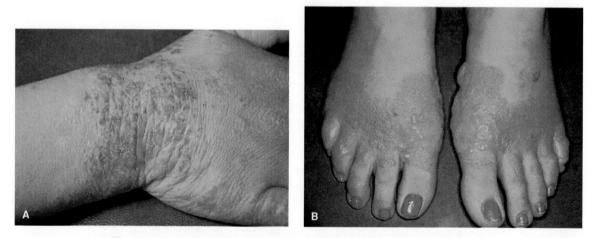

Figure 21-5 Dermatitis. (*A*) Eczema (atopic dermatitis) on an infant's wrist. (*B*) Contact dermatitis from shoe material. Note several fluid-filled bullae (see Box 21-2).

21

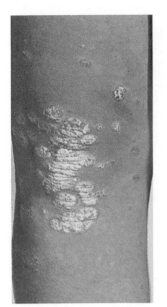

Figure 21-6 Psoriasis. Plaques with scales seen at the front of the knee (see *plaque*, Box 21-2).

Dermatologists treat psoriasis in the following ways depending on severity:

1. topical agents, including corticosteroids, immunosuppressants, vitamins A and D
2. phototherapy—exposure to ultraviolet light B (UVB); administration of the drug psoralen (P) to increase skin sensitivity to light followed by exposure to ultraviolet light A (UVA); laser treatment
3. systemic suppression of the immune system

Autoimmune Disorders

The diseases discussed below are caused, at least in part, by autoimmune reactions. They are diagnosed by biopsy of lesions and by antibody studies.

Pemphigus is characterized by the formation of bullae (blisters) in the skin and mucous membranes caused by a separation of epidermal cells from underlying layers (Fig. 21-7; see also, *bullae*, Box 21-2). Rupture of these lesions leaves deeper skin areas unprotected from infection and fluid loss, much as in cases of burns. The cause is an autoimmune reaction to epithelial cells. Pemphigus is fatal unless treated by suppressing the immune system.

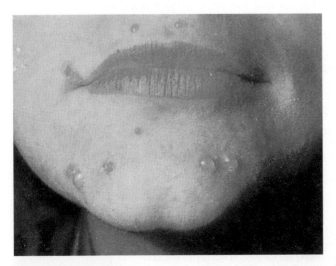

Figure 21-7 Pemphigus. Vesicles are shown on the chin (see *vesicle*. Box 21-2).

21

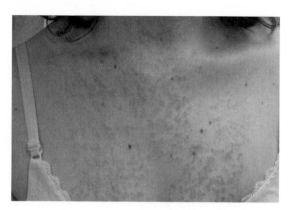

Figure 21-8 Discoid (cutaneous) lupus erythematosus. Erythematous papules and plaques in a typical sun-exposed distribution on the chest.

Lupus erythematosus (LE) is a chronic inflammatory autoimmune disease of connective tissue. The more widespread form of the disease, systemic lupus erythematosus (SLE), involves the skin and other organs. SLE is more prevalent in women than in men and has a higher incidence among Asians and blacks than in other populations.

The discoid form (DLE) involves only the skin. It is seen as rough, raised, erythematous papules that are worsened by exposure to the ultraviolet radiation in sunlight (Fig. 21-8). Lupus skin lesions are confined to the face and scalp and may form a typical butterfly-shaped rash across the nose and cheeks.

Scleroderma is a disease of unknown cause that involves thickening and tightening of the skin. There is gradual fibrosis of the dermis because of collagen overproduction. Sweat glands and hair follicles are also involved. A very early sign of scleroderma is Raynaud disease, in which blood vessels in the fingers and toes constrict in the cold, causing numbness, pain, coldness, and tingling. Skin symptoms first appear on the forearms and around the mouth. Internal organs become involved in a diffuse form of scleroderma called progressive systemic sclerosis (PSS).

Skin Cancer

Skin cancer is the most common type of human cancer. Its rate has been increasing in recent years, mainly because of the mutation-causing effects of sunlight's ultraviolet rays. **Squamous cell carcinoma** and **basal cell carcinoma** are both cancers of epithelial cells. Both appear in areas exposed to sunlight, such as the face and hands. Basal cell carcinoma constitutes more than 75 percent of all skin cancers. It usually appears as a smooth, pearly papule (Fig. 21-9; see also, *papules*, Box 21-2). Because these cancers are easily seen and do not metastasize, the cure rate after excision is greater than 95 percent.

Squamous cell carcinoma appears as a painless, firm, red nodule or plaque that may develop surface scales, ulceration, or crusting (Fig. 21-10; see also, Box 21-2). This cancer may invade underlying tissue but tends not to metastasize. It is treated by surgical removal and sometimes with x-irradiation or chemotherapy.

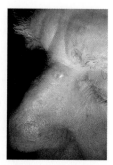

Figure 21-9 Basal cell carcinoma. An initial translucent nodule has spread, leaving a depressed center and a firm, elevated border (see *nodule*, Box 21-2).

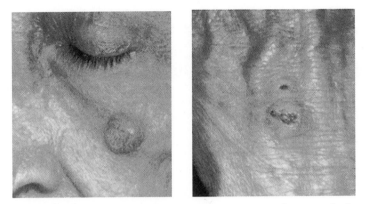

Figure 21-10 Squamous cell carcinoma. Lesions are shown on the face and the back of the hand, sun-exposed areas that are commonly affected.

21

Malignant melanoma results from an overgrowth of melanocytes, the pigment-producing cells in the epidermis. It is the most dangerous form of skin cancer because of its tendency to metastasize. This cancer appears as a lesion that is variable in color with an irregular border (Fig. 21-11). It may spread superficially for up to one or two years before it begins to invade the deeper skin tissues and to metastasize through blood and lymph. The prognosis for cure is good if the lesion is recognized and removed surgically before it enters this invasive stage.

Kaposi sarcoma, once considered rare, is now seen frequently in association with AIDS. It usually appears as distinct brownish areas on the legs. These plaques become raised and firm as the tumor progresses. In those with weakened immune systems, such as patients with AIDS, the cancer can metastasize.

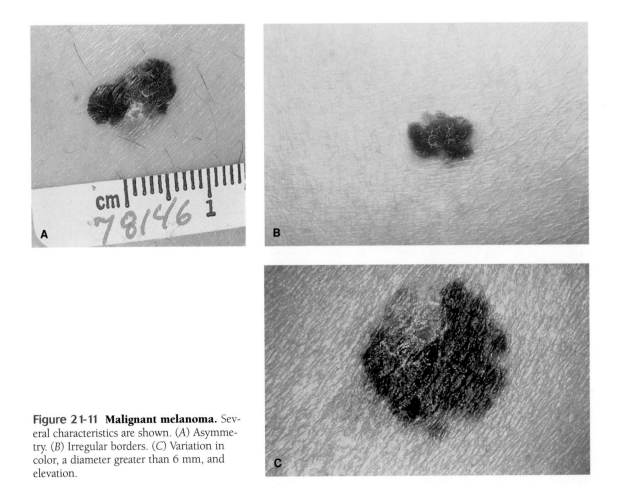

Figure 21-11 Malignant melanoma. Several characteristics are shown. (*A*) Asymmetry. (*B*) Irregular borders. (*C*) Variation in color, a diameter greater than 6 mm, and elevation.

TERMINOLOGY Key Terms

atopic dermatitis *a-TOP-ik der-ma-TĪ-tis*	Hereditary, allergic, chronic inflammation of the skin with pruritus (itching); eczema
basal cell carcinoma *BĀ-sal*	An epithelial tumor that rarely metastasizes and has a high cure rate with surgical removal
cicatrization *sik-a-tri-ZĀ-shun*	The process of scar formation; a scar is a cicatrix (*SIK-a-triks*)
débridement *da-brē-DMON*	Removal of dead or damaged tissue, as from a wound
dehiscence *dē-HIS-ens*	Splitting or bursting, as when the layers of a wound separate
dermatitis *der-ma-TĪ-tis*	Inflammation of the skin, often associated with redness and itching; may be caused by allergy, irritants (contact dermatitis), or a variety of diseases
dermatology *der-ma-TOL-ō-jē*	Study of the skin and diseases of the skin
dermatome *DER-ma-tōm*	Instrument for cutting thin sections of skin for skin grafting
eczema *EK-zē-ma*	A general term for an inflammation of the skin with redness, lesions, and itching; atopic dermatitis
erythema *er-i-THĒ-ma*	Diffuse redness of the skin
escharotomy *es-kar-OT-ō-mē*	Removal of scab tissue (eschar) resulting from burns or other skin injuries
evisceration *ē-vis-er-Ā-shun*	Protrusion of internal organs (viscera) through an opening, as through a wound
exudate *EKS-ū-dāt*	Material, which may include fluid, cells, pus, or blood, that escapes from damaged tissue
Kaposi sarcoma *KAP-ō-sē*	Cancerous lesion of the skin and other tissues seen most often in patients with AIDS
keloid *KĒ-loyd*	A raised, thickened scar caused by tissue overgrowth during scar formation
lupus erythematosus (LE) *LŪ-pus er-i-thē-ma-TŌ-sis*	A chronic, inflammatory, autoimmune disease of connective tissue that often involves the skin; types include the more widespread systemic lupus erythematosus (SLE) and a discoid form (DLE) that involves only the skin
malignant melanoma	A metastasizing pigmented tumor of the skin
pemphigus *PEM-fi-gus*	An autoimmune disease of the skin characterized by sudden, intermittent formation of bullae (blisters); may be fatal if untreated

TERMINOLOGY Key Terms

Continued

pressure ulcer	An ulcer caused by pressure to an area of the body, as from a bed or chair; decubitus (*dē-KŪ-bi-tus*) ulcer, bedsore, pressure sore
pruritus *prū-RĪ-tus*	Severe itching
psoriasis *so-RĪ-a-sis*	A chronic hereditary dermatitis with red lesions covered by silvery scales
rule of nines	A method for estimating the extent of body-surface area involved in a burn by assigning percentages in multiples of nine to various regions of the body
scleroderma *sklēr-ō-DER-ma*	A chronic disease that is characterized by thickening and tightening of the skin and that often involves internal organs in a form called progressive systemic sclerosis (PSS)
squamous cell carcinoma	An epidermal cancer that may invade deeper tissues but tends not to metastasize

Go to the pronunciation glossary in Chapter 21 on the CD-ROM to hear these words pronounced.

TERMINOLOGY Supplementary Terms

SYMPTOMS AND CONDITIONS

acne *AK-nē*	An inflammatory disease of the sebaceous glands and hair follicles usually associated with excess secretion of sebum; acne vulgaris
actinic *ak-TIN-ik*	Pertaining to the effects of radiant energy, such as sunlight, ultraviolet light, and x-rays
albinism *AL-bin-izm*	A hereditary lack of pigment in the skin, hair, and eyes
alopecia *al-ō-PĒ-shē-a*	Absence or loss of hair; baldness

Supplementary Terms

Beau lines *bō*	White lines across the fingernails; usually a sign of systemic disease or injury (Fig. 21-12)
bromhidrosis *brō-mi-DRŌ-sis*	Sweat that has a foul odor because of bacterial decomposition; also called bromidrosis
carbuncle *CAR-bung-kil*	A localized infection of the skin and subcutaneous tissue, usually caused by staphylococcus, and associated with pain and discharge of pus
comedo *KOM-e-dō*	A plug of sebum, often containing bacteria, in a hair follicle; a blackhead (plural: comedones)
dermatophytosis *der-ma-tō-fi-TŌ-sis*	Fungal infection of the skin, especially between the toes; athlete's foot (root: *phyt/o* means "plant")
diaphoresis *dī-a-fō-RĒ-sis*	Profuse sweating
dyskeratosis *dis-ker-a-TŌ-sis*	Any abnormality in keratin formation in epithelial cells
ecchymosis *ek-i-MŌ-sis*	A collection of blood under the skin caused by leakage from small vessels
erysipelas *er-i-SIP-e-las*	An acute infectious disease of the skin with localized redness and swelling and systemic symptoms
erythema nodosum *nō-DŌ-sum*	Inflammation of subcutaneous tissues resulting in tender, erythematous nodules; may be an abnormal immune response to a systemic disease, an infection, or a drug
exanthem *eks-AN-them*	Any eruption of the skin that accompanies a disease, such as measles; a rash
excoriation *eks-kō-rē-Ā-shun*	Lesion caused by scratching or abrasion (Fig. 21-13)
folliculitis *fō-lik-ū-LĪ-tis*	Inflammation of a hair follicle

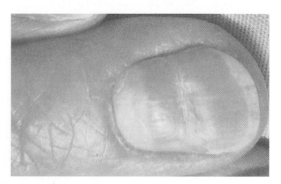

Figure 21-12 Beau lines. These transverse depressions in the nails are associated with acute severe illness.

TERMINOLOGY Supplementary Terms

Continued

furuncle *FŪ-rung-kil*	A painful skin nodule caused by staphylococci that enter through a hair follicle; a boil
hemangioma *hē-man-jē-Ō-ma*	A benign tumor of blood vessels; in the skin, called birthmarks or port wine stains
herpes simplex *HER-pēz SIM-pleks*	A group of acute infections caused by herpes simplex virus. Type I herpes simplex virus produces fluid-filled vesicles, usually on the lips, after fever, sun exposure, injury, or stress; cold sore, fever blister. Type II infections usually involve the genital organs.
hirsutism *HIR-sū-tizm*	Excessive growth of hair
ichthyosis *ik-thē-Ō-sis*	A dry, scaly condition of the skin (from the root *ichthy/o*, meaning "fish")
impetigo *im-pe-TĪ-gō*	A bacterial skin infection with pustules that rupture and form crusts; most commonly seen in children, usually on the face (Fig. 21-14; see also, *pustules*, Box 21-2)

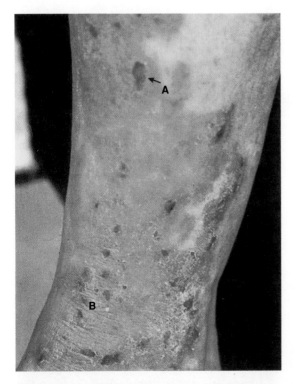

Figure 21-13 Skin lesions associated with dermatitis. (*A*) Excoriation. (*B*) Lichenification.

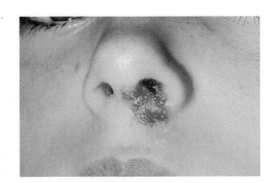

Figure 21-14 Impetigo. This bacterial skin infection, seen here on the nostril, causes pustules that rupture and form crusts (see *pustule*, Box 21-2).

21

keratosis *ker-a-TŌ-sis*	Any skin condition marked by thickened or horny growth. Seborrheic keratosis is a benign tumor, yellow or light brown in color, that appears in the elderly. Actinic keratosis is caused by exposure to sunlight and may lead to squamous cell carcinoma.
lichenification *lī-ken-i-fi-KĀ-shun*	Thickened marks caused by chronic rubbing, as seen in atopic dermatitis (a lichen is a flat, branching type of plant that grows on rocks and bark) (see Fig. 21-13)
mycosis fungoides *mī-KŌ-sis fun-GOY-dēz*	A rare malignant disease that originates in the skin and involves the internal organs and lymph nodes. There are large, painful, ulcerating tumors.
nevus *NĒ-vus*	A defined discoloration of the skin; a congenital vascular tumor of the skin; a mole, birthmark
paronychia *par-ō-NIK-ē-a*	Infection around a nail (Fig. 21-15). Caused by bacteria or fungi, and may affect multiple nails.
pediculosis *pe-dik-ū-LŌ-sis*	Infestation with lice
petechiae *pē-TĒ-kē-e*	Flat, pinpoint, purplish-red spots caused by bleeding within the skin or mucous membrane (singular, petechia)
photosensitization *fō-tō-sen-si-ti-ZĀ-shun*	Sensitization of the skin to light, usually from the action of drugs, plant products, or other substances
purpura *PUR-pū-ra*	A condition characterized by hemorrhages into the skin and other tissues
rosacea *rō-ZĀ-shē-a*	A condition of unknown cause involving redness of the skin, pustules, and overactivity of sebaceous glands, mainly on the face
scabies *SKĀ-bēz*	A highly contagious skin disease caused by a mite

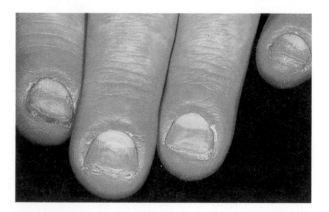

Figure 21-15 Paronychia.
Infection and inflammation of the proximal and lateral nail folds is shown.

TERMINOLOGY Supplementary Terms

Continued

21

senile lentigines *len-TIJ-i-nēz*	Brown macules that appear on sun-exposed skin in adults; liver spots
shingles	An acute eruption of vesicles along the path of a nerve; herpes zoster (*HER-pēz ZOS-ter*); caused by the same virus that causes chickenpox
tinea *TIN-ē-a*	A fungal infection of the skin; ringworm (Fig. 21-16)
tinea versicolor *VER-si-kol-or*	Superficial chronic fungal infection that causes varied pigmentation of the skin
urticaria *ur-ti-KĀ-rē-a*	A skin reaction marked by temporary, smooth, raised areas (wheals) associated with itching; hives (Fig. 21-17; see also, *wheals*, Box 21-2)
venous stasis ulcer	Ulcer caused by venous insufficiency and stasis of venous blood; usually forms near the ankle (Fig. 21-18; see also, *ulcer*, Box 21-2)
verruca *ver-RŪ-ka*	An epidermal tumor; a wart
vitiligo *vit-i-LĪ-gō*	Patchy disappearance of pigment in the skin; leukoderma (Fig. 21-19)
xeroderma pigmentosum *zē-rō-DER-ma pig-men-TŌ-sum*	A fatal hereditary disease that begins in childhood with discolorations and ulcers of the skin and muscle atrophy. There is increased sensitivity to the sun and increased susceptibility to cancer.

DIAGNOSIS AND TREATMENT

aloe *A-lō*	A plant (*Aloe vera*), the leaves of which contain a gel that is used in treatment of burns and minor skin irritations

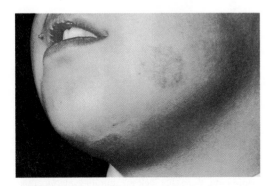

Figure 21-16 Tinea corporis (ringworm). This fungal infection is shown on the face.

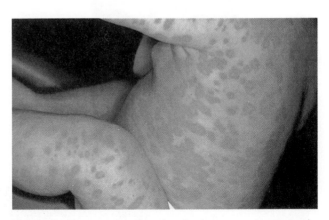

Figure 21-17 Urticaria (hives). Wheals associated with drug allergy are shown in an infant (see *wheal*, Box 21-2).

21

TERMINOLOGY Supplementary Terms
Continued

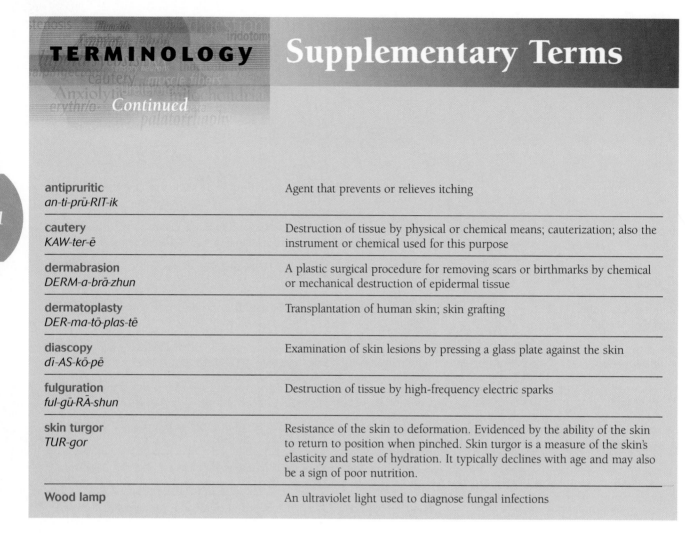

antipruritic *an-ti-prū-RIT-ik*	Agent that prevents or relieves itching
cautery *KAW-ter-ē*	Destruction of tissue by physical or chemical means; cauterization; also the instrument or chemical used for this purpose
dermabrasion *DERM-a-brā-zhun*	A plastic surgical procedure for removing scars or birthmarks by chemical or mechanical destruction of epidermal tissue
dermatoplasty *DER-ma-tō-plas-tē*	Transplantation of human skin; skin grafting
diascopy *dī-AS-kō-pē*	Examination of skin lesions by pressing a glass plate against the skin
fulguration *ful-gū-RĀ-shun*	Destruction of tissue by high-frequency electric sparks
skin turgor *TUR-gor*	Resistance of the skin to deformation. Evidenced by the ability of the skin to return to position when pinched. Skin turgor is a measure of the skin's elasticity and state of hydration. It typically declines with age and may also be a sign of poor nutrition.
Wood lamp	An ultraviolet light used to diagnose fungal infections

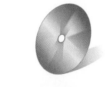

Go to the pronunciation glossary in Chapter 21 of the CD-ROM to hear these words pronounced.

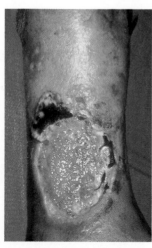

Figure 21-18 Venous stasis ulcer. Lesion on the ankle caused by venous insufficiency and blood stasis (see *ulcer*. Box 21-2).

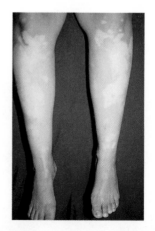

Figure 21-19 Vitiligo. Depigmented macules appear on the skin and may merge into large areas that lack melanin (see *macule*, Box 21-2). The brown pigment seen in the illustration is the person's normal skin color; the pale areas are caused by vitiligo.

TERMINOLOGY Abbreviations

BSA	Body-surface area		**SLE**	Systemic lupus erythematosus
DLE	Discoid lupus erythematosus		**SPF**	Sun protection factor
FTSG	Full-thickness skin graft		**STSG**	Split-thickness skin graft
LE	Lupus erythematosus		**UV**	Ultraviolet
PSS	Progressive systemic sclerosis		**UVA**	Ultraviolet A
PUVA	Psoralen ultraviolet A		**UVB**	Ultraviolet B
SCLE	Subacute cutaneous lupus erythematosus		**VAC**	Vacuum-assisted closure

21

CHAPTER REVIEW

LABELING EXERCISE
Cross Section of the Skin

Write the name of each numbered part on the corresponding line of the answer sheet.

21

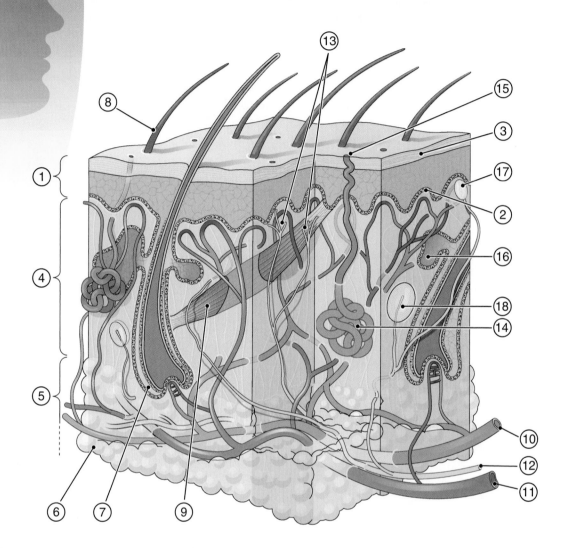

adipose tissue	1. _____
arrector pili muscle	2. _____
artery	3. _____
dermis (corium)	4. _____
epidermis	5. _____
hair	6. _____
hair follicle	7. _____
nerve	8. _____
nerve endings	9. _____

pore (opening of sweat gland)

10. _____

pressure receptor

11. _____

sebaceous (oil) gland

12. _____

stratum basale (growing layer)

13. _____

stratum corneum

14. _____

subcutaneous layer

15. _____

sudoriferous (sweat) gland

16. _____

touch receptor

17. _____

vein

18. _____

TERMINOLOGY

Multiple choice. Select the best answer and write the letter of your choice to the left of each number:

_____	1. hypodermis	**a.**	thickened layer of the epidermis
_____	2. stratum corneum	**b.**	growing layer of the epidermis
_____	3. sebum	**c.**	subcutaneous layer
_____	4. stratum basale	**d.**	sheath that contains a hair
_____	5. follicle	**e.**	oily secretion of the skin
_____	6. exudate	**a.**	excess scar tissue
_____	7. pruritus	**b.**	autoimmune disease with thickening of the skin
_____	8. scleroderma	**c.**	fluid that drains from a wound
_____	9. pressure ulcer	**d.**	severe itching
_____	10. keloid	**e.**	bedsore

Supplementary Terms

_____	11. nevus	**a.**	excess growth of hair
_____	12. hirsutism	**b.**	hives
_____	13. urticaria	**c.**	baldness
_____	14. alopecia	**d.**	blackhead
_____	15. comedo	**e.**	mole or birthmark
_____	16. tinea	**a.**	sweat with a foul odor
_____	17. rosacea	**b.**	infection around a nail

(continued on next page)

_____ 18. bromhidrosis   c. bacterial skin infection

_____ 19. impetigo   d. fungal skin infection

_____ 20. paronychia   e. condition causing redness and pustules, mainly on the face

Fill in the blanks:

21. The adjective *cutaneous* refers to the _____.

22. A sudoriferous gland produces _____.

23. The main pigment in skin is _____.

24. The oil-producing glands of the skin are the _____.

25. The protein that thickens the skin and makes up hair and nails is _____.

Eliminations. In each of the sets below, underline the word that does not fit in with the rest and explain the reason for your choice:

26. nodule – vesicle – cicatrix – macule – papule

_____

27. eczema – débridement – psoriasis – dermatitis – pemphigus

_____

28. SLE – PSS – SCLE – BSA – DLE

_____

True–False. Examine the following statements. If the statement is true, write T in the first blank. If the statement is false, write F in the first blank and correct the statement by replacing the <u>underlined</u> word in the second blank.

29. The skin and its associated structures makes up the <u>integumentary system</u>.   _____ _____

30. The <u>stratum basale</u> is the outermost layer of the epidermis.   _____ _____

31. The root *trich/o* refers to a <u>nail</u>.   _____ _____

32. The <u>dermis</u> is between the epidermis and the subcutaneous layer.   _____ _____

33. Diaphoresis is profuse <u>bleeding</u>.   _____ _____

34. Eczema is also called <u>atopic dermatitis</u>.   _____ _____

Define the following words:

35. melanocyte (*MEL-an-ō-sīt*) _____

36. percutaneous (*per-kū-TĀ-nē-us*) _____

37. keratogenic (*ker-a-tō-JEN-ik*) _____

38. pachyderma (*pak-ē-DER-ma*) _____

39. trichomycosis (*trik-ō-mī-KŌ-sis*) _____

40. onychia (*ō-NIK-ē-a*) _____

41. xeroderma (*zē-rō-DER-ma*) _____

Word building. Write words for the following definitions:

42. discharge of sebum   _____

43. excess production of melanin   _____

44. hardening of the skin _____

45. tumor containing melanin _____

46. study of hair _____

47. instrument for cutting the skin _____

48. loosening or separation of a nail _____

49. any disease of the skin _____

Use the word *hidrosis* (sweating) as an ending for words with the following meanings:

50. absence of sweating _____

51. excess sweating _____

52. excretion of colored (chrom/o) sweat _____

Word analysis. Define the following words, and give the meaning of the word parts in each. Use a dictionary if necessary.

53. onychocryptosis (*on-i-kō-krip-TŌ-sis*) _____

    a. onych/o _____

    b. crypt/o _____

    c. -sis _____

54. achromotrichia (*a-krō-mō-TRIK-ē-a*) _____

    a. a- _____

    b. chrom/o _____

    c. trich/o _____

    d. -ia _____

55. hidradenoma (*hī-drad-e-NŌ-ma*) _____

    a. hidr/o _____

    b. aden/o _____

    c. -oma _____

Go to the word exercises in Chapter 21 of the CD-ROM for additional review exercises.

CASE STUDY 21-1: Basal Cell Carcinoma

K.B., a 32-year-old fitness instructor, had noticed a "tiny hard lump" at the base of her left nostril while cleansing her face. The lesion had been present for about two months when she consulted a dermatologist. She had recently moved north from Florida, where she had worked as a lifeguard. She thought the lump might have been triggered by the regular tanning salon sessions she had used to retain her tan because it did not resemble the acne pustules, blackheads, or resulting scars of her adolescent years. Although dermabrasion had removed the obvious acne scars and left several areas of dense skin, this lump was brown-pigmented and different. K.B. was afraid it might be a malignant melanoma. On examination, the dermatologist noted a small pearly-white nodule at the lower portion of the left ala (outer flared portion of the nostril). There were no other lesions on her face or neck.

A plastic surgeon excised the lesion and was able to reapproximate the wound edges without a full-thickness skin graft. The pathology report identified the lesion as a basal cell carcinoma with clean margins of normal skin and subcutaneous tissue and stated that the entire lesion had been excised. K.B. was advised to wear SPF 30 sun protection on her face at all times and to avoid excessive sun exposure and tanning salons.

CASE STUDY 21-2: Cutaneous Lymphoma

L.C., a 52-year-old female research chemist, has had a history of T-cell lymphoma for eight years. She was initially treated with systemic chemotherapy with methotrexate, until she contracted stomatitis. Continued therapy with topical chemotherapeutic agents brought measurable improvement. She also had a history of hidradenitis.

A recent physical examination showed diffuse erythroderma with scaling and hyperkeratosis, plus alopecia. She had painful leukoplakia and ulcerations of the mouth and tongue. L.C. was hospitalized and given two courses of topical chemotherapy. She was referred to Dental Medicine for treatment of the oral lesions and was discharged in stable condition with an appointment for follow-up in four weeks. Her discharge medications included the application of 2 percent hydrocortisone ointment to the affected lesions q hs, Keralyt gel bid for the hyperkeratosis, and Dyclone and Benadryl for her mouth ulcers prn.

CASE STUDY 21-3: Pressure Ulcer

L.N., an elderly woman in failing health, had recently moved in with her daughter after her hospitalization for a stroke. The daughter reported to the home care nurse that her mother had minimal appetite and was confused and disoriented and that a blister had developed on her lower back since she had been confined to bed. The nurse noted that L.N. had lost weight since her last visit and that her skin was dry, with poor skin turgor. She was wearing an "adult diaper," which was wet. After examining L.N.'s sacrum, the nurse noted a nickel-sized open area, 2 cm in diameter and 1 cm in depth (stage II pressure ulcer), with a 0.5-cm reddened surrounding area with no drainage. L.N. moaned when the nurse palpated the lesion. The nurse also noted reddened areas on L.N.'s elbows and heels.

The nurse provided L.N.'s daughter with instructions for proper skin care, incontinence management, enhanced nutrition, and frequent repositioning to prevent pressure ischemia to the prominent body areas. However, six months later L.N.'s pressure ulcer had deteriorated to a class III. She was hospitalized under the care of a plastic surgeon and wound-ostomy care nurse. Surgery was scheduled to débride the sacral wound and close it with a full-thickness skin graft taken from her thigh. L.N. was discharged eight days later to a long-term–care facility with orders for an alternating pressure mattress, position change every 2 hours, supplemental nutrition, and meticulous wound care.

CASE STUDY QUESTIONS

Multiple choice. Select the best answer and write the letter of your choice to the left of each number:

_____ 1. K.B.'s basal cell carcinoma may have been caused by chronic exposure to the sun and use of an ultraviolet tanning bed. The scientific explanation for this is the:
  a. autoimmune response
  b. actinic effect
  c. allergic reaction
  d. sun block tanning lotion theory
  e. dermatophytosis

_____ 2. The characteristic pimples of adolescent acne are whiteheads and blackheads. The medical terms for these lesions are:
  a. vesicles and lymphotomes
  b. pustules and blisters
  c. pustules and comedones
  d. vitiligo and macules
  e. furuncle and sebaceous cyst

_____ 3. Which skin cancer is an overgrowth of pigment-producing epidermal cells?
  a. basal cell carcinoma
  b. Kaposi sarcoma
  c. cutaneous lymphoma
  d. melanoma
  e. erythema nodosum

_____ 4. Basal cell carcinoma involves:
  a. subcutaneous tissue
  b. hair follicles
  c. connective tissue
  d. adipose tissue
  e. epithelial cells

_____ 5. Hidradenitis is inflammation of a:
  a. sweat gland
  b. salivary gland
  c. sebaceous gland
  d. ceruminous gland
  e. meibomian gland

_____ 6. Leukoplakia is:
  a. baldness
  b. ulceration
  c. formation of white patches in the mouth
  d. formation of yellow patches on the skin
  e. formation of scales on the skin

_____ 7. Hydrocortisone is a(n):
  a. vitamin
  b. steroid
  c. analgesic
  d. lubricant
  e. diuretic

_____ 8. An example of a topical drug is a:
   a. systemic chemotherapeutic agent
   b. drug derived from rain forest plants
   c. subdermal allergy test antigens
   d. skin ointment
   e. Benadryl capsule, 25 mg

_____ 9. Stomatitis, a common side effect of systemic chemotherapy, is an inflammatory condition of the:
   a. mouth
   b. colostomy
   c. stomach
   d. teeth and hair
   e. nails

_____ 10. Skin turgor is an indicator of:
   a. elasticity
   b. hydration
   c. aging
   d. nutrition
   e. all of the above

_____ 11. Another name for a pressure ulcer is a:
   a. shearing force
   b. bedsore
   c. decubitus ulcer
   d. a and b
   e. b and c

_____ 12. An FTSG is usually harvested (taken) from another body area with a scalpel, whereas an STSG is harvested with an instrument called a(n) _____, which can cut a thinner graft.
   a. tissue slicer
   b. Keralyt
   c. erythroderm
   d. dermatome
   e. débridement

Write terms from the case studies with the following meanings:

13. skin sanding procedure _____

14. a solid raised lesion larger than a papule _____

15. physician who cares for patients with skin diseases _____

16. connective tissue and fat layer beneath the dermis _____

17. diffuse redness of the skin _____

18. increased production of keratin in the skin _____

19. removal of dead or damaged skin _____

20. reduced blood flow to the tissue _____

Abbreviations. Define the following abbreviations:

21. FTSG _____

22. STSG _____

23. SPF _____

24. hs _____

25. bid _____

The Skin

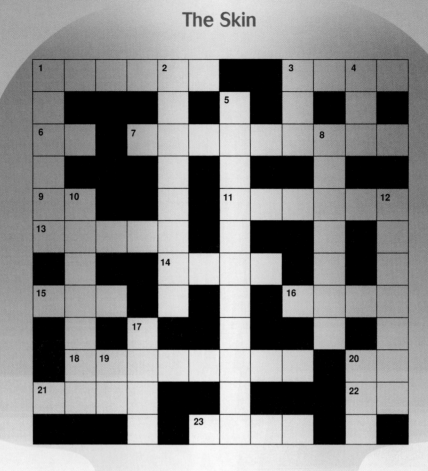

ACROSS

1. Horny layer of the skin: combining form
3. Inflammation of a sweat gland: _ _ _ _ adenitis
6. Autoimmune disease that affects the skin: abbreviation
7. Excess growth of hair
9. Within the skin: abbreviation
11. Viral disease that affects the skin
13. Skin: combining form
14. Sweat: combining form
15. Three: prefix
16. Scar: _ _ _ _ trix
18. Examination by pressing a glass plate against the skin
20. True, good, easy: prefix
21. Half: prefix
22. Part of a medical history: _ _ H: abbreviation
23. Under, below, decreased: prefix

DOWN

1. Raised, thickened scar
2. Pertaining to a hair
3. Measurement of packed red cells: abbreviation
4. Abnormal, painful: prefix
5. Removal of scab tissue
8. Bacterial skin infection common in children: _ _ _ _ _ _ _ o
10. Remove dead tissue, as from a wound
12. A layer, as of the skin
17. Meaning of the root *onych/o*
19. A route of injection: abbreviation
20. On, over: prefix

APPENDIX ONE

COMMONLY USED SYMBOLS

SYMBOL	MEANING	CHAPTER	SYMBOL	MEANING	CHAPTER
1°	primary	7	>	greater than	7
2°	secondary (to)	7	<	less than	7
Δ	change (Greek delta)	7	∧	above	7
Ⓛ	left	7	∨	below	7
Ⓡ	right	7	=	equal to	7
↑	increase(d)	7	≠	not equal to	7
↓	decrease(d)	7	±	doubtful, slight	7
♂	male	7	~	approximately	7
♀	female	7	×	times	7
°	degree	7	#	number, pound	7

APPENDIX TWO

ABBREVIATIONS AND THEIR MEANINGS

ABBREVIATIONS	MEANING	CHAPTER	ABBREVIATIONS	MEANING	CHAPTER
ā	before	8	ARF	acute respiratory failure	11
A, Acc	accommodation	18	ARF	acute renal failure	13
āā	of each	8	ART	assisted reproductive technology	15
A1c	glycated hemoglobin	16	ASA	acetylsalicylic acid (aspirin)	8
Ab	antibody	10	As, Ast	astigmatism	18
AB	abortion	15	AS	atrial stenosis; arteriosclerosis; left ear	9, 18
ABC	aspiration biopsy cytology	7	ASCVD	arteriosclerotic cardiovascular disease	9
ABG(s)	arterial blood gas(es)	11	ASD	atrial septal defect	9
ABR	auditory brainstem response	18	ASF	anterior spinal fusion	19
ac	before meals	8	ASHD	arteriosclerotic heart disease	9
AC	air conduction	18	ASHP	American Society of Health System Pharmacists	8
ACE	angiotensin-converting enzyme	9			
ACh	acetylcholine	17, 20	AT	atrial tachycardia	9
ACL	anterior cruciate ligament	19	ATN	acute tubular necrosis	13
ACTH	adrenocorticotropic hormone	16	AV	atrioventricular	9
ad lib	as desired	8			
AD	Alzheimer disease; right ear	17, 18	BAEP	brainstem auditory evoked potentials	17, 18
ADH	antidiuretic hormone	13			
ADHD	attention-deficit/hyperactivity disorder	17	BBB	bundle branch block	9
			BC	bone conduction	18
ADL	activities of daily living	7	BCG	bacille Calmette–Guérin (tuberculosis vaccine)	11
AE	above the elbow	19			
AED	automated external defibrillator	9	BE	barium enema; below the elbow	12; 19
AF	atrial fibrillation	9	bid	twice per day	8
AFB	acid-fast bacillus	11	BK	below the knee	19
AFP	alpha-fetoprotein	7, 15	BM	bowel movement	12
Ag	antigen	10	BMD	bone mineral density	19
AGA	appropriate for gestational age	15	BNO	bladder neck obstruction	14
AI	artificial insemination; aromatase inhibitor	15	BP	blood pressure	7, 9
			BPH	benign prostatic hyperplasia (hypertrophy)	14
AIDS	acquired immunodeficiency syndrome	10, 14			
AK	above the knee	19	bpm	beats per minute	7, 9
ALL	acute lymphoblastic (lymphocytic) leukemia	10	BRCA1	breast cancer gene 1	15
			BRCA2	breast cancer gene 2	15
ALS	amyotrophic lateral sclerosis	17, 20	BRP	bathroom privileges	7
AMA	against medical advice	7	BS	bowel sounds; breath sounds; blood sugar	7, 11, 16
AMB	ambulatory	7			
AMD	age-related macular degeneration	18	BSA	body-surface area	21
AMI	acute myocardial infarction	9	BSE	breast self-examination	15
AML	acute myeloblastic (myelogenous) leukemia	10	BSO	bilateral salpingo-oophorectomy	15
			BT	bleeding time	10
ANS	autonomic nervous system	17	BUN	blood urea nitrogen	13
AP	anteroposterior	7	BV	bacterial vaginosis	15
APAP	acetaminophen	8	bx	biopsy	7
APC	atrial premature complex	9			
APTT	activated partial thromboplastin time	10	c̄	with	8
aq	water, aqueous	8	C	Celsius (centigrade); compliance; cervical vertebra	7, 11, 19
AR	aortic regurgitation	9			
ARC	abnormal retinal correspondence	18			
ARDS	acute respiratory distress syndrome	11	C section	cesarean section	15

ABBREVIATIONS	MEANING	CHAPTER	ABBREVIATIONS	MEANING	CHAPTER
CA	cancer	6	DIFF	differential count	10
CABG	coronary artery bypass graft	9	DIP	distal interphalangeal	19
CAD	coronary artery disease	9	DJD	degenerative joint disease	19
CAM	complementary and alternative medicine	7	dL	deciliter	Appendix 8
			DLE	discoid lupus erythematosus	21
cap	capsule	8	DM	diabetes mellitus	16
CAPD	continuous ambulatory peritoneal dialysis	13	DNR	do not resuscitate	7
			DOE	dyspnea on exertion	9
CBC	complete blood count	10	DTaP	diphtheria, tetanus, acellular pertussis (vaccine)	11
CBD	common bile duct	12			
CBF	cerebral blood flow	17	DRE	digital rectal examination	14
CBR	complete bed rest	7	DS	double strength	8
cc	with correction	18	DSM	*Diagnostic and Statistical Manual of Mental Disorders*	17
CC	chief complaint	7			
CCPD	continuous cyclic peritoneal dialysis	13	DTR	deep tendon reflex(es)	17
CCU	coronary care unit, cardiac care unit	9	DUB	dysfunctional uterine bleeding	15
CF	cystic fibrosis	11	DVT	deep vein thrombosis	9
CFS	chronic fatigue syndrome	20	Dx	diagnosis	7
CHD	coronary heart disease	9			
CHF	congestive heart failure	9	EBL	estimated blood loss	7
Ci	Curie	7	EBV	Epstein–Barr virus	10
CIN	cervical intraepithelial neoplasia	15	ECMO	Extracorporeal membrane oxygenation	15
CIS	carcinoma in situ	6			
CJD	Creutzfeldt–Jakob disease	17	EDC	estimated date of confinement	15
CK	creatine kinase	20	EEG	electroencephalogram; electroencephalograph(y)	17
CK-MB	creatine kinase MB	9			
CLL	chronic lymphocytic leukemia	10	ECG (EKG)	electrocardiogram	9
cm	centimeter	Appendix 8	ELISA	enzyme-linked immunosorbent assay	10
CMG	cystometrography, cystometrogram	13	elix	elixir	8
CML	chronic myelogenous leukemia	10	EM	emmetropia	18
CNS	central nervous system	17	EMG	electromyography, electromyogram	20
c/o	complains of	7	ENG	electronystagmography	18
Co	coccyx; coccygeal	19	ENT	ear(s), nose, and throat	18
CO$_2$	carbon dioxide	11	EOM	extraocular movement, muscles	18
COLD	chronic obstructive lung disease	11	EOMI	extraocular muscles intact	7
COPD	chronic obstructive pulmonary disease	11	EPO	erythropoietin	10, 13
			ERCP	endoscopic retrograde cholangiopancreatography	12
CP	cerebral palsy	17			
CPAP	continuous positive airway pressure	11	ERG	electroretinography	18
CPD	cephalopelvic disproportion	15	ERV	expiratory reserve volume	11
C(P)K	creatine (phospho) kinase	20	ESR	erythrocyte sedimentation rate	10
CPR	cardiopulmonary resuscitation	9	ESRD	end-stage renal disease	13
CRF	chronic renal failure	13	ESWL	extracorporeal shock wave lithotripsy	13
crit	hematocrit	10	ET	esotropia	18
C&S	culture and sensitivity	7	ETOH	alcohol, ethyl alcohol	7
CSF	cerebrospinal fluid	17			
CSII	continuous subcutaneous insulin infusion	16	F	Fahrenheit	7
			FAP	familial adenomatous polyposis	12
CT	computed tomography	7	FBG	fasting blood glucose	16
CTS	carpal tunnel syndrome	20	FBS	fasting blood sugar	16
CVA	cerebrovascular accident	9, 17	FC	finger counting	18
CVD	cardiovascular disease; cerebrovascular disease	9, 17	FDA	Food and Drug Administration	8
			FEV	forced expiratory volume	11
CVI	chronic venous insufficiency	9	FFP	fresh frozen plasma	10
CVP	central venous pressure	9	FHR	fetal heart rate	15
CVS	chorionic villus sampling	15	FHT	fetal heart tone	15
CXR	chest x-ray	11	FMS	fibromyalgia syndrome	20
			FPG	fasting plasma glucose	16
D&C	dilatation and curettage	15	FRC	functional residual capacity	11
dB	decibel	18	FSH	follicle stimulating hormone	14, 15
dc, D/C	discontinue; discharge	7, 8	FTI	free thyroxine index	16
D&E	dilatation and evacuation	15	FTND	full-term normal delivery	15
DES	diethylstilbestrol	15	FTP	full-term pregnancy	15
DEXA	dual-energy x-ray absorptiometry (scan)	19	FTSG	full-thickness skin graft	21
			FUO	fever of unknown origin	6
DIC	disseminated intravascular coagulation	10	FVC	forced vital capacity	11
			Fx	fracture	19

A2

A2

ABBREVIATIONS	MEANING	CHAPTER
g	gram	Appendix 8
GA	gestational age	15
GAD	generalized anxiety disorder	17
GC	gonococcus	14, 15
GDM	gestational diabetes mellitus	16
GERD	gastroesophageal reflux disease	12
GFR	glomerular filtration rate	13
GH	growth hormone	16
GI	gastrointestinal	12
GIFT	gamete intrafallopian transfer	15
GTT	glucose tolerance test	16
gt(t)	drop(s)	8
GU	genitourinary	13, 14
GYN	gynecology	15
H&P	history and physical examination	7
HAV	hepatitis A virus	12
Hb, Hgb	hemoglobin	10
HbA1c	hemoglobin A1c; glycated hemoglobin	16
HBV	hepatitis B virus	12, 14
hCG	human chorionic gonadotropin	15
HCl	hydrochloric acid	12
Hct, Ht	hematocrit	10
HCV	hepatitis C virus	12
HDL	high-density lipoprotein	9
HDN	hemolytic disease of the newborn	10, 15
HDV	hepatitis D virus	12
HEV	hepatitis E virus	12
HEENT	head, eyes, ears, nose, and throat	7
HIV	human immunodeficiency virus	10, 14
HL	hearing level	18
HM	hand movements	18
HNP	herniated nucleus pulposus	19
h/o	history of	7
H & P	history and physical	7
HPI	history of present illness	7
HPS	*Hantavirus* pulmonary syndrome	11
HPV	human papillomavirus	15
HR	heart rate	7
HRT	hormone replacement therapy	15
hs	at bedtime	8
HSV	herpes simplex virus	14, 15
Ht, Hct	hemtocrit	10
HTN	hypertension	9
Hx	history	7
Hz	Hertz	18
131I	iodine-131	16
I&D	incision and drainage	7
I&O	intake and output	7
IABP	intraaortic balloon pump	9
IBD	inflammatory bowel disease	12
IBS	irritable bowel syndrome	12
IC	inspiratory capacity	11
ICD	implantable cardioverter-defibrillator	9
ICP	intracranial pressure	17
ICU	intensive care unit	7
ID	intradermal	8
I & D	incision and drainage	7
IF	intrinsic factor	10
IFG	impaired fasting blood glucose	16
Ig	immunoglobulin	10
IGT	impaired glucose tolerance	16
IM	intramuscular(ly); intramedullary	8, 19
INH	isoniazid	8, 11

ABBREVIATIONS	MEANING	CHAPTER
IOL	intraocular lens	18
IOP	intraocular pressure	18
IPPA	inspection, palpation, percussion, auscultation	7
IPPB	intermittent positive pressure breathing	11
IPPV	intermittent positive pressure ventilation	11
IRV	inspiratory reserve volume	11
ITP	idiopathic thrombocytopenic purpura	10
IU	international unit	8
IUD	intrauterine device	15
IV	intravenous(ly)	8
IVC	intravenous cholangiogram	12
IVCD	intraventricular conduction delay	9
IVDA	intravenous drug abuse	7
IVF	in vitro fertilization	15
IVP	intravenous pyelography	13
IVPB	intravenous piggyback	7
IVU	intravenous urography	13
JVP	jugular venous pulse	9
K	potassium	13
kg	kilogram	Appendix 8
km	kilometer	Appendix 8
KUB	kidney–ureter–bladder	13
KVO	keep vein open	7
L	lumbar vertebra	19
L	liter	Appendix 8
LA	long-acting	8
LAD	left anterior descending (coronary artery)	9
LAHB	left anterior hemiblock	9
LDL	low-density lipoprotein	9
LE	lupus erythematosus	21
LES	lower esophageal sphincter	12
LH	luteinizing hormone	14, 15
LL	left lateral	7
LLL	left lower lobe (of lung)	11
LLQ	left lower quadrant	5
LMN	lower motor neuron	17
LMP	last menstrual period	15
LOC	level of consciousness	17
LP	lumbar puncture	17
LUL	left upper lobe (of lung)	11
LUQ	left upper quadrant	5
LV	left ventricle	9
LVAD	left ventricular assist device	9
LVEDP	left ventricular end-diastolic pressure	9
LVH	left ventricular hypertrophy	9
lytes	electrolytes	10
μg	microgram	Appendix 8
μL	microliter	10, Appendix 8
μm	micrometer	Appendix 8
m	meter	Appendix 8
mcg	microgram	8, Appendix 8
mcL, mcl	microliter	10, Appendix 8
MAOI	monoamine oxidase inhibitor	17
MCH	mean corpuscular hemoglobin	10
MCHC	mean corpuscular hemoglobin concentration	10
MCP	metacarpophalangeal	19

ABBREVIATIONS	MEANING	CHAPTER	ABBREVIATIONS	MEANING	CHAPTER
MCV	mean corpuscular volume	10	ortho, ORTH	orthopedics	19
MDS	myelodysplastic syndrome	10	OS	left eye	18
MED(s)	medicine(s), medication(s)	8	OT	occupational therapy	20
MEFR	maximal expiratory flow rate	11	OTC	over-the-counter	8
MEN	multiple endocrine neoplasia	16	OU	both eyes; each eye	18
mEq	milliequivalent	10			
MET	metastasis	7	$\bar{p}$	after, post	8
mg	milligram	8, Appendix 8	P	pulse	7, 9
MG	myasthenia gravis	20	PA	posteroanterior; physician assistant	7
MI	myocardial infarction	9	PAC	premature atrial contraction	9
MID	multi-infarct dementia	17	$PaCO_2$	arterial partial pressure of carbon dioxide	11
mL	milliliter	Appendix 8			
mm	millimeter	Appendix 8	PACU	postanesthetic care unit	7
MMFR	maximum midexpiratory flow rate	11	PaO_2	arterial partial pressure of oxygen	11
mm Hg	millimeters of mercury	9	PAP	pulmonary arterial pressure	9
MMT	manual muscle test(ing)	20	pc	after meals	8
MN	myoneural	20	PCA	patient-controlled analgesia	7
MR	mitral regurgitation, reflux	9	PCI	percutaneous coronary intervention	9
MRI	magnetic resonance imaging	7	PCL	posterior cruciate ligament	19
MRSA	methicillin-resistant *Staphylococcus aureus*	6	PCOS	polycystic ovarian syndrome	15
			PCP	*Pneumocystis carinii* pneumonia; pneumocystic pneumonia	10, 11
MS	mitral stenosis; multiple sclerosis	9, 17			
MTP	metatarsophalangeal	19	PCV	packed cell volume	10
MUGA	multigated acquisition (scan)	9	PCWP	pulmonary capillary wedge pressure	9
MVP	mitral valve prolapse	9	PDA	patent ductus arteriosus	15
MVR	mitral valve replacement	9	PDD	pervasive developmental disorder	17
			PDR	*Physicians' Desk Reference*	8
Na	sodium	13	PE	physical examination	7
NAD	no apparent distress	7	PEEP	positive end-expiratory pressure	11
NB	newborn	15	PEFR	peak expiratory flow rate	11
NCCAM	National Center for Complementary and Alternative Medicine	7	PEG	percutaneous endoscopic gastrostomy (tube)	12
NG	nasogastric	12	PEP	protein electrophoresis	13
NGU	nongonococcal urethritis	14, 15	PERRLA	pupils equal, (regular) react to light and accommodation	7
NHL	non-Hodgkin lymphoma	10			
NICU	neonatal intensive care unit; neurologic intensive care unit	15, 17	PET	positron emission tomography	7, 17
			PFT	pulmonary function test(s)	11
NKDA	no known drug allergies	7	pH	scale for measuring hydrogen ion concentration (acidity or alkalinity)	10
NMJ	neuromuscular junction	20			
NPH	neutral protamine Hagedorn (insulin)	16	Ph	Philadelphia chromosome	10
NPH	normal pressure hydrocephalus	17	PICC	peripherally inserted central catheter	7
NPO	nothing by mouth	7	PID	pelvic inflammatory disease	15
NRC	normal retinal correspondence	18	PIH	pregnancy-induced hypertension	15
NREM	non–rapid eye movement (sleep)	17	PIP	peak inspiratory pressure	11
NS, N/S	normal saline	7	PIP	proximal interphalangeal	19
NSAID(s)	nonsteroidal antiinflammatory drug(s)	8, 19	PKU	phenylketonuria	15
			PMH	past medical history	7
NSR	normal sinus rhythm	9	PMI	point of maximal impulse	9
NSS	normal saline solution	7	PMN	polymorphonuclear (neutrophil)	10
NV	near vision	18	PMS	premenstrual syndrome	15
N/V, N&V, n&v	nausea and vomiting	12	PND	paroxysmal nocturnal dyspnea	11
N/V/D	nausea, vomiting, diarrhea	12	PNS	peripheral nervous system	17
			po	by mouth, orally	8
O_2	oxygen	11	poly, polymorph	neutrophil	10
OA	osteoarthritis	19	PONV	postoperative nausea and vomiting	12
OB	obstetrics	15	postop, post-op	postoperative	7
OCD	obsessive–compulsive disorder	17	pp	postprandial (after a meal)	8
OD	right eye	18	PPD	purified protein derivative (tuberculin)	11
ODS	Office of Dietary Supplements	8			
OGTT	oral glucose-tolerance test	16	PPI	proton pump inhibitor	12
OI	osteogenesis imperfecta	19	preop, pre-op	preoperative	7
OL	otolaryngology	18	PRICE	protection, rest, ice, compression, and elevation	20
OOB	out of bed	7			
OM	otitis media	18	prn	as needed	8
ORIF	open reduction internal fixation	19	PSA	prostate-specific antigen	14
ORL	otorhinolaryngology	18	PSF	posterior spinal fusion	19

A2

A2

ABBREVIATIONS	MEANING	CHAPTER
PSS	physiologic saline solution; progressive systemic sclerosis	7, 21
PSVT	paroxysmal supraventricular tachycardia	9
pt	patient	7
PT	physical therapy/therapist	20
PT, ProTime	prothrombin time	10
PTCA	percutaneous transluminal coronary angioplasty	9
PTSD	posttraumatic stress disorder	17
PTT	partial thromboplastin time	10
PUVA	psoralen ultraviolet A	21
PVC	premature ventricular contraction	9
PVD	peripheral vascular disease	9
PYP	pyrophosphate	9
qam	every morning	8
qd	every day	8
qh	every hour	8
q __ h	every __ hours	8
qid	four times per day	8
QNS	quantity not sufficient	7
qod	every other day	8
QS	quantity sufficient	7
R	respiration	7, 11
RA	rheumatoid arthritis	19
RAIU	radioactive iodine uptake	16
RAS	reticular activating system	17
RATx	radiation therapy	7
RBC	red blood cell; red blood (cell) count	10
RDS	respiratory distress syndrome	11
REM	rapid eye movement (sleep)	17
RIA	radioimmunoassay	16
RL	right lateral	7
RLL	right lower lobe (of lung)	11
RLQ	right lower quadrant	5
RLS	restless legs syndrome	20
RML	right middle lobe (of lung)	11
R/O	rule out	7
ROM	range of motion	20
ROS	review of systems	7
RSI	repetitive strain injury	20
RSV	respiratory syncytial virus	11
RTC	rotator cuff	20
RUL	right upper lobe (of lung)	11
RUQ	right upper quadrant	5
RV	residual volume	11
Rx	drug, prescription, therapy	7, 8
$\bar{s}$	without	8
S	sacrum; sacral	19
S_1	first heart sound	9
S_2	second heart sound	9
SA	sustained action; sinoatrial	8, 9
SARS	severe acute respiratory syndrome	11
SBE	subacute bacterial endocarditis	9
sc	without correction	18
SC, SQ, subcu.	subcutaneous(ly)	8
SCLE	subacute cutaneous lupus erythematosus	21
seg	neutrophil	10
SERM	selective estrogen receptor modulator	15, 19
SG	specific gravity	13

ABBREVIATIONS	MEANING	CHAPTER
SIADH	syndrome of inappropriate antidiuretic hormone	16
SIDS	sudden infant death syndrome	11
SITS	supraspinatus, infraspinatus, teres minor, subscapularis (muscles)	20
SK	streptokinase	9
SL	sublingual	8
SLE	systemic lupus erythematosus	10, 21
SPECT	single-photon emission-computed tomography	7
SPF	sun protection factor	21
SpO_2	oxygen percent saturation	11
SR	sustained release	8
$\overline{ss}$	half	8
SSEP	somatosensory evoked potentials	17
SSRI	selective serotonin reuptake inhibitor	17
ST	speech threshold	18
staph	staphylococcus	6
STAT	immediately	7
STD	sexually transmitted disease	14, 15
STI	sexually transmitted infection	14, 15
strep	streptococcus	6
STSG	split-thickness skin graft	21
supp	suppository	8
susp	suspension	8
SVD	spontaneous vaginal delivery	15
SVT	supraventricular tachycardia	9
T	temperature; thoracic vertebra	7, 19
T1DM	type 1 diabetes mellitus	16
T2DM	type 2 diabetes mellitus	16
T_3	triiodothyronine	16
T_4	thyroxine, tetraiodothyronine	16
T_7	free thyroxine index	16
T&A	tonsils and adenoids, tonsillectomy and adenoidectomy	11
tab	tablet	8
TAH	total abdominal hysterectomy	15
TB	tuberculosis	11
TBG	thyroxine-binding globulin	16
^{99m}Tc	technetium-99m	9
TCA	tricyclic antidepressant	17
TEE	transesophageal echocardiography	9
TGV	thoracic gas volume	11
THA	total hip arthroplasty	19
TIA	transient ischemic attack	17
tid	three times per day	8
tinct	tincture	8
TKA	total knee arthroplasty	19
TKO	to keep open	7
TLC	total lung capacity	11
Tm	maximal transport capacity; tubular maximum	13
TM	tympanic membrane	18
Tn	troponin	9
TNM	(primary) tumor, (regional lymph) nodes, (distant) metastases	7
TMJ	temporomandibular joint	19
tPA	tissue plasminogen activator	9
TPN	total parenteral nutrition	12
TPR	temperature, pulse, respiration	7
TPUR	transperineal urethral resection	14
TSE	testicular self-examination	14
TSH	thyroid-stimulating hormone	16
TSS	toxic shock syndrome	15

ABBREVIATIONS	MEANING	CHAPTER	ABBREVIATIONS	MEANING	CHAPTER
T(C)T	thrombin (clotting) time	10	VC	vital capacity	11
TTP	thrombotic thrombocytopenic purpura	10	VD	venereal disease	14, 15
			VDRL	Venereal Disease Research Laboratory	14
TTS	temporary threshold shift	18			
TUIP	transurethral incision of prostate	14	VEP	visual evoked potentials	17
TURP	transurethral resection of prostate	14	VF	ventricular fibrillation; visual field	9, 18
TV	tidal volume	11	v fib	ventricular fibrillation	9
Tx	traction	19	VLDL	very-low-density lipoprotein	9
			VPC	ventricular premature complex	9
U	units	8	VRSA	vancomycin-resistant *Staphylococcus aureus*	6
UA	urinalysis	13			
UAE	uterine artery embolization	15	VS	vital signs	7
UC	uterine contractions	15	VSD	ventricular septal defect	9
UG	urogenital	14	VT	ventricular tachycardia	9
UGI	upper gastrointestinal	12	VTE	venous thromboembolism	9
UMN	upper motor neuron	17	V_{TG}	thoracic gas volume	11
ung	ointment	8	vWF	von Willebrand factor	10
URI	upper respiratory infection	11			
USP	*United States Pharmacopeia*	8	WBC	white blood cell; white blood (cell) count	10
UTI	urinary tract infection	13, 14			
UTP	uterine term pregnancy	15	WD	well developed	7
UV	ultraviolet	7, 21	WNL	within normal limits	7
UVA	ultraviolet A	21	w/o	without	7
UVB	ultraviolet B	21	WPW	Wolff–Parkinson–White syndrome	9
VA	visual acuity	18	x	times	8
VAC	vacuum-assisted closure	21	XT	exotropia	18
VAD	ventricular assist device	9			
VBAC	vaginal birth after cesarean section	15	ZIFT	zygote intrafallopian transfer	15

A2

A3

WORD PART	MEANING	REFERENCE PAGE
a-	not, without, lack of, absence	37
ab-	away from	39
abdomin/o	abdomen	82
-ac	pertaining to	22
acous, acus	sound, hearing	536
acro-	extremity, end	82
ad-	toward, near	39
aden/o	gland	63
adip/o	fat	66
adren/o	adrenal gland, epinephrine	459
adrenal/o	adrenal gland	459
adrenocortic/o	adrenal cortex	459
aer/o	air, gas	134
-al	pertaining to	22
alg/o, algi/o, algesi/o	pain	105, 153
-algesia	pain	107, 532
-algia	pain	107
ambly-	dim	555
amnio	amnion	428
amyl/o	starch	66
an-	not, without, lack of, absence	37
andr/o	male	379
angi/o	vessel	188
an/o	anus	311
ante-	before	42
anti-	against	37, 153
aort/o	aorta	188
-ar	pertaining to	22
arter/o, arteri/o	artery	188
arteriol/o	arteriole	188
arthr/o	joint	579
-ary	pertaining to	22
-ase	enzyme	65
atel/o	incomplete	283
atlant/o	atlas	577
atri/o	atrium	187
audi/o	hearing	536
auto-	self	245
azo, azot/o	nitrogenous compounds	238
bacill/i, bacill/o	bacillus	110
bacteri/o	bacterium	110
balan/o	glans penis	389
bar/o	pressure	134
bi-	two, twice	34
bili	bile	312
blast/o, -blast	immature cell, productive cell, embryonic cell	65
blephar/o	eyelid	547
brachi/o	arm	82
brachy-	short	389

WORD PART	MEANING	REFERENCE PAGE
brady-	slow	106
bronch/o, bronch/i	bronchus	273
bronchiol	bronchiole	273
bucc/o	cheek	309
burs/o	bursa	579
calc/i	calcium	238
cali/o, calic/o	calyx	347
-capnia	carbon dioxide (level of)	272
carcin/o	cancer, carcinoma	105
cardi/o	heart	187
cec/o	cecum	310
-cele	hernia, localized dilation	107
celi/o	abdomen	82
centesis	puncture, tap	136
cephal/o	head	81
cerebell/o	cerebellum	493
cerebr/o	cerebrum	493
cervic/o	neck, cervix	81, 410
chem/o	chemical	153
cheil/o	lip	325
cholangi/o	bile duct	312
chol/e, chol/o	bile, gall	312
cholecyst/o	gallbladder	312
choledoch/o	common bile duct	312
chondr/o	cartilage	579
chori/o, choroid/o	choroid	548
chrom/o, chromat/o	color, stain	134
chron/o	time	134
circum-	around	83
clasis, -clasia	breaking	107
clitor/o, clitorid/o	clitoris	412
coccy, coccyg/o	coccyx	580
cochle/o	cochlea (of inner ear)	536
col/o, colon/o	colon	310
colp/o	vagina	411
contra-	against, opposite	37, 153
copro	feces	494
corne/o	cornea	547
cortic/o	outer portion, cerebral cortex	493
cost/o	rib	580
counter-	opposite, against	153
crani/o	skull, cranium	580
cry/o	cold	134
crypt/o	hidden	386
cus	sound, hearing	536
cyan/o-	blue	37
cycl/o	ciliary body, ciliary muscle (of eye)	548
cyst/o, cyst/i	filled sac or pouch, cyst, bladder, urinary bladder	105, 348
-cyte, cyt/o	cell	63

WORD PART	MEANING	REFERENCE PAGE	WORD PART	MEANING	REFERENCE PAGE
dacry/o	tear, lacrimal apparatus	547	gravida	pregnant woman	428
dacryocyst/o	lacrimal sac	547	gyn/o, gynec/o	woman	409
dactyl/o	finger, toe	82			
de-	down, without, removal, loss	38	hem/o, hemat/o	blood	236
dent/o, dent/i	tooth, teeth	309	hemi-	half, one side	34
derm/o, dermat/o	skin	645	-hemia	condition of blood	236
-desis	binding, fusion	136	hepat/o	liver	312
dextr/o-	right	43	hetero-	other, different, unequal	40
di-	two, twice	34	hidr/o	sweat, perspiration	645
dia-	through	39	hist/o, histi/o	tissue	63
dilation, dilatation	expansion, widening	109	homo-, homeo-	same, unchanging	40
dipl/o-	double	34	hydr/o	water, fluid	65
dis-	absence, removal, separation	38	hyper-	over, excess, increased, abnormally high	40
duoden/o	duodenum	310			
dys-	abnormal, painful, difficult	106	hypn/o	sleep	153
			hypo-	under, below, decreased, abnormally low	40
ec-	out, outside	43			
ectasia, ectasis	dilation, dilatation, distention	109	hypophys	pituitary, hypophysis	459
ecto-	out, outside	43	hyster/o	uterus	410
-ectomy	excision, surgical removal	136			
edema	accumulation of fluid, swelling	109	-ia	condition of	18
electr/o	electricity	134	-ian	specialist	20
embry/o	embryo	428	-ia/sis	condition of	18
emesis	vomiting	313	-iatrics	medical specialty	20
-emia	condition of blood	236	-iatr/o	physician	111
encephal/o	brain	493	-iatry	medical specialty	20
end/o-	in, within	43	-ic	pertaining to	22
endocrin/o	endocrine	459	-ical	pertaining to	22
enter/o	intestine	310	-ics	medical specialty	20
epi-	on, over	83	-ile	pertaining to	22
epididym/o	epididymis	382	ile/o	ileum	310
episi/o	vulva	412	ili/o	ilium	580
equi-	equal, same	40	im-	not	38
erg/o	work	134, 619	immun/o	immunity, immune system	237
erythr/o-	red, red blood cell	37, 236	in-	not	38
erythrocyt/o	red blood cell	236	infra-	below	83
esophag/o	esophagus	310	in/o	fiber, muscle fiber	619
-esthesia, -esthesi/o	sensation	532	insul/o	pancreatic islets	459
eu-	true, good, easy, normal	40	inter-	between	83
ex/o-	away from, outside	43	intra-	in, within	83
extra-	outside	83	ir, irit/o, irid/o	iris	548
			-ism	condition of	18
fasci/o	fascia	619	iso-	equal, same	40
fer	to carry	489	-ist	specialist	20
ferr/i, ferr/o	iron	238	-itis	inflammation	107
fet/o	fetus	428			
fibr/o	fiber	63	jejun/o	jejunum	310
-form	like, resembling	22	juxta-	near, beside	83
galact/o	milk	428	kali	potassium	238
gangli/o, ganglion/o	ganglion	492	kary/o	nucleus	63
gastr/o	stomach	310	kerat/o	cornea, keratin, horny layer of skin	548, 645
gen, genesis	origin, formation	65			
ger/e, ger/o	old age	34	kin/o, kine, kinesi/o, kinet/o	movement	619
-geusia	sense of taste	532			
gingiv/o	gum, gingiva	309	labi/o	lip	309
gli/o	neuroglia	492	labyrinth/o	labyrinth (inner ear)	536
glomerul/o	glomerulus	347	lacrim/o	tear, lacrimal apparatus	547
gloss/o	tongue	309	lact/o	milk	428
gluc/o	glucose	65	-lalia	speech, babble	494
glyc/o	sugar, glucose	65	lapar/o	abdominal wall	82
gnath/o	jaw	309	laryng/o	larynx	273
goni/o	angle	556, 596	lent/i	lens	548
-gram	record of data	135	-lepsy	seizure	494
-graph	instrument for recording data	135	leuk/o-	white, colorless, white blood cell	37, 236
-graphy	act of recording data	135			

A3

A3

WORD PART	MEANING	REFERENCE PAGE	WORD PART	MEANING	REFERENCE PAGE
leukocyt/o	white blood cell	236	olig/o-	few, scanty, deficiency of	40
-lexia	reading	494	-oma	tumor	107
lingu/o	tongue	309	onc/o	tumor	105
lip/o	fat, lipid	66	onych/o	nail	645
-listhesis	slipping	591	oo	ovum	409
lith	calculus, stone	105	oophor/o	ovary	409
-logy	study of	20	ophthalm/o	eye	547
lumb/o	lumbar region, lower back	82	-opia	eye, vision	549
lymphaden/o	lymph node	204	-opsia	vision	549
lymphangi/o	lymphatic vessel	205	opt/o	eye, vision	547
lymph/o	lymph, lymphatic system, lymphocyte	204, 237	orchid/o, orchi/o	testis	381
			or/o	mouth	309
lymphocyt/o	lymphocyte	237	ortho-	straight, correct, upright	41
-lysis	separation, loosening, dissolving, destruction	109	-ory	pertaining to	22
			osche/o	scrotum	381
-lytic	dissolving, reducing, loosening	153	-ose	sugar	65
			-o/sis	condition of	18
macro-	large, abnormally large	40	-osmia	sense of smell	532
mal-	bad, poor	106	oste/o	bone	579
malacia	softening	109	ot/o	ear	536
mamm/o	breast, mammary gland	412	-ous	pertaining to	22
-mania	excited state, obsession	494	ovari/o	ovary	409
mast/o	breast, mammary gland	412	ov/o, ovul/o	ovum	409
medull/o	inner part, medulla oblongata, spinal cord	493	-oxia	oxygen (level of)	272
			ox/y	oxygen, sharp, acute	238, 416
mega-, megalo-	large, abnormally large	41			
-megaly	enlargement	107	pachy-	thick	106
melan/o-	black, dark, melanin	37, 645	palat/o	palate	309
mening/o, meninge/o	meninges	492	palpebr/o	eyelid	547
men/o, mens	month, menstruation	409	pan-	all	40
mes/o-	middle	43	pancreat/o	pancreas	312
-meter	instrument for measuring	135	papill/o	nipple	63
metr/o	measure	549	para-	near, beside, abnormal	83, 532
metr/o, metr/i	uterus	410	para	woman who has given birth	428
-metry	measurement of	135	parathyr/o, parathyroid/o	parathyroid	459
micro-	small, one millionth	41			
-mimetic	mimicking, simulating	153	-paresis	partial paralysis	494
mon/o-	one	34	path/o, -pathy	disease, any disease of	105, 107
morph/o	form, structure	63	ped/o	foot, child	82, 592
muc/o	mucus, mucous membrane	63	pelvi/o	pelvis	580
multi-	many	35	-penia	decrease in, deficiency of	236
muscul/o	muscle	619	per-	through	39
myc/o	fungus, mold	110	peri-	around	83
myel/o	bone marrow, spinal cord	236, 492, 579	perine/o	perineum	412
my/o	muscle	619	periton, peritone/o	peritoneum	82
myring/o	tympanic membrane	536	-pexy	surgical fixation	136
myx/o	mucus	63	phac/o, phak/o	lens	548
			phag/o	eat, ingest	65
narc/o	stupor, unconsciousness	153, 493	pharm, pharmac/o	drug, medicine	153
nas/o	nose	273	pharyng/o	pharynx	273
nat/i	birth	428	-phasia	speech	494
natri	sodium	238	phil, -philic	attracting, absorbing	65
necrosis	death of tissue	109	phleb/o	vein	188
neo-	new	41	-phobia	fear	494
nephr/o	kidney	347	phon/o	sound, voice	134
neur/o, neur/i	nervous system, nerve	492	-phonia	voice	272
noct/i	night	138, 360	phot/o	light	134
non-	not	38	phren/o	diaphragm	274
normo-	normal	41	phrenic/o	phrenic nerve	274
nucle/o	nucleus	63	phyt/o	plant	152, 656
nyct/o	night, darkness	138	pituitar	pituitary, hypophysis	459
			plas, -plasia	formation, molding, development	65
ocul/o	eye	547	-plasty	plastic repair, plastic surgery, reconstruction	136
odont/o	tooth, teeth	309			
-odynia	pain	107	-plegia	paralysis	494
-oid	like, resembling	22	pleur/o	pleura	274

A3

WORD PART	MEANING	REFERENCE PAGE	WORD PART	MEANING	REFERENCE PAGE
-pnea	breathing	272	somat/o	body	63
pneum/o, pneumat/o	air, gas, lung, respiration	274	-some	body, small body	63
pneumon/o	lung	274	somn/i, somn/o	sleep	493
pod/o	foot	82	son/o	sound, ultrasound	134
-poiesis	formation, production	236	spasm	sudden contraction, cramp	109
poikilo-	varied, irregular	41	sperm/i	semen, spermatozoa	382
poly-	many, much	35	spermat/o	semen, spermatozoa	382
post-	after, behind	42	-spermia	condition of semen	382
pre-	before, in front of	42	spir/o	breathing	274
presby-	old	545	splen/o	spleen	205
prim/i-	first	34	spondyl/o	vertebra	580
pro-	before, in front of	42	staped/o, stapedi/o	stapes	536
proct/o	rectum	311	staphyl/o	grapelike cluster, staphylococcus	110
prostat/o	prostate	382	stasis	suppression, stoppage	109
prote/o	protein	66	steat/o	fatty	66
pseudo-	false	41	stenosis	narrowing, constriction	109
psych/o	mind	493	steth/o	chest	545
ptosis	dropping, downward displacement, prolapse	109	sthen/o	strength	545
			stoma, stomat/o	mouth	309
ptysis	spitting	284	-stomy	surgical creation of an opening	136
puer	child	437	strept/o-	twisted chain, streptococcus	110
pulm/o, pulmon/o	lung	274	sub-	below, under	83
pupill/o	pupil	548	super-	above, excess	40
pyel/o	renal pelvis	347	supra-	above	83
pylor/o	pylorus	310	syn-, sym-	together	43
py/o	pus	105	synov/i	synovial joint, synovial membrane	579
pyr/o, pyret/o	fever, fire	105, 153			
			tachy-	rapid	106
quadr/i-	four	35	tax/o	order, arrangement	626
			tel/e-, tel/o-	end	43
rachi/o	spine	580	ten/o, tendin/o	tendon	619
radicul/o	root of spinal nerve	492	terat/o	malformed fetus	436
radi/o	radiation, x-ray	134	test/o	testis, testicle	381
re-	again, back	41	tetra-	four	35
rect/o	rectum	311	thalam/o	thalamus	493
ren/o	kidney	347	therm/o	heat, temperature	134
reticul/o	network	63	thorac/o	chest, thorax	81
retin/o	retina	548	thromb/o	blood clot	237
retro-	behind, backward	83	thrombocyt/o	platelet, thrombocyte	237
rhabd/o	rod, muscle cell	627	thym/o	thymus gland	205
-rhage, -rhagia	bursting forth, profuse flow, hemorrhage	107	thyr/o, thyroid/o	thyroid	459
			toc/o	labor	428
-rhaphy	surgical repair, suture	136	-tome	instrument for incising (cutting)	137
-rhea	flow, discharge	107	-tomy	incision, cutting	137
-rhexis	rupture	108	ton/o	tone	619
rhin/o	nose	273	tonsill/o	tonsil	205
			tox/o, toxic/o	poison, toxin	105, 153
sacchar/o	sugar	66	toxin	poison	109
sacr/o	sacrum	580	trache/o	trachea	273
salping/o	tube, oviduct, eustachian (auditory) tube	409, 536	trans-	through	39
			tri-	three	35
-schisis	fissure, splitting	108, 580	trich/o	hair	645
scler/o	hard, sclera (of eye)	105, 547	-tripsy	crushing	137
sclerosis	hardening	109	trop,- tropic	act(ing) on, affect(ing)	65, 153
-scope	instrument for viewing or examining	135	troph/o, -trophy, -trophia	feeding, growth, nourishment	65
-scopy	examination of	135	tympan/o	tympanic cavity (middle ear), tympanic membrane	536
seb/o	sebum, sebaceous gland	645			
semi-	half, partial	34			
semin	semen	382	un-	not	38
sept/o	septum, dividing wall, partition	286	uni-	one	34
sial/o	saliva, salivary gland, salivary duct	309	-uresis	urination	349
sider/o	iron	238	ureter/o	ureter	348
sigmoid/o	sigmoid colon	311	urethr/o	urethra	348
sinistr/o	left	43	-uria	condition of urine, urination	349
-sis	condition of	18	ur/o	urine, urinary tract	348

WORD PART	MEANING	REFERENCE PAGE	WORD PART	MEANING	REFERENCE PAGE
urin/o	urine	348	vertebr/o	vertebra, spinal column	580
uter/o	uterus	409	vesic/o	urinary bladder	348
uve/o	uvea (of eye)	548	vesicul/o	seminal vesicle	382
uvul/o	uvula	309	vestibul/o	vestibule, vestibular apparatus (of ear)	536
vagin/o	sheath, vagina	411	vir/o	virus	110
valv/o, valvul/o	valve	187	vulv/o	vulva	412
varic/o	twisted and swollen vein, varix	200			
			xanth/o-	yellow	37
vascul/o	vessel	188	xen/o	foreign, strange	502
vas/o	vessel, duct, vas deferens	153, 188, 382	xero-	dry	106
ven/o, ven/i	vein	188			
ventricul/o	cavity, ventricle	187, 493	-y	condition of	18

Appendix Four

Meanings and Their Corresponding Word Parts

MEANING	WORD PART(S)	REFERENCE PAGE	MEANING	WORD PART(S)	REFERENCE PAGE
abdomen	abdomin/o, celi/o	82	binding	-desis	136
abdominal wall	lapar/o	82	birth	nat/i	428
abnormal	dys-, para-	106, 532	black	melan/o-	37, 645
abnormally high	hyper-	40	bladder	cyst/o, cyst/i	105, 348
abnormally large	macro-, mega-, megalo-	40, 41	bladder (urinary)	cyst/o, vesic/o	105
abnormally low	hypo-	40	blood	hem/o, hemat/o	236
above	super-, supra-	40, 83	blood (condition of)	-emia, -hemia	236
absence	a-, an-, dis-	37, 38	blood clot	thromb/o	236
absorb(ing)	phil, -philic	65	blue	cyan/o-	37
accumulation of fluid	edema	109	body	somat/o, -some	63
act of recording data	-graphy	135	bone	oste/o	579
act(ing) on	trop, -tropic	65, 153	bone marrow	myel/o	236, 492, 579
acute	ox/y	446	brain	encephal/o	493
adrenal gland	adren/o, adrenal/o	459	breaking	-clasis, -clasia	107
adrenaline	adren/o	459	breast	mamm/o, mast/o	412
adrenal	adren/o	459	breathing	-pnea, spir/o	272, 274
adrenal cortex	adrenocortic/o	459	bronchiole	bronchiol	273
affect(ing)	trop, -tropic	65	bronchus	bronch/i, bronch/o	273
after	post-	42	bursa	burs/o	579
again	re-	41	bursting forth	-rhage, -rhagia	107
against	anti-, contra-, counter-	37, 153			
air	aer/o, pneumat/o	134, 274	calcium	calc/i	238
all	pan-	40	calculus	lith	105
amnion, amniotic sac	amnio	428	calyx	cali/o, calic/o	347
angle	goni/o	556, 596	cancer	carcin/o	105
anus	an/o	311	carbon dioxide	-capnia	272
any disease of	-pathy	107	carcinoma	carcin/o	105
aorta	aort/o	188	carry	fer	489
arm	brachi/o	82	cartilage	chondr/o	579
around	circum-, peri-	83	cavity	ventricul/o	187, 493
arrangement	tax/o	626	cecum	cec/o	310
arteriole	arteriol/o	188	cell	-cyte, cyt/o	63
artery	arter/o, arteri/o	188	cerebellum	cerebell/o	493
atlas	atlant/o	577	cerebral cortex	cortic/o	493
atrium	atri/o	187	cerebrum	cerebr/o	493
attract(ing)	phil, -philic	65	cervix	cervic/o	410
away from	ab-, ex/o-	39, 43	chain (twisted)	strept/o	110
			cheek	bucc/o	309
babble	-lalia	494	chemical	chem/o	153
bacillus	bacill/i, bacill/o	110	chest	thorac/o, steth/o	81
back	re-	41	child	ped/o, puer	437, 592
backward	retro-	83	choroid	chori/o, choroid/o	548
bacterium	bacteri/o	110	ciliary body	cycl/o	548
bad	mal-	106	ciliary muscle	cycl/o	548
before	ante-, pre-, pro-	42	clitoris	clitor/o, clitorid/o	412
behind	post-, retro-	42, 83	clot	thromb/o	237
below	hypo-, infra-, sub-	40, 83	coccyx	coccy, coccyg/o	580
beside	para-, juxta-	83	cochlea	cochle/o	536
between	inter-	83	cold	cry/o	134
bile	bili, chol/e, chol/o	312	colon	col/o, colon/o	310
bile duct	cholangi/o	312	color	chrom/o, chromat/o	134

MEANING	WORD PART(S)	REFERENCE PAGE
colorless	leuk/o-	37
common bile duct	choledoch/o	312
condition of	-ia, -ia/sis, -ism, -o/sis, -sis, -y	18
condition of blood	-emia, -hemia	236
condition of urine, urination	-uria	349
condition of semen	-spermia	382
constriction	stenosis	109
contraction (sudden)	spasm	109
cornea	corne/o, kerat/o	547
correct	ortho-	41
cramp	spasm	109
cranium	crani/o	580
crushing	-tripsy	137
cutting	-tomy	137
cutting instrument	-tome	137
cyst	cyst/o, cyst/i	105
dark	melan/o-	37, 645
darkness	nyct/o	138
data	-gram	135
death of tissue	necrosis	109
decreased, decrease in	hypo-, -penia	40, 236
deficiency of	oligo-, -penia	40, 236
destruction	lysis	109
development	plas, -plasia	65
diaphragm	phren/o	274
different	hetero-	40
difficult	dys-	106
dilatation, dilation	ectasia, ectasis	109
distention	ectasia, ectasis	109
dim	ambly-	555
discharge	-rhea	107
disease	path/o, -pathy	105
dissolving	lysis, -lytic	153
distention	ectasia, ectasis	109
double	dipl/o-	34
down	de-	38
dropping, downward displacement	ptosis	109
drug	pharm, pharmac/o	153
dry	xero-	106
duct	vas/o	188
ductus deferens	vas/o	382
duodenum	duoden/o	310
ear	ot/o	536
easy	eu-	40
eat	phag/o	65
egg cell	oo, ov/o, ovul/o	409
electricity	electr/o	134
embryo	embry/o	428
embryonic cell	-blast, blast/o	65
end	tel/e, tel/o, acro	43, 82
endocrine	endocrin/o	459
enlargement	-megaly	107
enzyme	-ase	65
epididymis	epididym/o	382
epinephrine	adren/o	459
equal	iso-, equi-	40
erythrocyte	erythr/o, erythrocyt/o	236
esophagus	esophag/o	310
eustachian (auditory) tube, tube, oviduct	salping/o	536
examination of	-scopy	135

MEANING	WORD PART(S)	REFERENCE PAGE
excess	hyper-, super-	40
excision	-ectomy	136
excited state	mania	494
expansion	dilation, dilatation, ectasia, ectasis	109
extremity	acro	82
eye	ocul/o, ophthalm/o, opt/o, -opia	547
eyelid	blephar/o, palpebr/o	547
false	pseudo-	41
fascia	fasci/o	619
fat	adip/o, lip/o	66
fatty	steat/o	66
fear	-phobia	494
feces	copro	494
feeding	troph/o, -trophy, -trophia	65
fetus	fet/o	428
fetus (malformed)	terat/o	436
fever	pyr/o, pyret/o	105, 153
few	oligo-	40
fiber	fibr/o, in/o	63, 619
filled sac or pouch	cyst/o, cyst/i	105
finger	dactyl/o	82
fire	pyr/o, pyret/o	105
first	prim/i	34
fissure	-schisis	108, 580
fixation (surgical)	-pexy	136
flow	-rhea	107
fluid	hydr/o	65
foot	ped/o, pod/o	82
foreign	xen/o	502
form	morph/o	63
formation	gen, genesis, plas, -plasia, -poiesis	65, 236
four	quadr/i, tetra-	35
fungus	myc/o	110
fusion	-desis	136
gall	chol/e, chol/o	312
gallbladder	cholecyst/o	312
ganglion	gangli/o, ganglion/o	492
gas	aer/o, pneum/o, pneumon/o, pneumat/o	134, 274
gingiva (gum)	gingiv/o	309
gland	aden/o	63
glans penis	balan/o	389
glomerulus	glomerul/o	347
glucose	gluc/o, glyc/o	65
good	eu-	40
grapelike cluster	staphyl/o	110
growth	troph/o, -trophy, -trophia	65
gum, gingiva	gingiv/o	309
hair	trich/o	645
half	hemi-, semi-	34
hard	scler/o	105
hardening	sclerosis	109
head	cephal/o	81
hearing	acous, acus, audi/o, cus	536
heart	cardi/o	187
heat	therm/o	134
hemorrhage	-rhage, -rhagia	107
hernia	-cele	107
hidden	crypt/o	386
horny layer of skin	kerat/o	645
hypophysis	hypophys, pituitar	459

MEANING	WORD PART(S)	REFERENCE PAGE	MEANING	WORD PART(S)	REFERENCE PAGE
islets (pancreatic)	insul/o	459	many	multi-, poly-	35
ileum	ile/o	310	marrow	myel/o	236
ilium	ili/o	580	measure	metr/o	549
immature cell	blast/o, -blast	65	measuring instrument	-meter	134
immune system	immun/o	237	measurement of	-metry	135
immunity	immun/o	237	medical specialty	-ics, -iatrics, iatry	20
in	end/o-, intra-	43, 83	medicine	pharm, pharmac/o	153
in front of	pre-, pro-	42	medulla oblongata	medull/o	493
incision of	-tomy	137	melanin	melan/o	645
incomplete	atel/o-	283	meninges	mening/o, meninge/o	492
increased	hyper-	40	menstruation	men/o, mens	409
inflammation	-itis	107	middle	meso-	43
ingest	phag/o	65	milk	galact/o, lact/o	428
instrument for incising (cutting)	-tome	138	mimicking	-mimetic	153
			mind	psych/o	493
instrument for measuring	-meter	135	mold	myc/o	110
			molding	plas, -plasia	65
instrument for recording data	-graph	135	month	men/o, mens	409
			mouth	or/o, stoma, stomat/o	309
instrument for viewing or examining	-scope	135	movement	kin/o, kine, -kinesi/o, kinet/o	619
intestine	enter/o	310	much	poly-	35
iris	ir, irid/o, irit/o	548	mucus	muc/o, myx/o	63
iron	ferr/i, ferr/o, sider/o	238	mucous membrane	muc/o	63
irregular	poikilo-	41	muscle	my/o, muscul/o	619
			muscle cell	rhabd/o	627
jaw	gnath/o	309	muscle fiber	in/o	619
jejunum	jejun/o	310			
joint	arthr/o	579	nail	onych/o	645
			narrowing	stenosis	109
keratin	kerat/o	645	near	ad-, juxta-, para-	39, 83
kidney	nephr/o, ren/o	347	neck	cervic/o	81, 410
			nerve, nervous system, nervous tissue	neur/o, neur/i	492
labor	toc/o	428			
labyrinth	labyrinth/o	536	network	reticul/o	63
lack of	a-, an-	37	neuroglia	gli/o	492
lacrimal apparatus	dacry/o, lacrim/o	547	new	neo-	41
lacrimal sac	dacryocyst/o	547	night	noct/i, nyct/o	138, 360
large	macro-, mega-, megalo-	40, 41	nipple	papill/o	63
larynx	laryng/o	273	nitrogenous compounds	azo, azot/o	238
left	sinistr/o	43			
lens	lent/i, phac/o, phak/o	548	normal	eu-, normo-	40, 41
leukocyte	leuk/o, leukocyt/o	236	nose	nas/o, rhin/o	273
level of carbon dioxide	-capnia	272	not	a-, an-, in-, im-, non-, un-	37, 38
level of oxygen	-oxia	272	nourishment	troph/o, -trophy, -trophia	65
light	phot/o	134	nucleus	kary/o, nucle/o	63
like	-form, -oid	22			
lip	labi/o, cheil/o	309, 325	obsession	mania	494
lipid	lip/o	66	old	presby-	545
liver	hepat/o	312	old age	ger/e, ger/o	34
localized dilation	-cele	107	on	epi-	82
loosening	lysis, -lytic	109, 153	one	mon/o-, uni-	34
loss	de-	38	one side	hemi-	34
lumbar region, lower back	lumb/o	82	opening (created surgically)	-stomy	136
lung, lungs	pneum/o, pneumat/o, pneumon/o, pulm/o, pulmon/o	274	opposite	contra-, counter-	37, 153
			order	tax/o	626
lymph, lymphatic system	lymph/o	204	origin	gen, genesis	65
			other	hetero-	40
lymph node	lymphaden/o	204	out, outside	ec-, ecto-, ex/o, extra-	43, 83
lymphatic vessel	lymphangi/o	205	outer portion	cortic/o	493
lymphocyte	lympho, lymphocyt/o	237	ovary	ovari/o, oophor/o	409
			over	hyper-, epi-	40, 83
male	andr/o	379	oviduct	salping/o	410
malformed fetus	terat/o	436	ovum	oo, ov/o, ovul/o	409
mammary gland	mamm/o, mast/o	412	oxygen	ox/y, -oxia	238, 272

A4

A4

MEANING	WORD PART(S)	REFERENCE PAGE	MEANING	WORD PART(S)	REFERENCE PAGE
pain	-algia, -odynia	107	root of spinal nerve	radicul/o	492
pain	-algesia, alg/o, algi/o, algesi/o	105, 107, 153, 532	rupture	-rhexis	108
painful	dys-	106	sac (filled)	cyst/o, cyst/i	105
palate	palat/o	309	sacrum	sacr/o	580
pancreas	pancreat/o	312	saliva, salivary gland, salivary duct	sial/o	309
pancreatic islets	insul/o	459	same	equi-, homo-, homeo-, iso-	40
paralysis	-plegia	494	sclera (of eye)	scler/o	547
paralysis (partial)	-paresis	494	scanty	oligo-	40
parathyroid	parathyr/o, parathyroid/o	459	scrotum	osche/o	381
partial	semi-	34	sebum, sebaceous gland	seb/o	645
partial paralysis	-paresis	494	seizure	-lepsy	494
partition	sept/o	286	self	auto-	245
pelvis	pelvi/o	580	semen	semin, sperm/i, spermat/o	382
perineum	perine/o	412	semen, condition of	-spermia	382
peritoneum	periton, peritone/o	82	seminal vesicle	vesicul/o	382
perspiration	hidr/o	645	sensation	-esthesia, esthesi/o	532
pertaining to	-ac, -al, -ar, -ary, -ic, -ical, -ile, -ory, -ous	22	sense of smell	-osmia	532
pharynx	pharyng/o	273	sense of taste	-geusia	532
phrenic nerve	phrenic/o	274	separation	dis-, -lysis	38, 109
physician	iatr/o	111	septum	sept/o	286
pituitary	pituitary, hypophys	459	sharp	ox/y	446
plant	phyt/o	152, 656	short	brachy-	389
plastic repair, plastic surgery	-plasty	136	sigmoid colon	sigmoid/o	311
platelet	thrombocyt/o	237	simulating	-mimetic	153
pleura	pleur/o	274	skin	derm/o, dermat/o	645
poison	tox/o, toxic/o, toxin	105, 153	skull	crani/o	580
poor	mal-	106	sleep	hypn/o, somn/o, somn/i	153, 493
potassium	kali	238	slipping	-listhesis	591
pouch (filled)	cyst/o, cyst/i	105	slow	brady-	106
pregnant woman	gravida	428	small	micro-	41
pressure	bar/o	134	small body	-some	63
production	-poiesis	236	smell (sense of)	-osmia	532
productive cell	blast/o, -blast	65	sodium	natri	238
profuse flow	-rhage, -rhagia	107	softening	malacia	109
prolapse	ptosis	109	sound	phon/o, son/o, acous, acus, cus	134, 536
prostate	prostat/o	382	specialist	-ian, -ist, -logist	20
protein	prote/o	66	specialty	-ics, -iatrics, -iatry	20
puncture	centesis	136	speech	-phasia, -lalia	494
pupil	pupill/o	548	sperm, spermatozoa	sperm/i, spermat/o	382
pus	py/o	105	spinal column	vertebr/o	580
pylorus	pylor/o	310	spinal cord	myel/o, medull/o	492
			spinal nerve root	radicul/o	492
radiation	radi/o	134	spine	rachi/o	580
rapid	tachy-	106	spitting	ptysis	284
reading	-lexia	494	spleen	splen/o	205
reconstruction	-plasty	136	splitting	-schisis	108
record of data	-gram	135	stain	chrom/o, chromat/o	134
recording data (act of)	-graphy	135	stapes	staped/o, stapedi/o	536
rectum	rect/o, proct/o	311	staphylococcus	staphyl/o	110
red	erythr/o-	37	starch	amyl/o	66
red blood cell	erythr/o, erythrocyt/o	236	stomach	gastr/o	310
reducing	-lytic	153	stone	lith	105
removal	de-, dis-	38	stoppage	stasis	109
removal (surgical)	-ectomy	136	straight	ortho-	41
renal pelvis	pyel/o	347	strength	sthen/o	545
repair (plastic)	-plasty	136	streptococcus	strept/o	110
repair (surgical)	-rhaphy	136	structure	morph/o	63
respiration	pneum/o, pneumat/o	274	study of	-logy	20
resembling	-form, -oid	22	stupor	narc/o	153, 493
retina	retin/o	548	sugar	glyc/o, sacchar/o, -ose	65
rib	cost/o	580	sudden contraction	spasm	109
right	dextr/o-	43	suppression	stasis	109
rod	rhabd/o	627	surgery (plastic)	-plasty	136

MEANING	WORD PART(S)	REFERENCE PAGE
surgical creation of an opening	-stomy	136
surgical fixation	-pexy	136
surgical removal	-ectomy	136
surgical repair	-rhaphy	136
suture	-rhaphy	136
sweat	hidr/o	645
swelling	edema	109
synovial fluid, joint, membrane	synov/i	579
tap	centesis	136
taste (sense of)	-geusia	532
tear	dacry/o, lacrim/o	547
teeth	dent/o, denti, odont/o	309
temperature	therm/o	134
tendon	ten/o, tendin/o	619
testicle	test/o	381
testis	test/o, orchid/o, orchi/o	381
thalamus	thalam/o	493
thick	pachy-	106
thorax	thorac/o	81
three	tri-	35
thrombocyte	thrombocyt/o	237
through	dia-, per-, trans-	39
thymus gland	thym/o	205
thyroid	thyr/o, thyroid/o	459
time	chron/o	134
tissue	hist/o, histi/o	63
tissue death	necrosis	109
toe	dactyl/o	82
together	syn-, sym-	43
tone	ton/o	619
tongue	gloss/o, lingu/o	309
tonsil	tonsill/o	205
tooth	-dent/o, dent/i, odont/o	309
toward	ad-	39
toxin	tox/o, toxic/o	153
trachea	trache/o	273
true	eu-	40
tube	salping/o	410, 536
tumor	onc/o, -oma	105, 107
twice	bi-, di-	34
twisted chain	strept/o	110
twisted and swollen vein	varic/o	200
two	bi-, di-, dipl/o-	34
tympanic cavity	tympan/o	536
tympanic membrane	myring/o, tympan/o	536
ultrasound	son/o	134
unchanging	homo-, homeo-	40

MEANING	WORD PART(S)	REFERENCE PAGE
unconsciousness	narc/o	493
under	hypo-, sub-	40, 83
unequal	hetero-	40
upright	ortho-	41
ureter	ureter/o	348
urethra	urethr/o	348
urinary bladder	cyst/o, vesic/o	348
urine, urinary tract, urination	ur/o, -uria	348
urination	-uresis	349
urine	urin/o	348
uterus	hyster/o, metr/o, metr/i, uter/o	410
uvea	uve/o	548
uvula	uvul/o	309
vagina	colp/o, vagin/o	411
valve	valv/o, valvul/o	187
varicose vein, varix	varic/o	200
varied	poikilo-	41
vas deferens	vas/o	382
vein	ven/o, ven/i, phleb/o	188
vein (twisted, swollen)	varic/o	200
ventricle	ventricul/o	187, 493
vertebra	spondyl/o, vertebr/o	580
vessel	angi/o, vas/o, vascul/o	153, 188, 382
vestibular apparatus, vestibule	vestibul/o	536
virus	vir/o	110
vision	opt/o, -opia, -opsia	549
voice	phon/o, -phonia	134, 272
vomiting	emesis	321
vulva	episi/o, vulv/o	412
wall, dividing wall	sept/o	286
water	hydr/o	65
white	leuk/o-	37
white blood cell	leuk/o, leukocyt/o	236
widening	ectasia, ectasis, dilation, dilatation	109
within	end/o-, intra-	43, 83
without	a-, an-, de-	37, 38
woman	gyn/o, gynec/o	409
woman who has given birth	para	428
work	erg/o	134, 619
x-ray	radi/o	134
yellow	xanth/o-	37

A4

ROOT	MEANING	REFERENCE PAGE	ROOT	MEANING	REFERENCE PAGE
abdomin/o	abdomen	82	chem/o	chemical	153
acous, acus	sound, hearing	536	cholangi/o	bile duct	312
acro	extremity, end	82	chol/e, chol/o	bile, gall	312
aden/o	gland	63	cholecyst/o	gallbladder	312
adip/o	fat	66	choledoch/o	common bile duct	312
adren/o	adrenal gland, epinephrine	459	chondr/o	cartilage	579
adrenal/o	adrenal gland	459	copro	feces	494
adrenocortic/o	adrenal cortex	459	chori/o, choroid/o	choroid	548
aer/o	air, gas	134	chrom/o, chromat/o	color, stain	134
alg/o, algi/o, algesi/o	pain	105, 153	chron/o	time	134
amnio	amnion	428	clasis	breaking	107
amyl/o	starch	66	clitor/o, clitorid/o	clitoris	412
andr/o	male	379	coccy, coccyg/o	coccyx	580
angi/o	vessel	188	cochle/o	cochlea (of inner ear)	536
an/o	anus	311	col/o, colon/o	colon	310
aort/o	aorta	188	colp/o	vagina	411
arter/o, arteri/o	artery	188	corne/o	cornea	547
arteriol/o	arteriole	188	cortic/o	outer portion, cerebral cortex	493
arthr/o	joint	579	cost/o	rib	580
atel/o	incomplete	283	crani/o	skull, cranium	580
atlant/o	atlas	577	cry/o	cold	134
atri/o	atrium	187	crypt/o	hidden	386
audi/o	hearing	536	cus	sound, hearing	536
azo, azot/o	nitrogenous compounds	238	cycl/o	ciliary body, ciliary muscle (of eye)	548
			cyst/o, cyst/i	filled sac or pouch, cyst, bladder, urinary bladder	105, 348
bacill/i, bacill/o	bacillus	110			
bacteri/o	bacterium	110	cyt/o	cell	63
balan/o	glans penis	39			
bar/o	pressure	134	dacry/o	tear, lacrimal apparatus	547
bili	bile	312	dacryocyst/o	lacrimal sac	547
blast/o	immature cell, productive cell, embryonic cell	65	dactyl/o	finger, toe	82
			dent/o, dent/i	tooth, teeth	309
blephar/o	eyelid	547	derm/o, dermat/o	skin	645
brachi/o	arm	82	dilation, dilatation	expansion, widening	109
bronch/i, bronch/o	bronchus	273	duoden/o	duodenum	310
bronchiol	bronchiole	273			
bucc/o	cheek	309	ectasia, ectasis	dilation, dilatation, distention	109
burs/o	bursa	579	edema	accumulation of fluid, swelling	109
			electr/o	electricity	134
calc/i	calcium	238	embry/o	embryo	428
cali/o, calic/o	calyx	347	emesis	vomiting	321
carcin/o	cancer, carcinoma	105	encephal/o	brain	493
cardi/o	heart	187	endocrin/o	endocrine	459
cec/o	cecum	310	enter/o	intestine	310
celi/o	abdomen	82	epididym/o	epididymis	382
centesis	puncture, tap	136	episi/o	vulva	412
cephal/o	head	81	erg/o	work	134, 619
cerebell/o	cerebellum	493	erythr/o-	red, red blood cell	37, 236
cerebr/o	cerebrum	493	erythrocyt/o	red blood cell	236
cervic/o	neck, cervix	81, 410	esophag/o	esophagus	310
cheil/o	lip	325			

ROOT	MEANING	REFERENCE PAGE
fasci/o	fascia	619
fer	carry	489
ferr/i, ferr/o	iron	238
fet/o	fetus	428
fibr/o	fiber	63
galact/o	milk	428
gangli/o, ganglion/o	ganglion	492
gastr/o	stomach	310
gen	origin, formation	65
ger/e, ger/o	old age	34
gingiv/o	gum, gingiva	309
gli/o	neuroglia	492
glomerul/o	glomerulus	347
gloss/o	tongue	309
gluc/o	glucose	65
glyc/o	sugar, glucose	65
gnath/o	jaw	309
goni/o	angle	556, 596
gravida	pregnant woman	428
gyn/o, gynec/o	woman	409
hem/o, hemat/o	blood	236
hepat/o	liver	312
hidr/o	sweat, perspiration	645
hist/o, histi/o	tissue	63
hydr/o	water, fluid	65
hypn/o	sleep	153
hypophys	pituitary, hypophysis	459
hyster/o	uterus	410
iatr/o	physician	111
ile/o	ileum	310
ili/o	ilium	580
immun/o	immunity, immune system	237
in/o	fiber, muscle fiber	619
insul/o	pancreatic islets	459
ir, irit/o, irid/o	iris	548
jejun/o	jejunum	310
kali	potassium	238
kary/o	nucleus	63
kerat/o	cornea, keratin, horny layer of skin	548, 645
kin/o, kine, kinesi/o, kinet/o	movement	619
labi/o	lip	309
labyrinth/o	labyrinth (inner ear)	536
lacrim/o	tear, lacrimal apparatus	547
lact/o	milk	428
lapar/o	abdominal wall	82
laryng/o	larynx	273
lent/i	lens	548
leuk/o	white, colorless, white blood cell	37, 236
leukocyt/o	white blood cell	236
lingu/o	tongue	309
lip/o	fat, lipid	66
listhesis	slipping	591
lith	calculus, stone	105
lumb/o	lumbar region, lower back	82
lymphaden/o	lymph node	204
lymphangi/o	lymphatic vessel	205
lymph/o	lymph, lymphatic system, lymphocyte	205, 237

ROOT	MEANING	REFERENCE PAGE
lymph/o, lymphocyt/o	lymphocyte	237
lysis	separation, loosening, dissolving, destruction	109
malacia	softening	109
mamm/o	breast, mammary gland	412
mania	excited state, obsession	494
mast/o	breast, mammary gland	412
medull/o	inner part, medulla oblongata, spinal cord	493
melan/o	dark, black, melanin	37, 645
mening/o, meninge/o	meninges	492
men/o, mens	month, menstruation	409
metr/o	measure	549
metr/o, metr/i	uterus	410
morph/o	form, structure	63
muc/o	mucus, mucous membrane	63
muscul/o	muscle	619
myc/o	fungus, mold	110
myel/o	bone marrow, spinal cord	236, 492, 579
my/o	muscle	619
myring/o	tympanic membrane	536
myx/o	mucus	63
narc/o	stupor, unconsciousness	153, 493
nas/o	nose	273
nat/i	birth	428
natri	sodium	238
necrosis	death of tissue	109
nephr/o	kidney	347
neur/o, neur/i	nervous system, nerve	492
noct/i	night	138
nucle/o	nucleus	63
nyct/o	night, darkness	138
ocul/o	eye	547
odont/o	tooth, teeth	309
onc/o	tumor	105
onych/o	nail	645
oo	ovum	409
oophor/o	ovary	409
ophthalm/o	eye	547
opt/o	eye, vision	547
orchid/o, orchi/o	testis	381
or/o	mouth	309
osche/o	scrotum	381
oste/o	bone	579
ot/o	ear	536
ovari/o	ovary	409
ov/o, ovul/o	ovum	409
ox/y	oxygen, sharp, acute	238, 446
palat/o	palate	309
palpebr/o	eyelid	547
pancreat/o	pancreas	312
papill/o	nipple	63
para	woman who has given birth	428
parathyr/o, parathyroid/o	parathyroid	459
paresis	partial paralysis	494
path/o	disease, any disease of	100, 105
ped/o	foot, child	82, 592
pelvi/o	pelvis	580
perine/o	perineum	412
periton, peritone/o	peritoneum	82

A5

ROOT	MEANING	REFERENCE PAGE	ROOT	MEANING	REFERENCE PAGE
phac/o, phak/o	lens	548	spermat/o	semen, spermatozoa	382
phag/o	eat, ingest	65	spir/o	breathing	274
pharm, pharmac/o	drug, medicine	153	splen/o	spleen	205
pharyng/o	pharynx	273	spondyl/o	vertebra	580
phil	attracting, absorbing	65	staped/o, stapedi/o	stapes	536
phleb/o	vein	188	staphyl/o	grapelike cluster, staphylococcus	110
phobia	fear	494	stasis	suppression, stoppage	109
phon/o	sound, voice	134	steat/o	fatty	66
phot/o	light	134	stenosis	narrowing, constriction	109
phren/o	diaphragm	274	steth/o	chest	545
phrenic/o	phrenic nerve	274	sthen/o	strength	545
phyt/o	plant	152, 656	stoma, stomat/o	mouth	309
pituitar	pituitary, hypophysis	459	synov/i	synovial joint, synovial membrane	579
plas	formation, molding, development	65			
pleur/o	pleura	274	tax/o	order, arrangement	626
pneum/o, pneumat/o	air, gas, lung, respiration	274	ten/o, tendin/o	tendon	619
pneumon/o	lung	274	terat/o	malformed fetus	436
pod/o	foot	82	test/o	testis, testicle	381
proct/o	rectum	311	thalam/o	thalamus	493
prostat/o	prostate	382	therm/o	heat, temperature	134
prote/o	protein	66	thorac/o	chest, thorax	81
psych/o	mind	493	thromb/o	blood clot	237
ptosis	dropping, downward displacement, prolapse	109	thrombocyt/o	platelet, thrombocyte	237
			thym/o	thymus gland	205
ptysis	spitting	284	thyr/o, thyroid/o	thyroid	459
puer	child	437	toc/o	labor	428
pulm/o, pulmon/o	lung	274	ton/o	tone	619
pupill/o	pupil	548	tonsill/o	tonsil	205
pyel/o	renal pelvis	347	tox/o, toxic/o	poison, toxin	105, 153
pylor/o	pylorus	310	trache/o	trachea	273
py/o	pus	105	trich/o	hair	645
pyr/o, pyret/o	fever, fire	105, 153	trop	act(ing) on, affect(ing)	65, 153
			troph/o	feeding, growth, nourishment	65
rachi/o	spine	580	tympan/o	tympanic cavity (middle ear), tympanic membrane	536
radicul/o	root of spinal nerve	492			
radi/o	radiation, x-ray	134			
rect/o	rectum	311	ureter/o	ureter	348
ren/o	kidney	347	urethr/o	urethra	348
reticul/o	network	63	ur/o	urine, urinary tract	348
retin/o	retina	548	urin/o	urine	348
rhabd/o	rod, muscle cell	627	uter/o	uterus	410
rhin/o	nose	273	uve/o	uvea (of eye)	548
			uvul/o	uvula	309
racchar/o	sugar	66			
sacchar/o	sugar	66	vagin/o	sheath, vagina	411
sacr/o	sacrum	580	valv/o, valvul/o	valve	187
salping/o	tube, oviduct, eustachian (auditory) tube	410, 536	varic/o	twisted and swollen vein, varix	200
schisis	fissure	580	vascul/o	vessel	188
scler/o	hard, sclera (of eye)	105, 547	vas/o	vessel, duct, vas deferens	153, 188, 382
sclerosis	hardening	109	ven/o, ven/i	vein	188
seb/o	sebum, sebaceous gland	645	ventricul/o	cavity, ventricle	187, 493
semin	semen	382	vertebr/o	vertebra, spinal column	580
sept/o	septum, partition, dividing wall	286	vesic/o	urinary bladder	348
sial/o	saliva, salivary gland, salivary duct	309	vesicul/o	seminal vesicle	382
sider/o	iron	238	vestibul/o	vestibule, vestibular apparatus (of ear)	536
sigmoid/o	sigmoid colon	311	vir/o	virus	110
somat/o	body	63	vulv/o	vulva	412
somn/i, somn/o	sleep	493			
son/o	sound, ultrasound	134	xen/o	foreign, strange	502
spasm	sudden contraction, cramp	109			
sperm/i	semen, spermatozoa	382			

A5

APPENDIX SIX ∘ SUFFIXES

SUFFIX	MEANING	REFERENCE PAGE
-ac	pertaining to	22
-al	pertaining to	22
-algesia	pain	107, 532
-algia	pain	107
-ar	pertaining to	22
-ary	pertaining to	22
-ase	enzyme	65
-blast	immature cell, productive cell, embryonic cell	65
-capnia	carbon dioxide (level of)	272
-cele	hernia, localized dilation	107
-centesis	puncture, tap	136
-clasis, -clasia	breaking	107
-cyte	cell	63
-desis	binding, fusion	136
-dilation, -dilatation	expansion, widening	109
-ectasia,- ectasis	dilation, dilatation, distention	109
-ectomy	excision, surgical removal	136
-edema	accumulation of fluid, swelling	109
-emia	condition of blood	236
-esthesia, -esthesi/o	sensation	532, 593
-form	like, resembling	22
-gen, -genesis	origin, formation	65
-geusia	sense of taste	532
-gram	record of data	135
-graph	instrument for recording data	135
-graphy	act of recording data	135
-hemi	half, one side	34
-hemia	condition of blood	236
-ia	condition of	18
-ian	specialist	20
-ia/sis	condition of	18
-iatrics	medical specialty	20
-iatry	medical specialty	20
-ic	pertaining to	22
-ical	pertaining to	22
-ics	medical specialty	20
-ile	pertaining to	22
-ism	condition of	18
-ist	specialist	20
-itis	inflammation	107

SUFFIX	MEANING	REFERENCE PAGE
-lalia	speech, babble	494
-lepsy	seizure	494
-lexia	reading	494
-logy	study of	20
-lysis	separation, loosening, dissolving, destruction	109
-lytic	dissolving, reducing, loosening	153
-malacia	softening	109
-mania	excited state, obsession	494
-megaly	enlargement	107
-meter	instrument for measuring	135
-metry	measurement of	135
-mimetic	mimicking, simulating	153
-necrosis	death of tissue	109
-odynia	pain	107
-oid	like, resembling	22
-oma	tumor	107
-opia	eye, vision	549
-opsia	vision	549
-ory	pertaining to	22
-ose	sugar	65
-o/sis	condition of	18
-osmia	sense of smell	532
-ous	pertaining to	22
-oxia	oxygen (level of)	272
-paresis	partial paralysis	494
-pathy	disease, any disease of	107
-penia	decrease in, deficiency of	236
-pexy	surgical fixation	136
-phasia	speech	494
-philic	attracting, absorbing	65
-phobia	fear	494
-phonia	voice	272
-plasia	formation, molding, development	65
-plasty	plastic repair, plastic surgery, reconstruction	136
-plegia	paralysis	494
-pnea	breathing	272
-poiesis	formation, production	236
-ptosis	dropping, downward displacement, prolapse	109
-rhage, -rhagia	bursting forth, profuse flow, hemorrhage	107
-rhaphy	surgical repair, suture	136

691

A6

SUFFIX	MEANING	REFERENCE PAGE	SUFFIX	MEANING	REFERENCE PAGE
-rhea	flow, discharge	107	-stomy	surgical creation of an opening	136
-rhexis	rupture	108			
			-tome	instrument for incising (cutting)	137
-schisis	fissure, splitting	108	-tomy	incision, cutting	137
-sclerosis	hardening	109	-toxin	poison	109
-scope	instrument for viewing or examining	135	-tripsy	crushing	137
			-tropic	act(ing) on, affect(ing)	153
-scopy	examination of	135	-trophy, -trophia	feeding, growth, nourishment	65
-sis	condition of	18			
-some	body, small body	63	-uresis	urination	349
-spasm	sudden contraction, cramp	109	-uria	condition of urine, urination	349
-stasis	suppression, stoppage	109			
-spermia	condition of semen	382	-y	condition of	18
-stenosis	narrowing, constriction	109			

PREFIX	MEANING	REFERENCE PAGE	PREFIX	MEANING	REFERENCE PAGE
a-	not, without, lack of, absence	37	iso-	equal, same	40
ab-	away from	39			
acro-	extremity, end	82	juxta-	near, beside	83
ad-	toward, near	39			
ambly-	dim	555	leuk/o	white, colorless, white blood cell	37, 236
an-	not, without, lack of, absence	37			
ante-	before	42	macro-	large, abnormally large	40
anti-	against	37, 153	mal-	bad, poor	106
atel/o	incomplete	283	mega-, megalo-	large, abnormally large	41
auto-	self	245	melan/o-	black, dark, melanin	37, 613
			mes/o-	middle	43
bi-	two, twice	34	micro-	small, one millionth	41
brachy-	short	389	mon/o-	one	34
brady-	slow	106	multi-	many	35
circum-	around	83	neo-	new	41
contra-	against, opposite	37, 153	non-	not	38
counter-	opposite, against	153	normo-	normal	41
cyan/o-	blue	37			
			olig/o-	few, scanty, deficiency of	40
de-	down, without, removal, loss	38	ortho-	straight, correct, upright	41
dextr/o-	right	43			
di-	two, twice	34	pachy-	thick	106
dia-	through	39	pan-	all	40
dipl/o-	double	34	para-	near, beside, abnormal	83, 532
dis-	absence, removal, separation	38	per-	through	39
dys-	abnormal, painful, difficult	106	peri-	around	83
			poikilo-	varied, irregular	41
ec-	out, outside	43	poly-	many, much	35
ecto-	out, outside	43	post-	after, behind	42
end/o-	in, within	43	pre-	before, in front of	42
epi-	on, over	83	presby-	old	545
equi-	equal, same	40	prim/i-	first	34
eu-	true, good, easy, normal	40	pro-	before, in front of	42
ex/o-	away from, outside	43	pseudo-	false	41
extra-	outside	83			
			quadr/i-	four	35
hemi-	half, one side	34			
hetero-	other, different, unequal	40	re-	again, back	41
homo-, homeo-	same, unchanging	40	retro-	behind, backward	83
hyper-	over, excess, increased, abnormally high	40			
			semi-	half, partial	34
hypo-	under, below, decreased, abnormally low	40	sinistr/o-	left	43
			staphyl/o-	grapelike cluster, staphylococcus	110
			strept/o-	twisted chain, streptococcus	110
im-	not	38	sub-	below, under	83
in-	not	38	super-	above, excess	40
infra-	below	83	supra-	above	83
inter-	between	83	syn-, sym-	together	43

A7

PREFIX	MEANING	REFERENCE PAGE	PREFIX	MEANING	REFERENCE PAGE
tachy-	rapid	106	un-	not	38
tel/e-, tel/o-	end	43	uni-	one	34
tetra-	four	35			
trans-	through	39	xanth/o-	yellow	37
tri-	three	35	xero-	dry	106

METRIC MEASUREMENTS

UNIT	ABBREVIATION	METRIC EQUIVALENT	U.S. EQUIVALENT
Units of Length			
kilometer	km	1000 meters	0.62 miles; 1.6 km/mile
meter*	m	100 cm; 1000 mm	39.4 inches; 1.1 yards
centimeter	cm	1/100 m; 0.01 m	0.39 inches; 2.5 cm/inch
millimeter	mm	1/1000 m; 0.001 m	0.039 inches; 25 mm/inch
micrometer	μm	1/1000 mm; 0.001 mm	
Units of Weight			
kilogram	kg	1000 g	2.2 lb
gram*	g	1000 mg	0.035 oz; 28.5 g/oz
milligram	mg	1/1000 g; 0.001 g	
microgram	μg, mcg	1/1000 mg; 0.001 mg	
Units of Volume			
liter*	L	1000 mL	1.06 qt
deciliter	dL	1/10 L; 0.1 L	
milliliter	mL	1/1000 L; 0.001 L	0.034 oz; 29.4 mL/oz
microliter	μL, mcL, mcl	1/1000 mL; 0.001 mL	

*Basic unit

A8

APPENDIX NINE
Stedman's Medical Dictionary At a Glance

A9

an·ti·bod·y (an'tē-bod'e) *Avoid the jargonsitic use of the plural antibodies when the reference is to a single antibody species.* An immunoglobulin molecule produced by B-lymphoid cells that combine specifically with an immunogen or antigen. A.'s may be present naturally, their specificity is determined through gene rearrangement or somatic replacement or may be synthesized in response to stimulus provided by the introduction of an antigen; a.'s are found in the blood and body fluids, although the basic structure of the molecule consists of two light and two heavy chains, a.'s may also be found as dimers, trimers, or pentamers. After binding antigen, some a.'s may fix, complement, bind to surface receptors on immune cells, and in some cases may neutralize microorganisms, SEE ALSO immunoglobulin. SYN immune protein, protective protein, sensitizer (2).

Usage notes appear in italics before definition

Large header for entries with numerous subentries

ANTIGEN

Pronunciation

Main entry

Indicates term is illustrated

an·ti·gen (Ag) (an'ti-jen). Any substance that, as a result of coming in contact with appropriate cells, induces a state of sensitivity or immune responsiveness and that reacts in a demonstrable way with antibodies or immune cells of the sensitized subject in vivo or in vitro. Modern usage tends to retain the broad meaning of a., employing the terms "antigenic determinant" or "determinant group" for the particular chemical group of a molecule that confers antigenic specificity. SEE ALSO hapten, SYN immunogen. [anti-body) + G, -gen, producing.]

Subentry

Etymologies appear in brackets

Australia a. [MIM*209800], an a. so called because first recognized in an Australian aborigine, but now known to be a subunit of the hepatitis B virus surface antigen. SYN Au a. (2), Aus a.

Abbreviation

carcinoembryonic a. (CEA), a glycoprotein constituent of the glycocalyx of embryonic endodermal epithelium, which may be elevated in the serum of some patients with colon cancer and certain other cancers and in serum of long-term tobacco smokers.

Cross references in blue indicate where to find the defined / preferred term. In multi-word terms, the italicized term indicates the main entry under which the term can be found.

Main word is abbreviated in subentries

conjugated a., SYN conjugated *hapten.*

High profile terms (entries) with broad significance to the practice of medicine and to the world appear in blue boxes

prostate-specific a. (PSA), a single-chain, 31-kD glycoprotein with 240 amino acid residues and 4 carbohydrate side-chains; a kallikrein protease produced by prostatic epithelial cells and normally found in seminal fluid and circulating blood. Elevations of serum PSA are highly organ-specific but occur in both cancer (adenocarcinoma) and benign disease (e.g. benign prostatic hyperplasia, prostatitis). A significant number of patients with organ-confined cancer have normal PSA values. SEE carcinoma of the prostate. SYN human glandular kallikrein 3.

Cross references

KEY

♻	Combining Forms
🛈	Indicates term is illustrated, *see Illustration Index*
SYN	Synonym
Cf.	Compare
[NA]	Nomina Anatomica
[TA]	Terminologia Anatomica
☆	Official alternate Terminologia Anatomica term
[MIM]	Mendelian Inheritance in Man
C.I.	*Color Index*

696

ANSWER KEY

Chapter 1

Pretest

1. root
2. prefix
3. suffix
4. Greek/Latin
5. k
6. s

Chapter Review

1. suffix
2. combining form
3. diarrhea
4. cardiology
5. c
6. b
7. c
8. d
9. *dis-LEK-sē-a*
10. *RŪ-ma-tizm*
11. *nu-MŌ-nē-a*
12. *kē-mō-THER-a-pē*
13. FAR-ma-sist
14. cardiac
15. hydrogen
16. ocular
17. interface
18. rheumatic

Case Study Questions

1. c
2. d
3. b
4. d
5. a
6. hem/o, hemat/o
7. Chapter 7
8. in; within
9. intra-

10. ear; nose; larynx
11. g
12. computed tomography

Chapter 2

Pretest

1. ing
2. nouns
3. adjectives
4. like, resembling
5. study of
6. ova
7. phenomenon

Chapter Exercises

EXERCISE 2-1

1. -ia
2. -y
3. -ism
4. -sis, iasis
5. -ia
6. -ism
7. -sis, -osis
8. -y
9. -sis, -esis

EXERCISE 2-2

1. -ist
2. -logy
3. -iatrics
4. -logy
5. -ian
6. dermatologist
7. pediatrician
8. radiologist
9. podiatrist
10. anatomist
11. technologist; also, technician

Exercise 2-3

1. -ary
2. -al
3. -ic
4. -ous
5. -form
6. -oid
7. -al, -ical
8. -ile
9. -al, -ical
10. -ar
11. -ary
12. -ory
13. -ic

Exercise 2-4

1. patell*ae* (*pa-TEL-ē*)
2. gangli*a* (*GANG-lē-a*)
3. oment*a* (*ō-MEN-ta*)
4. test*es* (*TES-tēz*)
5. matri*ces* (*MĀ-tri-sēz*)
6. ov*a* (*Ō-va*)
7. protozo*a* (*prō-tō-ZŌ-a*)
8. meni*nges* (*me-NIN-jēz*)
9. fung*i* (*FUN-jī*)
10. spermatozo*on* (*sper-ma-tō-ZŌ-on*)
11. appendi*x*
12. adeno*ma* (*ad-e-NŌ-ma*)
13. embol*us* (*EM-bō-lus*)
14. pelvi*s* (*PEL-vis*)
15. forame*n* (*fō-RĀ-men*)
16. curricul*um* (*kur-RIK-ū-lum*)

Chapter Review

1. -ism
2. -ia
3. -sis, -osis
4. -y
5. -sis
6. -ia
7. -iatry
8. -ics
9. -ist
10. -ian
11. -ist
12. -logy
13. pediatrician
14. dermatologist
15. cardiologist
16. obstetrician
17. -ic
18. -al
19. -ous
20. -oid
21. -ar
22. -ic
23. -ary
24. -al
25. -oid
26. -ile
27. -al, -ical
28. -ar
29. -ory
30. gingivae
31. diagnoses
32. bacteria
33. foramina
34. criteria
35. larynges
36. vertebrae
37. focus
38. nucleus
39. apex
39. ganglion
40. lumen
41. testis
42. carcinoma

Case Study Questions

1. b
2. a
3. a
4. -sis, -osis
5. -y
6. -ia
7. -ile
8. -ical
9. -ic
10. patella
11. ovum
12. protozoon
13. viral
14. necrosis
15. archeologist
16. internist
17. abdominal

Chapter 3

Pretest

1. at the beginning
2. before

3. micro-
4. -ic
5. numbers
6. colors
7. hypoglycemia
8. prenatal, antenatal

Chapter Exercises

EXERCISE 3-1
1. b. uni-; d. bi-; a. tri-; c. tetra-
2. one
3. four
4. one
5. half
6. two
7. four
8. three
9. two
10. bi-
11. multi-
12. semi-
13. uni-

EXERCISE 3-2
1. d
2. c
3. a
4. b
5. e

EXERCISE 3-3
1. a-; not, without, lack of, absence
2. anti-; against, opposite
3. a-; not, without (root *mnem/o* means "memory")
4. dis-; absence, removal, separation
5. contra-; against
6. in-; not
7. de-; down, without, removal, loss
8. non-; not
9. unconscious
10. insignificant
11. disinfect
12. unusual
13. nonspecific
14. decongestant
15. incompatible

EXERCISE 3-4
1. dia-; through
2. per-; through
3. ad-; toward, near
4. ab-; away from

5. dia-; through
6. trans-; through

EXERCISE 3-5
1. c
2. e
3. d
4. b
5. a

EXERCISE 3-6
1. d
2. e
3. c
4. b
5. a
6. homeo-; same, unchanging
7. equi-; equal, same
8. ortho-; straight, correct, upright
9. re-; again, back
10. eu-; true, good, easy, normal
11. neo-; new
12. mega-; large, abnormally large
13. iso-; equal, same
14. normo-; normal
15. heterogeneous (*het-er-ō-JĒ-nē-us*)
16. macroscopic (*mak-rō-SKOP-ik*)

EXERCISE 3-7
1. c
2. a
3. e
4. b
5. d
6. pre-; before, in front of
7. post-; after, behind
8. pro-; before, in front of
9. pre- before, in front of
10. ante-; before

EXERCISE 3-8
1. e
2. c
3. a
4. b
5. d
6. sym-; together
7. ex-; away from, outside
8. ecto-; out, outside
9. syn-; together
10. endo-; in, within
11. endogenous (*en-DOJ-e-nus*)
12. sinistromanual (*sin-is-trō-MAN-ū-al*)
13. endoderm (*EN-dō-derm*)

Chapter Review

1. e
2. c
3. d
4. b
5. a
6. d
7. c
8. a
9. b
10. e
11. e
12. d
13. a
14. b
15. c
16. e
17. a
18. b
19. c
20. d
21. one
22. four
23. left
24. two
25. opposite
26. four
27. hyper-; over, excess, abnormally high, increased
28. trans-; through
29. dis-; absence, removal, separation
30. re-; again, back
31. ex-; away from, outside
32. ad-; toward, near
33. un-; not
34. de-; down, without, removal, loss
35. semi-; half, partial
36. pre-; before, in front of
37. per-; through
38. dia-; through
39. anti-; against
40. micro-; small
41. dis-; absence, removal, separation
42. ecto-; out, outside
43. sym-; together
44. pro-; before, in front of
45. in-; not
46. T
47. F; one
48. T
49. F; right
50. F; four
51. T
52. dehumidify
53. adduct
54. impermeable
55. homogeneous
56. endotoxin
57. microscopic
58. hyperventilation
59. presynaptic
60. hypersensitivity
61. microcyte
62. prenatal
63. equilateral

Case Study Questions

1. pre-; before, in front of
2. an-; not, without, lack of, absence
3. dis-; absence, removal, separation
4. re-; again, back
5. bi-; two, twice
6. hemi-; half, one side
7. de-; down, without, removal, loss
8. hyper-; over, excess, abnormally high, increased
9. a-; not, without, lack, absence
10. poly-; many, much
11. syn-; together
12. condition of
13. pertaining to, like, resembling
14. preoperative
15. postoperative
16. abduction
17. melanoma

Chapter 4

Pretest

1. cyt/o
2. hist/o
3. nucleus
4. mitosis
5. enzymes
6. DNA
7. organs

Chapter Exercises

Exercise 4-1

1. fiber
2. tissues
3. forms
4. nucleus
5. nucleus
6. gland

7. nipple
8. mucus
9. network
10. mucus
11. body
12. morphology (*mor-FOL-ō-jē*)
13. cytology (*sī-TOL-ō-jē*)
14. histology (*his-TOL-ō-jē*)

Exercise 4-2
1. d
2. c
3. e
4. b
5. a
6. d
7. c
8. e
9. b
10. a
11. gen; origin, formation
12. phag/o; eat, ingest
13. blast; immature cell, productive cell, embryonic cell
14. plas; formation, molding, development
15. troph; feeding, growth, nourishment

Exercise 4-3
1. sugars
2. sugar
3. water
4. starch
5. lipid, fat
6. glucose
7. fat, lipid
8. steat/o; fatty
9. lip/o; lipid, fat
10. glyc/o; sugar, glucose
11. gluc/o; glucose

Chapter Review

Labeling Exercise
Generalized Animal Cell
1. plasma membrane
2. nucleus
3. nuclear membrane
4. nucleolus
5. cytosol
6. smooth endoplasmic reticulum (ER)
7. rough endoplasmic reticulum (ER)
8. ribosomes
9. mitochondrion
10. Golgi apparatus
11. lysosome

12. vesicle
13. peroxisome
14. centriole
15. microvilli
16. cilia

Terminology
1. b
2. d
3. e
4. a
5. c
6. e
7. c
8. b
9. a
10. d
11. d
12. a
13. b
14. c
15. e
16. e
17. a
18. c
19. b
20. d
21. d
22. c
23. a
24. e
25. b
26. b
27. e
28. a
29. d
30. c
31. b
32. c
33. d
34. a
35. e
36. metabolism
37. epithelial, connective, muscle, nervous
38. glucose
39. nucleus
40. enzyme
41. cells
42. water
43. lipid, fat
44. mucus
45. F; lipid, fat
46. F; water

47. T
48. T
49. T
50. morphology
51. histology
52. cytogenesis
53. amylase

Case Study Questions

1. c
2. d
3. d
4. a
5. mono-; one
6. pro-; before, in front of
7. neo-; new
8. a-; not, without, lack of, absence
9. leuk/o-; white, colorless
10. neutrophils, eosinophils, basophils
11. thromboplastin, neoplasm, dysplasia
12. lymphocytes, monocytes, cytology, leukocyte

Chapter 5

Pretest

1. anterior
2. sagittal plane
3. thoracic cavity
4. dorsal
5. head
6. arm
7. around
8. near

Chapter Exercises

EXERCISE 5-1

1. abdominal (*ab-DOM-i-nal*)
2. cervical (*SER-vi-kal*)
3. thoracic (*thō-RAS-ik*)
4. lumbar (*LUM-bar*)
5. cephalic (*se-FAL-ik*)
6. peritoneum
7. abdomen
8. head

EXERCISE 5-2

1. extremities (hands and feet)
2. arms
3. fingers or toes
4. arms and head
5. foot

EXERCISE 5-3

1. circumoral
2. subscapular
3. perivascular
4. infracostal
5. circumorbital
6. suprapatellar
7. intracellular
8. suprascapular
9. near the nose
10. behind the peritoneum
11. above the abdomen
12. within the uterus
13. above the ankle
14. between the buttocks
15. around the navel (umbilicus)
16. near the sacrum
17. within the chest (thorax)

Chapter Review

LABELING EXERCISE
Directional Terms

1. superior (cranial)
2. inferior (caudal)
3. anterior (ventral)
4. posterior (dorsal)
5. medial
6. lateral
7. proximal
8. distal

Planes of Division

1. frontal (coronal) plane
2. sagittal plane
3. transverse (horizontal) plane

Body Cavities, Lateral View

1. dorsal cavity
2. cranial cavity
3. spinal cavity (canal)
4. ventral cavity
5. thoracic cavity
6. diaphragm
7. abdominopelvic cavity
8. abdominal cavity
9. pelvic cavity

The Nine Regions of the Abdomen

1. epigastric (*ep-i-GAS-trik*) region
2. umbilical (*um-BIL-i-kal*) region
3. hypogastric (*hī-pō-GAS-trik*) region
4. right hypochondriac (*hī-pō-KON-drē-ak*) region
5. left hypochondriac region

6. right lumbar (*LUM-bar*) region
7. left lumbar region
8. right iliac (*IL-ē-ak*) region; also inguinal (*ING-gwi-nal*) region
9. left iliac region; also, inguinal region

Chapter Review

1. e
2. b
3. d
4. c
5. a
6. d
7. e
8. b
9. c
10. a
11. b
12. c
13. d
14. a
15. e
16. F; dorsal
17. T
18. T
19. F; frontal, coronal
20. F; superior
21. T
22. F; prone
23. T
24. finger or toe
25. neck
26. head
27. back of knee
28. arm
29. abdomen
30. below the umbilicus (navel)
31. behind the peritoneum
32. under the tongue
33. between the ribs
34. having two feet
35. periocular
36. inframammary
37. posterior
38. ventral
39. microcephaly
40. extracellular
41. proximal
42. superior
43. suprapubic
44. deep, internal
45. spinal cavity; The spinal cavity is a dorsal cavity; the others are ventral cavities.

46. cephalic region; *Cephalic* refers to the head; the others are abdominal regions.
47. sagittal; *Sagittal* refers to a plane of division; the others are body positions.
48. lumb/o; The root *lumb/o* refers to the small of the back; the others refer to the extremities.

Case Study Questions

1. b
2. c
3. e
4. d
5. b
6–15. See diagram.

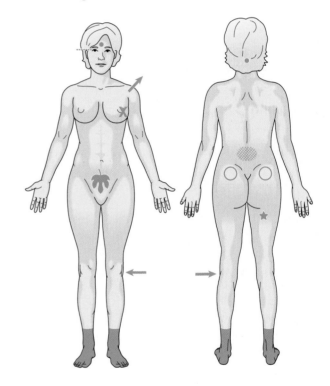

Chapter 6

Pretest

1. microorganism
2. acute
3. neoplasia
4. cocci
5. protozoa
6. inflammation

Chapter Exercises

EXERCISE 6-1

1. pyr/o; fever
2. path/o; disease
3. py/o; pus

4. tox/o; poison
5. cancer, carcinoma
6. calculus, stone
7. pus
8. fever
9. disease
10. hardening
11. poison, toxin
12. pain
13. tumor

EXERCISE 6-2

1. b
2. a
3. e
4. d
5. c
6. mal-; bad, poor
7. dys-; abnormal, painful, difficult
8. xero-; dry

EXERCISE 6-3

1. c
2. a
3. e
4. b
5. d
6. d
7. a
8. e
9. b
10. c
11. pain in a muscle
12. rupture of a muscle
13. any disease of muscle
14. tumor of muscle
15. pain in a muscle

EXERCISE 6-4

1. e
2. d
3. b
4. a
5. c
6. substance poisonous or harmful to the spleen
7. dropping or prolapse of the spleen
8. softening of the spleen

EXERCISE 6-5

1. bacteria
2. fungus
3. bacilli
4. grapelike cluster
5. twisted chain
6. bacteriology (bak-tēr-ē-OL-ō-jē)

7. virology (vī-ROL-ō-jē)
8. mycology (mī-KOL-ō-jē)

Chapter Review

1. a
2. c
3. e
4. b
5. d
6. d
7. c
8. e
9. a
10. b
11. e
12. d
13. b
14. a
15. c
16. d
17. b
18. c
19. e
20. a
21. e
22. c
23. b
24. d
25. a
26. d
27. e
28. a
29. c
30. b
31. inflammation
32. neoplasm
33. metastasis
34. hernia
35. toxins; poisons
36. necrosis
37. tumor
38. T
39. F; streptococci
40. F; acute
41. T
42. F; bradycardia
43. T
44. helminths; *Helminths* are worms, the others are types of bacteria
45. pathogen; A *pathogen* is a disease-causing microorganism, the others are terms related to neoplasia.

46. metastatic; *Metastatic* refers to the spread of cancer; the others are terms describing infections.
47. carcinogenesis
48. pyogenesis
49. pathogenesis
50. oncogenesis
51. bronchospasm (*BRONG-kō-spazm*)
52. bronchitis (*brong-KĪ-tis*)
53. bronchostenosis (*brong-kō-sten-Ō-sis*)
54. bronchorrhea (*brong-kō-RĒ-a*)
55. osteonecrosis (*os-tē-ō-ne-KRŌ-sis*)
56. osteomalacia (*os-tē-ō-ma-LĀ-shē-a*)
57. osteoclasis (*os-tē-OK-la-sis*)
58. osteoma (*os-tē-Ō-ma*)
59. osteolysis (*os-tē-OL-i-sis*)

Case Study Questions

1. c
2. b
3. c
4. d
5. a
6. d
7. c
8. b
9. a
10. e
11. hernia
12. gland
13. bacillus
14. sarcoma
15. malignant hyperpyrexia (also, hyperthermia)
16. human immunodeficiency virus
17. purified protein derivative
18. electrocardiogram
19. acid-fast bacillus

Chapter 7

Pretest

1. diagnosis
2. vital signs
3. systolic and diastolic
4. prognosis
5. cancer; metastasis
6. surgical removal of the appendix
7. surgical incision of the trachea

Chapter Exercises

EXERCISE 7-1

1. e
2. b

3. d
4. c
5. a
6. son/o; sound
7. aer/o; air (oxygen)
8. chrom/o; color
9. therm/o; heat, temperature
10. chron/o; time
11. erg/o; work
12. pressure
13. cold
14. light
15. electricity
16. sound

EXERCISE 7-2

1. b
2. d
3. e
4. a
5. c
6. b
7. a
8. d
9. e
10. c

EXERCISE 7-3

1. c
2. e
3. b
4. a
5. d
6. cystostomy (*sis-TOS-tō-mē*)
7. cystorrhaphy (*sis-TOR-a-fē*)
8. cystoplasty (*SIS-tō-plas-tē*)
9. cystotomy (*sis-TOT-ō-mē*)
10. cystopexy (*SIS-tō-pek-sē*)
11. arthrocentesis (*ar-thrō-sen-TĒ-sis*)
12. arthroplasty (*AR-thrō-plas-tē*)
13. arthrodesis (*ar-THROD-e-sis*)
14. arthrotome (*AR-thrō-tōm*)
15. arthrotomy (*ar-THROT-ō-mē*)
16. colostomy (*kō-LOS-tō-mē*)
17. tracheotomy (*trā-kē-OT-ō-mē*)
18. gastropexy (*GAS-trō-pek-sē*)

Chapter Review

1. c
2. a
3. b
4. e
5. d

6. c

7. e

8. b

9. d

10. a

11. b

12. a

13. d

14. e

15. c

16. b

17. d

18. a

19. e

20. c

21. e

22. c

23. b

24. a

25. d

26. chron/o; time

27. therm/o; heat, temperature

28. son/o; sound

29. erg/o; work

30. radi/o; radiation, x-ray

31. aer/o; air, gas

32. hepatorrhaphy (*hep-a-TOR-a-fē*)

33. hepatotomy (*hep-a-TOT-ō-mē*)

34. hepatopexy (*HEP-a-tō-pek-sē*)

35. hepatectomy (*hep-a-TEK-tō-mē*)

36. T

37. F; radiograph

38. F; prognosis

39. T

40. T

41. F; pressure

42. remission.   *Remission* is the lessening of disease symptoms; the others are examining methods.

43. syncope.   *Syncope* is fainting; the others are examination instruments.

44. prodrome.   A *prodrome* is a symptom indicating an approaching disease; the others are surgical instruments.

45. TNM.   *TNM* is an abbreviation for a system of staging cancer; the others are abbreviations for imaging techniques.

46. simultaneous occurrence of two events
    a. together
    b. time
    c. condition of

47. test that records the heart's sounds
    a. sound
    b. heart
    c. act of recording

48. Formation of color or pigment
    a. color
    b. origin, formation
    c. condition of

Case Study Questions

1. sequelae

2. palpation

3. normocephalic

4. paracentesis

5. biopsy

6. diagnostic laparoscopy

7. hyperabduction

8. c

9. b

10. d

11. c

12. a

13. history of present illness

14. cancer

15. temperature, pulse, respiration

16. beats per minute

17. within normal limits

18. discontinue

19. normal saline solution

Chapter 8

Pretest

1. Food and Drug Administration (FDA)

2. contraindication

3. trade name, brand name

4. prescription

5. pharm, pharmac/o

6. intravenous(ly)

Chapter Exercises

Exercise 8-1

1. -lytic; dissolving, reducing, loosening

2. -tropic; acting on

3. -mimetic; mimicking, simulating

4. antiinflammatory

5. contraindicated

6. antiseptic

7. counteract

8. antitoxin

9. antipyretic

10. hypn/o; sleep

11. tox, toxic/o; poison

12. algesi/o; pain

13. chem/o; chemical

14. narc/o; stupor
15. widening of a vessel
16. study of drugs
17. dissolving mucus
18. acting on the gonads (sex glands)

Chapter Review

1. c
2. a
3. b
4. e
5. d
6. e
7. a
8. b
9. d
10. c
11. c
12. a
13. e
14. b
15. d
16. c
17. d
18. a
19. e
20. b
21. e
22. c
23. e
24. d
25. a
26. b
27. tolerance
28. pain
29. vein
30. plants
31. skin
32. antineoplastics.   An *antineoplastic* kills cancer cells; the others are cardiac drugs.
33. adrenergic.   An *adrenergic* is a sympathomimetic, which mimics the effects of the sympathetic nervous system; the others are drugs to eliminate sensation and relieve pain.
34. lozenge.   A *lozenge* is a tablet or disk; the others are forms of liquid solutions.
35. hypolipidemic.   A *hypolipidemic* reduces cholesterol; the others are respiratory agents.
36. reducing anxiety
37. under the tongue
38. acting on the mind
39. widening of the bronchi
40. anticoagulant

41. vasoconstriction
42. anticonvulsant
43. counterbalance
44. contraindicated
45. antitoxin
46. toxicologist
47. thrombolytic
48. pharmacology
49. antipyretic
50. international unit
51. *United States Pharmacopeia*
52. as desired
53. nonsteroidal antiinflammatory drugs
54. prescription
55. milligram
56. Food and Drug Administration
57. Activated by or secreting adrenaline (epinephrine)
    a. adrenaline
    b. work
    c. pertaining to
58. Movement of drugs within the body as affected by biologic function
    a. drug
    b. movement
    c. pertaining to

Case Study Questions

1. a
2. c
3. d
4. d
5. e
6. c
7. b
8. d
9. a
10. d
11. b
12. a
13. e
14. e
15. b
16. c

Chapter 9

Pretest

1. cardiovascular system
2. myocardium
3. ventricles
4. artery
5. lymphatic system

6. myocardial infarction
7. atherosclerosis

Chapter Exercises

Exercise 9-1

1. heart
2. atrium
3. ventricle
4. valve
5. cardiac (*KAR-dē-ak*)
6. myocardial (*mī-ō-KAR-dē-al*)
7. atrial (*Ā-trē-al*)
8. valvular (*VAL-vū-lar*); also valvar
   (*VAL-var*)
9. ventricular (*ven-TRIK-ū-lar*)
10. pericardial (*per-i-KAR-dē-al*)
11. endocarditis (*en-dō-kar-DĪ-tis*)
12. myocarditis (*mī-ō-kar-DĪ-tis*)
13. pericarditis (*per-i-kar-DĪ-tis*)
14. cardiology (*kar-dē-OL-ō-jē*)
15. interventricular (*in-tra-ven-TRIK-ū-lar*)
16. atrioventricular (*ā-trē-ō-ven-TRIK-ū-lar*)
17. cardiomegaly (*kar-dē-ō-MEG-a-lē*)
18. valvotomy (*val-VOT-ō-mē*); also, valvulotomy
   (*val-vū-LOT-ō-mē*)

Exercise 9-2

1. vessel
2. artery
3. arteriole
4. vessels
5. aorta
6. vein
7. vessels
8. inflammation of a vessel or vessels
9. pertaining to the heart and vessels
10. rupture of an artery
11. within the aorta
12. inflammation of a vein
13. angiogram
14. aortogram
15. phlebogram; venogram
16. angiopathy (*an-jē-OP-a-thē*)
17. angiectasis (*an-jē-EK-ta-sis*); also, hemangiectasis (*hē-man-jē-EK-ta-sis*)
18. angioplasty (*AN-jē-ō-plas-tē*)
19. angiogenesis (*an-jē-ō-JEN-e-sis*)
20. aortosclerosis (*ā-or-tō-skle-RŌ-sis*)
21. phlebectomy (*fle-BEK-tō-mē*); venectomy
   (*vē-NEK-tō-mē*)

22. arteriotomy (*ar-tēr-ē-OT-ō-mē*)
23. intravenous (*in-tra-VĒ-nus*)

Exercise 9-3

1. lymph
2. lymph node
3. lymphatic vessels
4. spleen
5. thymus gland
6. tonsils
7. lymphangi/o; lymphatic vessel
8. lymphaden/o; lymph node
9. splen/o; spleen
10. thym/o; thymus gland
11. tonsill/o; tonsil
12. lymphangitis (*lim-fan-JĪ-tis*); also, lymphangiitis (*lim-fan-jē-Ī-tis*)
13. lymphoma (*lim-FŌ-ma*)
14. lymphadenopathy (*lim-fad-e-NOP-a-thē*)
15. splenomegaly (*splē-nō-MEG-a-lē*)
16. thymic (*THĪ-mik*)
17. tonsillitis (*ton-si-LĪ-tis*)

Chapter Review

Labeling Exercise
The Cardiovascular System

1. right atrium
2. right ventricle
3. left pulmonary artery
4. left lung
5. right lung
6. left pulmonary vein
7. left atrium
8. left ventricle
9. aorta
10. head and arms
11. superior vena cava
12. internal organs
13. legs
14. inferior vena cava

The Heart and Great Vessels

1. superior vena cava
2. inferior vena cava
3. right atrium
4. right AV (tricuspid) valve
5. right ventricle
6. pulmonary valve
7. pulmonary artery
8. right pulmonary artery (branches)
9. left pulmonary artery (branches)
10. left pulmonary veins

11. right pulmonary veins
12. left atrium
13. left AV (mitral) valve
14. left ventricle
15. aortic valve
16. ascending aorta
17. aortic arch
18. brachiocephalic artery
19. left common carotid artery
20. left subclavian artery
21. apex
22. interventricular septum
23. endocardium
24. myocardium
25. epicardium

Location of Lymphoid Tissue

1. nodes
2. tonsils
3. thymus gland
4. spleen
5. appendix
6. Peyer patches (in intestine)

TERMINOLOGY

1. d
2. a
3. b
4. e
5. c
6. d
7. b
8. a
9. e
10. c
11. d
12. c
13. e
14. a
15. b
16. c
17. e
18. d
19. b
20. a
21. b
22. e
23. d
24. a
25. c
26. sinoatrial (SA) node
27. ventricle

28. myocardium
29. capillaries
30. aorta
31. left atrium
32. thymus
33. common iliac (*IL-ē-ak*) arteries
34. jugular (*JUG-ū-lar*)
35. varicose vein, varix
36. vein
37. subclavian veins
38. F; tricuspid
39. F; pulmonary circuit
40. F; artery
41. T
42. F; left ventricle
43. T
44. T
45. T
46. apex. The *apex* is the pointed lower region of the heart; the others are part of the heart's conduction system.
47. murmur. A *murmur* is an abnormal heart sound; the others are terms associated with blood pressure.
48. S₁. S_1 symbolizes the first heart sound; the others are waves of the ECG.
49. cusp. A *cusp* is a flap of a heart valve; the others are lymphoid tissue.
50. incision of an atrium
51. without vessels
52. inflammation of lymph nodes
53. excision of the spleen
54. above a ventricle
55. dilatation of a vein
56. plastic repair of a vessel
57. cardiologist
58. arteriorrhaphy
59. splenopexy
60. valvotome; valvulotome
61. lymphostasis
62. lymphadenectomy
63. aortoptosis
64. aortostenosis
65. aortogram
66. preaortic
67. atrial
68. thymic
69. venous
70. septal
71. sclerotic
72. splenic; splenetic
73. thrombi

74. varices
75. stenoses
76. septa
77. automated external defibrillator
78. left ventricular assist device
79. deep vein thrombosis
80. ventricular fibrillation
81. bundle branch block
82. percutaneous transluminal coronary angioplasty
83. excision of the inner layer of an artery thickened by atherosclerosis
    a. within
    b. artery
    c. out
    d. to cut
84. Permanent dilation of small blood vessels causing small, local red lesions
    a. end
    b. vessel
    c. dilation
85. Inflammation of lymphatic vessels and veins
    a. lymphatic system
    b. vessel
    c. vein
    d. inflammation

Case Study Questions

1. diaphoresis
2. sublingual
3. stress test
4. cardiovascular disease
5. endarterectomies
6. murmur
7. cyanosis
8. stenosis
9. interatrial
10. substernal
11. d
12. b
13. c
14. e
15. a
16. e
17. a
18. coronary/cardiac care unit
19. acute myocardial infarction
20. coronary artery disease
21. left anterior descending
22. congestive heart failure
23. transesophageal echocardiogram
24. mitral valve replacement

Crossword Puzzle

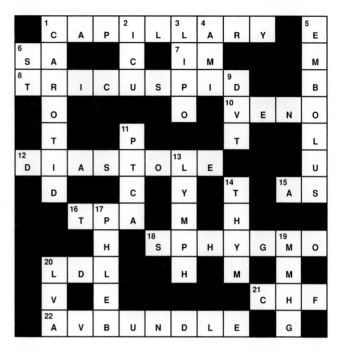

Chapter 10

Pretest

1. erythrocytes
2. leukocytes
3. blood clotting; coagulation
4. lymphocytes
5. antibodies
6. anemia
7. leukemia

Chapter Exercises

EXERCISE 10-1

1. decreased protein in the blood
2. excess albumin in the blood
3. deficiency of red blood cells (erythrocytes)
4. presence of toxins (poisons) in the blood
5. presence of bacteria in the blood
6. production of erythrocytes (red blood cells)
7. pyemia (pī-Ē-mē-a)
8. viremia (vī-RĒ-mē-a)
9. leukemia (lū-KĒ-mē-a)

EXERCISE 10-2

1. myel/o; bone marrow
2. thromb/o; blood clot
3. immun/o; immunity
4. hem/o; blood
5. blood

6. erythrocytes; red blood cells
7. platelets; thrombocytes
8. leukocytes; white blood cells
9. immunity
10. blood cells
11. bone marrow
12. lymphocytes
13. lymphoblast (*LIM-fō-blast*)
14. myeloma (*mī-e-LŌ-ma*)
15. erythropenia (*e-rith-rō-PĒ-nē-a*); also, erythrocytopenia
16. thrombolysis (*throm-BOL-i-sis*)
17. myelopoiesis (*mī-e-lō-poy-Ē-sis*)
18. granulocytosis (*gran-ū-lō-sī-TŌ-sis*)
19. lymphocytosis (*lim-fō-sī-TŌ-sis*)
20. erythrocytosis (*e-rith-rō-sī-TŌ-sis*)
21. monocytosis (*mon-ō-sī-TŌ-sis*)
22. thrombocytosis (*throm-bō-sī-TŌ-sis*)

EXERCISE 10-3
1. iron
2. potassium
3. nitrogenous compounds
4. oxygen
5. iron
6. calcium
7. kalemia (*ka-LĒ-mē-a*)
8. azotemia (*az-ō-TĒ-mē-a*)
9. natremia (*nā-TRĒ-mē-a*)
10. calcemia (*kal-SĒ-mē-a*)

Chapter Review

LABELING EXERCISE
Blood Cells
1. platelet
2. leukocyte
3. erythrocyte

Leukocytes (white blood cells)
1. neutrophil
2. eosinophil
3. basophil
4. lymphocyte
5. monocyte

TERMINOLOGY
1. b
2. e
3. c
4. a
5. d
6. c
7. d
8. a
9. e

10. b
11. b
12. e
13. a
14. d
15. c
16. b
17. e
18. d
19. a
20. c
21. d
22. c
23. a
24. e
25. b
26. phagocytosis
27. hemoglobin
28. electrolyte
29. platelets (thrombocytes)
30. antigen
31. blood cells
32. oxygen
33. blood
34. anemia
35. bone marrow
36. F; thrombocyte
37. T
38. T
39. T
40. F; neutrophil
41. T
42. increase in eosinophils in the blood
43. increase in erythrocytes (red blood cells) in the blood
44. increase in thrombocytes (platelets) in the blood
45. increase in neutrophils in the blood
46. increase in monocytes in the blood
47. lymphoblast; lymphocytoblast
48. thrombocytopenia
49. leukopoiesis
50. pyemia
51. immunologist
52. hemorrhage
53. basophilic (*bā-sō-FIL-ik*)
54. lymphocytic (*lim-fō-SIT-ik*)
55. leukemic (*lū-KĒ-mik*)
56. septicemic (*sep-ti-SĒ-mik*)
57. hemolytic (*hē-mō-LIT-ik*)
58. thrombotic (*throm-BOT-ik*)
59. a toxin (poison) to bone marrow
60. presence of viruses in the blood
61. deficiency of neutrophils
62. immunity to one's own tissue

63. deficiency of oxygen in the blood
64. thrombolysis.   *Thrombolysis* is lysis of a blood clot; the others pertain to formation of a blood clot.
65. CD4.   *CD4* refers to a type of lymphocyte that is infected by HIV (the virus that causes AIDS); the others are abbreviations for blood tests.
66. reticulocyte.   A *reticulocyte* is an immature red blood cell; the others are types of leukocytes.
67. immunodeficiency.   *Immunodeficiency* is a failure in the immune system; the others are terms associated with immune responses.
68. increase in the number of red cells in the blood
    a. many
    b. cell
    c. blood
    d. condition of
69. deposit of iron-containing pigment in tissues causing bronzing of the skin and other symptoms
    a. blood
    b. color
    c. condition of
70. presence in the blood of erythrocytes showing excessive variation in size
    a. not
    b. equal
    c. cell
    d. condition of
71. pertaining to dysfunctional bone marrow
    a. bone marrow
    b. abnormal
    c. formation
    d. condition of

Case Study Questions

1. b
2. c
3. d
4. b
5. b
6. e
7. d
8. d
9. c
10. a
11. c
12. e
13. b
14. b
15. c
16. d
17. e
18. b
19. a

20. immunoglobulin
21. hemoglobin
22. hematocrit
23. fresh frozen plasma
24. prothrombin time
25. partial thromboplastin time
26. disseminated intravascular coagulation

Crossword Puzzle

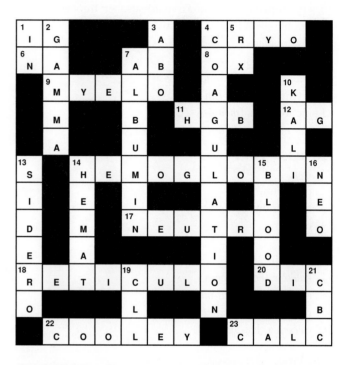

Chapter 11

Pretest

1. oxygen
2. carbon dioxide
3. alveoli
4. bronchi
5. pneumonia; pneumonitis
6. pleurisy; pleuritis

Chapter Exercises

EXERCISE 11-1

1. apnea (*AP-nē-a*)
2. bradypnea (*brad-ip-NĒ-a*)
3. dyspnea (*disp-NĒ-a*)
4. eupnea (*ūp-NĒ-a*)
5. apneic (*ap-NĒ-ik*)
6. bradypneic (*brad-ip-NĒ-ik*)
7. dyspneic (*disp-NĒ-ik*)
8. eupneic (*ūp-NE-ik*)
9. hypocapnia (*hī-pō-KAP-nē-a*)
10. anoxia (*an-OK-sē-a*)

11. eucapnia (*ū-KAP-nē-a*)

12. aphonia (*a-FŌ-nē-a*)

EXERCISE 11-2

1. rhinoplasty (*RĪ-nō-plas-tē*)
2. pharyngeal (*fa-RIN-jē-al*)
3. pharyngitis (*far-in-JĪ-tis*)
4. laryngoscopy (*lar-ing-GŌS-kō-pē*)
5. laryngoplasty (*la-RING-gō-plas-tē*)
6. tracheotomy (*trā-kē-OT-ō-mē*)
7. bronchostenosis (*brong-ko-ste-NŌ-sis*)
8. bronchiolitis (*brong-kē-ō-LĪ-tis*)
9. within the nose
10. within the trachea
11. pertaining to the nose and pharynx
12. around a bronchus
13. dilatation of a bronchus
14. pertaining to the bronchioles

EXERCISE 11-3

1. pain in the pleura
2. pertaining to the pleura and lungs
3. inflammation of the lungs
4. plastic repair of the lungs
5. study of the lungs
6. absence of a lung
7. intrapleural (*in-tra-PLŪ-ral*)
8. supraphrenic (*sū-pra-FREN-ik*)
9. pleurocentesis (*plū-rō-sen-TĒ-sis*)
10. pneumonopathy (*nu-mō-NOP-a-thē*)
11. phrenicotomy (*fren-i-KOT-ō-mē*)
12. spirogram (*SPĪ-rō-gram*)

Chapter Review

LABELING EXERCISE
Respiratory System

1. frontal sinus
2. sphenoidal sinus
3. nasal cavity
4. nasopharynx
5. oropharynx
6. laryngeal pharynx
7. larynx and vocal cords
8. epiglottis
9. esophagus
10. trachea
11. right lung
12. left lung
13. mediastinum
14. right bronchus
15. terminal bronchiole
16. alveolar duct
17. alveoli

18. capillaries
19. diaphragm

TERMINOLOGY

1. d
2. b
3. e
4. c
5. a
6. b
7. a
8. e
9. c
10. d
11. d
12. e
13. a
14. b
15. c
16. c
17. d
18. a
19. e
20. b
21. d
22. a
23. e
24. b
25. c
26. carbon dioxide
27. diaphragm
28. smell
29. pleura
30. alveoli
31. bronchi
32. lungs
33. tuberculosis
34. upright
35 tidal volume
36. coughing
37. mucus
38. septum
39. apnea
40. residual volume
41. T
42. T
43. F; larynx
44. F; three
45. T
46. T
47. phrenicotomy (*fren-i-KOT-ō-mē*)
48. pleurocele (*PLŪ-rō-sēl*)
49. pharyngitis (*far-in-JĪ-tis*)

50. bronchiolitis (*brong-kē-ō-LĪ-tis*)
51. tracheostomy (*tra-kē-OS-tō-mē*)
52. accumulation of air or gas in the pleural space
53. accumulation of blood in the pleural space
54. accumulation of pus in the pleural space
55. accumulation of fluid in the pleural space
56. pain in the pleura
57. deficiency of oxygen in the tissues
58. any disease of the lungs
59. slow rate of respiration
60. dilatation of the bronchi
61. within the lungs
62. plastic repair of the nose
63. dryness of the throat
64. spir/o; breathing
65. pulmon/o; lung
66. py/o; pus
67. phren/o; diaphragm
68. pneum/o; pertaining to air or gas
69. hypercapnia
70. expiration
71. bradypnea
72. extubation
73. alveolar
74. laryngeal
75. pleural
76. nasal
77. tracheal
78. bronchial
79. nares
80. pleurae
81. alveoli
82. conchae
83. bronchi
84. mediastinum; The *mediastinum* is the space between the lungs; the others are parts of the nose.
85. sinus; A *sinus* is a cavity or channel; the others are parts of the larynx.
86. asthma; *Asthma* is a chronic breathing problem caused by allergy and other factors; the others are infectious diseases.
87. URI; *URI* is an abbreviation for "upper respiratory infection"; the others are abbreviations for lobes of the lung.
88. incomplete expansion of the alveoli
    a. incomplete
    b. expansion, dilation
89. presence of air or gas in a blood vessel of the heart
    a. air, gas
    b. heart
    c. condition of

CASE STUDY QUESTIONS
1. b
2. c

3. d
4. b
5. d
6. e
7. wheezing
8. bronchodilator
9. lobectomy
10. diaphoresis
11. thoracotomy
12. thoracoscopy
13. hemithorax
14. mediastinoscopy
15. ventilation
16. chronic obstructive pulmonary disease
17. forced vital capacity
18. arterial blood gas
19. acute respiratory distress syndrome
20. do not resuscitate

Crossword Puzzle

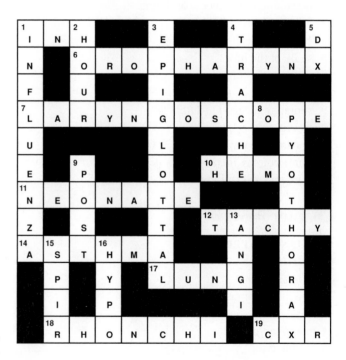

Chapter 12

Pretest

1. esophagus
2. gastr; gastr/o
3. colon
4. intestine
5. absorption
6. liver
7. gallbladder

Chapter Exercises

EXERCISE 12-1

1. oral (*OR-al*); stomal (*STŌ-mal*)
2. dental (*DEN-tal*)
3. gingival (*JIN-ji-val*)
4. lingual (*LING-gwal*); glossal (*GLOS-sal*)
5. buccal (*BUK-al*)
6. labial (*LĀ-bē-al*)
7. jaw
8. tongue
9. mouth
10. mouth
11. salivary
12. teeth
13. teeth
14. under the tongue
15. suture of the palate
16. inflammation of the gums
17. pertaining to the lip and teeth
18. under the tongue
19. outside the cheek
20. dropping of the uvula

EXERCISE 12-2

1. gastric (*GAS-trik*)
2. enteric (*en-TER-ik*)
3. pyloric (*pī-LOR-ik*)
4. colic (*KOL-ik*); also, colonic (*kō-LON-ik*)
5. duodenal (*dū-ō-DĒ-nal*)
6. jejunal (*je-JUN-al*)
7. ileal (*IL-ē-al*)
8. cecal (*SĒ-kal*)
9. anal (*Ā-nal*)
10. gastroenterology (*gas-trō-en-ter-OL-ō-jē*)
11. esophagitis (*ē-sof-a-JĪ-tis*)
12. gastropexy (*GAS-trō-pek-sē*)
13. pyloroptosis (*pī-lor-ō-TŌ-sis*)
14. ileectomy (*il-ē-EK-tō-mē*)
15. duodenoscopy (*dū-ō-de-NOS-kō-pē*)
16. jejunostomy (*je-jū-NOS-tō-mē*)
17. anorectal (*ā-nō-REK-tal*)
18. colostomy (*kō-LOS-tō-mē*)
19. colopexy (*KŌ-lō-pek-sē*)
20. colitis (*kō-LĪ-tis*)
21. colocentesis (*kō-lō-sen-TĒ-sis*)
22. colonopathy (*kō-lō-NOP-a-thē*)
23. colonoscopy (*kō-lon-OS-kō-pē*)
24. esophagogastrostomy (*ē-sof-a-gō-gas-TROS-tō-mē*)
25. gastroenterostomy (*gas-trō-en-ter-OS-tō-mē*)
26. gastrojejunostomy (*gas-trō-je-jū-NOS-tō-mē*)
27. duodenoileostomy (*dū-ō-dē-nō-il-ē-OS-tō-mē*)
28. sigmoidoproctostomy (*sig-moy-dō-prok-TOS-tō-mē*)

EXERCISE 12-3

1. hepatic (*he-PAT-ik*)
2. cholecystic (*kō-lē-SIS-tik*)
3. pancreatic (*pan-krē-AT-ik*)
4. hepatography (*hep-a-TOG-ra-fē*)
5. cholecystography (*kō-lē-sis-TOG-ra-fē*)
6. cholangiography (*kō-lan-jē-OG-ra-fē*)
7. pancreatography (*pan-krē-a-TOG-ra-fē*)
8. choledocholithiasis (*kō-led-o-kō-li-THĪ-a-sis*)
9. pancreatolithiasis (*pan-krē-a-tō-li-THĪ-a-sis*)
10. liver
11. gallstone; biliary calculus
12. bile
13. common bile duct
14. hepatitis (*hep-a-TĪ-tis*)
15. pancreas
16. bile duct
17. gallbladder

Chapter Review

LABELING EXERCISE
The Digestive System

1. mouth
2. pharynx
3. esophagus
4. stomach
5. duodenum (of small intestine)
6. small intestine
7. cecum
8. ascending colon
9. transverse colon
10. descending colon
11. sigmoid colon
12. rectum
13. anus
14. parotid salivary glands
15. sublingual salivary glands
16. submandibular salivary glands
17. liver (cut)
18. gallbladder
19. pancreas

Accessory Organs of Digestion

1. liver
2. common hepatic duct
3. gallbladder
4. cystic duct
5. common bile duct
6. pancreas
7. pancreatic duct
8. duodenum
9. spleen
10. diaphragm

TERMINOLOGY

1. e
2. a
3. b
4. c
5. d
6. b
7. e
8. d
9. a
10. c
11. c
12. d
13. e
14. a
15. b
16. c
17. a
18. d
19. e
20. b
21. d
22. e
23. a
24. c
25. b
26. palate
27. teeth
28. tongue
29. cheek
30. intestine
31. cecum
32. liver
33. bile
34. liver
35. gallbladder
36. pylorus; The *pylorus* is the distal part of the stomach; the others are parts of the mouth.
37. spleen; The *spleen* is a lymphatic organ; the others are parts of the large intestine.
38. villi; The *villi* are tiny projections in the lining of the small intestine that aid in the absorption of nutrients; the others are accessory organs of digestion.
39. peristalsis; *Peristalsis* is wavelike movement of organ walls; the others are disorders of the digestive tract.
40. F; above
41. F; jejunum
42. F; saliva
43. T
44. T
45. T
46. periodontist

47. gastrectomy
48. palatorrhaphy
49. pylorostenosis
50. pancreatitis
51. ileocecal
52. rectocele; proctocele
53. gastroenterologist
54. colostomy
55. gastroduodenostomy
56. ileitis
57. intrahepatic
58. diverticula
59. gingivae
60. calculi
61. anastomoses
62. total parenteral nutrition
63. gastroesophageal reflux disease
64. gastrointestinal
65. hydrochloric acid
66. percutaneous endoscopic gastrostomy (tube)
67. hepatitis A virus
68. pertaining to the muscular coat of the intestine
    a. muscle
    b. intestine
    c. pertaining to
69. radiography of the biliary tract and gallbladder using radionuclides
    a. bile
    b. spark (radiation)
    c. act of recording data
70. referring to any route other than the alimentary canal
    a. beside
    b. intestine
    c. pertaining to

Case Study Questions

1. c
2. d
3. a
4. e
5. d
6. a
7. c
8. b
9. c
10. d
11. b
12. e
13. b
14. endoscopic retrograde cholangiopancreatography
15. right upper quadrant
16. nasogastric

17. inflammatory bowel disease
18. duodenal
19. mesenteric
20. focal
21. exudate
22. occult blood
23. icterus
24. antiemetic
25. cholelithiasis
26. laparoscopic cholecystectomy
27. cholecystitis
28. cholangiogram
29. sphincter
30. biopsy

Crossword Puzzle

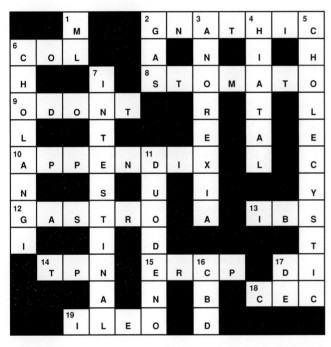

Chapter 13

Pretest

1. kidneys
2. urethra
3. red blood cells; erythrocytes
4. urination; voiding of urine
5. urinary bladder
6. glomeruli and kidney
7. dialysis

Chapter Exercises

EXERCISE 13-1

1. postrenal (*pōst-RĒ-nal*)
2. intrarenal (*in-tra-RĒ-nal*)
3. suprarenal (*sū-pra-RĒ-nal*)

4. perirenal (*per-i-RĒ-nal*); circumrenal (*sir-kum-RĒ-nal*)
5. nephrectomy (*ne-FREK-tō-mē*)
6. nephrology (*ne-FROL-ō-jē*)
7. nephromalacia (*nef-rō-ma-LĀ-shē-a*)
8. nephrotoxic (*nef-rō-TOK-sik*)
9. nephropathy (*ne-FROP-a-thē*)
10. glomerulitis (*glō-mer-ū-LĪ-tis*)
11. caliectasis (*kā-lē-EK-ta-sis*; calicectasis (*kal-i-SEK-ta-sis*)
12. pyelogram (*PĪ-e-lō-gram*)
13. pyeloplasty (*pī-e-lō-PLAS-tē*)
14. renography (*rē-NOG-ra-fē*); nephrography (*ne-FROG-ra-fē*)
15. glomerulosclerosis (*glo-mer-ū-lō-skle-RŌ-sis*)
16. pyelonephritis (*pi-e-lō-nef-RĪ-tis*)

EXERCISE 13-2

1. urology (*ū-ROL-ō-jē*)
2. urography (*ū-ROG-ra-fē*)
3. urolith (*Ū-rō-lith*)
4. uremia (*ū-RĒ-mē-a*)
5. anuria (*an-Ū-rē-a*)
6. dysuria (*dis-Ū-rē-a*)
7. polyuria (*pol-ē-Ū-rē-a*)
8. cyturia (*sī-TŪ-rē-a*)
9. hematuria (*hē-ma-TŪ-rē-a*)
10. diuresis (*dī-ū-RĒ-sis*)
11. anuresis (*an-ū-RĒ-sis*)
12. natriuresis (*nā-trē-ū-RĒ-sis*)
13. kaliuresis (*kā-lē-ū-RĒ-sis*)
14. urethroscopy (*ū-rē-THROS-kō-pē*)
15. ureterolith (*ū-RĒ-ter-ō-lith*)
16. ureterostomy (*ū-rē-ter-OS-tō-mē*)
17. urethropexy (*ū-RĒ-thrō-pek-sē*)
18. cystitis (*sis-TĪ-tis*)
19. cystopexy (*SIS-tō-pek-sē*)
20. cystoscope (*SIS-tō-skōp*)
21. cystotomy (*sis-TOT-ō-mē*)
22. intravesical (*in-tra-VES-i-kal*)
23. urethrovesical (*ū-rē-thrō-VES-i-kal*)
24. through the urethra
25. surgical incision of the ureter
26. pain in the urinary bladder
27. formation of urine

Chapter Review

LABELING EXERCISE
Urinary System

1. right kidney
2. adrenal gland
3. abdominal aorta
4. renal artery
5. common iliac artery

6. common iliac vein
7. renal vein
8. inferior vena cava
9. right ureter
10. urinary bladder
11. urethra
12. prostate gland

The Kidney

1. renal capsule
2. renal cortex
3. renal medulla
4. pyramids of medulla
5. nephrons
6. calyx
7. hilum
8. renal pelvis
9. ureter

The Urinary Bladder

1. ureter
2. smooth muscle
3. openings of ureters
4. trigone
5. urethra
6. internal urethral sphincter
7. external urethral sphincter
8. prostate

TERMINOLOGY

1. b
2. c
3. a
4. e
5. d
6. c
7. e
8. b
9. a
10. d
11. d
12. e
13. c
14. b
15. a
16. b
17. e
18. d
19. c
20. a
21. nephron
22. glomerulus
23. urination; voiding of urine
24. urinalysis

25. urea
26. cast
27. T
28. F; kidney
29. T
30. F; medulla
31. F; urethra
32. T
33. T
34. F; potassium
35. before or in front of the kidney
36. painful or difficult urination
37. acting on the kidney
38. near the glomerulus
39. pertaining to a calyx
40. narrowing of a urethra
41. nephropathy
42. cystourethrogram
43. cystectomy
44. nephromalacia
45. pyelonephritis
46. ureteropyeloplasty
47. ureterosigmoidostomy
48. pyelocaliectasis; pyelocalicectasis
49. trigone; The *trigone* is a triangle at the base of the bladder; the others are parts of the kidney.
50. prostate; The *prostate* is a gland below the bladder in males; the others are parts of a nephron.
51. hydronephrosis; *Hydronephrosis* is collection of urine in the renal pelvis due to obstruction; the others are pretreatment procedures for the urinary tract.
52. dehydration
53. hypervolemia
54. antidiuretic
55. hyponatremia
56. anuresis
57. vesical
58. urologic
58. uremic
60. diuretic
61. nephrotic
62. ureteral
63. urethral
64. glomeruli
65. calyces
66. pelves
67. intravenous pyelography
68. antidiuretic hormone
69. erythropoietin
70. intravenous urography
71. sodium
72. glomerular filtration rate
73. urinalysis

74. test that measures and records bladder function
    a. urinary bladder
    b. measure
    c. act of recording data
75. surgical creation of a new passage between a ureter and the bladder
    a. ureter
    b. new
    c. bladder
    d. surgical creation of an opening

Case Study Questions

1. c
2. d
3. a
4. a
5. d
6. IV urogram
7. oliguria
8. nocturia
9. ureteral laser lithotripsy
10. kidney transplant
11. lithotomy
12. urinary tract infection
13. continuous ambulatory peritoneal dialysis
14. blood urea nitrogen
15. end-stage renal disease
16. human immunodeficiency virus
17. cystometrogram
18. physiologic saline solution
19. extracorporeal shock-wave lithotripsy

Crossword Puzzle

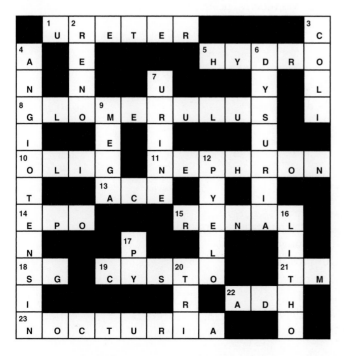

Chapter 14

Pretest

1. spermatozoon, sperm cell
2. testis
3. testosterone
4. semen
5. prostate
6. hernia
7. testis

Chapter Exercises

EXERCISE 14-1

1. any disease of a testis
2. pain in the prostate
3. plastic repair of the scrotum
4. excision of the epididymis
5. pain in the testis
6. pertaining to semen
7. inflammation of the testis and epididymis
8. orchiotomy (*or-kē-OT-ō-mē*); also, orchidotomy (*or-ki-DOT-ō-mē*)
9. orchioplasty (*OR-kē-ō-plas-tē*); also, orchidoplasty (*OR-ki-dō-plas-tē*)
10. orchiopexy (*or-kē-ō-PEK-sē*); also, orchidopexy (*or-ki-dō-PEK-sē*)
11. spermatogenesis (*sper-ma-tō-JEN-e-sis*)
12. spermatocyte (*sper-MA-tō-sīt*)
13. spermatorrhea (*sper-ma-to-RĒ-a*)
14. spermatolysis (*sper-ma-TOL-i-sis*)
15. spermaturia (*sper-ma-TŪ-rē-a*)
16. aspermia (*a-SPER-mē-a*)
17. hemospermia (*hē-mō-SPER-mē-a*); also, hematospermia (*hem-at-ō-SPER-mē-a*)
18. pyospermia (*pī-ō-SPER-mē-a*)
19. oligospermia (*ol-i-gō-SPER-mē-a*)
20. vasectomy (*va-SEK-tō-mē*)
21. vesiculitis (*ve-sik-ū-LĪ-tis*)
22. prostatectomy (*pros-ta-TEK-tō-mē*)
23. oscheoma (*os-kē-Ō-ma*)
24. vesiculography (*ve-sik-ū-LOG-ra-fē*)
25. vasorrhaphy (*vas-OR-a-fē*)
26. epididymitis (*ep-i-did-i-MĪ-tis*)

Chapter Review

LABELING EXERCISE
Male Reproductive System

1. testis
2. epididymis
3. scrotum
4. ductus (vas) deferens

5. ejaculatory duct
6. urethra
7. penis
8. glans penis
9. prepuce (foreskin)
10. seminal vesicle
11. prostate
12. bulbourethral (Cowper) gland
13. kidney
14. ureter
15. urinary bladder
16. peritoneal cavity
17. rectum
18. anus

TERMINOLOGY

1. e
2. d
3. a
4. b
5. c
6. d
7. e
8. b
9. a
10. c
11. b
12. e
13. a
14. d
15. c
16. d
17. e
18. b
19. c
20. a
21. testis
22. scrotum
23. semen
24. testosterone
25. inguinal canal
26. epididymis
27. T
28. F; scrotum
29. T
30. T
31. F; urethra
32. T
33. suture of the vas deferens
34. absence of a testis
35. tumor of the scrotum
36. incision of the seminal vesicle
37. instrument for measuring the prostate

38. presence of blood in the semen
39. vesiculitis
40. prostatotomy
41. oscheolith
42. orchiopexy; orchidopexy
43. oscheoplasty
44. vasovasostomy
45. spermatic cord; The *spermatic cord* suspends the testis in the scrotum and contains the ductus deferens, nerves, and vessels; the others are the glands that contribute to semen.
46. semen; *Semen* is the secretion that transports spermatozoa; the others are hormones active in reproduction.
47. hernia; A *hernia* is a protrusion of tissue through an abnormal body opening; the others are sexually transmitted infections.
48. seminal
49. prostatic
50. penile
51. urethral
52. scrotal
53. sexually transmitted infection
54. transurethral incision of prostate
55. gonococcus
56. prostate-specific antigen
57. genitourinary
58. digital rectal examination
59. undescended testes
    a. hidden
    b. testis
    c. condition of
60. inflammation of the ductus deferens and seminal vesicle
    a. vas (ductus) deferens
    b. seminal vesicle
    c. inflammation

Case Study Questions

1. d
2. a
3. c
4. d
5. c
6. a
7. c
8. bilateral inguinal herniorrhaphy
9. strangulated hernia
10. prostatitis
11. intravesical
12. balanitis
13. phimosis
14. benign prostatic hyperplasia

15. transurethral resection of the prostate
16. bladder neck obstruction
17. urinary tract infection

Crossword Puzzle

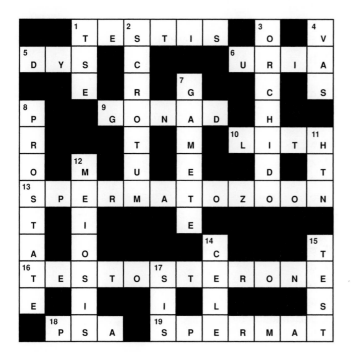

Chapter 15

Pretest

1. ovary
2. estrogen and progesterone
3. contraception
4. embryo
5. placenta
6. lactation
7. woman
8. uterus
9. congenital

Chapter Exercises

EXERCISE 15-1

1. any disease of women
2. before menstruation
3. formation of an ovum
4. without ovulation
5. pertaining to an ovary
6. inflammation of an ovary
7. gynecologist (gī-ne-KOL-ō-jist)
8. postovulatory (PŌST-ov-ū-la-tō-rē)
9. menorrhagia (men-ō-RĀ-jē-a)

10. dysmenorrhea (DIS-men-ō-rē-a)
11. amenorrhea (a-men-ō-RĒ-a)
12. oligomenorrhea (ol-i-gō-men-ō-RĒ-a)
13. ovariocentesis (ō-var-ē-ō-sen-TĒ-sis)
14. ovariocele (o-VAR-ē-ō-sēl)
15. ovariorrhexis (ō-var-ē-ō-REK-sis)
16. oophorotomy (ō-of-ō-ROT-ō-mē)
17. oophoroma (ō-of-ō-RŌ-ma)

EXERCISE 15-2

1. excision of an oviduct
2. endoscopic examination of the uterus
3. softening of the uterus
4. pertaining to the uterus and bladder
5. within the cervix
6. plastic repair of the vagina
7. pain in the vagina
8. salpingopexy (sal-PING-gō-pek-sē)
9. salpingography (sal-ping-GOG-ra-fē)
10. pyosalpinx (pī-ō-SAL-pinx)
11. hydrosalpinx (hī-drō-SAL-pinx)
12. salpingo-oophorectomy (sal-ping-gō-ō-of-ō-REK-tō-mē); also, salpingo-ovariectomy (sal-ping-gō-ō-var-ē-EK-tō-me)
13. uterine (Ū-ter-in)
14. hysterosalpingogram (his-ter-ō-sal-PING-gō-gram)
15. hysteropexy (his-ter-ō-PEK-sē)
16. metroptosis (mē-trō-TŌ-sis)
17. metrostenosis (mē-trō-ste-NŌ-sis)
18. transcervical (trans-SER-vi-kal)
18. intracervical (in-tra-SER-vi-kal)
19. vaginitis (vaj-i-NĪ-tis)
20. colpocele (KOL-pō-sēl)

EXERCISE 15-3

1. vulvopathy (vul-VOP-a-thē)
2. episiorrhaphy (e-piz-ē-OR-a-fē)
3. vaginoperineal (vaj-i-nō-per-i-NĒ-al)
4. clitoritis (klit-o-RĪ-tis)
5. mammogram (MAM-ō-gram)
6. mastitis (mas-TĪ-tis)
7. mastectomy (mas-TEK-tō-mē); also, mammectomy (ma-MEK-tō-mē)

EXERCISE 15-4

1. formation of an embryo
2. before birth
3. pertaining to a newborn
4. developing in one amniotic sac
5. endoscopic examination of the fetus
6. excess secretion of milk
7. lack of milk production
8. amniotomy (am-nē-OT-ō-mē)
9. amniorrhexis (am-nē-ō-REK-sis)
10. amniocyte (AM-nē-ō-sīt)

11. embryology (*em-brē-OL-ō-jē*)
12. fetoscope (*FĒ-tō-skōp*)
13. embryopathy (*em-brē-OP-a-thē*)
14. neonatology (*nē-ō-nā-TOL-ō-jē*)
15. postnatal (*pōst-NĀ-tal*)
16. primigravida (*pri-mi-GRAV-i-da*)
17. multigravida (*mul-ti-GRAV-i-da*)
18. nullipara (*nul-IP-a-ra*)
19. primipara (*pri-MIP-a-ra*)
20. xerotocia (*zē-rō-TŌ-sē-a*)
21. bradytocia (*brad-ē-TŌ-sē-a*)
22. galactocele (*ga-LAK-to-sēl*); also, lactocele (*LAK-tō-sēl*)
23. galactorrhea (*ga-lak-tō-RE-a*); also, lactorrhea (*lak-tō-RE-a*)

Chapter Review

LABELING EXERCISE
Female Reproductive System

1. ovary
2. fimbriae
3. oviduct (fallopian tube)
4. uterus
5. cervix
6. posterior fornix
7. vagina
8. clitoris
9. labium minus
10. labium majus
11. urinary bladder
12. urethra
13. rectum
14. anus
15. peritoneal cavity
16. cul-de-sac

Ovulation and Fertilization

1. ovary
2. fimbriae
3. ovum
4. sperm cells (spermatozoa)
5. oviduct (fallopian tube)
6. implanted embryo
7. corpus (body) of uterus
8. cervix
9. vagina
10. greater vestibular (Bartholin) gland

TERMINOLOGY

1. c
2. d
3. e
4. a
5. b
6. e
7. c
8. b
9. a
10. d
11. c
12. a
13. b
14. e
15. d
16. e
17. d
18. c
19. a
20. b
21. c
22. b
23. a
24. e
25. d
26. ovary
27. ovum (egg cell)
28. placenta
29. lactation
30. abortion
31. uterus
32. breasts (mammary glands)
33. T
34. T
35. F; endometrium
36. F; corpus luteum
37. F; oviduct
38. T
39. F; embryo
40. labia majora; The *labia majora* are part of the vulva; the others are associated with pregnancy.
41. colostrum; *Colostrum* is the breast fluid released before milk is produced; the others are hormones involved in reproduction.
42. measles; *Measles* is an infectious disease; the others are hereditary disorders.
43. candidiasis; *Candidiasis* is a fungal infection; the others are procedures used to diagnose fetal abnormalities.
44. spina bifida; Spina bifida is a congenital spinal defect; the others are disorders of pregnancy.
45. softening of the uterus
46. behind the uterus
47. any disease of the uterus
48. narrowing of the vagina
49. pus in the oviduct
50. without ovulation

51. below the breasts
52. after birth
53. outside the embryo
54. woman who has never been pregnant
55. woman who has given birth three times
56. causing fetal abnormalities
57. metrostenosis
58. hysterosalpingectomy
59. episiorrhaphy
60. mammography
61. salpingocele
62. cervicitis
63. amniorrhexis
64. embryology
65. fetometry
66. dystocia
67. newborn
68. primipara
69. nulligravida
70. postpartum
71. prenatal
72. eutocia
73. ovulatory
74. cervical
75. uterine
76. perineal
77. vaginal
78. embryonic
79. amniotic
80. ova
81. cervices
82. fimbriae
83. labia
84. toxic shock syndrome
85. intrauterine device
86. dysfunctional uterine bleeding
87. last menstrual period
88. gamete intrafallopian transfer
89. gestational age
90. fetal heart rate
91. vaginal birth after cesarean section
92. excessive development of the mammary glands in the male, even to the secretion of milk
    a. woman
    b. breast
    c. condition of
93. extreme rapidity of labor
    a. sharp, acute
    b. labor
    c. condition of
94. A deficiency of amniotic fluid
    a. few, scanty
    b. fluid
    c. amnion

Case Study Questions

1. b
2. d
3. b
4. a
5. e
6. d
7. c
8. e
9. prolapsed
10. zygote
11. pelvimetry
12. fundus
13. Apgar score
14. placenta
15. dilatation and curettage
16. bilateral salpingo oophorectomy
17. pelvic inflammatory disease
18. hormone replacement therapy
19. in vitro fertilization
20. cephalopelvic disproportion
21. obstetrics
22. gynecology
23. genitourinary

Crossword Puzzle

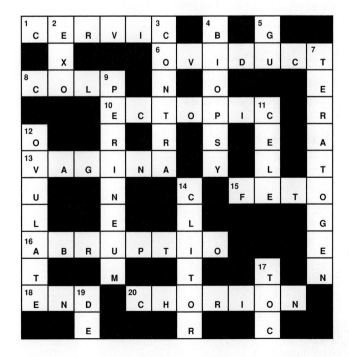

Chapter 16

Pretest
1. hormones
2. pituitary (hypophysis)
3. adrenals
4. pancreas (pancreatic islets)
5. thyroid

Chapter Exercises

EXERCISE 16-1
1. any disease of the endocrine glands or system
2. pertaining to the hypophysis (pituitary gland)
3. acting on the thyroid gland
4. condition of underactivity of the adrenal gland
5. inflammation of the pancreatic islets
6. hypothyroidism (*hī-pō-THĪ-royd-izm*)
7. hypoparathyroidism (*hī-pō-par-a-THĪ-royd-izm*)
8. hyperadrenalism (*hī-per-a-DRĒ-nal-izm*)
9. hyperadrenocorticism (*hī-per-a-drē-nō-KOR-ti-sizm*)
10. hypopituitarism (*hī-pō-pi-TŪ-i-ta-rizm*)
11. endocrinologist (*en-dō-kri-NOL-ō-jist*)
12. thyrotomy (*thī-ROT-ō-mē*); also, thyroidotomy (*thī-roy-DOT-ō-mē*)
13. adrenalopathy (*a-drē-na-LOP-a-thē*); also, adrenopathy (*a-drē-NOP-a-thē*)
14. adrenalitis (*a-drē-nal-Ī-tis*); also, adrenitis (*a-dre-NĪ-tis*)
15. insuloma (*in-sū-LŌ-ma*)

Chapter Review

LABELING EXERCISE
The Endocrine Glands
1. pineal
2. pituitary (hypophysis)
3. thyroid
4. parathyroids
5. thymus
6. adrenals
7. pancreatic islets
8. ovaries
9. testes

TERMINOLOGY
1. c
2. e
3. d

4. b
5. a
6. d
7. b
8. e
9. a
10. c
11. b
12. d
13. e
14. c
15. a
16. c
17. e
18. d
19. a
20. b
21. d
22. c
23. e
24. a
25. b
26. pituitary (hypophysis)
27. thyroid
28. adrenals
29. diabetes mellitus
30. hyperglycemia
31. T
32. F; cortex
33. F; calcium
34. F; thyroid
35. T
36. T
37. T
38. ADH; *ADH* is from the posterior pituitary; the others are hormones produced by the anterior pituitary.
39. dwarfism; *Dwarfism* is caused by hyposecretion of growth hormone: the others are caused by hypersecretion of hormones.
40. TBG; *TBG* is a test of thyroid function; the others are abbreviations associated with diabetes mellitus.
41. larynx; The *larynx* is above the trachea and is part of the respiratory system; the others are endocrine glands.
42. pertaining to the hypophysis (pituitary)
43. condition caused by underactivity of the pituitary gland
44. any disease of the adrenal gland
45. excision of the thyroid
46. physician who specializes in study and treatment of endocrine disorders

47. enlargement of the adrenal gland
48. hypophysitis
49. insuloma
50. adrenocortical
51. thyroiditis
52. hemithyroidectomy
53. parathyroidectomy
54. hyperadrenalism
55. thyrotropic
56. thyrolytic
57. thyropathy
58. normal function of the thyroid gland
    a. true, good, normal
    b. thyroid gland
    c. condition of
59. condition of complete underactivity of the pituitary gland
    a. all
    b. under, abnormally low
    c. pituitary gland
    d. condition of
60. a toxic condition caused by hyperactivity of the thyroid gland
    a. thyroid
    b. poisonous
    c. condition of

Case Study Questions

1. b
2. a
3. d
4. a
5. c
6. d
7. a
8. b
9. c
10. e
11. jaundice
12. lipase
13. nephrectomy
14. adenoma
15. ampule
16. hyperglycemia
17. nothing by mouth/non per os
18. nasogastric
19. blood urea nitrogen
20. within normal limits
21. neutral protamine Hagedorn
22. continuous subcutaneous insulin
    infusion

Crossword Puzzle

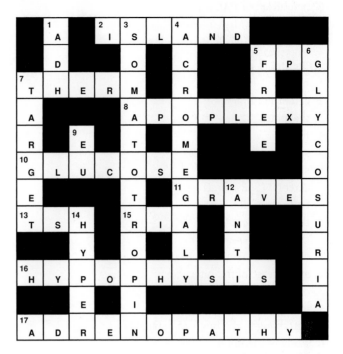

Chapter 17

Pretest

1. neuron
2. cerebrum
3. brainstem
4. autonomic nervous system
5. reflex
6. epilepsy
7. electroencephalograph (EEG)
8. phobia

Chapter Exercises

EXERCISE 17-1

1. pertaining to a nerve or the nervous system
2. pertaining to neuroglia, glial cells
3. pertaining to a ganglion
4. pertaining to the meninges
5. pertaining to a spinal nerve root
6. spinal cord
7. nervous system, nervous tissue
8. meninges
9. spinal nerve roots
10. destruction of a nerve or nervous tissue
11. radiographic study of the spinal cord
12. tumor of the meninges
13. any disease of a spinal nerve root
14. ganglioma (*gang-glē-Ō-ma*)

15. myelitis (*mī-e-LĪ-tis*)
16. neuralgia (*nū-RAL-jē-a*)
17. myelogram (*MĪ-e-lō-gram*)
18. neuropathy (*nū-ROP-a-thē*)

EXERCISE 17-2

1. brain
2. cerebrum, brain
3. thalamus
4. mind
5. stupor, unconsciousness
6. sleep
7. cerebral (*SER-e-bral*)
8. cortical (*KOR-ti-kal*)
9. thalamic (*tha-LAM-ik*)
10. cerebellar (*ser-e-BEL-ar*)
11. ventricular (*ven-TRIK-ū-lar*)
12. any disease of the brain
13. outside the medulla
14. incision of a ventricle
15. pertaining to the brain and spinal cord
16. study of the mind
17. lack of sleep, inability to sleep
18. encephalitis (*en-sef-a-LĪ-tis*)
19. intracerebellar (*in-tra-ser-e-BEL-ar*)
20. corticothalamic (*kor-ti-kō-tha-LAM-ik*)
21. ventriculogram (*ven-TRIK-ū-lō-gram*)
22. extracerebral (*eks-tra-SER-e-bral*)

EXERCISE 17-3

1. speech
2. seizures
3. partial paralysis
4. read
5. tetraplegia (*tet-ra-PLĒ-jē-a*)
6. lack of speech communication
7. slowness of reading
8. obsession with fire
9. fear of women
10. bradylalia (*brad-ē-LĀ-lē-a*)
11. hemiplegia (*hem-i-PLĒ-jē-a*)
12. cardioplegia (*kar-dē-ō-PLĒ-jē-a*)
13. noctiphobia (*nok-ti-FŌ-bē-a*); also, nyctophobia (*nik-tō-FŌ-bē-a*)
14. photophobia (*fō-tō-FŌ-bē-a*)

Chapter Review

LABELING EXERCISE
Anatomic Divisions of the Nervous System

1. brain
2. spinal cord
3. central nervous system
4. cranial nerves
5. spinal nerves
6. peripheral nervous system

Motor Neuron

1. cell body
2. nucleus
3. dendrites
4. axon covered with myelin sheath
5. axon branch
6. myelin
7. muscle

External Surface of the Brain

1. sulci
2. gyri
3. frontal lobe
4. parietal lobe
5. occipital lobe
6. temporal lobe
7. pons
8. medulla oblongata
9. cerebellum
10. spinal cord

Spinal Cord, Lateral View

1. brain
2. brainstem
3. spinal cord
4. cervical enlargement
5. lumbar enlargement
6. cervical nerves
7. thoracic nerves
8. lumbar nerves
9. sacral nerves
10. coccygeal nerve

Spinal Cord, Cross Section

1. white matter
2. gray matter
3. dorsal horn
4. ventral horn
5. central canal
6. dorsal root of spinal nerve
7. dorsal-root ganglion
8. ventral root of spinal nerve
9. spinal nerve

Reflex Pathway

1. receptor
2. sensory neuron
3. spinal cord (CNS)
4. motor neuron
5. effector

TERMINOLOGY

1. c
2. e
3. d
4. a
5. b
6. c
7. e
8. a
9. d
10. b
11. d
12. c
13. e
14. a
15. b
16. a
17. d
18. b
19. c
20. e
21. b
22. d
23. a
24. e
25. c
26. c
27. a
28. d
29. b
30. e
31. neuron
32. synapse
33. reflex
34. meninges
35. autonomic nervous system (ANS)
36. neurotransmitter
37. cerebellum
38. T
39. T
40. F; white
41. F; axon
42. T
43. T
44. F; dura
45. lumbar puncture; *Lumbar puncture* is a diagnostic procedure for sampling CSF; the others are vascular disorders.
46. hematoma; *Hematoma* is a local collection of clotted blood; the others are neoplasms.
47. mania; *Mania* is a state of elation; the others are parts of the brain.

48. CNS; *CNS* is the central nervous system; the others are behavioral disorders.
49. absence of a brain
50. pertaining to the cerebral cortex and thalamus
51. inflammation of many nerves
52. treatment of mental disorders
53. softening of the brain
54. partial paralysis of half the body
55. total paralysis
56. pertaining to a spinal nerve root
57. sleep disorder
58. neuropathy
59. neurology
60. myelomeningitis
61. ganglionectomy; gangliectomy
62. ventriculostomy
63. intracerebellar
64. hemiplegia
65. dyslexia
66. hydrophobia
67. extramedullary
68. contralateral
69. postganglionic
70. tachylalia
71. sensory
72. dorsal
73. efferent
74. ganglionic
75. cortical
76. dural
77. meningeal
78. psychotic
79. ganglia
80. ventricles
81. meninges
82. gyri
83. abnormal development of the spinal cord
    a. spinal cord
    b. abnormal
    c. development
    d. condition of
84. inflammation of many nerves and nerve roots
    a. many
    b. nerve
    c. spinal nerve root
    d. inflammation
85. disturbance of muscle coordination
    a. abnormal, difficult
    b. together
    c. work
    d. condition of

Case Study Questions

1. e
2. b
3. a
4. b
5. c
6. e
7. b
8. e
9. astrocytoma
10. craniotomy
11. seizure
12. hemiparesis
13. aphasia
14. meningitis
15. subdural hematoma
16. paranoia
17. antispasmodic
18. neuroleptics
19. psychiatrist
20. computed tomography
21. lumbar puncture
22. neurological intensive care unit (also means neonatal intensive care unit)
23. intracranial pressure
24. cerebrospinal fluid
25. cerebrovascular accident
26. transient ischemic attack
27. level of consciousness

Crossword Puzzle

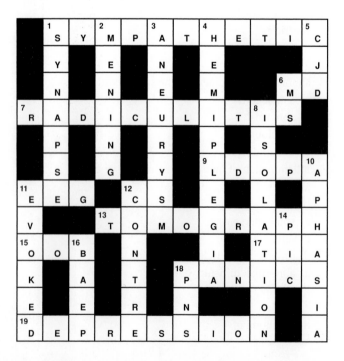

Chapter 18

Pretest

1. olfaction
2. hearing and equilibrium
3. inflammation of the ear
4. retina
5. sclera
6. cataract

Chapter Exercises

Exercise 18-1

1. abnormal sensation
2. false sense of smell
3. lack of taste sensation
4. anesthesia (*an-es-THĒ-zē-a*)
5. pseudogeusia (*sū-dō-GŪ-zē-a*)
6. thermesthesia (*ther-mes-THĒ-zē-a*)
7. hyperalgesia (*hī-per-al-JĒ-zē-a*)
8. dysgeusia (*dis-GŪ-zē-a*)
9. myesthesia (*MĪ-es-thē-zē-a*)

Exercise 18-2

1. hearing
2. sound
3. ear
4. pertaining to hearing
5. pertaining to the ear
6. pertaining to the labyrinth (inner ear)
7. pertaining to the vestibule or vestibular apparatus
8. pertaining to the cochlea
9. pertaining to the stapes
10. audiometry (*aw-dē-OM-e-trē*)
11. otalgia (*ō-TAL-jē-a*)
12. tympanoplasty (*tim-PAN-ō-plas-tē*)
13. myringotomy (*mir-in-GOT-ō-mē*); also, tympanotomy (*tim-pan-OT-ō-mē*)
14. stapedectomy (*stā-pē-DEK- ō-mē*)
15. vestibulocochlear (*ves-tib-ū-lō-KOK-lē-ar*)
16. labyrinthotomy (*lab-i-rin-THOT-ō-mē*)
17. salpingoscopy (*sal-ping-GOS-kō-pē*)
18. endocochlear (*en-dō-KOK-lē-ar*); intracochlear (*in-tra-KOK-lē-ar*)
19. instrument used to measure hearing
20. any disease of the vestibule or vestibular apparatus
21. pertaining to the eustachian (auditory) tube and pharynx
22. instrument used to examine the eardrum
23. inflammation of the ear

Exercise 18-3

1. excision of a lacrimal sac
2. paralysis of the eyelid
3. between the eyelids

4. pertaining to the nose and lacrimal apparatus
5. blepharospasm (*BLEF-a-rō-spasm*)
6. dacryorrhea (*dak-rē-ō-RĒ-a*)
7. dacryocystitis (*dak-rē-ō-sis-TĪ-tis*)

Exercise 18-4

1. eye
2. lens
3. cornea
4. vision
5. lens
6. ophthalm/o; eye
7. pupill/o; pupil
8. lent/i; lens
9. uve/o; uvea
10. phac/o; lens
11. irid/o; iris
12. opt/o; eye, vision
13. retinopexy (*ret-i-nō-PEK-sē*)
14. uveoscleritis (*ū-vē-ō-skle-RĪ-tis*)
15. pupillary (*PU-pi-ler-ē*)
16. phacomalacia (*fak-ō-ma-LĀ-shē-a*)
17. cyclitis (*sī-KLĪ-tis*)
18. ophthalmoscope (*of-THAL-mō-skōp*)
19. ophthalmology (*of-thal-MOL-ō-jē*)
20. iridectomy (*ir-i-DEK-tō-mē*)
21. iridoplegia (*ir-id-ō-PLĒ-jē-a*)
22. pertaining to the eye or vision
23. splitting of the retina
24. instrument used to incise the sclera
25. pertaining to the lens
26. inflammation of the sclera
27. incision of the ciliary muscle
28. inflammation of the iris and ciliary body
29. pertaining to the choroid and retina
30. pertaining to the right eye

Exercise 18-5

1. macropsia (*ma-KROP-sē-a*)
2. achromatopsia (*a-krō-ma-TOP-sē-a*)
3. diplopia (*dip-LŌ-pē-a*)
4. presbyopia (*pres-bē-Ō-pē-a*)
5. ametropia (*am-e-TRŌ-pē-a*)
6. heterometropia (*het-er-ō-me-TRŌ-pē-a*); also, anisometropia (*an-ī-sō-me-TRŌ-pē-a*)

Chapter Review

Labeling Exercise
The Ear

1. outer ear
2. pinna
3. external auditory canal
4. tympanic membrane
5. ossicles of middle ear
6. malleus
7. incus
8. stapes
9. eustachian (auditory) tube
10. inner ear
11. vestibule
12. semicircular canals
13. cochlea

The Eye

1. sclera
2. cornea
3. conjunctival sac
4. choroid
5. ciliary muscle
6. lens
7. iris
8. aqueous humor
9. vitreous body
10. retina
11. fovea
12. optic disk (blind spot)
13. optic nerve

Terminology

1. d
2. e
3. a
4. c
5. b
6. b
7. a
8. e
9. d
10. c
11. d
12. c
13. e
14. b
15. a
16. e
17. c
18. b
19. a
20. d
21. b
22. a
23. d
24. e
25. c
26. d

27. b

28. a

29. c

30. e

31. sclera

32. ear wax

33. proprioception

34. stapes

35. refraction

36. retina

37. cornea

38. tympanic membrane

39. taste; *Taste* is a special sense; the others are general senses.

40. pinna; The *pinna* is part of the outer ear; the others are parts of the inner ear.

41. incus; The *incus* is an ossicle of the ear; the others are structures that protect the eye.

42. presbycusis; *Presbycusis* is loss of hearing due to age; the others are disorders of the eye.

43. F; constrict

44. T

45. T

46. F; taste

47. T

48. T

49. F; tympanic membrane

50. F; tears

51. specialist in the study and treatment of hearing disorders

52. absence of a lens

53. below the sclera

54. instrument for measuring the eye

55. inflammation of the cornea and iris

56. incision of the iris

57. around the lens

58. pertaining to the choroids and retina

59. excess flow of tears

60. incision of the tympanic membrane

61. vestibulocochlear

62. stapedectomy

63. otoplasty

64. analgesia

65. blepharoptosis

66. retinopathy

67. pupillometry

68. tympanosclerosis; myringosclerosis

69. lacrimal

70. salpingoscopy

71. cyclectomy

72. cochlear

73. palpebral

74. vestibular

75. uveal

76. corneal

77. scleral

78. pupillary

79. miosis

80. exotropia

81. cc

82. myopia

83. hyperesthesia

84. OD

85. unequal refractive powers in the two eyes
   a. not, without
   b. equal
   c. measure
   d. vision

86. weakness or tiring of the eyes
   a. lack of
   b. strength
   c. vision

87. study and treatment of the ear, nose, and throat (ENT)
   a. ear
   b. nose
   c. throat
   d. study of

Case Study Questions

1. a

2. a

3. d

4. c

5. e

6. d

7. b

8. d

9. e

10. b

11. tympanogram

12. aural

13. otitis media

14. otitis externa

15. ophthalmologist

16. intraocular

17. miosis

18. midazolam

19. hertz

20. brainstem auditory evoked potentials

21. right eye

22. intraocular lens

Crossword Puzzle

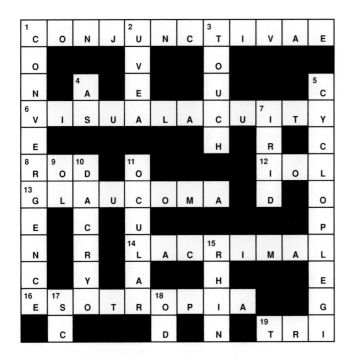

Chapter 19

Pretest

1. bone
2. bone marrow
3. vertebra
4. ilium
5. carpals
6. femur
7. arthritis
8. cartilage

Chapter Exercises

Exercise 19-1

1. bone, bone tissue
2. bone marrow
3. joint
4. cartilage
5. bursa
6. dissolving or destruction of bone
7. formation of bone marrow
8. tumor of cartilage
9. surgical puncture of a joint
10. inflammation of a bursa
11. pertaining to or resembling bone marrow
12. osteomyelitis (*os-tē-ō-mī-e-LĪ-tis*)
13. osteopenia (*os-tē-ō-PĒ-nē-a*)
14. arthroplasty (*AR-thrō-plas-tē*)
15. myeloma (*mī-e-LŌ-ma*)
16. bursotomy (*bur-SOT-ō-mē*)
17. synovitis (*si-nō-VĪ-tis*)
18. arthroscope (*AR-thrō-skōp*)
19. chondroid (*KON-droyd*)
20. arthropathy (*ar-THROP-a-thē*)
21. hyperostosis (*hī-per-os-TŌ-sis*)
22. dysostosis (*dis-os-TŌ-sis*)

Exercise 19-2

1. cranial
2. costal
3. pelvic
4. iliac
5. vertebral
6. sacral
7. incision of the cranium (skull)
8. near the vertebrae or spinal column
9. pain in a vertebra
10. above the pelvis
11. cranioschisis (*krā-nē-OS-ki-sis*)
12. spondylitis (*spon-di-LĪ-tis*)
13. costectomy (*kos-TEK-tō-mē*)
14. rachiocentesis (*rā-kē-ō-sen-TĒ-sis*); also, rachicentesis (*rā-kē-sen-TĒ-sis*)
15. sacroiliac (*sā-krō-IL-ē-ak*)
16. craniosacral (*krā-nē-ō-SĀ-kral*)
17. pelvimetry (*pel-VIM-e-trē*)
18. presacral (*prē-SĀ-kral*)
19. coccygectomy (*kok-si-JEK-tō-mē*)
20. iliococcygeal (*il-ē-ō-kok-SIJ-ē-al*)
21. infracostal (*in-fra-KOS-tal*); subcostal (*sub-KOS-tal*)

Chapter Review

Labeling Exercise
The Skeleton

1. cranium
2. facial bones
3. mandible
4. vertebral column
5. sacrum
6. sternum
7. ribs
8. clavicle
9. scapula
10. humerus
11. radius
12. ulna
13. carpals
14. metacarpals
15. phalanges
16. pelvis
17. ilium
18. femur

19. patella
20. fibula
21. tibia
22. tarsals
23. calcaneus
24. metatarsals
25. phalanges

Skull from the Left

1. frontal
2. parietal
3. occipital
4. temporal
5. sphenoid
6. lacrimal
7. nasal
8. zygomatic
9. maxilla
10. mandible
11. hyoid

Vertebral Column

1. cervical vertebrae
2. thoracic vertebrae
3. lumbar vertebrae
4. sacrum
5. coccyx
6. intervertebral disk
7. body of vertebra

The Pelvic Bones

1. ilium
2. ischium
3. pubis
4. pubic symphysis
5. acetabulum
6. sacrum

Structure of a Long Bone

1. proximal epiphysis (*e-PIF-i-sis*)
2. diaphysis (*dī-AF-i-sis*)
3. distal epiphysis
4. cartilage
5. epiphyseal line (growth line)
6. spongy bone (containing red marrow)
7. compact bone
8. medullary (marrow) cavity
9. artery and vein
10. yellow marrow
11. periosteum (*per-ē-OS-tē-um*)

TERMINOLOGY

1. d
2. a
3. e
4. c
5. b
6. d
7. a
8. e
9. c
10. b
11. c
12. d
13. e
14. a
15. b
16. d
17. c
18. e
19. b
20. a
21. orthopedics
22. cartilage
23. ligament
24. sacrum
25. bursa
26. synovial fluid; synovia
27. joint
28. cartilage
29. vertebrae
30. spine
31. F; diaphysis
32. T
33. T
34. F; appendicular
35. F; cervical
36. T
37. T
38. F; lordosis
39. T
40. hyoid; The *hyoid* is the bone below the mandible (lower jaw); the others are bone markings.
41. coronal; *Coronal* refers to a suture or plane at right angles to the midline; the others are bones of the skull.
42. cost/o; *Cost/o* refers to a rib; the others are roots pertaining to the spine.
43. sciatic; *Sciatic* refers to the sciatic nerve that travels through the leg; the others are types of bone fractures.
44. RA; *RA* is an abbreviation for rheumatoid arthritis; the others are abbreviations for spinal regions.
45. originating in bone marrow
46. inflammation of bone
47. fusion of a joint
48. excision of a synovial membrane
49. within a bone
50. around a bursa
51. pain in a vertebra

52. pertaining to many joints
53. below a rib
54. pertaining to the coccyx
55. chondrogenesis
56. osteonecrosis
57. craniotomy
58. osteochondroma
59. arthrostenosis
60. chondrectomy
61. bursolith
62. arthroclasis
63. arthrotome
64. pelvimetry
65. arthroscopy
66. sacroiliac
67. osteolysis
68. coccygectomy
69. parasacral
70. cranial
71. iliac
72. coccygeal
73. pelvic
74. vertebral
75. benign tumor of cartilage-forming cells
    a. cartilage
    b. immature, productive cell
    c. tumor
76. surgical fusion (ankylosis) between vertebrae
    a. vertebra
    b. together
    c. fusion, binding
77. decreased growth of cartilage in the growth plate of long bones resulting in dwarfism
    a. lack of
    b. cartilage
    c. formation, molding

Case Study Questions

1. c
2. b
3. c
4. e
5. c
6. a
7. d
8. b
9. zygomatic
10. periosteum
11. meniscus
12. bilateral
13. arthroplasty
14. idiopathic
15. scapulectomy

16. fracture
17. osteotomies
18. degenerative joint disease
19. magnetic resonance imaging
20. nonsteroidal antiinflammatory drugs
21. computed tomography
22. normal saline solution
23. temporomandibular joint
24. osteogenesis imperfecta
25. open reduction internal fixation
26. posterior spinal fusion
27. estimated blood loss

Crossword Puzzle

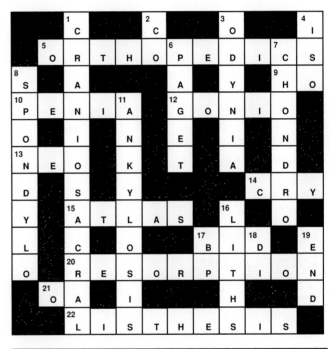

Chapter 20

Pretest

1. nerve; neuron
2. insertion
3. thigh
4. supination
5. tendon
6. muscles

Chapter Exercises

EXERCISE 20-1

1. pertaining to muscle
2. pertaining to fascia
3. pertaining to a tendon
4. pertaining to movement
5. pertaining to tone
6. muscle

7. work
8. tone
9. movement; motion
10. fascia
11. fibers
12. muscle
13. muscle; smooth muscle
14. lack of muscle tone
15. binding or fusion of a tendon
16. abnormality of movement
17. pain in a muscle
18. pertaining to muscle and tendon
19. inflammation of a tendon
20. excess muscle tone
21. treatment using movement
22. suture of fascia
23. producing or generating work
24. pertaining to muscle and fascia
25. plastic repair of tendon and muscle
26. polymyositis (pol-ē-mī-ō-SĪ-tis)
27. myopathy (mī-OP-a-thē)
28. fasciectomy (fash-ē-EK-tō-mē)
29. kinesiology (ki-nē-sē-OL-ō-jē)
30. tenotomy (ten-OT-ō-mē)
31. myotenositis (mī-ō-ten-ō-SĪ-tis)

Chapter Review

LABELING EXERCISE
Superficial Muscles, Anterior View

1. temporalis
2. orbicularis oculi
3. orbicularis oris
4. masseter
5. sternocleidomastoid
6. trapezius
7. deltoid
8. pectoralis major
9. serratus anterior
10. biceps brachii
11. brachioradialis
12. flexor carpi
13. extensor carpi
14. external oblique
15. internal oblique
16. rectus abdominis
17. intercostals
18. sartorius
19. adductors of thigh
20. quadriceps femoris
21. gastrocnemius
22. soleus

23. peroneus longus
24. tibialis anterior

Superficial Muscles, Posterior View

1. sternocleidomastoid
2. trapezius
3. deltoid
4. teres minor
5. teres major
6. latissimus dorsi
7. triceps brachii
8. gluteus medius
9. gluteus maximus
10. hamstring group
11. gastrocnemius
12. peroneus longus

TERMINOLOGY

1. d
2. b
3. e
4. a
5. c
6. c
7. a
8. d
9. b
10. e
11. d
12. c
13. b
14. a
15. e
16. d
17. b
18. e
19. a
20. c
21. c
22. e
23. d
24. b
25. a
26. acetylcholine
27. fascia
28. two
29. flexor
30. tendon
31. Achilles tendon
32. abduction
33. osteoblast; An *osteoblast* is a bone cell; the others are related to muscle structure.
34. soleus; The *soleus* is a calf muscle; the others are muscles of the arm.

35. intercostals; The *intercostals* are between the ribs; the others are quadriceps muscles in the anterior thigh.
36. actin; *Actin* is a type of muscle filament involved in contraction; the others are types of movement.
37. EMG; *EMG* is electromyography, a method for studying the electrical energy in muscles; the others are diseases that involve muscles.
38. F; insertion
39. F; posterior
40. T
41. T
42. F; four
43. T
44. pain in a muscle
45. pertaining to muscle and fascia
46. plastic repair of a tendon (also, tendinoplasty)
47. inflammation of fibers (fibrous tissue)
48. decreased muscle tone
49. abnormally increased movement
50. myology
51. myonecrosis
52. fasciotomy
53. atony
54. fasciitis, also fascitis
55. kinesiology
56. tenorrhaphy
57. tendinous
58. antagonist
59. insertion
60. adduction
61. supination
62. flexion
63. ataxic
64. athetotic
65. spastic, spasmodic
66. clonic
67. electromyography, electromyogram
68. acetylcholine
69. occupational therapy
70. neuromuscular junction
71. creatine kinase
72. lack of smooth or accurate muscle movement because coordination between muscle components is lacking
    a. abnormal
    b. together
    c. work
    d. condition of
73. pertaining to muscle wasting, atrophy
    a. lack of
    b. muscle
    c. nourishment
    d. pertaining to
74. muscular weakness

a. muscle
b. lack of
c. strength
d. condition of

Case Study Questions

1. b
2. d
3. e
4. a
5. b
6. d
7. c
8. a
9. c
10. d
11. b
12. c
13. c
14. e
15. brachial
16. orthopedic
17. flexion
18. plantar flexion
19. physical therapy
20. range of motion
21. rule out
22. electromyogram
23. somatosensory evoked potentials
24. postanesthetic care unit

Crossword Puzzle

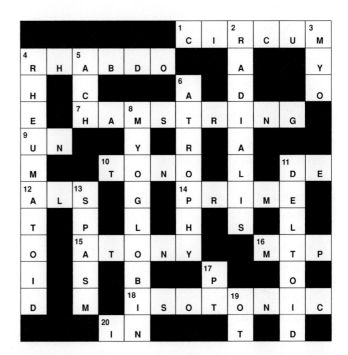

Chapter 21

Pretest

1. epidermis
2. follicle
3. sebaceous glands
4. burns
5. melanoma
6. sweat, perspiration
7. nail

Chapter Exercises

Exercise 21-1

1. derm/o; skin
2. melan/o; melanin
3. seb/o; sebum
4. kerat/o; keratin, horny layer of the skin
5. hidr/o; sweat
6. onych/o; nail
7. trich/o; hair
8. skin
9. keratin
10. melanin
11. sweat, perspiration
12. nail
13. hair
14. skin
15. dermatome (DER-ma-tōm)
16. keratogenesis (ker-a-tō-JEN-e-sis)
17. melanoma (mel-a-NŌ-ma)
18. dermatolysis (der-ma-TOL-i-sis); dermolysis (der-MOL-i-sis)
19. trichology (trik-OL-ō-jē)
20. hyperhidrosis (hī-per-hī-DRŌ-sis)
21. onychomalacia (on-i-kō-ma-LĀ-shē-a)
22. dermatology (der-ma-TOL-ō-jē)
23. scleroderma (sklēr-ō-DER-ma)
24. pyoderma (pī-ō-DER-ma)

Chapter Review

Labeling Exercise
Cross Section of the Skin

1. epidermis
2. stratum basale (growing layer)
3. stratum corneum
4. dermis (corium)
5. subcutaneous layer
6. adipose tissue
7. hair follicle
8. hair
9. arrector pili muscle
10. artery

11. vein
12. nerve
13. nerve endings
14. sudoriferous (sweat) gland
15. pore (opening of sweat gland)
16. sebaceous (oil) gland
17. touch receptor
18. pressure receptor

Terminology

1. c
2. a
3. e
4. b
5. d
6. c
7. d
8. b
9. e
10. a
11. e
12. a
13. b
14. c
15. d
16. d
17. e
18. a
19. c
20. b
21. skin
22. sweat, perspiration
23. melanin
24. sebaceous glands
25. keratin
26. cicatrix; A cicatrix is a scar; the others are types of skin lesions.
27. débridement; Débridement is removal of dead or damaged tissue; the others are types of skin diseases.
28. BSA; BSA is an abbreviation for body-surface area; the others are abbreviations for skin diseases (mainly forms of lupus).
29. T
30. F; stratum corneum
31. F; hair
32. T
33. F; sweating
34. T
35. a cell that produces melanin
36. through the skin
37. producing keratin
38. thickening of the skin
39. fungal infection of the hair

40. infection of a nail and nail bed
41. dryness of the skin
42. seborrhea
43. hypermelanosis
44. scleroderma; dermatosclerosis
45. melanoma
46. trichology
47. dermatome
48. onycholysis
49. dermatopathy; dermopathy
50. anhidrosis
51. hyperhidrosis
52. chromhidrosis
53. ingrown toenail
     a. nail
     b. hidden
     c. condition of
54. lack of color or graying of the hair
     a. lack of
     b. color
     c. hair
     d. condition of
55. benign tumor of a sweat gland
     a. sweat
     b. gland
     c. tumor

Case Study Questions

1. b
2. c
3. d
4. e
5. a
6. c
7. b
8. d
9. a
10. e

11. e
12. d
13. dermabrasion
14. nodule
15. dermatologist
16. subcutaneous tissue
17. erythema/erythroderma
18. hyperkeratosis
19. débridement
20. ischemia
21. full-thickness skin graft
22. split-thickness skin graft
23. sun protection factor
24. at bedtime
25. twice per day

Crossword Puzzle

¹K	E	R	A	²T	O			H	I	⁴D		R
E				R		⁵E		C		Y		
⁶L	E		⁷H	I	R	S	U	T	⁸I	S		M
O				C		C			M			
⁹I	¹⁰D			H		¹¹H	E	R	P	E		¹²S
¹³D	E	R	M	O		A			E			T
	B		¹⁴I	D	R	O			T			R
¹⁵T	R	I		D		O		¹⁶C	I	C		A
	I		¹⁷N			T		G				T
¹⁸D	¹⁹I	A	S	C	O	P	Y			²⁰E		U
²¹S	E	M	I			M				P		M
			L		²³H	Y	P	O		I		

FIGURE CREDITS

FIGURE 1-3	■	Cohen B. Memmler's *The Human Body in Health and Disease*. 10th ed. Baltimore: Lippincott Williams & Wilkins, 2005.
FIGURE 2-2	■	Smeltzer SC, Bare B. *Medical-Surgical Nursing*. 10th ed. Philadelphia: Lippincott Williams & Wilkins, 2004.
FIGURE 2-3	■	Taylor C, Lillis C, LeMone P. *Fundamentals of Nursing*. 5th ed. Philadelphia: Lippincott Williams & Wilkins, 2005.
FIGURE 2-4	■	Taylor C, Lillis C, LeMone P. *Fundamentals of Nursing*. 5th ed. Philadelphia: Lippincott Williams & Wilkins, 2005.
FIGURE 2-5	■	Taylor C, Lillis C, LeMone P. *Fundamentals of Nursing*. 5th ed. Philadelphia: Lippincott Williams & Wilkins, 2005.
FIGURE 2-6	■	Cormack DH. *Essential Histology*. 2nd ed. Philadelphia: Lippincott Williams & Wilkins, 2001.
FIGURE 2-7	■	Cohen B. Memmler's *The Human Body in Health and Disease*. 10th ed. Baltimore: Lippincott Williams & Wilkins, 2005.
FIGURE 2-8	■	Cohen B. Memmler's *The Human Body in Health and Disease*. 10th ed. Baltimore: Lippincott Williams & Wilkins, 2005.
FIGURE 2-9	■	Cormack DH. *Essential Histology*. 2nd ed. Philadelphia: Lippincott Williams & Wilkins, 2001.
FIGURE 2-10	■	Cohen B. Memmler's *The Human Body in Health and Disease*. 10th ed. Baltimore: Lippincott Williams & Wilkins, 2005.
FIGURE 3-1	■	Cohen B. Memmler's *The Human Body in Health and Disease*. 10th ed. Baltimore: Lippincott Williams & Wilkins, 2005.
FIGURE 3-2	■	Cohen B. Memmler's *The Human Body in Health and Disease*. 10th ed. Baltimore: Lippincott Williams & Wilkins, 2005.
FIGURE 3-3	■	Koneman EW, et al. *Diagnostic Microbiology*. 4th ed. Philadelphia: Lippincott Williams & Wilkins, 1992.
FIGURE 3-4	■	Bickley LS. Bates' *Guide to Physical Examination and History Taking*. 8th ed. Philadelphia: Lippincott Williams & Wilkins, 2003.
FIGURE 3-5	■	Cohen B. Memmler's *The Human Body in Health and Disease*. 10th ed. Baltimore: Lippincott Williams & Wilkins, 2005.
FIGURE 3-6	■	Taylor C, Lillis C, LeMone P. *Fundamentals of Nursing*. 5th ed. Philadelphia: Lippincott Williams & Wilkins, 2005.
FIGURE 3-7	■	Cohen B. Memmler's *The Human Body in Health and Disease*. 10th ed. Baltimore: Lippincott Williams & Wilkins, 2005.
FIGURE 3-8	■	Cohen B. Memmler's *The Human Body in Health and Disease*. 10th ed. Baltimore: Lippincott Williams & Wilkins, 2005.
FIGURE 4-1	■	Cohen B. Memmler's *The Human Body in Health and Disease*. 10th ed. Baltimore: Lippincott Williams & Wilkins, 2005.
FIGURE 4-2	■	Cohen B. Memmler's *The Human Body in Health and Disease*. 10th ed. Baltimore: Lippincott Williams & Wilkins, 2005.
FIGURE 4-3	■	Cohen B. Memmler's *The Human Body in Health and Disease*. 10th ed. Baltimore: Lippincott Williams & Wilkins, 2005.
FIGURE 4-5	■	Cohen B. Memmler's *The Human Body in Health and Disease*. 10th ed. Baltimore: Lippincott Williams & Wilkins, 2005.
FIGURE 4-6	■	Parts A and B: Mills SE. *Histology for Pathologists*. 3rd ed. Philadelphia: Lippincott Williams & Wilkins, 2006; Part C: Gartner LP, Hiatt JL. *Color Atlas of Histology*. 4th ed. Baltimore: Lippincott Williams & Wilkins, 2005
FIGURE 4-7	■	Part A: Cormack DH: *Essential Histology*. 2nd ed. Baltimore: Lippincott Williams & Wilkins, 2001. Part B: Gartner LP, Hiatt JL. *Color Atlas of Histology*. 4th ed. Baltimore: Lippincott Williams & Wilkins, 2005

FIGURE 4-8 ■ Cohen B. Memmler's *The Human Body in Health and Disease*. 10th ed. Baltimore: Lippincott Williams & Wilkins, 2005.

FIGURE 4-9 ■ Cohen B. Memmler's *The Human Body in Health and Disease*. 10th ed. Baltimore: Lippincott Williams & Wilkins, 2005.

FIGURE 4-10 ■ Cohen B. Memmler's *The Human Body in Health and Disease*. 10th ed. Baltimore: Lippincott Williams & Wilkins, 2005.

FIGURE 5-1 ■ Cohen B. Memmler's *The Human Body in Health and Disease*. 10th ed. Baltimore: Lippincott Williams & Wilkins, 2005.

FIGURE 5-2 ■ Cohen B. Memmler's *The Human Body in Health and Disease*. 10th ed. Baltimore: Lippincott Williams & Wilkins, 2005.

FIGURE 5-3 ■ Cohen B. Memmler's *The Human Body in Health and Disease*. 10th ed. Baltimore: Lippincott Williams & Wilkins, 2005.

FIGURE 5-4 ■ Cohen B. Memmler's *The Human Body in Health and Disease*. 10th ed. Baltimore: Lippincott Williams & Wilkins, 2005.

FIGURE 5-5 ■ Cohen B. Memmler's *The Human Body in Health and Disease*. 10th ed. Baltimore: Lippincott Williams & Wilkins, 2005.

FIGURE 6-1 ■ Cohen B. Memmler's *The Human Body in Health and Disease*. 10th ed. Baltimore: Lippincott Williams & Wilkins, 2005.

FIGURE 6-2 ■ Cohen B. Memmler's *The Human Body in Health and Disease*. 10th ed. Baltimore: Lippincott Williams & Wilkins, 2005.

FIGURE 6-3 ■ Cohen B. Memmler's *The Human Body in Health and Disease*. 10th ed. Baltimore: Lippincott Williams & Wilkins, 2005.

FIGURE 6-4 ■ Bickley LS. Bates' *Guide to Physical Examination and History Taking*. 8th ed. Philadelphia: Lippincott Williams & Wilkins, 2003.

FIGURE 6-5 ■ Cohen B. Memmler's *The Human Body in Health and Disease*. 10th ed. Baltimore: Lippincott Williams & Wilkins, 2005.

FIGURE 7-1 ■ Taylor C, Lillis C, LeMone P. *Fundamentals of Nursing*. 5th ed. Philadelphia: Lippincott Williams & Wilkins, 2005.

FIGURE 7-2 ■ Taylor C, Lillis C, LeMone P. *Fundamentals of Nursing*. 5th ed. Philadelphia: Lippincott Williams & Wilkins, 2005.

FIGURE 7-3 ■ Taylor C, Lillis C, LeMone P. *Fundamentals of Nursing*. 5th ed. Philadelphia: Lippincott Williams & Wilkins, 2005.

FIGURE 7-4 ■ Taylor C, Lillis C, LeMone P. *Fundamentals of Nursing*. 5th ed. Philadelphia: Lippincott Williams & Wilkins, 2005.

FIGURE 7-5 ■ Taylor C, Lillis C, LeMone P. *Fundamentals of Nursing*. 5th ed. Philadelphia: Lippincott Williams & Wilkins, 2005.

FIGURE 7-6 ■ Taylor C, Lillis C, LeMone P. *Fundamentals of Nursing*. 5th ed. Philadelphia: Lippincott Williams & Wilkins, 2005.

FIGURE 7-8 ■ Erkonen WE. *Radiology 101*. Philadelphia: Lippincott Williams & Wilkins, 1998.

FIGURE 7-9 ■ Erkonen WE. *Radiology 101*. Philadelphia: Lippincott Williams & Wilkins, 1998.

FIGURE 7-10 ■ Pilletteri A. *Maternal and Child Health Nursing*. 4th ed. Philadelphia: Lippincott Williams & Wilkins, 2003.

FIGURE 7-12 ■ Taylor C, Lillis C, LeMone P. *Fundamentals of Nursing*. 5th ed. Philadelphia: Lippincott Williams & Wilkins, 2005.

FIGURE 7-13 ■ Smeltzer SC, Bare B. *Medical-Surgical Nursing*. 10th ed. Philadelphia: Lippincott Williams & Wilkins, 2004.

FIGURE 7-14 ■ Taylor C, Lillis C, LeMone P. *Fundamentals of Nursing*. 5th ed. Philadelphia: Lippincott Williams & Wilkins, 2005.

FIGURE 8-1 ■ Rosedahl CB, Kowalski MT. *Textbook of Basic Nursing*. 8th ed. Philadelphia: Lippincott Williams & Wilkins, 2002.

FIGURE 8-4 ■ Taylor C, Lillis C, LeMone P. *Fundamentals of Nursing*. 5th ed. Philadelphia: Lippincott Williams & Wilkins, 2005.

FIGURE 9-1 ■ Cohen B. Memmler's *The Human Body in Health and Disease*. 10th ed. Baltimore: Lippincott Williams & Wilkins, 2005.

FIGURE 9-2 ■ Cohen B. Memmler's *The Human Body in Health and Disease*. 10th ed. Baltimore: Lippincott Williams & Wilkins, 2005.

FIGURE 9-3 ■ Cohen B. Memmler's *The Human Body in Health and Disease*. 10th ed. Baltimore: Lippincott Williams & Wilkins, 2005.

FIGURE 9-4 ■ Smeltzer SC, Bare B. *Medical-Surgical Nursing*. 10th ed. Philadelphia: Lippincott Williams & Wilkins, 2004.

FIGURE 9-7 ■ Bickley LS. Bates' *Guide to Physical Examination and History Taking*. 8th ed. Philadelphia: Lippincott Williams & Wilkins, 2003.

FIGURE 9-8 ■ Cohen B. Memmler's *The Human Body in Health and Disease*. 10th ed. Baltimore: Lippincott Williams & Wilkins, 2005.

FIGURE 9-11 ■ Smeltzer SC, Bare B. *Medical-Surgical Nursing*. 10th ed. Philadelphia: Lippincott Williams & Wilkins, 2004.

FIGURE 9-16A ■ Cohen B. Memmler's *The Human Body in Health and Disease*. 10th ed. Baltimore: Lippincott Williams & Wilkins, 2005.

FIGURE 9-16B ■ Porth CM. *Pathophysiology*. 7th ed. Philadelphia: Lippincott Williams & Wilkins, 2005.

FIGURE 9-17 ■ Bickley LS. Bates' *Guide to Physical Examination and History Taking*. 8th ed. Philadelphia: Lippincott Williams & Wilkins, 2003.

FIGURE 9-18 ■ Cohen B. Memmler's *The Human Body in Health and Disease*. 10th ed. Baltimore: Lippincott Williams & Wilkins, 2005.

FIGURE 9-19 ■ Cohen B. Memmler's *The Human Body in Health and Disease*. 10th ed. Baltimore: Lippincott Williams & Wilkins, 2005.

FIGURE 9-20 ■ Cohen B. Memmler's *The Human Body in Health and Disease*. 10th ed. Baltimore: Lippincott Williams & Wilkins, 2005.

FIGURE 9-21 ■ Bickley LS. Bates' *Guide to Physical Examination and History Taking*. 8th ed. Philadelphia: Lippincott Williams & Wilkins, 2003.

FIGURE 10-1 ■ Cohen B. Memmler's *The Human Body in Health and Disease*. 10th ed. Baltimore: Lippincott Williams & Wilkins, 2005.

FIGURE 10-2 ■ Cohen B. Memmler's *The Human Body in Health and Disease*. 10th ed. Baltimore: Lippincott Williams & Wilkins, 2005.

FIGURE 10-3 ■ Cohen B. Memmler's *The Human Body in Health and Disease*. 10th ed. Baltimore: Lippincott Williams & Wilkins, 2005.

FIGURE 10-4 ■ Cohen B. Memmler's *The Human Body in Health and Disease*. 10th ed. Baltimore: Lippincott Williams & Wilkins, 2005.

FIGURE 10-5 ■ Gartner LP, Hiatt JL. *Color Atlas of Histology*. 3rd ed. Philadelphia: Lippincott Williams & Wilkins, 2000.

FIGURE 10-6 ■ Gartner LP, Hiatt JL. *Color Atlas of Histology*. 3rd ed. Philadelphia: Lippincott Williams & Wilkins, 2000.

FIGURE 10-7 ■ Cohen B. Memmler's *The Human Body in Health and Disease*. 10th ed. Baltimore: Lippincott Williams & Wilkins, 2005.

FIGURE 10-8 ■ Cohen B. Memmler's *The Human Body in Health and Disease*. 10th ed. Baltimore: Lippincott Williams & Wilkins, 2005.

FIGURE 10-12 ■ Rubin E, Farber JL. *Pathology*. 4th ed. Philadelphia: Lippincott Williams & Wilkins, 2005.

FIGURE 10-13 ■ Rubin R, Strayes DS. *Rubin's Pathology: Clinicopathologic Foundations of Medicine*. 5th ed. Baltimore: Lippincott Williams & Wilkins, 2007.

FIGURE 10-14 ■ Rubin E, Farber JL. *Pathology*. 4th ed. Philadelphia: Lippincott Williams & Wilkins, 2005.

FIGURE 10-15 ■ Rubin E, Farber JL. *Pathology*. 4th ed. Philadelphia: Lippincott Williams & Wilkins, 2005.

FIGURE 10-16 ■ Rubin E, Farber JL. *Pathology*. 4th ed. Philadelphia: Lippincott Williams & Wilkins, 2005.

BOX 10-6 ■ Cormack DH. *Essential Histology*. 2nd ed. Philadelphia: Lippincott Williams & Wilkins, 2001.

FIGURE 11-1 ■ Cohen B. Memmler's *The Human Body in Health and Disease*. 10th ed. Baltimore: Lippincott Williams & Wilkins, 2005.

FIGURE 11-2 ■ Cohen B. Memmler's *The Human Body in Health and Disease*. 10th ed. Baltimore: Lippincott Williams & Wilkins, 2005.

FIGURE 11-3 ■ Cohen B. Memmler's *The Human Body in Health and Disease*. 10th ed. Baltimore: Lippincott Williams & Wilkins, 2005.

FIGURE 11-4 ■ Cohen B. Memmler's *The Human Body in Health and Disease*. 10th ed. Baltimore: Lippincott Williams & Wilkins, 2005.

FIGURE 11-5 ■ Cohen B. Memmler's *The Human Body in Health and Disease*. 10th ed. Baltimore: Lippincott Williams & Wilkins, 2005.

FIGURE 11-6 ■ Cohen B. Memmler's *The Human Body in Health and Disease*. 10th ed. Baltimore: Lippincott Williams & Wilkins, 2005.

FIGURE 11-8 ■ Rubin E, Farber JL. *Pathology*. 4th ed. Philadelphia: Lippincott Williams & Wilkins, 2005.

FIGURE 11-12 ■ Taylor C, Lillis C, LeMone P. *Fundamentals of Nursing*. 5th ed. Philadelphia: Lippincott Williams & Wilkins, 2005.

FIGURE 11-13 ■ Cohen B. Memmler's *The Human Body in Health and Disease*. 10th ed. Baltimore: Lippincott Williams & Wilkins, 2005.

FIGURE 11-14 ■ Taylor C, Lillis C, LeMone P. *Fundamentals of Nursing*. 5th ed. Philadelphia: Lippincott Williams & Wilkins, 2005.

FIGURE 12-1 ■ Cohen B. Memmler's *The Human Body in Health and Disease*. 10th ed. Baltimore: Lippincott Williams & Wilkins, 2005.

FIGURE 12-2 ■ Cohen B. Memmler's *The Human Body in Health and Disease*. 10th ed. Baltimore: Lippincott Williams & Wilkins, 2005.

FIGURE 12-3 ■ Cohen B. Memmler's *The Human Body in Health and Disease*. 10th ed. Baltimore: Lippincott Williams & Wilkins, 2005.

FIGURE 12-4 ■ Cohen B. Memmler's *The Human Body in Health and Disease*. 10th ed. Baltimore: Lippincott Williams & Wilkins, 2005.

FIGURE 12-5 ■ Cohen B. Memmler's *The Human Body in Health and Disease*. 10th ed. Baltimore: Lippincott Williams & Wilkins, 2005.

FIGURE 12-10 ■ Rubin E, Farber JL. *Pathology*. 4th ed. Philadelphia: Lippincott Williams & Wilkins, 2005.

FIGURE 12-11 ■ Erkonen WE. *Radiology 101*. Philadelphia: Lippincott Williams & Wilkins, 1998.

FIGURE 12-12 ■ Bickley LS. Bates' *Guide to Physical Examination and History Taking*. 8th ed. Philadelphia: Lippincott Williams & Wilkins, 2003.

FIGURE 12-13 ■ Erkonen WE. *Radiology 101*. Philadelphia: Lippincott Williams & Wilkins, 1998.

FIGURE 12-16 ■ Stedman's *Medical Dictionary for the Health Professions and Nursing*. 5th ed. Baltimore: Lippincott Williams & Wilkins, 2005.

FIGURE 12-17B ■ Erkonen WE. *Radiology 101*. Philadelphia: Lippincott Williams & Wilkins, 1998.

FIGURE 13-1 ■ Cohen B. Memmler's *The Human Body in Health and Disease*. 10th ed. Baltimore: Lippincott Williams & Wilkins, 2005.

FIGURE 13-2 ■ Cohen B. Memmler's *The Human Body in Health and Disease*. 10th ed. Baltimore: Lippincott Williams & Wilkins, 2005.

FIGURE 13-3 ■ Cohen B. Memmler's *The Human Body in Health and Disease*. 10th ed. Baltimore: Lippincott Williams & Wilkins, 2005.

FIGURE 13-4 ■ Cohen B. Memmler's *The Human Body in Health and Disease*. 10th ed. Baltimore: Lippincott Williams & Wilkins, 2005.

FIGURE 13-6 ■ Porth CM. *Pathophysiology*. 7th ed. Philadelphia: Lippincott Williams & Wilkins, 2005.

FIGURE 13-9 ■ Rubin E, Farber JL. *Pathology*. 4th ed. Philadelphia: Lippincott Williams & Wilkins, 2005.

FIGURE 13-12 ■ Erkonen WE. *Radiology 101*. Philadelphia: Lippincott Williams & Wilkins, 1998.

FIGURE 13-13 ■ Rubin E, Farber JL. *Pathology*. 4th ed. Philadelphia: Lippincott Williams & Wilkins, 2005.

FIGURE 13-15 ■ Rubin E, Farber JL. *Pathology*. 4th ed. Philadelphia: Lippincott Williams & Wilkins, 2005.

FIGURE 13-16 ■ Rubin E, Farber JL. *Pathology*. 4th ed. Philadelphia: Lippincott Williams & Wilkins, 2005.

FIGURE 14-1 ■ Cohen B. Memmler's *The Human Body in Health and Disease*. 10th ed. Baltimore: Lippincott Williams & Wilkins, 2005.

FIGURE 14-3 ■ Cohen B. Memmler's *The Human Body in Health and Disease*. 10th ed. Baltimore: Lippincott Williams & Wilkins, 2005.

FIGURE 14-4 ■ Cohen B. Memmler's *The Human Body in Health and Disease*. 10th ed. Baltimore: Lippincott Williams & Wilkins, 2005.

FIGURE 14-6 ■ Rubin E, Farber JL. *Pathology*. 4th ed. Philadelphia: Lippincott Williams & Wilkins, 2005

FIGURE 15-1 ■ Cohen B. Memmler's *The Human Body in Health and Disease*. 10th ed. Baltimore: Lippincott Williams & Wilkins, 2005.

FIGURE 15-2 ■ Cohen B. Memmler's *The Human Body in Health and Disease*. 10th ed. Baltimore: Lippincott Williams & Wilkins, 2005.

FIGURE 15-3 ■ Cohen B. Memmler's *The Human Body in Health and Disease*. 10th ed. Baltimore: Lippincott Williams & Wilkins, 2005.

FIGURE 15-4 ■ Cohen B. Memmler's *The Human Body in Health and Disease*. 10th ed. Baltimore: Lippincott Williams & Wilkins, 2005.

FIGURE 15-7 ■ Rubin E, Farber JL. *Pathology*. 4th ed. Philadelphia: Lippincott Williams & Wilkins, 2005.

FIGURE 15-10 ■ Erkonen WE. *Radiology 101*. Philadelphia: Lippincott Williams & Wilkins, 1998.

FIGURE 15-12 ■ Cohen B. Memmler's *The Human Body in Health and Disease*. 10th ed. Baltimore: Lippincott Williams & Wilkins, 2005.

FIGURE 15-13 ■ Pilletteri A. *Maternal and Child Health Nursing*. 4th ed. Philadelphia: Lippincott Williams & Wilkins, 2003.

FIGURE 15-14 ■ Cohen B. Memmler's *The Human Body in Health and Disease*. 10th ed. Baltimore: Lippincott Williams & Wilkins, 2005.

FIGURE 15-15 ■ Cohen B. Memmler's *The Human Body in Health and Disease.* 10th ed. Baltimore: Lippincott Williams & Wilkins, 2005.

FIGURE 15-17 ■ Pilletteri A. *Maternal and Child Health Nursing.* 4th ed. Philadelphia: Lippincott Williams & Wilkins, 2003.

FIGURE 15-18 ■ Pilletteri A. *Maternal and Child Health Nursing.* 4th ed. Philadelphia: Lippincott Williams & Wilkins, 2003.

FIGURE 15-19 ■ Pilletteri A. *Maternal and Child Health Nursing.* 4th ed. Philadelphia: Lippincott Williams & Wilkins, 2003.

FIGURE 15-20 ■ Erkonen WE. *Radiology 101.* Philadelphia: Lippincott Williams & Wilkins, 1998.

FIGURE 16-1 ■ Cohen B. *Memmler's The Human Body in Health and Disease.* 10th ed. Baltimore: Lippincott Williams & Wilkins, 2005.

FIGURE 16-2 ■ Cohen B. *Memmler's The Human Body in Health and Disease.* 10th ed. Baltimore: Lippincott Williams & Wilkins, 2005.

FIGURE 16-3 ■ Cohen B. *Memmler's The Human Body in Health and Disease.* 10th ed. Baltimore: Lippincott Williams & Wilkins, 2005.

FIGURE 16-5 ■ Cohen B. *Memmler's The Human Body in Health and Disease.* 10th ed. Baltimore: Lippincott Williams & Wilkins, 2005.

FIGURE 16-6 ■ Courtesy of Sandoz Pharmaceutical Corporation, Princeton, NJ.

FIGURE 16-7 ■ Rubin E, Farber JL. *Pathology.* 4th ed. Philadelphia: Lippincott Williams & Wilkins, 2005.

FIGURE 17-1 ■ Cohen B. Memmler's *The Human Body in Health and Disease.* 10th ed. Baltimore: Lippincott Williams & Wilkins, 2005.

FIGURE 17-2 ■ Cohen B. Memmler's *The Human Body in Health and Disease.* 10th ed. Baltimore: Lippincott Williams & Wilkins, 2005.

FIGURE 17-3 ■ Cohen B. Memmler's *The Human Body in Health and Disease.* 10th ed. Baltimore: Lippincott Williams & Wilkins, 2005.

FIGURE 17-4 ■ Cohen B. Memmler's *The Human Body in Health and Disease.* 10th ed. Baltimore: Lippincott Williams & Wilkins, 2005.

FIGURE 17-5 ■ Cohen B. Memmler's *The Human Body in Health and Disease.* 10th ed. Baltimore: Lippincott Williams & Wilkins, 2005.

FIGURE 17-6 ■ Cohen B. Memmler's *The Human Body in Health and Disease.* 10th ed. Baltimore: Lippincott Williams & Wilkins, 2005.

FIGURE 17-7 ■ Cohen B. Memmler's *The Human Body in Health and Disease.* 10th ed. Baltimore: Lippincott Williams & Wilkins, 2005.

FIGURE 17-8 ■ Cohen B. Memmler's *The Human Body in Health and Disease.* 10th ed. Baltimore: Lippincott Williams & Wilkins, 2005.

FIGURE 17-9 ■ Cohen B. Memmler's *The Human Body in Health and Disease.* 10th ed. Baltimore: Lippincott Williams & Wilkins, 2005.

FIGURE 17-10 ■ Cohen B. Memmler's *The Human Body in Health and Disease.* 10th ed. Baltimore: Lippincott Williams & Wilkins, 2005.

FIGURE 17-11 ■ Sheldon D. Boyd's *Introduction to the Study of Disease.* 11th ed. Philadelphia: Lea & Febiger, 1992.

FIGURE 17-12 ■ Rubin E, Farber JL. *Pathology.* 4th ed. Philadelphia: Lippincott Williams & Wilkins, 2005.

FIGURE 17-14 ■ Smeltzer SC, Bare B. *Medical-Surgical Nursing.* 10th ed. Philadelphia: Lippincott Williams & Wilkins, 2004.

FIGURE 17-15 ■ Erkonen WE. *Radiology 101.* Philadelphia: Lippincott Williams & Wilkins, 1998.

FIGURE 17-16 ■ Rubin E, Farber JL. *Pathology.* 4th ed. Philadelphia: Lippincott Williams & Wilkins, 2005.

FIGURE 17-17 ■ Porth CM. *Pathophysiology.* 7th ed. Philadelphia: Lippincott Williams & Wilkins, 2005.

FIGURE 17-18 ■ Erkonen WE. *Radiology 101.* Philadelphia: Lippincott Williams & Wilkins, 1998.

FIGURE 18-1 ■ Cohen B. *Memmler's The Human Body in Health and Disease.* 10th ed. Baltimore: Lippincott Williams & Wilkins, 2005.

FIGURE 18-2 ■ Cohen B. *Memmler's The Human Body in Health and Disease.* 10th ed. Baltimore: Lippincott Williams & Wilkins, 2005.

FIGURE 18-3 ■ Image provided by Anatomical Chart Co.

FIGURE 18-4 ■ Cohen B. Memmler's *The Human Body in Health and Disease.* 10th ed. Baltimore: Lippincott Williams & Wilkins, 2005.

FIGURE 18-5 ■ Smeltzer SC, Bare B. *Medical-Surgical Nursing.* 10th ed. Philadelphia: Lippincott Williams & Wilkins, 2004.

FIGURE 18-6 ■ Smeltzer SC, Bare B. *Medical-Surgical Nursing.* 10th ed. Philadelphia: Lippincott Williams & Wilkins, 2004.

FIGURE 18-7 ■ Bickley LS. Bates' *Guide to Physical Examination and History Taking.* 8th ed. Philadelphia: Lippincott Williams & Wilkins, 2003.

FIGURE 18-9	■	Cohen B. Memmler's *The Human Body in Health and Disease*. 10th ed. Baltimore: Lippincott Williams & Wilkins, 2005.
FIGURE 18-10	■	Cohen B. Memmler's *The Human Body in Health and Disease*. 10th ed. Baltimore: Lippincott Williams & Wilkins, 2005.
FIGURE 18-11	■	Cohen B. Memmler's *The Human Body in Health and Disease*. 10th ed. Baltimore: Lippincott Williams & Wilkins, 2005.
FIGURE 18-12	■	Moore KL, Dalley AF. *Clinically Oriented Anatomy*. 4th ed. Philadelphia: Lippincott Williams & Wilkins, 1999.
FIGURE 18-13	■	Cohen B. Memmler's *The Human Body in Health and Disease*. 10th ed. Baltimore: Lippincott Williams & Wilkins, 2005.
FIGURE 18-14	■	Smeltzer SC, Bare B. *Medical-Surgical Nursing*. 10th ed. Philadelphia: Lippincott Williams & Wilkins, 2004.
FIGURE 18-15	■	Smeltzer SC, Bare B. *Medical-Surgical Nursing*. 10th ed. Philadelphia: Lippincott Williams & Wilkins, 2004.
FIGURE 18-16	■	Rubin E, Farber JL. *Pathology*. 4th ed. Philadelphia: Lippincott Williams & Wilkins, 2005.
FIGURE 19-1	■	Cohen B. Memmler's *The Human Body in Health and Disease*. 10th ed. Baltimore: Lippincott Williams & Wilkins, 2005.
FIGURE 19-2	■	Cohen B. Memmler's *The Human Body in Health and Disease*. 10th ed. Baltimore: Lippincott Williams & Wilkins, 2005.
FIGURE 19-3	■	Cohen B. Memmler's *The Human Body in Health and Disease*. 10th ed. Baltimore: Lippincott Williams & Wilkins, 2005.
FIGURE 19-4	■	Cohen B. Memmler's *The Human Body in Health and Disease*. 10th ed. Baltimore: Lippincott Williams & Wilkins, 2005.
FIGURE 19-5	■	Cohen B. Memmler's *The Human Body in Health and Disease*. 10th ed. Baltimore: Lippincott Williams & Wilkins, 2005.
FIGURE 19-6	■	Rubin R, Strayer DS. *Rubin's Pathology: Clinicopathologic Foundations of Medicine*. 5th ed. Baltimore: Lippincott Williams & Wilkins, 2007.
FIGURE 19-7	■	Cohen B. Memmler's *The Human Body in Health and Disease*. 10th ed. Baltimore: Lippincott Williams & Wilkins, 2005.
FIGURE 19-8	■	Erkonen WE. *Radiology 101*. Philadelphia: Lippincott Williams & Wilkins, 1998.
FIGURE 19-10	■	Rubin E, Farber JL. *Pathology*. 4th ed. Philadelphia: Lippincott Williams & Wilkins, 2005.
FIGURE 19-11	■	Erkonen WE. *Radiology 101*. Philadelphia: Lippincott Williams & Wilkins, 1998.
FIGURE 19-13	■	Rubin E, Farber JL. *Pathology*. 4th ed. Philadelphia: Lippincott Williams & Wilkins, 2005.
FIGURE 19-15	■	Rubin E, Farber JL. *Pathology*. 4th ed. Philadelphia: Lippincott Williams & Wilkins, 2005.
FIGURE 19-16	■	Erkonen WE. *Radiology 101*. Philadelphia: Lippincott Williams & Wilkins, 1998.
FIGURE 19-17B	■	Erkonen WE. *Radiology 101*. Philadelphia: Lippincott Williams & Wilkins, 1998.
FIGURE 20-2	■	Cohen B. Memmler's *The Human Body in Health and Disease*. 10th ed. Baltimore: Lippincott Williams & Wilkins, 2005.
FIGURE 20-3	■	Cohen B. Memmler's *The Human Body in Health and Disease*. 10th ed. Baltimore: Lippincott Williams & Wilkins, 2005.
FIGURE 20-4	■	Cohen B. Memmler's *The Human Body in Health and Disease*. 10th ed. Baltimore: Lippincott Williams & Wilkins, 2005.
FIGURE 20-5	■	Cohen B. Memmler's *The Human Body in Health and Disease*. 10th ed. Baltimore: Lippincott Williams & Wilkins, 2005.
FIGURE 20-6	■	Cohen B. Memmler's *The Human Body in Health and Disease*. 10th ed. Baltimore: Lippincott Williams & Wilkins, 2005.
FIGURE 20-7	■	Cohen B. Memmler's *The Human Body in Health and Disease*. 10th ed. Baltimore: Lippincott Williams & Wilkins, 2005.
FIGURE 20-8	■	Adapted from Frontera WR, Silver JS. *Essentials of Physical Medicine and Rehabilitation*. Philadelphia: Hanley and Belfus, 2002.
FIGURE 20-9	■	Stedman's *Medical Dictionary*. 28th ed. Baltimore: Lippincott Williams & Wilkins, 2006.
FIGURE 21-1	■	Cohen B. Memmler's *The Human Body in Health and Disease*. 10th ed. Baltimore: Lippincott Williams & Wilkins, 2005.
FIGURE 21-2A	■	Bickley LS. Bates' *Guide to Physical Examination and History Taking*. 8th ed. Philadelphia: Lippincott Williams & Wilkins, 2003.
FIGURE 21-2B	■	Cohen B. Memmler's *The Human Body in Health and Disease*. 10th ed. Baltimore: Lippincott Williams & Wilkins, 2005.
FIGURE 21-3	■	Rubin E, Farber JL. *Pathology*. 4th ed. Philadelphia: Lippincott Williams & Wilkins, 2005.

FIGURE 21-4	■	Cohen B. Memmler's *The Human Body in Health and Disease.* 10th ed. Baltimore: Lippincott Williams & Wilkins, 2005.
FIGURE 21-5	■	Hall JC. Sauer's *Manual of Skin Diseases.* 10th ed. Philadelphia: Lippincott Williams & Wilkins, 1999.
FIGURE 21-6	■	Bickley LS. Bates' *Guide to Physical Examination and History Taking.* 8th ed. Philadelphia: Lippincott Williams & Wilkins, 2003.
FIGURE 21-7	■	Bickley LS. Bates' *Guide to Physical Examination and History Taking.* 8th ed. Philadelphia: Lippincott Williams & Wilkins, 2003.
FIGURE 21-8	■	Hall JC. Sauer's *Manual of Skin Diseases.* 8th ed. Baltimore: Lippincott Williams & Wilkins, 1999.
FIGURE 21-9	■	Bickley LS. Bates' *Guide to Physical Examination and History Taking.* 8th ed. Philadelphia: Lippincott Williams & Wilkins, 2003.
FIGURE 21-10	■	Bickley LS. Bates' *Guide to Physical Examination and History Taking.* 8th ed. Philadelphia: Lippincott Williams & Wilkins, 2003.
FIGURE 21-11	■	The American Cancer Society, American Academy of Dermatology.
FIGURE 21-12	■	Bickley LS. Bates' *Guide to Physical Examination and History Taking.* 8th ed. Philadelphia: Lippincott Williams & Wilkins, 2003.
FIGURE 21-13	■	Bickley LS. Bates' *Guide to Physical Examination and History Taking.* 8th ed. Philadelphia: Lippincott Williams & Wilkins, 2003.
FIGURE 21-14	■	Smeltzer SC, Bare B. *Medical-Surgical Nursing.* 10th ed. Philadelphia: Lippincott Williams & Wilkins, 2004.
FIGURE 21-15	■	Bickley LS. Bates' *Guide to Physical Examination and History Taking.* 8th ed. Philadelphia: Lippincott Williams & Wilkins, 2003.
FIGURE 21-16	■	Smeltzer SC, Bare B. *Medical-Surgical Nursing.* 10th ed. Philadelphia: Lippincott Williams & Wilkins, 2004.
FIGURE 21-17	■	Bickley LS. Bates' *Guide to Physical Examination and History Taking.* 8th ed. Philadelphia: Lippincott Williams & Wilkins, 2003.
FIGURE 21-18	■	Smeltzer SC, Bare B. *Medical-Surgical Nursing.* 10th ed. Philadelphia: Lippincott Williams & Wilkins, 2004.
FIGURE 21-19	■	Bickley LS. Bates' *Guide to Physical Examination and History Taking.* 8th ed. Philadelphia: Lippincott Williams & Wilkins, 2003.

INDEX

-ia, -ism, -sis, -y

-ac, -al, -ar, -ary, -ial,
-ic, -ile, -ory, -ous

-logy

cyan/o

erythr/o

leuk/o

a-, an-

in-, -im-, non-, un-

meaning

pertaining to

meaning

condition of

meaning

blue

meaning

study of

meaning

white, colorless

meaning

red

meaning

not

meaning

not, without, lack of, absence

dia-, per-, trans-

hyper-

hypo-

eu-

ante-, pre-, pro-

post-

ec-, ecto-, ex/o-

end/o-

meaning

**over, excess,
abnormally high,
increased**

meaning

through

meaning

good, true, easy

meaning

**under, below,
abnormally low,
decreased**

meaning

after, behind

meaning

before, in front of

meaning

in, within

meaning

out, outside

morph/o

cyt/o, –cyte

hist/o, histi/o

aden/o

gen, genesis

phag/o

–ase

hydr/o

meaning

cell

meaning

form

meaning

gland

meaning

tissue

meaning

eat, ingest

meaning

origin, formation

meaning

water, fluid

meaning

enzyme

cervic/o

thorac/o

supra-

intra-

inter-

infra-

alg/o, algi/o, algesi/o, -algia, -algesia, -odynia

carcin/o

meaning

chest, thorax

meaning

neck, cervix

meaning

in, within

meaning

above

meaning

below

meaning

between

meaning

cancer, carcinoma

meaning

pain

cyst/o, cyst/i

onc/o

py/o

tox/o, toxic/o

dys–

mal

–cele

mega–, megal/o, –megaly

meaning

tumor

meaning

filled sac or pouch,
cyst, bladder,
urinary bladder

meaning

poison, toxin

meaning

pus

meaning

bad, poor

meaning

abnormal, painful,
difficult

meaning

large, abnormally large,
enlargement

meaning

hernia,
localized dilatation

-oma

path/o, -pathy

ectasia, ectasis

therm/o

-ectomy

-pexy

-rhaphy

-stomy

meaning

**disease,
any disease of**

meaning

tumor

meaning

heat, temperature

meaning

**dilation, dilatation,
distention**

meaning

surgical fixation

meaning

excision, surgical removal

meaning

**surgical creation
of an opening**

meaning

surgical repair, suture

-penia

-poiesis

thromb/o

-pnea

-oxia

pneumon/o, pneum/o, pneumat/o, pulm/o, pulmon/o

gastr/o

enter/o

meaning

formation, production

meaning

decrease in, deficiency of

meaning

breathing

meaning

blood clot

meaning

lung

meaning

level of oxygen

meaning

intestine

meaning

stomach

col/o, colon/o

rect/o, proct/o

hepat/o

bili, chol/e, chol/o

cholecyst/o

ren/o, nephr/o

ur/o

test/o, orchi/o,
orchid/o

meaning

rectum

meaning

colon

meaning

bile, gall

meaning

liver

meaning

kidney

meaning

gallbladder

meaning

testis, testicle

meaning

urine, urinary tract

gyn/o, gynec/o

ovari/o, oophor/o

salping/o

uter/o, metr/o, metr/i, hyster/o

vagin/o, colp/o

mamm/o, mast/o

insul/o

neur/o, neur/i

meaning

ovary

meaning

woman

meaning

uterus

meaning

tube, oviduct, eustachian (auditory) tube

meaning

breast, mammary gland

meaning

vagina

meaning

nervous system, nervous tissue, nerve

meaning

pancreatic islets

Ch. 17 word part	Ch. 17 word part
myel/o	medull/o
Ch. 17 word part	Ch. 17 word part
cortic/o	psych/o
Ch. 17 word part	Ch. 18 word part
-plegia	-phobia
Ch. 17 word part	Ch. 18 word part
-mania	acous, acus, cus

meaning

**medulla oblongata,
spinal cord,
inner part**

meaning

**spinal cord,
bone marrow**

meaning

mind

meaning

**cerebral cortex,
outer portion**

meaning

persistent, irrational fear

meaning

paralysis

meaning

sound, hearing

meaning

excited state, obsession

ot/o

myring/o, tympan/o

ocul/o, ophthalm/o

corne/o, kerat/o

lent/i, phak/o, phac/o

ir, irit/o, irid/o

oste/o

chondr/o

meaning

tympanic membrane

meaning

ear

meaning

cornea

meaning

eye

meaning

iris

meaning

lens

meaning

cartilage

meaning

bone

Ch. 19 word part	Ch. 19 word part
arthr/o	**spondyl/o, vertebr/o**
Ch. 19 word part	Ch. 20 word part
cost/o	**my/o, muscul/o**
Ch. 20 word part	Ch. 21 word part
kin/o, kine, kinesi/o, kinet/o	**derm/o, dermat/o**
Ch. 20 word part	Ch. 21 word part
melan/o	**hidr/o**

meaning

vertebra

meaning

joint

meaning

muscle

meaning

rib

meaning

skin

meaning

movement

meaning

sweat, perspiration

meaning

dark, black, melanin